Instant Clinical Diagnosis in Ophthalmology

Pediatric Ophthalmology

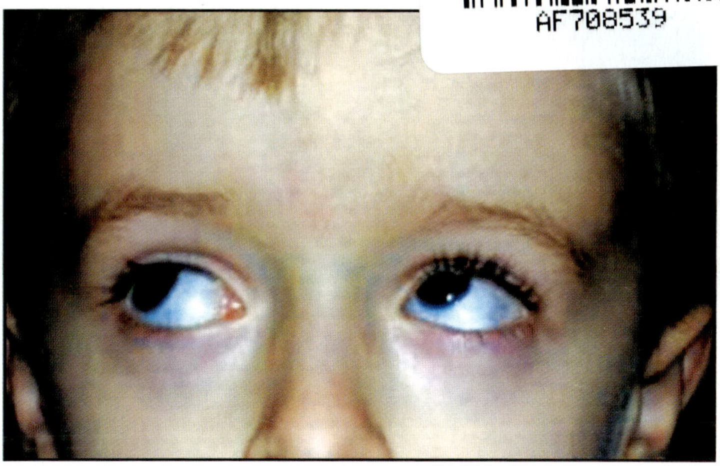

Instant Clinical Diagnosis in Ophthalmology

Pediatric Ophthalmology

Series Editors

Ashok Garg MS PhD FIAO (Bel)
FRSM FAIMS ADM FICA
International and National Gold Medalist
Chairman and Medical Director
Garg Eye Institute and Research Centre
235-Model Town, Dabra Chowk
Hisar-125 005, India

Emanuel Rosen MD
Medical Director
Rosen Eye Associates
Harbour City, Salford Quays
M50 3 BH
United Kingdom

Editors

Shui H Lee MD FRCS FAAO
Medical Director
Sunray Outpatient Aesthetic
Multispecialty Surgical Center
Medical Director
Central Square Medical Eye Clinic
Unit 255-4231 Hazel Bridge Way
Richmond B.C. V6X 3L7, Canada

Eric R Crouch MD
Assistant Professor
Pediatric Ophthalmology
Eastern Virginia Medical School
880 Kemphsville Road
Suite 2500, Norflock
Virginia 23502, USA

Ewa Oleszczynska Prost MD PhD
Director
Center for Pediatric Ophthalmology
Hertza 9, 04-603
Warsaw, Poland

Rupal H Trivedi MD PhD
Research Assistant Professor
Storm Eye Institute
Medical University of
South Carolina (MUSC)
Charleston, USA

Foreword

Nicola Freeman

Jaypee Brothers

McGraw Hill Medical

First published in India in 2009 by

Jaypee Brothers Medical Publishers (P) Ltd.

Corporate Office
4838/24 Ansari Road, Daryaganj, **New Delhi** - 110002, India, +91-11-43574357

Registered Office
B-3 EMCA House, 23/23B Ansari Road, Daryaganj, **New Delhi** 110 002, India
Phones: +91-11-23272143, +91-11-23272703, +91-11-23282021,
+91-11-23245672, Rel: +91-11-32558559 Fax: +91-11-23276490, +91-11-23245683
e-mail: jaypee@jaypeebrothers.com, Website: www.jaypeebrothers.com

First published in USA by The McGraw-Hill Companies, 2 Penn Plaza, New York, NY 10121. Exclusively worldwide distributor except South Asia (India, Nepal, Sri Lanka, Bhutan, Pakistan, Bangladesh, Malaysia).

ISBN-13: 978-0-07-174948-0
ISBN-10: 0-07-174948-9

To

- My Respected Param Pujya Guru Sant Gurmeet Ram Rahim Singh Ji for his blessings and motivation
- My Respected Parents, Teachers, my wife Dr Aruna Garg, son Abhishek and daughter Anshul for their constant support and patience during all these days of hard work
- My dear friend Dr Amar Agarwal, a renowned International Ophthalmologist for his constant support, guidance and expertise

— Ashok Garg

The memory of my step daughter Nicola Ross who enjoyed benefits from refractive surgery were cut short by a tragic fatal illness

— Emanuel Rosen

- My parents for their inspiration, teaching and motivation
- My brother Peter for his continued support, guidance and inspiration in my professional career

— Shui H Lee

My patients

— Eric R Crouch

My parents, husband and son for patience and understanding

— Ewa Oleszczynska Prost

My mentor, Dr Abhay R Vasavada, in deep appreciation for his unending encouragement and direction of my academic and research career in ophthalmology

— Rupal H Trivedi

Contributors

A Azimzadeh MD
Ophthalmology Department
Labbafinejad Medical Centre
Pesdaran Avenue
Boostan 9 Street
Tehran-16666 (Iran)

Abhiyan Kumar MD
Dr RP Center for Ophthalmic Sciences
All India Institute of Medical Sciences
(AIIMS), Ansari Nagar
New Delhi-110029, India

Ahmad K Khalil MD PhD
Medical Director
Saridar Clinic Building
92, Tahrir St
Dokki, Cairo
Egypt

Ajay Aurora MS
Senior Vitreoretina Consultant and
Director, Delhi Retina Centre
Chaudhary Eye Centre and Laser Vision
4802, Bharat Ram Road
24, Darya Ganj
New Delhi, India

Ali Saeed Odadi Assiri
Department of Ophthalmology
Cairo University, Cairo
Egypt

Anjli Hussain MS
Medical Retina and ROP Specialist
LV Prasad Eye Institute
LV Prasad Marg
Banjara Hills, Hyderabad
India

Ankur Sinha
Senior Resident
Dr RP Center for Ophthalmic Sciences
All India Institute of Medical Sciences
(AIIMS), Ansari Nagar
New Delhi-110029, India

Antonio Marinho MD PhD
Professor of Ophthalmology
University of Porto
Portugal

Arif Adenwala MS
Consultant
Aditya Jyot Eye Hospital Pvt Ltd
Plot No. 153, Road No.9
Major Parmeshwaran Road
Wadala, Mumbai-400031
India

Arturo Perez Arteaga MD
Medical Director
Centro Oftalmologico Tlalnepantla
Dr Perez - Arteaga Vallarta No.42
Tlalnepantla, Centro, Estado de Mexico
54000, Mexico

Anita Panda MD
Professor of Ophthalmology
Dr RP Centre for Ophthalmic Sciences
All India Institute of Medical Sciences
(AIIMS), New Delhi-110029, India

Ashok Garg MS PhD FRSM
Chairman and Medical Director
Garg Eye Institute and Research Centre
235-Model Town, Dabra Chowk
Hisar-125005
India

Ashok K Grover MD FRCS
Chairman
Department of Ophthalmology
Sir Ganga Ram Hospital
Rajinder Nagar
New Delhi-110060
Director, Vision Eye Clinic
12/27, West Patel Nagar
Near Arya Samaj Mandir
New Delhi-110008, India

Ashok Sharma MS
Director
Dr Ashok Sharma's Cornea Centre
SCO 833-34 (2nd Floor)
Sector 22-A, Opp. Parade Ground
Near Bus Stand, Chandigarh-160022
India

Belquiz A Nassaralla MD PhD
Goiania Eye Institute
Department of Cornea and Refractive
Surgery, Goiania, GO, Brazil

Berdine M Burger MD
Department of Ophthalmology
Storm Eye Institute
Medical University of South Carolina
167, Ashley Avenue
Charleston SC 29425, USA

Bhuvan Chanana MD
Dr RP Centre for Ophthalmic Sciences
All India Institute of Medical Sciences
(AIIMS), Ansari Nagar
New Delhi-110029, India

Bojan Pajic MD
Chief of the Cornea and Refractive
Surgery Department
Klinik Pallas
Louis Giroud-Str. 20
4600 Olten
Switzerland

Cyres K Mehta MS FSVH FAGE
Director and Consultant
Mehta International Eye Institute
Seaside, 147, Colaba Road
Mumbai-400005
India

Debraj Shome MS
Consultant
Aditya Jyot Eye Hospital Pvt Ltd
Plot No. 153, Road No. 9
Major Parmeshwaran Road
Opp. SIWS College, Gate No. 3
Wadala, Mumbai-400031
India

D Godts CO
Department of Ophthalmology
University Hospital
Antwerp
Belgium

Dimitrii Dementiev MD
Chief and Medical Director
Blue Eye Centro di
Michro Chirurgia Oculare Eye Clinic
Arese 20020 (MI)
Via Campo Gallo 21/10
Italy

Emanuel Rosen MD FRCS
Rosen Eye Associates
Harbour City
Salford Quays
M50 3 BH
UK

Eric R Crouch MD
Assistant Professor of Pediatric
Ophthalmology
Eastern Virginia Medical School
880 Kemphsville Road
Suite 2500, Norflock
Virginia 23502
USA

Essam EL Toukhy MD FRCOph
Assistant Professor of Ophthalmology
Consultant, International Eye Hospital
14-A El Sobki Street # 23
Dokki, Cairo
Egypt-12311

Ewa Oleszczynska Prost MD PhD
Director
Center for Pediatric Ophthalmology
Hertza 9, 04-603
Warsaw, Poland

Frederic Hehn MD
Centre de La Vision
Nations - Vision
23, Boulevard de l' Europe
54500, Vandoeuvre
France

Geeta Behera MD
Dr RP Center for Ophthalmic Sciences
All India Institute of Medical Sciences
(AIIMS), Ansari Nagar
New Delhi-110029
India

Hala M Elhilaly MD
Professor of Ophthalmology
Department of Ophthalmology
Cairo University, Cairo
Egypt

Harinder Singh Sethi MS DNB FRCS
Senior Research Associate
Dr RP Centre for Ophthalmic
Sciences, All India Institute of Medical
Sciences (AIIMS), Ansari Nagar
New Delhi-110029
India

Hoda MH Mostafa MD
Lecturer of Ophthalmology
Department of Ophthalmology
Cairo University, Cairo
Egypt

Ibrahim Mosad MD
Department of Ophthalmology
Cairo University, Cairo
Egypt

I De Veuster MD
Department of Ophthalmology
University Hospital
Antwerp, Belgium

Jerome Bovet MD
Consultant Ophthalmic Surgeon, FMH
Clinique de I' Oeil
15, Avenue du Bois-de-la-Chapelle
CH-1213 Onex
Switzerland

Joao J Nassaralla Jr MD PhD
Faculty of Health Sciences
University of Brasilia, DF
Goiania Eye Institute
Department of Retina and Vitreous
Goiania, GO, Brazil

Jörg Müller MS
Surgery Department
Klinik Pallas
Louis Giroud-Str. 20
4600 Olten, Switzerland

Kali Bliss Cole MD (Mph)
Department of Ophthalmology
Storm Eye Institute
Medical University of South Carolina
167, Ashley Avenue
Charleston SC 29425, USA

Keiki R Mehta MS DO FIOS
Chairman and Medical Director
Mehta International Eye Institute
147, Shahid Bhagat Singh Road
Colaba Road, Mumbai-400005, India

L Gobin PhD
Department of Ophthalmology
University Hospital, Antwerp
Belgium

Mahesh Dalvi MS
Consultant
Pediatric Ophthalmology
Tejomay Eye Hospital
Kohlapur, Maharashtra, India

Malvika Bansal MS
Department of Ophthalmology
Sir Ganga Ram Hospital
Old Rajinder Nagar, New Delhi, India

Marek E Prost MD
Professor of Ophthalmology and
Director
Center for Pediatric Ophthalmology
Hertza 9, 04-603, Warsaw
Military Institute of Aviation Medicine
Kransinskiego 54, 01-755 Warsaw
Poland

Maria Da Luz Freitas MD
R Crasto, 708 4150-243 Porto
Portugal

Marie Jose Tassignon MD PhD FEBO
Professor and Head
Department of Ophthalmology
University Hospital of Antwerp
Antwerp, Belgium

Masoud Soheilian MD
Ophthalmology Department
Labbafinejad Medical Centre
Pesdaran Avenue, Boostan 9 Street
Tehran-16666 (Iran)

Mayur Moreker MS
Fellow
LV Prasad Eye Institute
Banjara Hills, Hyderabad
India

M Edward Wilson MD
Pierre Gautier Jenkins
Professor and Chairman
Department of Ophthalmology
Director
Albert Florens Storm Eye Institute
Medical University of South Carolina
Charleston, SC, USA 29425

Milind Kirtane MS
Consultant
PD Hinduja National Hospital and
MRC, Veer Savarkar Marg, Mahim
Mumbai-400016, India

Milind Navlakhe MS
Associate Professor
Department of Ophthalmology
KEM Hospital
Mumbai, India

Mohamed El Badri
Specialist Ophthalmologist
National Eye Center
Egypt

Mohammad Mehdi Sadoughi MD
Ophthalmology Department
Labbafinejad Medical Centre
Pesdaran Avenue, Boostan 9 Street
Tehran-16666, Iran

Rezaei Kanavi MD
Ophthalmology Department
Labbafinejad Medical Centre
Pesdaran Avenue, Boostan 9 Street
Tehran-16666, Iran

Nazimul Hussain MS DNB
Consultant Vitreoretina Specialist
Al Zahra Pvt Hospital
Sharjah/Dubai, UAE

Neeraj Sanduja MD
Consultant Vitreoretinal Surgeon
Dr Chaudhary Eye Centre and
Laser Vision, 4802, Bharat Ram Road
24, Daryaganj, New Delhi
India

Nicola Freeman MBChB DO FCOphth
Senior Consultant Ophthalmic
Surgeon - Paediatric Clinics
Department of Ophthalmology
Faculty of Health Sciences
University of Stellenbosch
Tygerberg Academic Hospital
Cape Town
South Africa

Nikoloz Labauris MS
Aditya Jyot Eye Hospital Pvt Ltd
Plot No. 153, Road No. 9
Major Parmeshwaran Road
Opp. SIWS College, Gate No. 3
Wadala, Mumbai-400031
India

Peter WT de Waard MD
The Rotterdam Eye Hospital
Schiedamse Vest 180
3011, BH-Rotterdam
Netherlands

Priyanka Doctor MS
Aditya Jyot Eye Hospital Pvt Ltd
Plot No. 153, Road No. 9
Major Parmeshwaran Road
Opp. SIWS College, Gate No. 3
Wadala, Mumbai-400031
India

Rajpal Vohra MD
Professor of Ophthalmology
Dr RP Centre for Ophthalmic Sciences
AIIMS, New Delhi-110029
India

Rajvardhan Azad MD
Professor of Ophthalmology
Dr RP Centre for Ophthalmic Sciences
All India Institute of Medical Sciences
(AIIMS), New Delhi-110029, India

Ramesh Murthy MD
Ophthalmic Plastic Services
LV Prasad Eye Institute
LV Prasad Marg
Banjara Hills
Hyderabad-500034
India

Rania El Essawy MD FRCSEd
Assistant Professor of Ophthalmology
Department of Ophthalmology
Cairo University, Cairo
Egypt

Roberto Bellucci MD
Chief of Ophthalmic Unit
Hospital of Verona
University of Verona
Italy

Rohit Saxena
Additional Professor
Dr RP Centre for Ophthalmic Sciences
All India Institute of Medical Sciences
(AIIMS), New Delhi-110029, India

Ronald GW Teed MD
Assistant Professor
Department of Ophthalmology
Storm Eye Institute
Medical University of South Carolina
167, Ashley Avenue
Charleston SC 29425
USA

Roshmi Gupta MD
Consultant
Ophthalmic Plastic and Ocular
Oncology Services
LV Prasad Eye Institute
Vishakapatnam
India

Rupal H Trivedi MD MSCR
Assistant Professor
MUSC Storm Eye Institute
167, Ashley Avenue
Charleston SC-29425
USA

Santosh G Honavar MD FACS
Director
Ophthalmic Plastics and Ocular Oncology
Services
LV Prasad Eye Institute, LV Prasad Marg
Banjara Hills, Hyderabad-500034
India

Savari Desai MD
Ophthalmic Plastics and Ocular Oncology
Services
LV Prasad Eye Institute
LV Prasad Marg, Banjara Hills
Hyderabad-500034
India

Simonetta Morselli MD
Director of Anterior Segment Surgery
Ophthalmic Unit
Hospital of Verona
University of Verona
Italy

Shaloo Bageja MS
Consultant
Department of Ophthalmology
Sir Ganga Ram Hospital
Rajinder Nagar
New Delhi
India

Saurabh Patwardhan MD
Registrar
Dr RP Centre for Ophthalmic Sciences
All India Institute of Medical Sciences (AIIMS), Ansari Nagar
New Delhi-110029, India

Shui H Lee MD FRCS FAAO
Medical Director
Sunray Outpatient Aesthetic
Multispecialty Surgical Center
Medical Director
Central Square Medical Eye Clinic
Unit 255-4231 Hazel Bridge Way
Richmond B.C. V6X 3L7, Canada

Soumen Mondal MS
Aditya Jyot Eye Hospital Pvt Ltd
Plot No. 153, Road No. 9
Major Parmeshwaran Road
Opp. SIWS College, Gate No.3
Wadala, Mumbai-400031, India

S Natarajan MS FRVS
Chairman and Medical Director
Aditya Jyot Eye Hospital Pvt Ltd
Plot No. 153, Road No. 9
Major Parmeshwaran Road
Opp. SIWS College, Gate No. 3
Wadala, Mumbai-400031, India

Susannah Mistr MD
Miles Center for Pediatric Ophthalmology
Storm Eye Institute
Department of Ophthalmology
Medical University of South Carolina
Charleston, SC, USA

Sunil Moreker MD
Consultant Ophthalmologist
PD Hinduja National Hospital and
Medical Research Centre
Veer Savarkar Marg, Mahim
Mumbai-400016
India

Supriya Dabir MS
Aditya Jyot Eye Hospital Pvt Ltd
Plot No. 153, Road No. 9
Major Parmeshwaran Road
Opp. SIWS College, Gate No.3
Wadala, Mumbai-400031
India

Swati Phuljhele
Senior Resident
Dr RP Centre for Ophthalmic Sciences
All India Institute of Medical Sciences
(AIIMS), Ansari Nagar
New Delhi-110029
India

Foreword

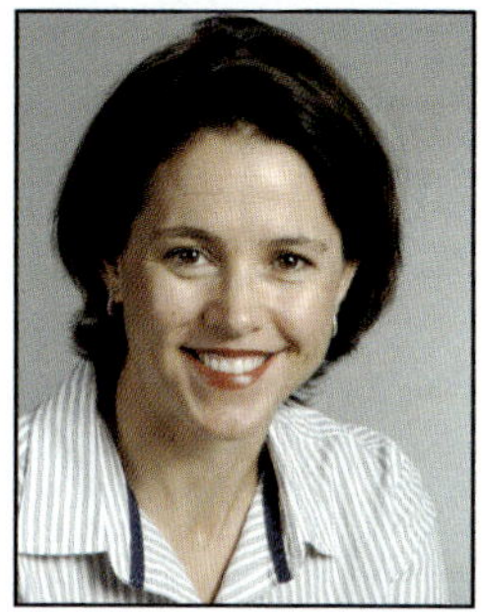

In most countries, pediatric eye care cannot be met by the relatively limited number of trained pediatric ophthalmologists available.

This book presents the essence of pediatric ophthalmology in a succinct and didactic format that can be accessed readily and rapidly. Topical and controversial issues have also been included to make readers aware of the debates. The goal is not to replace the main comprehensive textbooks, but rather to provide a reference that can be used in the busy practice when posed with a pediatric eye problem or question. It is likely to become the trusted clinic friend that stimulates further reading.

Safeguarding and actively promoting the vision of growing children is crucial to the future of any nation. Dr Ashok Garg and Dr Emanuel Rosen must be commended on a much needed publication which provides ophthalmologists "instant" textbook information, thus hopefully improving pediatric eye care in as many corners of the earth as possible.

Nicola Freeman
MBChB (SA) DipOphth (SA) FCOphth (SA)
Senior Consultant Ophthalmologist
Tygerberg Pediatric Hospital and
Department of Ophthalmology
Tygerberg Academic Hospital and
University of Stellenbosch
Cape Town, South Africa
Email: drfree@sun.ac.za

Preface

In modern day, busy and fast life ophthalmologists are glued to their clinical and surgical practice and have little time to read large volume books. The need of the hour is to have pocket size ready reckoner enriched with complete and uptodate information of the diseases in a most comprehensive manner. At present, very few quality Ready Reference books are available at an International level.

After detailed research and according to the need of ophthalmologists, we have developed a series of 10 Volume Ready Reference Books termed as *Instant Clinical Diagnosis in Ophthalmology*. This series covers Oculoplastic and Reconstructive Surgery, Retina, Lens, Glaucoma, Refractive Surgery, Pediatric Ophthalmology, Strabismus, Anterior Segment Diseases, Cornea and Neuro-ophthalmology. This present series has been designed to provide uptodate information of concerned disease in a comprehensive and lucid manner along with high quality clinical photographs in an easy-to-read format. International Masters of concerned subject have contributed chapters in this series covering pathophysiology, clinical signs and symptoms, investigations, differential diagnosis, treatment and prognosis in a simiplified manner.

This volume deals with Pediatric Ophthalmology which is an exciting and challenging branch of Ophthalmology. Fifty-six chapters of this volume cover all clinical, medical and surgical aspects of Pediatric Ophthalmology specially Pediatric Lens Diseases, Cornea and External Eye Diseases, Anterior Segment Diseases, Strabismus and Neuro-ophthalmology, Pediatric Refractive Surgery, Pediatric Retinal Diseases and recent advances. This comprehensive handbook on Pediatric Ophthalmology is the first of its kind in ophthalmic field which shall provide a deep and instant insight into pediatric problems in a simplified and concise manner.

We are highly thankful to M/s Jaypee Brothers Medical Publishers (P) Ltd, New Delhi, especially Shri Jitendar P Vij (Chairman and Managing Director), Mr Tarun Duneja (Director-Publishing) and all staff members for their dedication and hard efforts put in the preparation of high quality series of Instant Clinical Books.

We hope this 10 volume set of ready reference pocket size books shall provide complete and useful clinical information to ophthalmologists all around the world and shall help them to accurately and precisely diagnose, treat and manage their clinical cases confidently to the satisfaction and expectations of their valued patients. We also hope this Ready Reckoner shall serve as useful companion on every clinician's desk.

Editors

Contents

Section 1
Anterior Segment

Section 2
Posterior Segment

Section 1

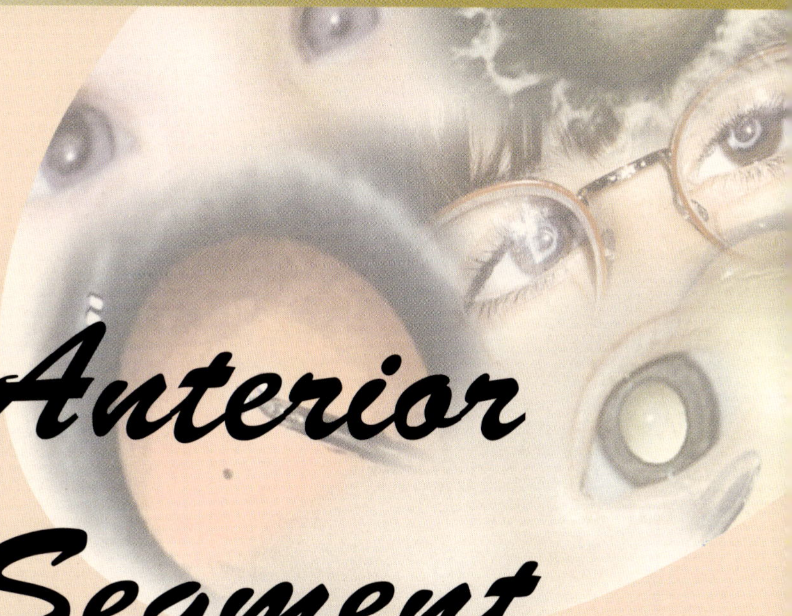

Anterior Segment

Chapter 1

Visual Acuity Assessment in Children

Saurabh Patwardhan
Harinder S Sethi (India)

Introduction

Single important clinical examination required in ophthalmology is that of visual acuity assessment. Unlike in adults where visual acuity assessment can be usually comfortably done with Snellen's charts or near charts, visual acuity assessment in children requires patience, need good observation and some special equipment. Good and reliable visual acuity assessment helps in proper diagnosis, management and follow-up of child.

A communication barrier exists between the practitioner and very young patients. With different methods and levels of communication, the adult ophthalmologist and infant patient are not easily able to understand each other. A range of techniques has been developed in an attempt to overcome the communication barrier between adult practitioners and young patients.

It is necessary to assess visual acuity in pediatric age group to:

1. Detect refractive errors, structural anomalies and amblyopia
2. Proceed with further investigations
3. Early visual rehabilitation of child
4. Baseline for particular age
5. When adult visual acuity level is attained

What is Visual Acuity?

Two points are discriminable as long as they stimulate two separate cones. Width of a foveal cone is 2.5 micron (30 sec angular separation). Individual part of 6/6 letter is equal to 1min angle at fovea. There are different ways in which visual acuity can be measured.

Minimum Visibles

It is ability to detect presence or absence of target. Simple example can be to detect presence of line in a field. Best threshold is 1 sec arc.

Minimum Discriminable (Hyperacuity)

It is ability to discriminate relative location of two or more features, e.g. is the upper line to right or left of lower line. Best threshold is 2 sec arc.

Minimum Resolvable/Recognizable

It is ability to distinguish more than one feature of a target.

This is the usual visual acuity that is checked using Snellen's charts.

Visual Development in Humans

Rods and cones do not attain adult like dimensions until 4 months after birth. Myelination of visual pathways is complete by 1 month, increases upto 2 years

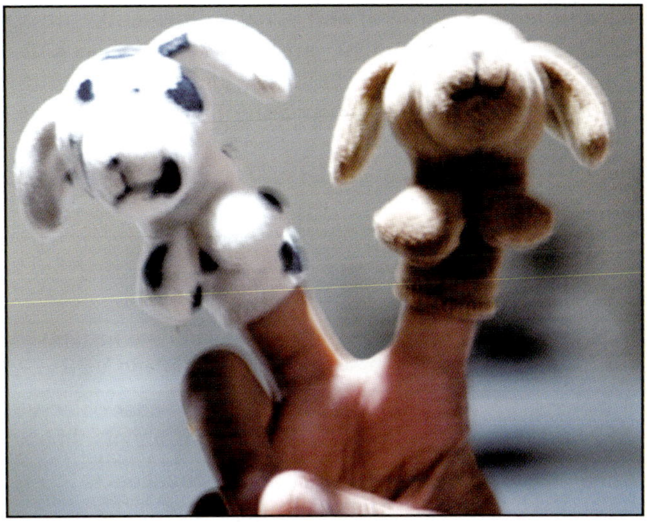

Figure 1: Toys

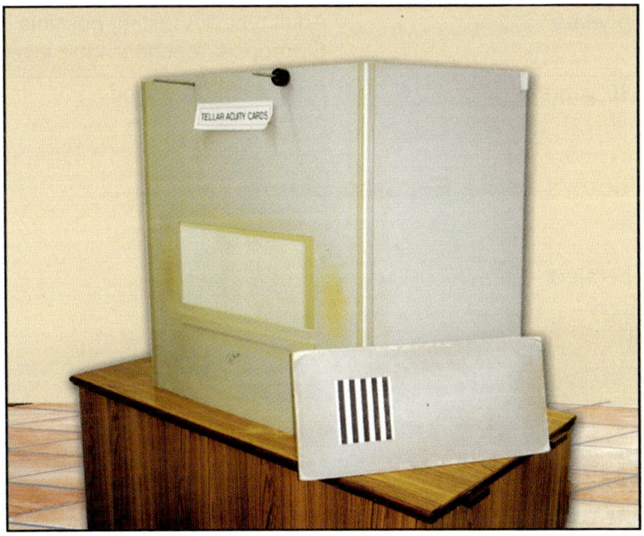

Figure 2: Teller's acuity cards (TAC)

Cortical neuronal dendritic growth and synapse formation are active in first 2 years. Still the visual development can be clinically detectable upto 10 to 12 years of age. This period is the period of visual plasticity during which probability of developing as well as recovering from amblyopia is present.

Table 1: Visual milestones

Age	*Visual milestones*
29 weeks	Pupillary light reflex
30 weeks	Dislikes bright light
At birth	Visual fixation (Intermittent) Following (OKN and VOR+)
3 months	Fixates well on near objects Following movements smooth
4 months	Full accommodation +
5 months	Menace reflex + Onset of stereopsis
6 months	Fixates well on distant objects VEP acuity reaches adult level
18 months	VA on TAC reaches adult level
3 years	Subjective VA testing possible VA tumbling E/HOTV = 6/9-6/6
5 years	Adult type VA testing possible Stereopsis reaches adult level
10 years	End of critical period

Various Factors to be Ensured before Testing

Child

- Should be alert
- Not hungry
- Relaxed

Examiner

- Should be gentle
- Friendly
- observant

Indirect assessment of vision is also important. Simple observations can predict the vision of the child. It is recommended to keep few attractive toys which help in acuity assessment and also attracts the child's attention.

- Simple observation
  - o Near objects preferred
  - o Occlusion of one eye strongly objected

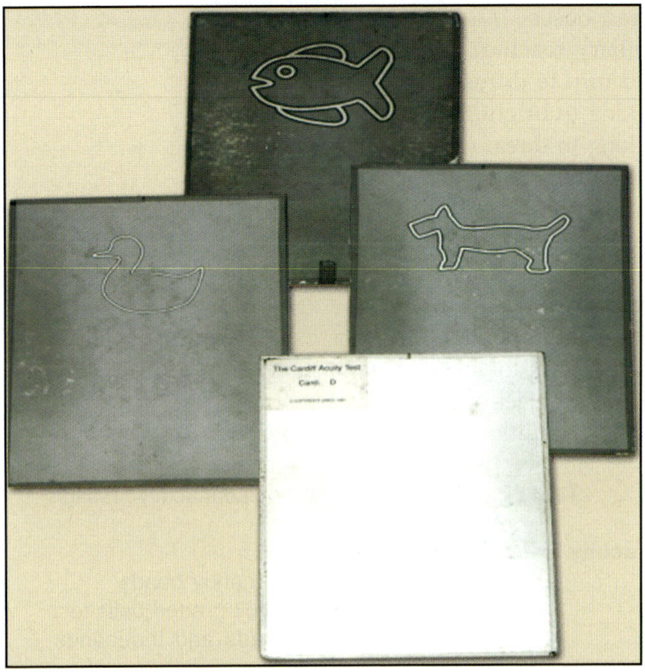

Figure 3: Cardiff acuity cards

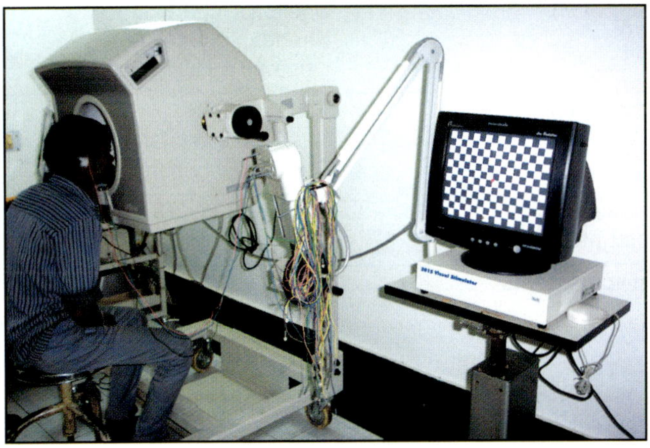

Figure 4: VEP

- Reflex responses
  - o Pupillary reaction
  - o Head turn to diffuse light source
  - o Blinking to bright light
  - o Blinking to threat (Menace reflex)
- Fixation pattern
  - o Fixation preference for moving, pattern, high contrast stimuli
  - o Ideal fixation target human face

Different methods of visual acuity testing are given in **Table 2**. The methods can also be classified as

1. Tests based on preferential looking, e.g. TAC , CAC
2. Tests based on optokinetic nystagmus e.g. OKNOVIS, Catford drum
3. Tests based on electrophysiology, e.g. VEP
4. Subjective recognition tests, e.g. Snellen's charts.

Table 2: Various methods for visual acuity testing

Detection acuity tests	
	Boeck candy beads STYCAR graded balls test Hundreds and thousands
Recognition acuity tests	
Direction identification	Landolt's C Snellen's E Sjögren's hand test Arrows
Letter identification	Snellen's chart Sheridan's letter test Lippman's HOTV test
Picture identification	Allen's cards Sheridan's miniature toys Cardiff acuity cards
Picture identification on behavioral pattern	OKNOVIS
Resolution acuity tests	
	OKN drum Preferential looking (PL) tests Pattern VEP

Since different tests tend to give different values of visual acuity at different ages, it is advisable to follow-up a child on single type of test. Though, different types of tests can be used to confirm the findings in case of doubt. Various important methods are mentioned here.

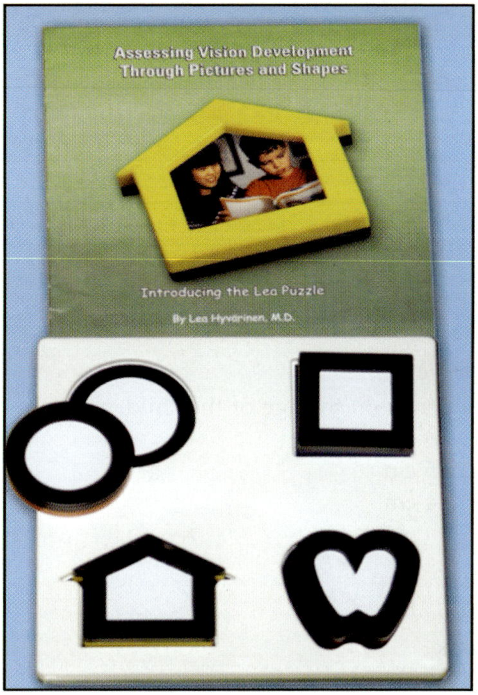

Figure 5: Lea puzzle

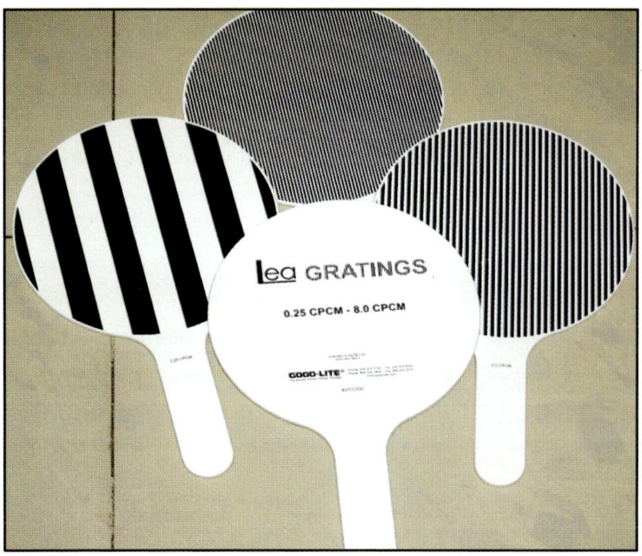

Figure 6: Lea gratings

Table 3: Visual acuity—according to age

Method	*Birth*	*1 month*	*6 month*	*6/6 achieved (months)*
OKN	6/120	6/120	6/30	20-30
PLT(TAC)	6/240	6/120	6/30	24-36
VEP	—	6/120	6/6-6/12	6-12

TAC (Teller's Acuity Cards)

Testing distance depends on the age of the child.

0-6 months	38 cm
7 months - 3 yr	55 cm
> 3 yr	84 cm

Responses

- Consistent look
- Inconsistent look
- Refusal to look

It is based on the principal of preferential looking. Black and white stripes exposed to a child over a homogenous gray luminance area. Childs score calculated on the resolution of the pattern he/she fixates on and for what time. Seventeen cards of 25.5 × 51 cm are there. Fifteen of these have 12.5 × 12.5 cm patches of square wave grating. The gratings have spatial frequency — stripe width from 38 to 0.32 cycles/cm. One low vision card (25.5*23 cm, 0.23 cycle/cm) and one black card.

For a child with very poor acuity test at near distance (19 cm) without screen or test with "low vision" card.

For a child with convergent squint test at closest distance (38 cm).

Table 4: TAC—Snellen's equivalent

Cycle/cm at 55 cm	*Snellen's equivalent*	
	Based 20 ft	*Based 6 m*
38	20/16	6/5
19	20/32	6/9
9.8	20/63	6/18
6.5	20/94	6/30
3.2	20/190	6/60
0.86	20/710	6/200
0.32	20/1900	6/600

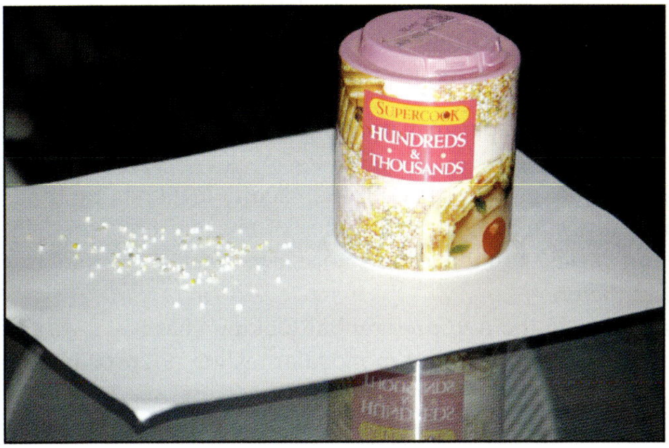

Figure 7: Hundreds and thousands test

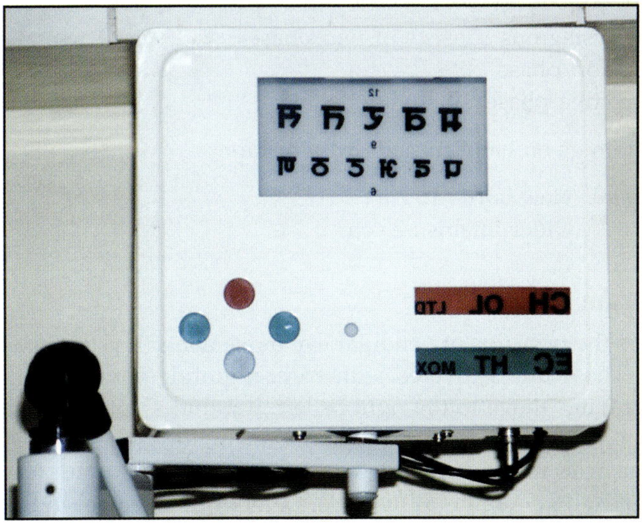

Figure 8: Snellen's chart

Drawbacks

- Test only near acuity (can miss mild myopia)
- Overestimates VA (Can miss amblyopia)

Cardiff Acuity Cards (CAC)

It is based on the principal of vanishing optotypes. Adoh and Woodhouse introduced it in 1992.

It consists of a set of 33 cards with each acuity level having three cards. The visual acuity values are given in minutes of arc and converted into Snellens equivalent and varies with the test distance, e.g. 6/6 to 6/60 for 1 m and 6/12 to 6/120 for 1/2 meter.

Comparison between the two preferential looking charts – TAC and CAC

- Both applicable for infants but monocular testing not possible in < 6 months with CAC
- Between 1-2 yr variance more with CAC due to variation in object learning in children
- Testing timeless with CAC
- CAC easy to conduct and enjoyable to children, attention span is more

Optokinetic Nystagmus (OKN), e.g. Catford Drum

Optokinetic nystagmus consists of two phases:

- Slow fixation phase
- Fast corrective phase

Stimulus: Gratings on hand turned drum or tape

Testing distance: New born : 15 cm
Older infants : 25 cm

Catford Drum

It is based on the principal of pendular eye movements. It is devised by Catford and Oliver. The drum is covered with vertical grating pattern, so that when it spins, the gratings move to the right or left. It induces optokinetic nystagmus. The drum may be presented at a range of viewing distances so that a range of spatial frequencies may be presented, using gratings of constant width. In very young (one- to three-month-old) infants, OKN eye movement in the temporal-to-nasal direction (for example, leftward movement when testing the right eye) is evident, but nasal-to-temporal movement is weak or absent.

Visual Evoked Potential (VEP)

It is nothing but EEG taken from occipital lobe. Primary electrode is taped over occipital pole.

Depending on stimulus it is classified as:

- Flash VEP

- Pattern VEP
- Sweep VEP.

Responses

- Transient
- Steady state.

Response Parameters

Amplitude: 10-25 microvolts (mass conduction)

Latency: 100-135 m sec (conduction time)

The striate cortex, first cortical center for most visual pathway fibers, is situated in the occipital lobe. The topography of the striate cortex is such that nerve fibers originating in the central retina are positioned most posteriorly (nearest to the scalp surface) and those originating in more peripheral retina are positioned more anteriorly. In addition, a disproportionate amount of cortical tissue is devoted to signals from the central retina. Thus, the VEP recorded at the scalp surface is usually dominated by signals arising from stimuli in the central visual field.

Retinal responses (such as the ERG) may be used in conjunction with the VEP to make an assessment of visual pathway function. The ERG tells us about retinal function and the VEP tells us about function of the retino-striate visual pathway as a whole. As an objective technique, the VEP requires no behavioral or subjective response from the observer, who is required only to attend to a visual stimulus. The stimulus is changing overtime, so that electrical signals should be generated regularly in response to each change. The stimulus change may involve pattern appearance and disappearance, for example, in which case a pattern and a uniform field (of equal space-average luminance) are alternated overtime. If the visual system is unable to distinguish the pattern, no regular response is expected, because visual system activity will be identical during the pattern appearance and disappearance phases and will remain unchanged overtime.

Clinical Uses in Children

- Visual potential in the eye with corneal opacities
- Detection of amblyopia
- Monitor occlusion and other amblyopia treatment modalities

Few other tests like Lea puzzle can be very good tool in less attentive children. Lea gratings are alternative to TAC with hand held cards. Hundreds and thousands test consists of multiple tiny beads of different sizes and can estimate visual acuity well in infants.

Different Tests Useful According to Age

1-2 Years of Age

- TAC
- CAC
- Hundreds and thousands
- Boeck candy test
- STYCAR graded ball test
- Worth ivory ball test (Ivory balls from 0.5 to 1.5 inches are rolled in front of child and the child is asked to retrieve them)
  VA in decimal = 0.3 * object distance (in meters)/Object size in mm.

2-3 Years

Language skills sufficient to name pictures

- Hundreds and thousands
- Allen's picture cards
- Sheridan's miniature toy test
- Kay's picture test
- Coin test
- Dot VA test
- Bailey-Hall, cereal test.

3-5 Years of Age

Able to take matching of letter optotypes

- Tumbling E or illiterate E
- Sheridan-Gardener's test
- Lippman's HOTV test
- Landolt's C test.

> 6 Years

For distance

- Snellen's letter charts
- ETDRS charts.

For near

- Reduced Snellen letter charts
- Jaeger's test types
- N's types (Times Roman).

Chapter 2

Congenital Cataract

SH Lee (Canada)

Introduction

A *cataract* is an opacification of the lens.

Congenital cataracts usually are diagnosed at birth. If a cataract goes undetected in an infant, permanent visual loss may ensue. Not all cataracts are visually significant. If a lenticular opacity is in the visual axis, it is considered visually significant and may lead to blindness. If the cataract is small, in the anterior portion of the lens, or in the periphery, no visual loss may be present.

Unilateral cataracts are usually isolated sporadic incidents. They can be associated with ocular abnormalities (e.g. posterior lenticonus, persistent hyperplastic primary vitreous, anterior segment dysgenesis, posterior pole tumors), trauma, or intrauterine infection, particularly rubella.

Bilateral cataracts are often inherited and associated with other diseases. They require a full metabolic, infectious, systemic, and genetic workup. The common causes are hypoglycemia, trisomy (e.g. Down, Edward, and Patau's syndromes), myotonic dystrophy, infectious diseases (e.g. toxoplasmosis, rubella, cytomegalovirus, and herpes simplex [TORCH]), and prematurity.

Clinical Features of Rubella's Syndrome

1. *Congenital heart disease* is commonly *patent ductus arteriosus* or peripheral pulmonary artery stenosis.
2. Eye defects include *cataracts, congenital glaucoma, pigmentary retinopathy* (50%—so-called "salt and pepper"), severe myopia, micro-ophthalmia.
3. Microcephaly.

Pathophysiology

The lens forms during the invagination of surface ectoderm overlying the optic vesicle. The embryonic nucleus develops by the sixth week of gestation. Surrounding the embryonic nucleus is the fetal nucleus. At birth, the embryonic and fetal nuclei make-up most of the lens. Postnatally, cortical lens fibers are laid down from the conversion of anterior lens epithelium into cortical lens fibers.

The Y-sutures are an important landmark because they identify the extent of the fetal nucleus. Lens material peripheral to the Y-sutures is lens cortex, whereas lens material within and including the Y-sutures is nuclear. At the slit lamp, the anterior Y-suture is oriented upright, and the posterior Y-suture is inverted.

Any insult (e.g. infectious, traumatic, metabolic) to the nuclear or lenticular fibers may result in an opacity (cataract) of the clear lenticular media. The location and pattern of this opacification may be used to determine the timing of the insult as well as the etiology.

Normal, clear lens　　　　Lens clouded by cataract

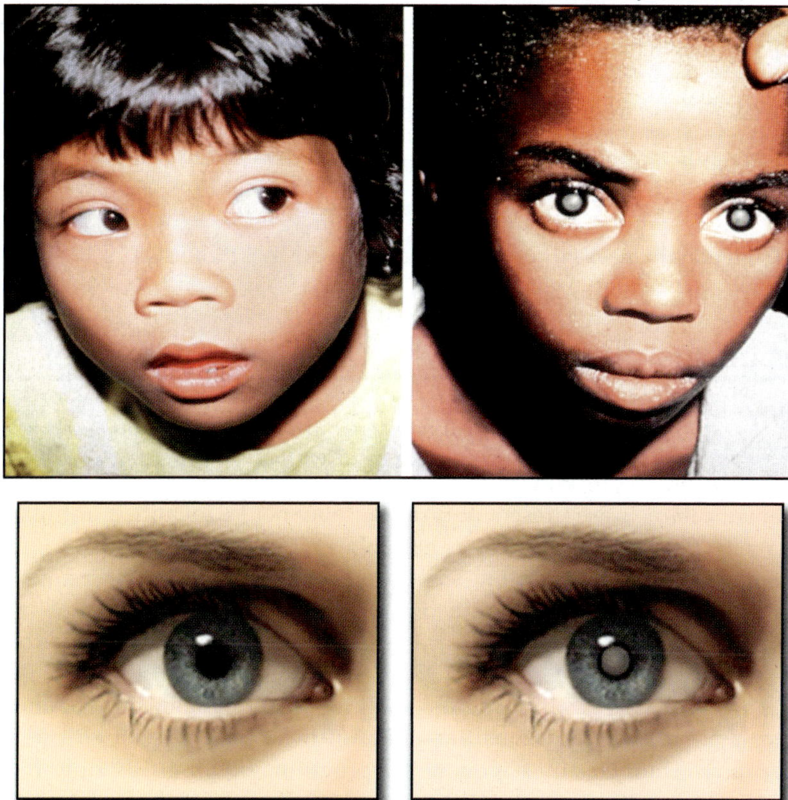

A cataract is an opacity (clouding) of the normally clear lens which may develop as a result of aging, metabolic disorders, trauma or heredity

Figure 1: Child in left picture with bilateral congenital cataracts

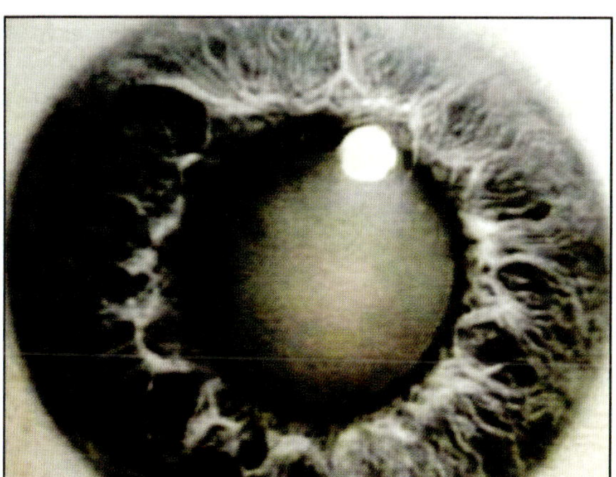

Figure 2: Clinical picture of cataract

Mortality/Morbidity

Visual morbidity may result from deprivation amblyopia, refractive amblyopia, glaucoma (as many as 10% post surgical removal), and retinal detachment.

Metabolic and systemic diseases are found in as many as 60% of bilateral cataracts.

Mental retardation, deafness, kidney disease, heart disease, and other systemic involvement may be part of the presentation.

Age: Congenital cataracts usually are diagnosed in newborns.

Symptoms and Signs

Symptoms

By large, the principal symptom of cataract is **blur of vision** when it affects the visual axis. As infant and child usually do not complain visual symptom, congenital cataracts are present at birth but may not be identified until later in life. Prenatal and family history is helpful.

Some cataracts are static, but some are progressive. This explains why not all congenital cataracts are identified at birth.

Anterior polar cataract and nuclear cataract are usually static, although they may rarely progress.

Cataracts that typically progress include posterior lenticonus, persistent hyperplastic primary vitreous, lamellar, sutural, and anterior or posterior subcapsular. They usually have a better prognosis because they only usually begin to obstruct the vision after the critical period of visual development has passed.

Not all cataracts are visually significant. If a lenticular opacity is in the visual axis, it usually is considered visually significant and requires removal.

Cataracts in the center of the visual axis that are greater than 3 mm in diameter are generally considered visually significant. This principle is furthermore correlated with the clinical ophthalmological examination of the patient.

A study by the Department of Pediatric Ophthalmology of the Wills Eye Hospital concluded that, in terms of the risk factor for *amblyopia*, more important than the cataract size is the anisometropia induced by the congenital anterior lens opacities. Patients with congenital anterior lens opacities who have anisometropia of 1 diopter (D) or more are 6.5 times more likely to develop amblyopia.

Signs

A lenticular opacity is called a cataract. Not all cataracts are visually significant.

Description of a congenital cataract must include location, color, density, and shape for purposes of identification.

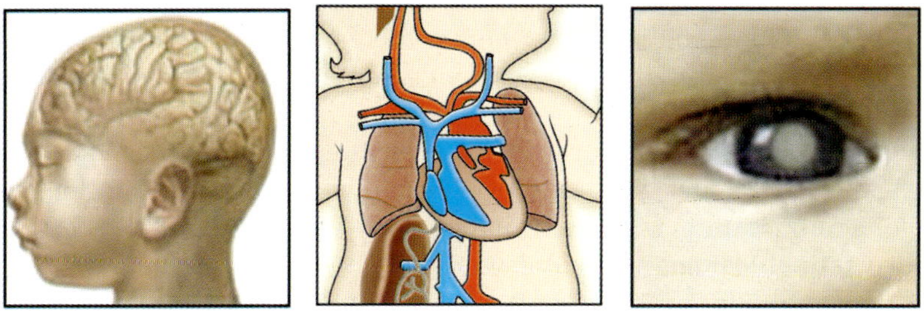

Microcephaly PDA Cataracts

Figure 3: Congenital cataract with Rubella's syndrome

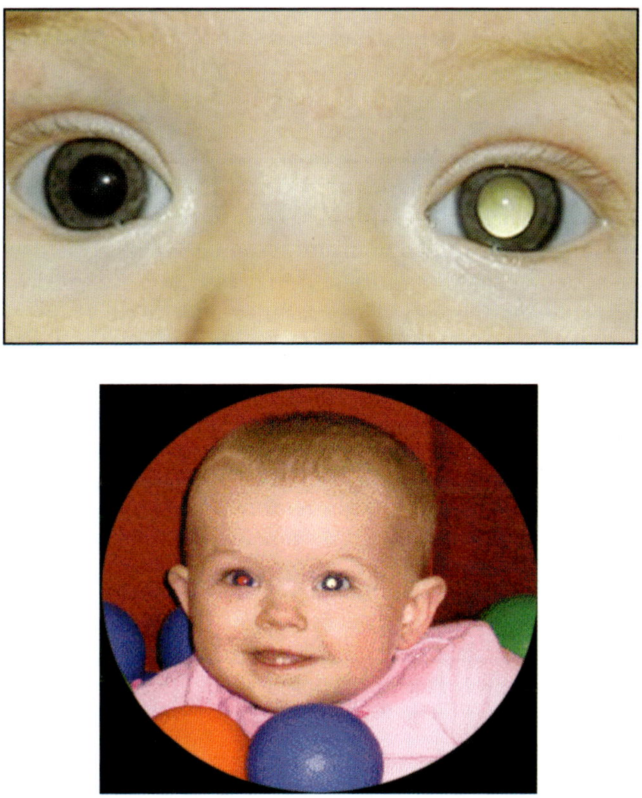

Figure 4: Child with left retinoblastoma

An irregular red reflex is the hallmark of visual problems. If an irregular red reflex is detected at the initial screening, this is usually an indication that a congenital cataract might be present and an ophthalmology consultation is warranted.

Leukocoria or white reflex can be the presenting sign of a cataract. In fact, in a 2008 study by Haider et al, 60% of patients who presented with leukocoria had congenital cataracts (18% unilateral and 42% bilateral). Other causes included **retinoblastoma** (11% unilateral and 7% bilateral), retinal detachment (2.8% unilateral and 1.4% bilateral), bilateral persistent **hyperplastic primary vitreous** (4.2%), and **unilateral coats disease** (4.2%).

Slit-lamp examination of both eyes (dilated pupil) not only may confirm the presence of a cataract but also may identify the time when the insult occurred *in utero* and if there is other systemic or metabolic involvement.

Dilated fundus examination is recommended as part of the ocular examination for both unilateral cataract cases and bilateral cataract cases.

Etiology

The most common etiology includes intrauterine infections, metabolic disorders, and genetically transmitted syndromes. One third of pediatric cataracts are sporadic; they are not associated with any systemic or ocular diseases. However, they may be spontaneous mutations and may lead to cataract formation in the patient's offspring. As many as 23% of congenital cataracts are familial. The most frequent mode of transmission is autosomal dominant with complete penetrance. This type of cataract may appear as a total cataract, polar cataract, lamellar cataract, or nuclear opacity. All close family members should be examined.

Infectious causes of cataracts include rubella (the most common), rubeola, chickenpox, cytomegalovirus, herpes simplex, herpes zoster, poliomyelitis, influenza, Epstein-Barr virus, syphilis, and toxoplasmosis.

Differential Diagnosis

The most important one is **Retinoblastoma**

Other Problems to be Considered

Corneal opacity (ulcer, scar, dermoid)

Other Differential Diagnosis

Persistent hyperplastic primary vitreous
Retinal detachment
Lenticular coloboma

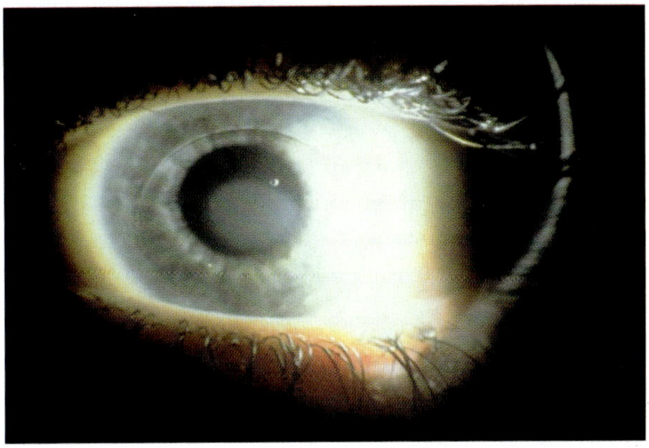

Figure 5: Child with congenital corneal opacity

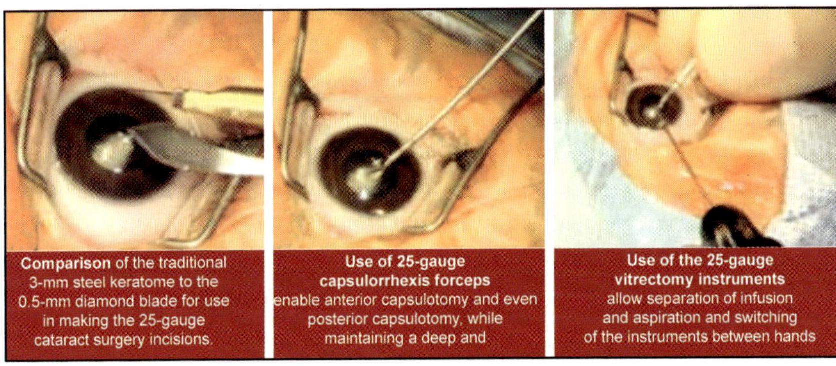

Figure 6: Procedure for extracting the congenital cataract and anterior vitrectomy or posterior capsulectomy

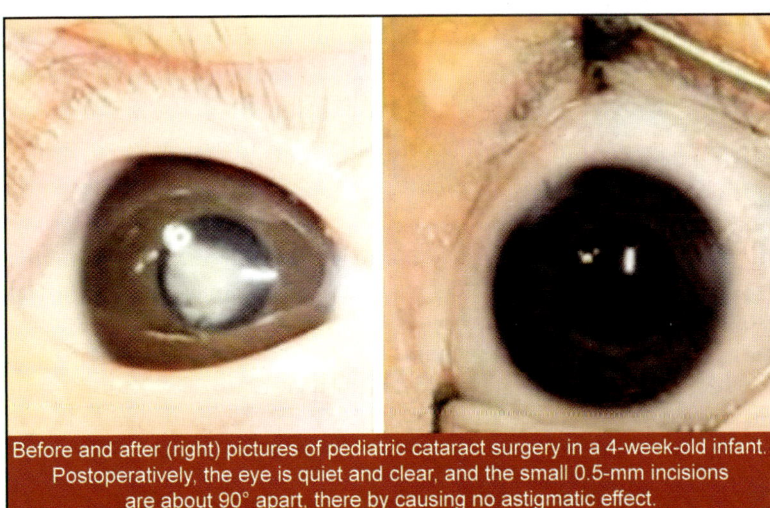

Figure 7: Congenital cataract before and after surgery

Diagnosis

Lab Studies

For unilateral cataracts, laboratory studies include TORCH titers for herpex simplex, and venereal disease research laboratory (VDRL) test.

For bilateral cataracts, laboratory studies include CBC, BUN, TORCH titers, VDRL, urine for reducing substances, red cell galactokinase, urine for amino acids, calcium, and phosphorus.

Imaging Studies

CT scan of brain to rule out any cranial developmental abnormalities.

Other Tests

Hearing test to rule out birth defect such as child with Rubella's syndrome.

Treatment

Medical Care

Medical therapy is directed at the prevention of amblyopia.

Surgical Care

Cataract surgery is the treatment of choice and should be performed when patients are younger than 17 weeks to ensure minimal or no visual deprivation. Most ophthalmologists opt for surgery much earlier, ideally when patients are younger than 2 months, to prevent irreversible amblyopia and sensory nystagmus in the case of bilateral congenital cataracts. The delay in surgery is because of glaucoma. Since glaucoma occurs in 10% of congenital cataract surgery, many surgeons delay the cataract surgery.

Unfortunately, the improved surgical techniques of the 1990s have not lowered the incidence of glaucoma from the series published in the 1980s. The development of glaucoma (which occurs in later years) only occurs in cataract eyes that undergo surgery. This may be in part due to the immaturity of the angle at the time of surgery. A delay of a few weeks allows the angle of the immature eye to develop.

Koc and colleagues concluded that early age at cataract extraction and microcornea are risk factors for delayed-onset glaucoma.

Extracapsular cataract extraction with primary posterior capsulectomy and anterior vitrectomy is the procedure of choice (via limbal or pars plana approach). Intracapsular cataract extraction in children is contraindicated because of vitreous traction and loss at the Wieger capsulohyaloid ligament. Vitrectomy instrumentation is the preferred method since the lens material is very soft. The whole procedure can be performed using one intraocular instrument. Young eyes develop capsular opacification very quickly, necessitating primary capsulectomy at the time of cataract extraction.

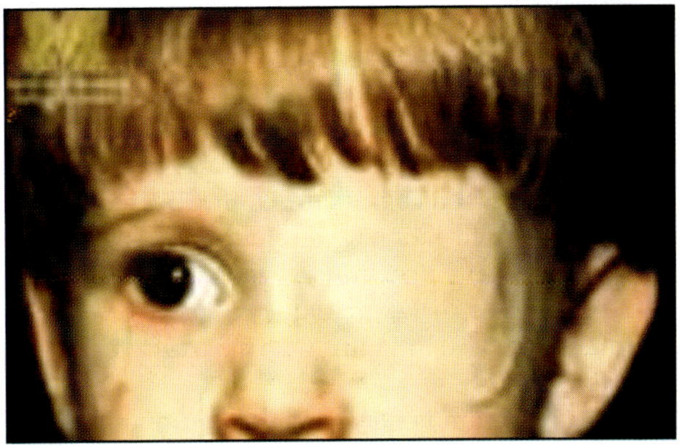

Figure 8: Child with eye patch therapy to the left normal eye after right congenital cataract surgery. Child, 1 year and 6 months has right congenital cataract surgery and secondary glaucoma and left normal eye and had EUA with following pictures, data and management

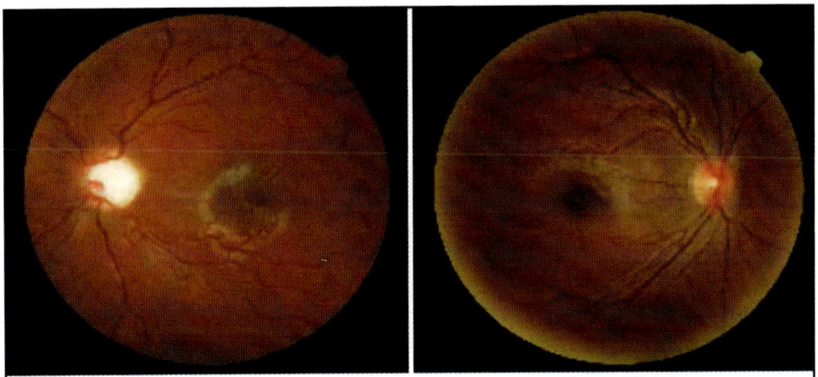

Increased cupping	Normal fundus

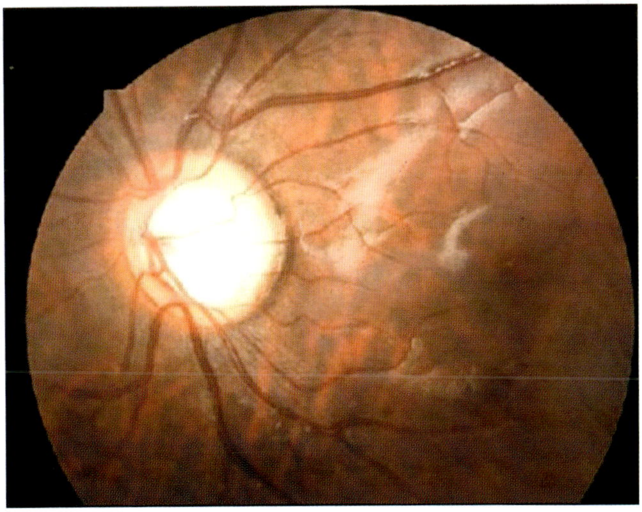

Figure 9: Increased cupping of the optic nerve

A study by the Retina Foundation of the Southwest in Texas compared intraocular lens (IOL) implantation with aphakic contact lenses (CLs) after the extraction of a unilateral cataract. Patients were as young as 6 months. They concluded that IOLs and aphakic CLs support similar visual acuity development after surgery for a unilateral cataract. IOLs may support better visual acuity development when compliance with CL wear is moderate to poor or when a cataract is extracted in a patient older than 1 year.

A study with promising preliminary results concerns the primary implantation of flexible IOLs in infants younger than 1 year. The population studied includes infants aged 3-11 months who have different forms of unilateral congenital cataracts.

A 2008 study by Capozzi and colleagues showed that in the first 42 months of age, corneal power (Km) and axial length (AL) values are significantly different according to age. These findings have implications for the calculation of IOL power. Km values were significantly greater, and AL readings were shorter, in younger children ($p < 0.001$). No differences according to gender were found. As a group, eyes from unilateral cataract cases had significantly longer AL readings than those from bilateral cataract cases ($p = 0.029$). In a small subgroup of unilateral cataract cases, for which readings from the clear lens eye were available (n. 39), Km values of the affected eye were significantly greater than that of the fellow healthy eye ($p = 0.007$).

Further Consideration

A red reflex is essential not only in the newborn nursery but also in all office visits.

Frequent eye examinations help in the prevention of amblyopia.

Frequent glaucoma screenings are needed throughout the patient's lifetime.

Complications of Surgical Treatment

Loss of vision even with aggressive surgical and optical treatment
Amblyopia

Secondary Glaucoma of Right Eye

EUA (Exam under anesthesia) of the child in Figure 8 at 1.5 years finding:
Corneal diameter : OD 12.25 mm, O.S. 9.75 mm
IOP OD 29 mm Hg, OS 20 mm Hg
C/D OD 0.95, OS 0.5
Refractive error OD +24.00, OS + 1.00
Goniotomy OD
Medical therapy—antiglaucomatous medications, e.g. eyedrop pilocarpine 4%

Other Complications to Monitor

1. Strabismus
2. Retinal detachment

Prognosis

Of persons with unilateral congenital cataracts, 40% develop visual acuity of 20/60 or better.

Of persons with bilateral congenital cataracts, 70% develop visual acuity of 20/60 or better.

The prognosis is poorer in persons with other ocular or systemic involvement.

Patient Education

Removal of the cataract is only the beginning. Visual rehabilitation requires many years of refractive correction (e.g. contact lenses, aphakic glasses), possible patching for amblyopia, possible strabismus surgery, and glaucoma screenings.

Patients must be made aware of the risk of potential visual loss from amblyopia, retinal detachment, or glaucoma.

Repeated surgical procedures, including a secondary lens implant, if other modalities of refractive correction fail, may be needed.

If this is a de novo chromosomal change or a familial abnormality, all siblings and future offspring are at risk.

Of persons with bilateral congenital cataracts, 70% develop visual acuity of 20/60 or better.

The prognosis is poorer in persons with other ocular or systemic involvement.

Chapter 3

Pediatric Cataract

Rupal H Trivedi, M Edward Wilson (USA)

Introduction

Cataract remains one of the most important causes of treatable blindness in children. A propensity for increased postoperative inflammation and capsular opacification, constantly changing refraction due to growth of the eye, difficulty in documenting anatomic and refractive changes due to poor compliance, and a tendency to develop amblyopia are among the factors that make cataract surgery in the child different from that in the adult.

Clinical Signs and Symptoms

A chief complaint from the parents may be a white spot in the pupil, visual inattentiveness, nystagmus, strabismus or ocular injury. Specific information should be gathered on age; birth weight; evidence of maternal infection, rash or febrile illness during pregnancy, age at onset of visual symptoms, etc.

The method of evaluating visual function will vary according to the level of cooperation. The red reflex test using the retinoscope or direct ophthalmoscope can be used to detect the density and extent of the opacity. Details on strabismus and nystagmus mainly help when explaining prognosis to the parents.

External examination of the eye with a suspected cataract usually consists of a penlight evaluation of eyelids, eyelashes, conjunctiva, sclera, cornea, and iris. A slit-lamp evaluation should be carried out if the child is cooperative. Lens subluxation, iridodonesis, aniridia, band-shaped keratopathy, posterior synechiae, or anterior lenticonus may be associated findings. A sudden onset of total cataract may be an indication of unsuspected trauma, diabetic cataract or spontaneous rupture of the anterior (reported in anterior lenticonus) or posterior capsule (reported in posterior lentiglobus). Finally, if possible a slit-lamp examination of both parents, helps to establish the presence of familial cataracts, which can have variable expressivity.

Investigations

As compared to unilateral cataract, laboratory investigation of bilateral cases is more rewarding. Exhaustive lists of laboratory investigations for a child with cataract can be found in several textbooks, however, in an otherwise healthy child, most physicians do not advise extensive laboratory and genetic investigations. Based on history and examination, customized laboratory investigations can be advised. Examination under anesthesia is generally required for detailed evaluation of eye including: IOP, keratometry, examine the eye using the operating microscope, A-scan, corneal diameter, and a fundus examination.

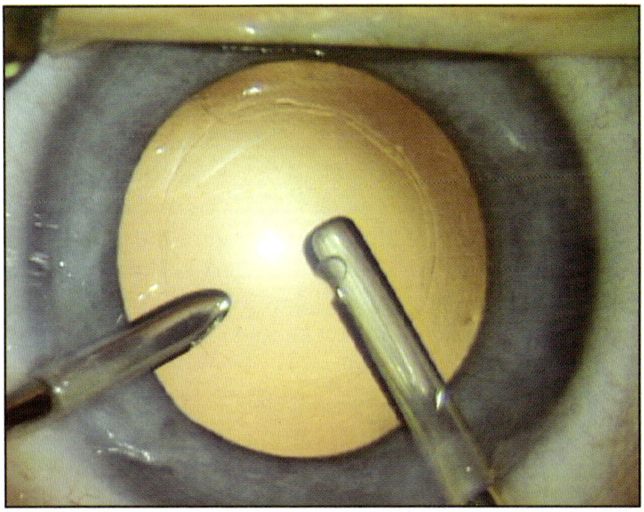

Figure 1: Anterior and posterior capsulorhexis in 3 month old child

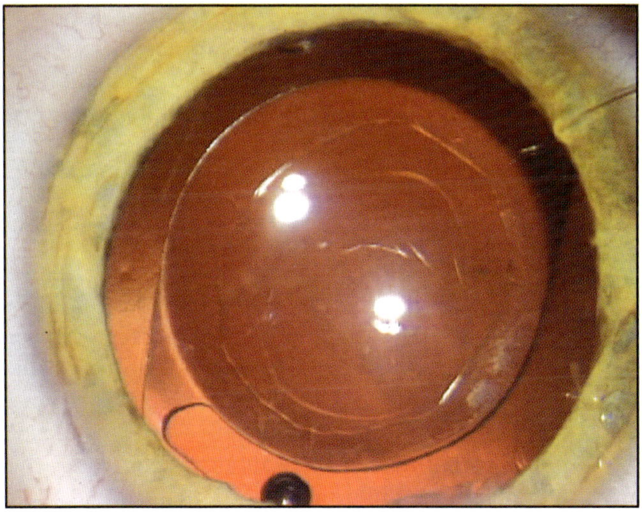

Figure 2: In-the-bag single piece AcrySof IOL implantation

Differential Diagnosis

Retinoblastoma, PFV, corneal opacity, iris cyst, retinal detachment, lenticular coloboma

Treatment

The aim of pediatric cataract surgery is to provide and maintain a clear visual axis and a focused retinal image. Cataract surgery in children is but one-step in the long road to visual rehabilitation, not the end of the journey.

Deciding on the appropriate timing of surgery is most critical during early infancy. Dense unilateral cataract present at birth can be removed within 4-6 weeks of age while bilateral cataract should be removed before 10 weeks of age. In children beyond the amblyopic age, surgery can more appropriately be decided based on convenience and other logistic issues.

The surgeon should strictly adhere to the principles of a closed-chamber technique. Proper wound construction and a tight fit around the instruments helps assure chamber stability throughout phacoaspiration. The anterior capsule in children is highly elastic and poses challenges in the creation of the capsulotomy. While a manual CCC is ideal for adults, it is more difficult to perform in young eyes. Overall, the vitrectorhexis is commonly used for infantile eyes. Manual CCC is used most often in children beyond infancy.

Since visual axis opacification (VAO) is one of the most frequent postoperative complications in pediatric cataract surgery, meticulous removal of the lens substance is a crucial step in the management of pediatric cataracts. Hydrodissection and bimanual irrigation/aspiration are helpful achieving the goal. Separate irrigation and aspiration help maintain the anterior chamber stability, decrease fluctuations of the anterior chamber and help thorough removal of lens substance. The addition of 0.5 ml of adrenaline to the infusion bottle helps to maintain mydriasis.

In young children who undergo pediatric cataract surgery, posterior capsule opacification (PCO) is rapid and virtually inevitable if the posterior capsule is left intact. As of today, primary posterior capsulectomy and anterior vitrectomy is common practice while managing younger children with cataract. An important question that remains is, when should the posterior capsule be left intact? We answer this question looking at several factors (age, association of posterior capsule plaque or defect, availability of YAG Laser, expected cooperation of child approximately 12-24 months after cataract surgery for YAG). As a rough guideline, in children below 5 years of age, we prefer to do primary posterior capsulectomy and vitrectomy. In children, 5-8 years of age, we will do a posterior capsulectomy with or without vitrectomy, as needed. In children above 8 years of age, we keep an intact posterior capsule more often.

Intraocular lens implantation (IOL) in children has the benefit of reducing dependency on compliance with aphakic glasses and contact lenses and provide at least a partial optical correction. These are important advantages to the visual development in amblyopia-prone eyes. However, concerns about primary IOL implantation are the technical difficulties of implanting an IOL in the eyes of children, selecting an appropriate IOL power, and the risk of VAO after implantation. Despite performing primary posterior capsulectomy and vitrectomy, the rate of VAO is higher in pseudophakic infantile eyes as compared with aphakic infantile eyes. On the other hand, although it is possible for an eye with a unilateral infantile cataract to achieve good visual outcome following contact lens correction, it has continued to be the exception rather than the rule. A general consensus exists that IOL implantation is appropriate for most older children undergoing cataract surgery. In contrast, the advisability of IOL implantation during the first year of life is still being questioned. Both IOLs and aphakic contact lenses may support similar VA after surgery for unilateral cataract in the presence of good compliance with contact lens. However, IOLs support better VA when compliance with contact lens wear is moderate or poor. For bilateral cataracts, aphakic glasses and/or contact lens use may be a reasonable option. However, for unilateral cataracts in infancy, the issue of when to implant an IOL is unresolved.

Implantation of a fixed-power IOL into an eye that is still growing makes it difficult to choose the IOL power to implant. IOL implantation at the calculated emmetropic power helps to fight amblyopia during childhood, but risks significant myopia at ocular maturity. Ideal IOL power should balance the best help to amblyopia management in childhood with the least possible refractive error in adulthood. Several nomograms have been published in the literature. However, we do not recommend the use of any published table alone for deciding IOL power. These tables are only meant to help as a starting point toward appropriate IOL power selection, which is a multifactorial decision customized for each child based on many variables [age, laterality (one eye or both), amblyopia status (dense or mild), likely compliance with glasses, and family history of myopia].

When placing an IOL in a child's eye, in-the-bag implantation is strongly recommended. The AcrySof® hydrophobic acrylic IOL (Alcon Laboratories, Ft Worth, Texas) has been shown to be very biocompatible for the pediatric eyes. The one-piece AcrySof® is especially suited for small soft eyes and can be inserted into the capsular bag with ease.

Suturing the wounds in children is the norm. The recommended closure material is a 10-0 synthetic absorbable suture. The use of non-absorbable sutures occasionally calls for an EUA for suture removal. Even when economic issues are a deciding factor in choice of suture material, it is better to use absorbable sutures rather than subject the child to additional anesthesia.

Prognosis

When cataract surgery is required in the early years of life, complications such as glaucoma and VAO are frequent. Eyes operated during first year of life and with associated ocular anomalies (e.g. anterior segment dysgenesis, iris hypoplasia, or persistent fetal vasculature) are at higher risk for developing VAO and glaucoma. Median visual acuity of 20/30 is reported but late surgery and poor follow-up can lead to very disappointing results. Amblyopia is the major cause of residual visual deficit. In bilateral cataracts, sensory nystagmus is a sign that the visual outcome will be markedly reduced.

Chapter 4

Pearls and Tricks in Congenital Cataract Surgery

Simonetta Morselli, Roberto Bellucci (Italy)

Introduction

The definition of congenital cataract is the evolutive opacification of the crystalline lens that causes limitation of the visual acuity. This type of opacity can be present at birth or it can develop in the first three months of life. This type of cataract is called "early developmental" cataract. The incidence of the congenital cataract is 0.4 % of the total population. It is an important blindness factor for babies, that accounts from 20 to 38% of the total blindness. The management of this disorder has long challenged clinicians, but the past few decades have seen significant changes in the approach and in the management, due to the information gathered from basic scientific and clinical research. The most important visual loss is mainly attributable to amblyopia, that is caused from stimulus deprivation with the additional factor of ocular rivalry in unilateral disease. Thus, enhanced understanding of critical periods of visual development led to surgical intervention for dense cataract being deemed necessary within the first 3 months of life, and possibly as early as the first 6 weeks in unilateral disease. The need to ensure early detection and to allow prompt treatment, has resulted in the implementation of various strategies, it is recommended to carry out population screening examinations of newborn examination in many countries.

Diagnosis

The diagnosis is very easy when a complete cataract is present at birth because of the visible leukocoria. When the cataract is posterior and not progressing to the anterior lens layers, the white colour of the pupil cannot be detected easily and the diagnosis can be very late, when nistagmus or strabismus appears. Unfortunately, the visual deprivation in the first month of life creates a sensorial obstacle that causes amblyopia, nistagmus and strabismus.

Preoperative Pearls

Pupil Dilation

The dilation of the pupil is a very important factor for congenital cataract surgery. The mydriasis is very difficult to obtain and to maintain during surgery. In our experience this type of mixture works very well:
1 ml of phenylephrine 10% and tropicamide 0.5% + 1 ml of atropine 1% diluted in the same syringe with 8 cc of saline water. Apply 1 drop every 15 min, starting two hours before surgery and until the pupil is dilated. To maintain the mydriasis inject 0.5 ml of adrenaline into the 500 ml BSS bottle used during surgery.

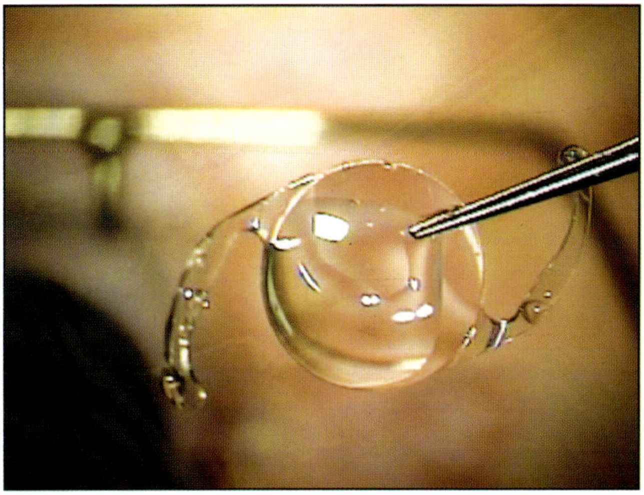

Figure 1: AcrySof SA30AL IOL is available. This model has a 12.5 mm overall diameter and 5.5 mm optic diameter

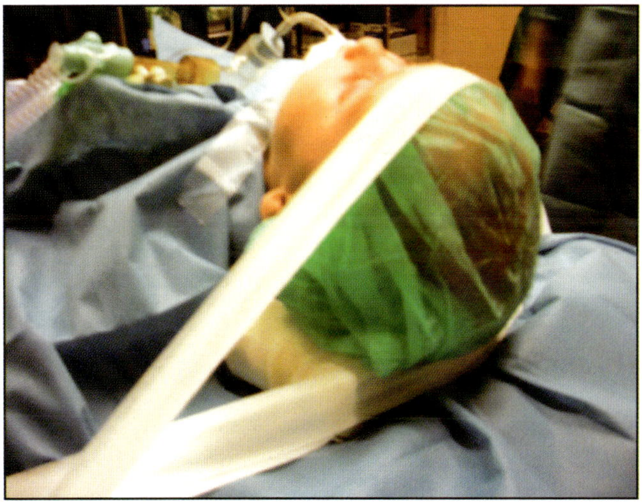

Figure 2: The baby head must be fixed with an adhesive strip to the operating bed

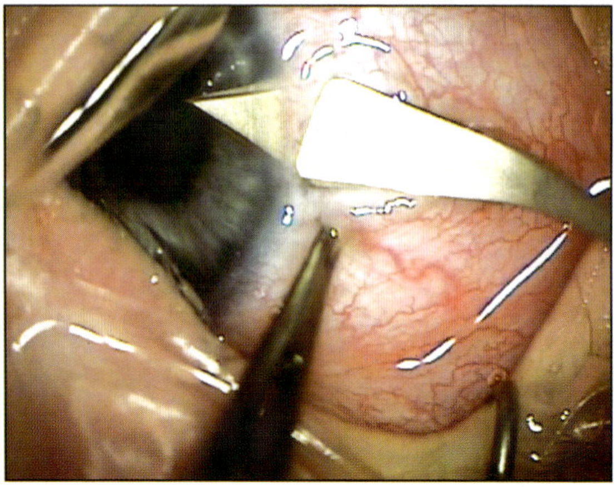

Figure 3: The incision is created at 12 o'clock under a conjunctival flap

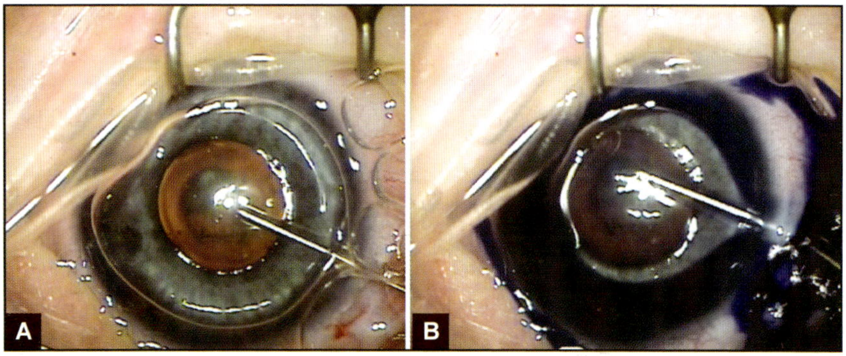

Figures 4A and B: Aspirate 1 ml of methylene blue in an insulin syringe with an air bubble, inject the air bubble first and then methylene blue, with the same syringe through the sideport incision

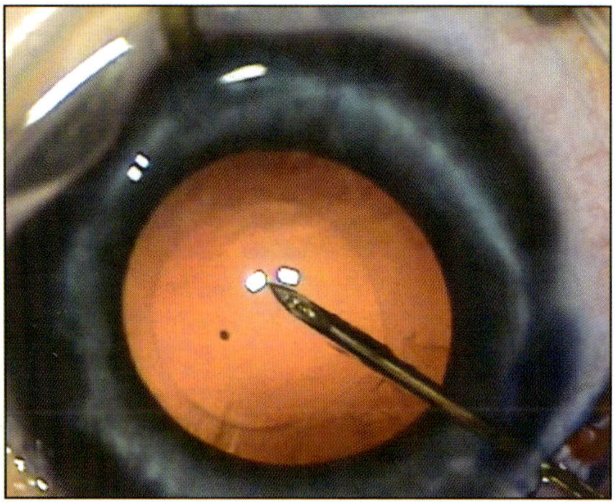

Figure 5: A small hole in the center of the posterior capsular bag with a needle

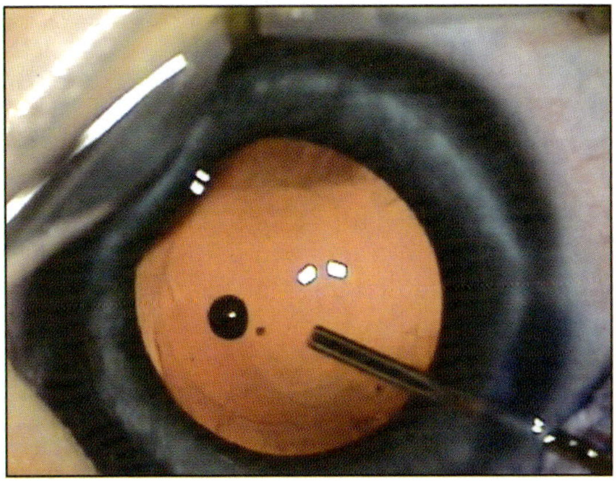

Figure 6: Inject the viscoelastic between the anterior surface of hyaloid and the posterior surface of the capsular bag

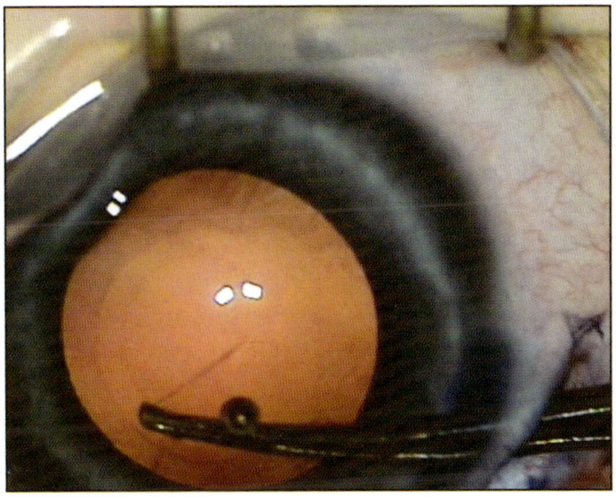

Figure 7: The capsulorhexis is completed with 'Coridon's forceps'

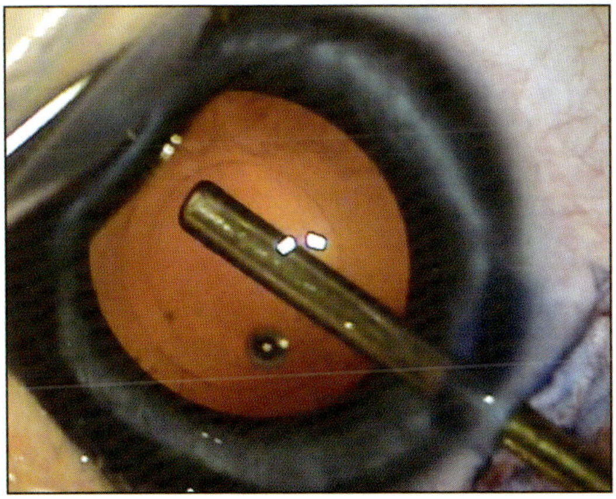

Figure 8: Anterior vitrectomy is mandatory

IOL Implantation

We plan to implant in babies from birth and onwards, because we had negative experiences in the compliance with glasses or with contact lenses after surgery. The type of IOL implantation at the time of cataract surgery is one of the most critical points in congenital cataract surgery. Polymethylmethacrylate (PMMA) IOLs have been successful in pediatric eyes; however, the capsular and inflammatory responses remain a problem. Now, the AcrySof IOLs made of flexible hydrophobic acrylic material are available(Alcon Laboratories, Forth Worth, Texas), with favourable outcome when used in children. Out of the AcrySof family, the 5.5 mm optic lens seems the most apt to small babies. Until recently, the 5.5 mm optic AcrySof IOL was available only in a 3-piece design with PMMA haptics (MA30 BM), with a total diameter of 12.5 mm. Now also the single piece AcrySof SA30AL IOL is produced, with the same optic diameter and overall length.

IOL Power Calculation

Preoperative values of axial length and corneal curvature are rarely available in patients with congenital cataracts. Therefore these values have to be obtained under general anesthesia immediately before surgery. K readings are not easy to obtain even under general anesthesia because a portable corneal topographer is necessary. In addition, the K readings can change during the growth of the eye. Therefore, it could be convenient to base the IOL power calculation not on the K readings but only on the axial length. We select the IOL power with reference to the rules of Dr Dahan for babies less than one year old. If the axial length is about 20 mm we select a +25 D IOL, if it is about 19 mm we implant a +26 D, if the length is about 18 mm we implant a +28 D IOL. If the axial length is between 21 mm and 23 mm the power of the IOL will be equal to the axial length value +1D per mm exceeding 21. If the axial length is longer than 24 mm the power implanted will be equal to the axial length value–1 D per mm exceeding 24.

General Anesthesia

The anesthesiologist must be skilled in general anesthesia in very young patients. The use of curare is mandatory to have the eye in natural position and not in the "Bell phenomenon position". The baby's head must be fixed with an adhesive strip to the operating bed; two rolled cloths help to immobilize the head.

Surgical Pearls and Tricks

We pass a suture through the superior rectus muscle and fix it with 'Pean forceps' to modulate the position of the eye as the surgeon requires during the various steps of the surgery.

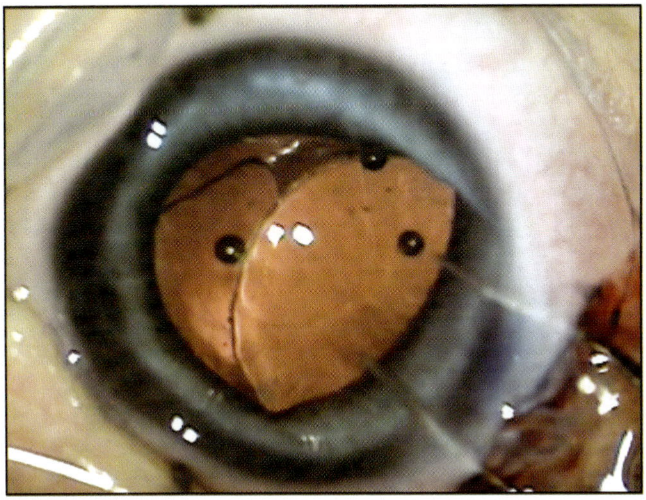

Figure 9: The IOL is inserted with the injector or with the forceps trying to inject the first in the sulcus

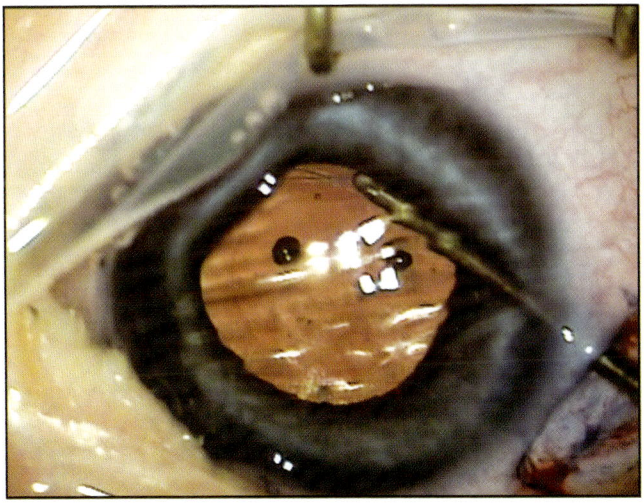

Figure 10: The optical plate of the IOL is incarcerated behind the two capsules

The main incision is created at 12 o'clock under a conjunctival flap.

At least one side-port incision is also created. At the end of the surgery it is mandatory to close the incisions with 10/0 vicryl.

The use of methylene blue under an air bubble is very helpful to color the anterior capsule before performing anterior capsulorhexis. Aspirate 0.5 ml of the methylene blue dye into an insulin syringe, followed by 0.5 ml of filtered air. Inject the air bubble first and then the methylene blue, to avoid any collapse of the anterior chamber: The air will empty the anterior chamber and the dye will be injected onto the capsule without touching the endothelium.

Use high molecular weight and cohesive viscoelastic substance to help performing capsulorhexis. The newborn capsule is very elastic and needs to be perforated by a 30G needle. The rhexis tear tends to escape toward the equator because of this elasticity, like it happens in pig eyes in wet-labs.

Posterior capsulorhexis is easier if you do not overfill the capsular bag with viscoelastic substance. A small hole in the center of the posterior capsule with a 30G needle helps creating space to inject allows viscoelastic injection between the anterior hyaloid surface and the posterior surface of the posterior capsule.

The posterior capsulorhexis is completed with 'Corydon forceps'.

Anterior vitrectomy is mandatory.

The IOL is inserted with the injector or with the forceps trying to inject the first loop into the ciliary sulcus.

This is usually difficult because the operated eye is very soft at this moment. The second loop is positioned in the sulcus with a manipulator. The optical plate is then pushed under the posterior capsulorhexis, so while the loops remain in the sulcus, the optical plate is incarcerated behind the two capsules.

Doing this maneuver the capsular bag remains closed and there is less opportunity for the remaining lens cells to proliferate and to create secondary cataract. The IOL remains stable and centered into the eye. The vitreous body stays behind the IOL and the capsular bag. With this method of IOL implantation, we experienced less inflammation and less synechiae between the IOL and the iris. In the postoperative, it is mandatory to maintain the pupil dilated with omatropine applied twice a day at least for one month to reduce inflammation and to prevent posterior synechiae.

Chapter 5

Bimanual Microphaco in Children

Jerome Bovet (Switzerland)

Introduction

Most of the adult cataract surgeon has to be familiar with the technique of pediatric cataract because in Europe, Africa and Asia there are very few ophthalmologist even less pediatric ophthalmologist. If you work in an eye camp or in a bush hospitals to do cataract surgery you will discover all kind of cataract and you will have not the possibility to say no to a children with a double white cataract.

Childhood cataract is the major preventable cause of lifelong visual impairment. In recent years technical and technological advances in adult surgery have helped pediatric cataract. Most of the surgeon agree now to implant at once as a mode of amblyopia rehabilitation. The aim of pediatric cataract surgery is to provide and maintain a clear visual axis and a focused retinal image. The long term visual outcome is often negatively affected by the development of amblyopia secondary to the cataract itself or owing to postoperative reopacification of the ocular media. One of the major challenges for pediatric cataract intraocular lens (IOL) surgery has been the adaptation of a techniques used for adult cataract –IOL surgery. The propensity for increased postoperative inflammation and capsular opacition, a refractive state that is constantly changing due to growth of the eye, a tendency to develop amblyopia are the factors that make cataract surgery in the child different from that in the adult.

The management of pediatric cataracts is far more complex than the management of cataracts in adults.

The use of Bimanual microphaco technique with 2 paracentesis has revolutionized cataract surgery. Most importantly it allows secure placement of the IOL within the confines of the capsular bag and limits its contact with the reactive uveal tissue.Minimal wound is also critical to the sucess of cataract surgery and can be achieved by the creation of a sutureless incision.

As we start doing bimanual phaco technique in 2001 we were surprise how easily this techniqe can be apply with very little change to pediatric cataract. This three next chapter will describe our bimanual phacotechnique apply to pediatrique cataract

I warmly recommend every surgeon to read the excellent textbook on pediatric cataract surgery by M Edward Wilson, Jr Rupal H Trivedi and Suresh K Pandey which is the reference textbook on the subject.

History

Phacoemulsification was used in pediatric cataract surgery for the first time in 1970 by Hiles et al and Callahan recommended phacoemulsification as a useful extension of the aspiration technique in children since the softness of the lens material can vary greatly from case to case.

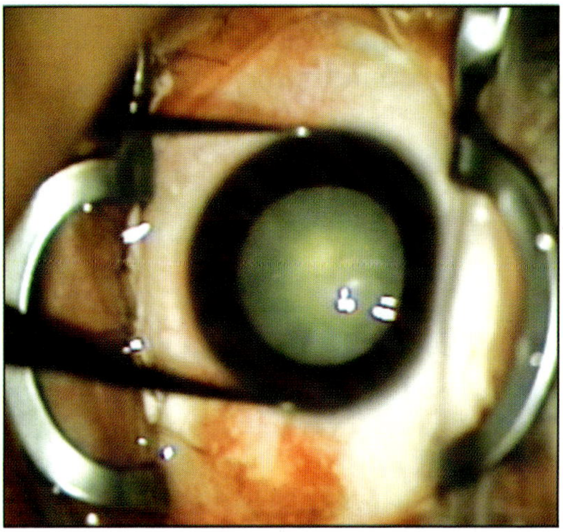

Figure 1: Measuring the white to white

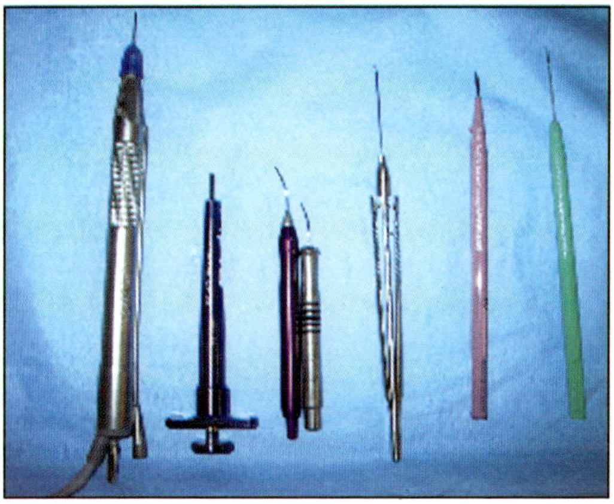

Figure 2: Instruments

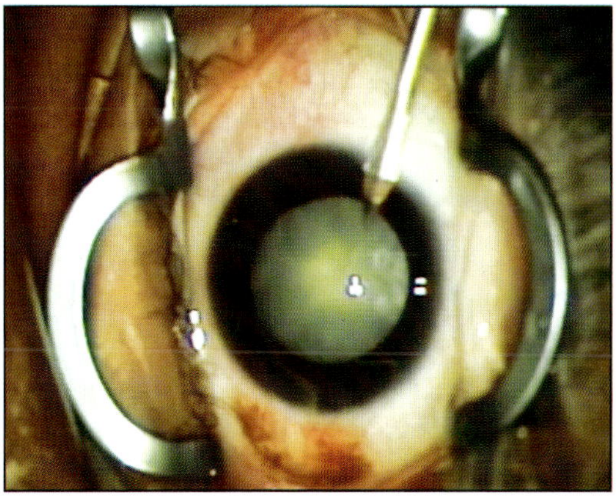

Figure 3: First paracentesis 19G

History Bimanual Phaco

To know who started the bimanual procedure we have to come back quit late the first which work with bimanual was de Dardenne in Bonn Germany he has one of the first the idea to take out the crystalline of a baby with a bimanual aspiration irrigation. Brauweiller come back with the technique with phaco and bimanual aspiration irrigation which is far more easier than with the monocannula. 1982 Steven P Shearing started to do phacoemulsification bimanual with a sleeweless tip.

Amar Agrawal restarted the technique of phakonit which mean phaco with a needle inside the hole. The reason the technique start this time that we found new lens which can be insert under an incision of 1.7 mm.

Pediatric cataract can be removed through a relatively small wound as the lens has no hard nuclei. That is why we propose to applicate the bimanual microphaco technique which is the last and the best technique for adult cataract to children with certain modifications which is necessary to fit to children.

Bimanual Microphacoemulsification Technique

We first measure the white to white distance to secure that we will have enough room to place a soft adult hydrophilic acrylic lens inside the bag at the end of the proceduren.

We use exactly the same Instruments for adult or pediatric Bimanual Microphaco phaco: probe sleveless 0.9 mm tip, bimanual irrigation-aspiration tip, shooter, capsulorhexis forceps, paracentesis 19G and 20G, we reserve for all children a bimanual vitrector with any vacuum pump machine to do an anterior vitrectomy

Anesthesia

The technique we generally use for a right eye is under general anesthesia.

Paracentesis

We started for a right eye by 2 paracentesis at 10 and 2 o'clock create a 20 gauge respectively a 19 G opening. We always control the width of the incision.

Dye of the Capsule

Injection of a buble of air and just after injection of trypan blue after 60 sec the excessive dye is washed out with the viscoelastic.

Viscous

Injection of high viscous acid hyaluronique, like healon GV or Healon 5.

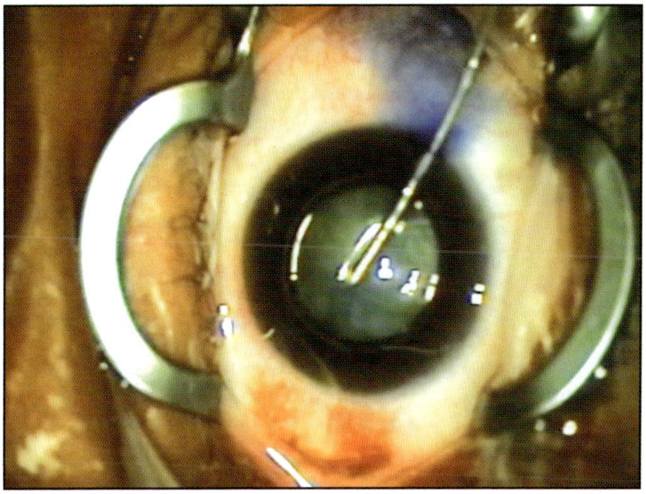

Figure 4: Dye the anterior capsule with trypan blue

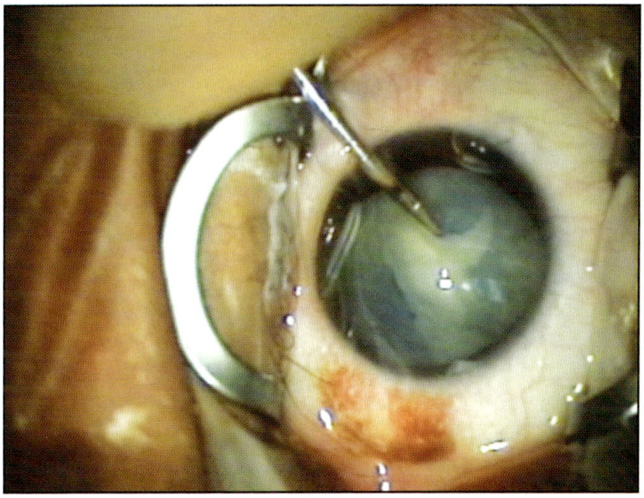

Figure 5: Rupture of the anterior capsule

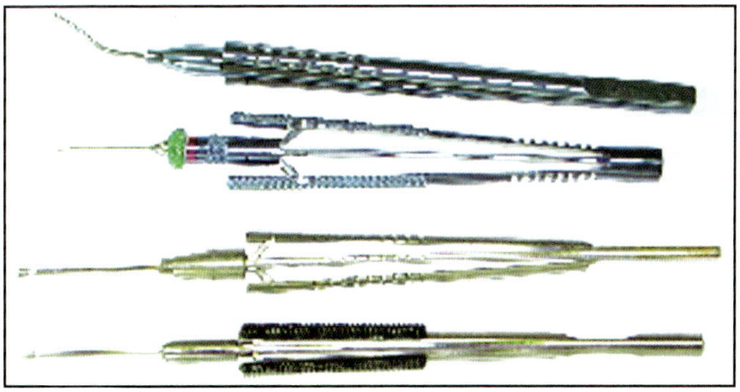

Figure 6: Capsulorhexis forceps

Capsulorhexis

Capsulorhexis with a double curve special 20 G forceps if the cutting force are centrifuge instead of centripet we repeat the procedure somewherelse if it's not possible we finish with a tin can opening that is does not mean that you will change the procedure.

You have to try many different forceps to find your cup of tea the most rigid, straight on used for vitrectomies are the worst, my best choice are the doubble curve first from the top.

Hydrodelineation-hydrodissection

For pediatric cataract we generally do not do any hydrodelineation because the nucleus is too soft. The hydrodissection of the cortex is more useful to detach the cortex from the capsule which is often sticky.

Phacoemulsification of the Nucleus

Bimanual microphaco technique change with the hardness of the cataract. We use most of the time very few phaco power because the pediatric cataract is very soft we aspirate most of the time the nucleus.

To succeed to your bimanual microphaco you have to change your fluidic systeme. You have to change the diameter of your irrigation from 20 gauge to a 19 gauge to increase the inflow in the anterior chamber to compensate the leak and the surge the outflow has to reach 30-35 cc/min to cool down the phacotip, the paracentesis have to be 1mm and for the phaco tip of 1,2 mm. To have the same efficacity during the phacotime we have to increase the vacuum to a level of 300 mmHg of vacuum.

Phacomachine manufacturers have devise numerous sophisticated strategies for minimizing the surge. The goal has been to provide surgeons the advantages with high vacuum without the danger . The simpliest and most efficacy to reach this target is to increase the flow inside the eye in increasing the lumen of the irrigating tip.

To prevent a surge the surgeon has to verify every session that the inflow is always superior has the outflow. For examples if you regulate your outflow to 35 cc/min and you have a 60 cc/min of inflow you will never have a surge even you have a vacuum of 500 mmHg that the secret of the 19 G technique. You have to play with the pedal like with the pedal of a piano not to give to much and to longer phacopower if you do not want to burn your cornea.

Epinucleus Removal if Exist

As progressively the soft nucleus is remove the posterior capsule is exposed to the phaco tip and the chamber stability becomes crucial. The vacuum has to be lower during the phase of aspirating the epinucleus but not to much. This phase is facilitate by a bimanual microphaco technique. The irrigating tip pass behind the epinucleus lo lift it in the anterior chamber.

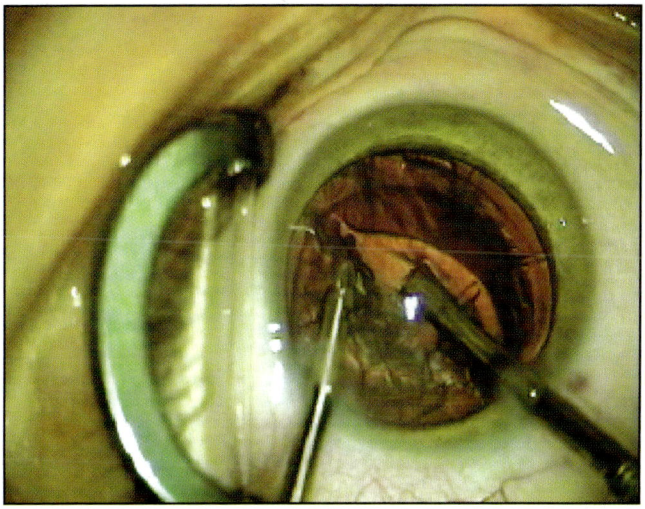

Figure 7: Bimanual MicroPhaco

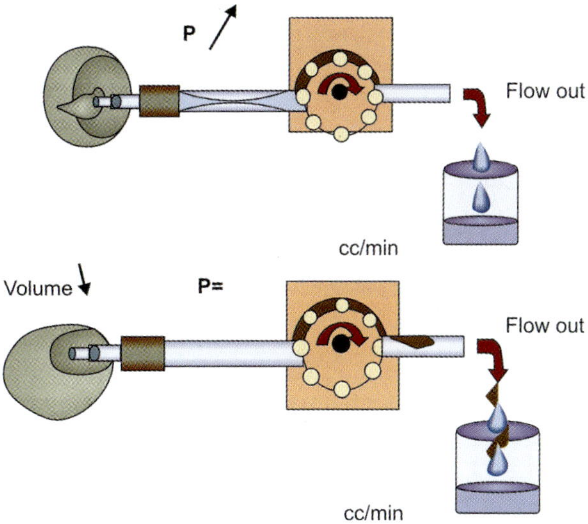

Figure 8: Vacuum with a Peristaltique pump

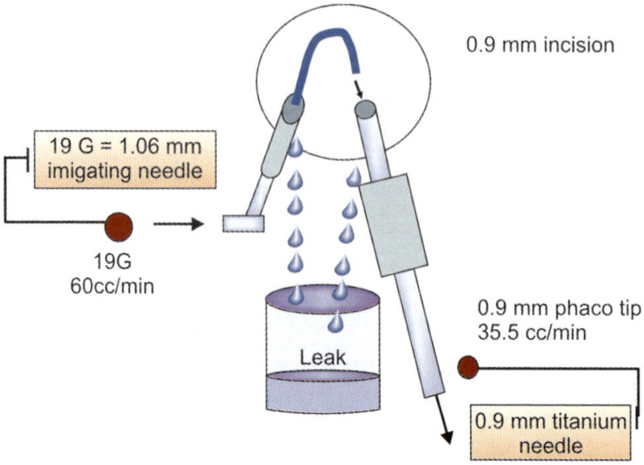

Figure 9: Inflow-Outflow=Leak

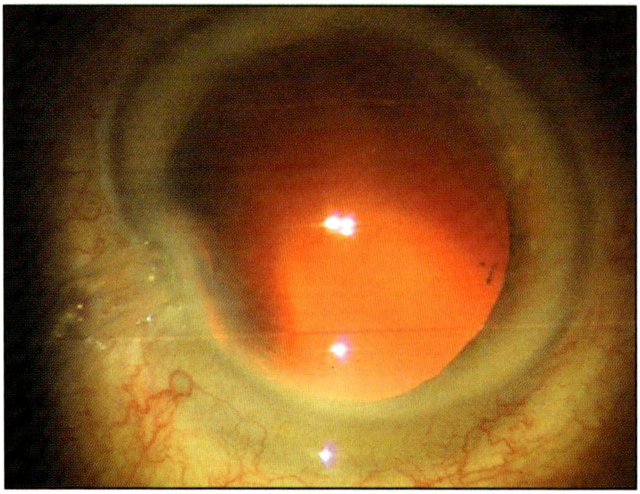

Figure 10: Injection a lens on a 1.7 mm incision

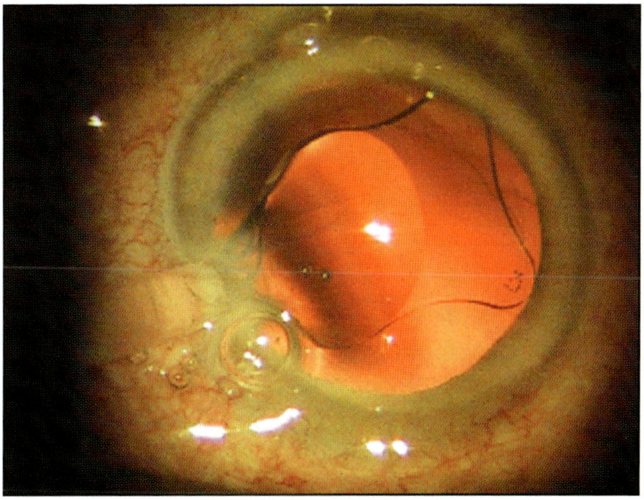

Figure 11: Insertion of an Acri Smart 36 A the catridge stay outside

Table 1: Setting bimanual Microphaco

Type of machine	*Amo Gemini*	*Amo Gemini*	*Amo Gemini*
Technique	Phaco chop Bimanual	Phaco chop Bimanual	Phaco chop Bimanual
Stage	Sculpting	Chopping	Epinucleus
Inflow cc/min	60.0	60.0	60.0
Real Bottle height cmH_2O	55	55	55
Pressure mmHg inside the eye	34.5	34.5	34,5
Outflow cc/min	36.5	36.5	36.5
Vacuum mmHg	100	300	200
Ultrasond % Linear,no pulse,no burst	30%	30%	30%

Irrigation-aspiration the Cortex

During this phase the vacuum has to be lower and the ultrasound switch off. We change the phacoemulsification probe by the irrigation-aspiration Duet systeme and we try to polish the anterior, posterior and equatorial capsule as much as we can to avoid a rapid posterior capsular opacity.

Lens

Only a few lens can be injected through an incision less than 2 mm for this purpose we have to put end to end the catridge and the corneal incision, then we have to shoot the lens like suppository inside the anterior chamber, we use most of the time the Acrismart 36 or 48 because of is stability and is accuracy with our biometry.The lens acrismart from Acritec is a acrylic hydrophilic-coated hydrophobic platelette lens. This lens has a very good reaction and the placement inside the bag is optimal.

Conclusion

The difference with a conventional phaco is the sleveless tip, the diameter of the bimanual irrigation-aspiration and the injector with a new catridge which permit to inject the lens without going inside the anterior chamber with the cartridge.

With pediatric cataract the 19G bimanual phacotechnique allowed the surgeon to switch from the phacoemulsification probe to the vitrector probe without changing any parameter and avoiding any surge of the anterior chamber which is one difficulties when we have to do an anterior vitrectomy or posterior vitrector capsulectomy.

The examples below give you an idea of what settings are being used at the beginning of the changing technique from coaxial to bimanual microphaco.

Chapter 6

Secondary Intraocular Lens Implantation in Children

Rupal H Trivedi, M Edward Wilson, Susannah Mistr (USA)

Introduction

The use of primary intraocular lenses (IOLs) in children has become increasingly common in recent years and accepted for children undergoing cataract surgery beyond their first birthday. Nevertheless, the implantation of an IOL at the time of cataract surgery in children younger than 1 year remains controversial. It is very likely that many of these patients will later require a secondary IOL implantation. Secondary implantation of an IOL is recommended when spectacle or contact lens correction of aphakia is unsuccessful. At times, teenagers will request a secondary implantation for cosmetic reasons.

Each surgeon faces a few important questions while deciding for or against secondary IOL implantation: Should this eye receive an implant? If yes, the surgeon must answer two important questions: *What is the best site for implant fixation?* and *What type of lens implant material should be chosen?* This chapter attempts to address these questions and to review the literature available on outcome of secondary IOL implantation for children.

Preoperative Evaluation

A complete ophthalmic examination including uncorrected and best corrected visual acuity (BCVA), slit-lamp biomicroscopy, and fundus examination after mydriasis should be performed. In children who do not permit reliable examination in the office, anesthesia may be required for examinations. Presence or absence of posterior synechiae, vitreous in the anterior chamber (AC) and associated ocular anomalies should be documented.

Capsular Support

The technical success of secondary implantation depends mainly on how much capsular support remained at the time of the primary cataract surgery. Visualization of 360 degrees of fused edge of an anterior and posterior capsulectomy from the primary surgery increases the chance of achieving a successful posterior segment implantation of an IOL. Hence, leaving an adequate portion of peripheral anterior and posterior capsule when performing cataract surgery without IOL implantation is particularly important. This will help subsequent secondary IOL placement if needed. An approximate 4.5 mm central anterior and posterior capsulectomy is usually adequate to prevent visual axis opacification (VAO) while assuring an adequate rim of support if a secondary IOL implantation is elected.

When adequate capsular support is not available to fixate an IOL in-the-bag or in the sulcus, implantation of an IOL is not recommended unless every contact lens and spectacle option has been fully explored. If the posterior capsule edge is not visible, depression should be performed posterior to the limbus using blunt-tipped forceps. Sometimes, examination through a peripheral iridectomy (if present) is useful to look for capsular remnants. The recent literature has also reported using high frequency ultrasound (HFU) for assessment of capsular

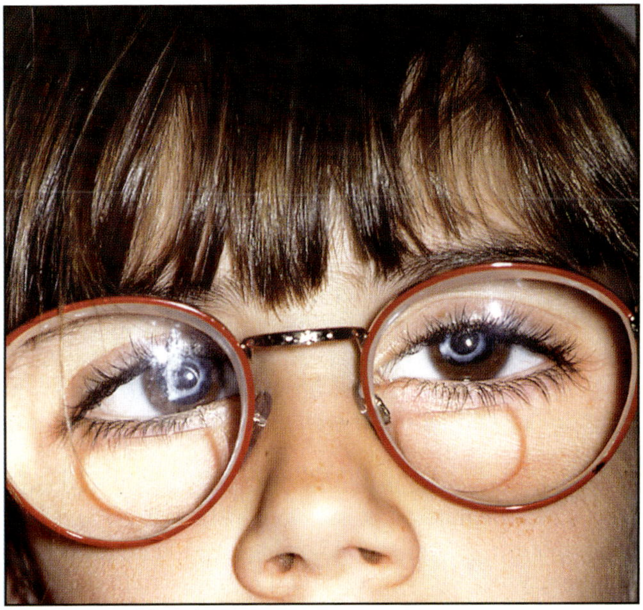

Figure 1: Eight years old girl operated for bilateral cataract at 3.2 year of age. Note the dense Soemmering's ring

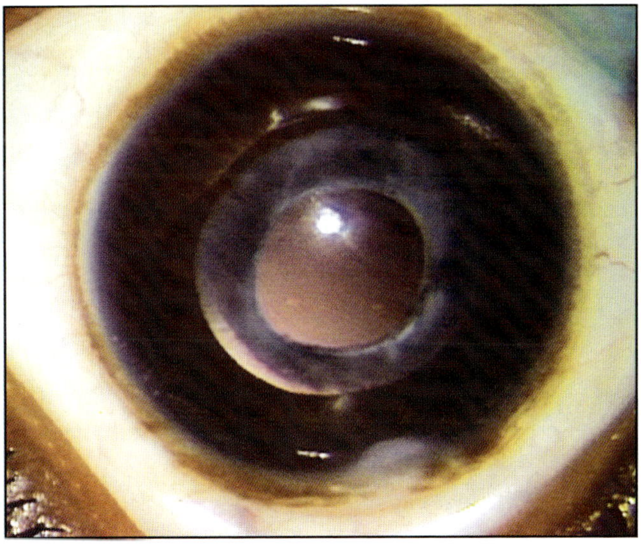

Figure 2: Fused anterior and posterior capsule edge increases the chances of achieving in-the-bag fixation

support for these eyes. The authors noted that in those patients in whom inadequate dilation precludes the detection of capsular support, HFU can be a useful tool to assess capsular support.

In a patient with bilateral aphakia, a clever strategy may be to operate first on the eye with the worse capsular support. In the rare instance if it is not feasible to safely achieve implantation, the end still will be bilateral aphakia. In the reverse situation, a less desirable scenario may happen: an IOL in one eye and aphakia in the other eye.

IOL Power Calculation

1. We use axial length (AL) and keratometry (K) readings to calculate IOL power with an "aphakic setting" on the A-scan ultrasound machine. Errors in keratometry readings can occur after wearing hard contact lense since their use affects corneal curvature. Resultant IOL calculations are variable. IOL calculations should be made well after discontinuation of hard contact lens wear.
2. McClatchey and Hofmeister recommend the following method to calculate IOL power using a pediatric IOL calculator: that is, they add the child's age, the A-constant of the IOL, K and AL values. Put in a power of "0" for "IOL power", and the program will tell you the predicted "resulting refraction". Next, adjust the AL value until the "resulting refraction" equals the measured refraction for that eye. Finally, put in your "goal refraction" and the resulting "IOL to use" output should be accurate. The pediatric IOL calculator can be downloaded from the American Association for Pediatric Ophthalmology and Strabismus website.
3. In the absence of AL measurements, some researchers recommends using aphakic refraction of an eye to calculate an IOL power. Axial length can be estimated from its aphakic refraction (spherical equivalent) using a previously-described method .

Many of these eyes undergoing secondary IOL implantation will not receive in-the-bag fixation. Appropriate correction of an IOL power needs to be done according to the site of IOL fixation. Remember, ciliary sulcus fixation of an IOL is 0.5 to 1.5 D less than bag fixation of an IOL. The higher the power of an IOL, the more the subtraction needs to be.

Site of Fixation of an IOL

In the Presence of Sufficient Capsular Support

In the presence of sufficient capsular support, pediatric secondary IOLs are commonly implanted into the ciliary sulcus. A lens placed in the ciliary sulcus may be a reasonably safe and effective option to treat pediatric aphakia. Awad and colleagues performed ultrabiomicroscopy on the ciliary sulcus in 10 eyes after secondary IOL implantation. No gross haptic erosion into the sclera, ciliary body or sulcus was seen. The structure of the sulcus in the implanted eye

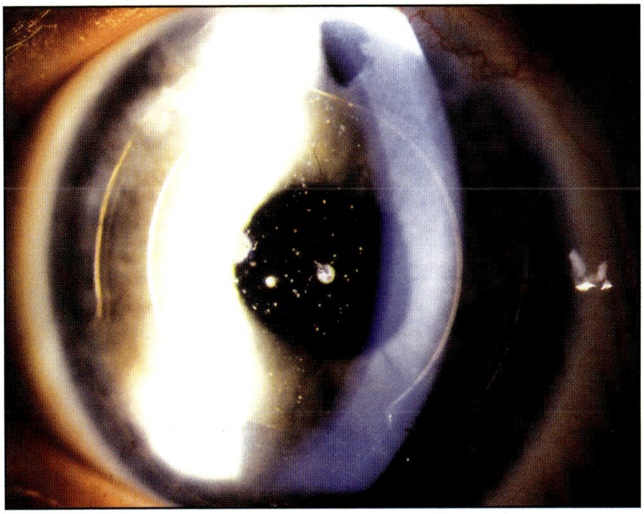

Figure 3: Note pigment dispersion

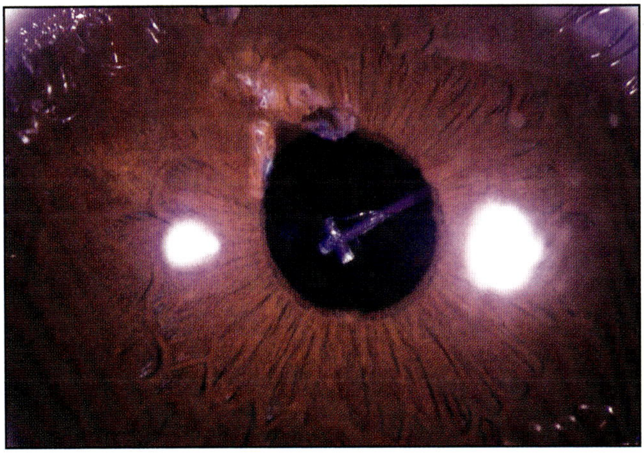

Figure 4: Clinically significant decentration of AcrySof IOL

appeared similar to the sulcus in the contralateral normal eye. However, ciliary-sulcus- fixated IOLs are more prone to develop complications such as pupillary capture, pigment dispersion, ciliary body erosion, decentration, unstable loop fixation, and lens tilt than bag-fixated IOL.

Amino and Yamakawa report in their study of adult eyes, that even more than 2-years after cataract surgery, AC flare counts in eyes with sulcus-to-sulcus IOL fixation were significantly higher than in eyes with in-the-bag fixation. In-the-bag implantation is the best position as it sequesters the IOL from the highly reactive uveal tissues and maintains optimum centration of the IOL. The technique of reopening the capsular bag for in-the-bag secondary IOL implantation in children has been reported by one of us (MEW). In young children, the process of equatorial epithelial cell proliferation produces a ring of cortex trapped between the lens equator and the fused anterior and posterior capsulectomy edges. Therefore, a potential space for in-the-bag placement of an IOL may be maintained between the anterior and posterior capsular leaflets. In-the-bag fixation is more consistently achieved in eyes made primarily aphakic during early infancy. Eyes operated in the first 6 months of life have much more exuberant cortex proliferation within the capsular bag remnant than children operated on at a later age. This material helps to maintain a potential space for IOL implantation. In older children, the anterior and posterior capsule leaflets often fuse together from the central opening far into the equator. It is important to assess if it is possible to reopen the capsular bag leaflets. The key is to locate one area in which the anterior capsule edge is not strongly adherent to the posterior capsule. Using that as the entry point, an ophthalmic viscosurgical device can be used to separate the capsular leaflets. If the adhesions are very strong, alternative dissecting techniques (with iris reposition and/or microvitreoretinal knife) need to be used. Surgeon should remove the Soemmering's ring by bimanual irrigation/aspiration and place a secondary IOL into the capsular bag whenever possible. Secondary in-the-bag fixation is more consistently achieved with foldable IOLs – either three-piece or single-piece.

Optic capture through fused anterior and posterior capsule and haptics in the bag is another viable option for secondary IOL implantation. It helps to achieve centration of the IOL.

Absence of Sufficient Capsular Support

In the absence of sufficient capsular support, choosing the best site for the IOL is more difficult and controversial. Sutured IOL, iris claw IOL or AC IOLs can be used depending on the surgeon's preference, ocular condition and availability of the IOL. Several reports of sutured IOL outcomes in the pediatric population have appeared in the literature. Various techniques have been suggested over the years for suturing an IOL. A scleral-fixated posterior chamber IOL can be sutured by passing the needles from outside of the eye inward (*ab-externo*) or inside out (*ab-interno*). The *ab-externo* approach is usually preferred over the *ab-interno* approach. Adequate anterior vitrectomy is mandatory before placement of sutures and the IOL. Scleral fixation of posterior chamber IOLs in children have been well tolerated according to some recent studies, but complications such as pupillary capture, suture erosion and refractive error from lens tilt or anterior/posterior displacement can occur.

Fixation of an IOL into the AC is another option for eyes with insufficient capsular support. It is stated that AC-IOLs are easy to insert but difficult to insert correctly. The three most common mistakes made during insertion are incorrect sizing, insufficient steps to avoid iris tuck, and inattention to the location of iridectomies and the capacity of haptics to rotate through them. Complications of AC-IOLs include corneal endothelial cell loss and subsequent corneal decompensation, iris sphincter erosion, glaucoma, and hyphema. AC-IOLs are not usually recommended in eyes with preexisting glaucoma, peripheral anterior synechiae, shallow AC or iris defects. Experience with AC-IOL implantation in children is limited. At present, no consensus exists on the indications as well as on the relative safety and efficacy of these different options available while implanting in an eye with insufficient capsular support.

Outcome of Secondary IOL Implantation

In the Presence of Sufficient Capsular Support

We have reported our experience and the outcome of secondary IOL implantation in children. A total of 77 eyes were reported, with a minimum follow-up of 6-months. Most commonly, secondary IOL implantation in our patients was performed between 2 to 4 years of age. Contact lens compliance can be difficult to achieve in this age-group, yet there is still hope to reverse amblyopia. Secondary IOLs were also commonly implanted in patients 12-14 years of age. Most of cases were bilaterally aphakic patients who requested IOL implantation for cosmetic purposes. Complications included clinically significant decentration (5.2%), VAO (5.2%), dislocation of the IOL (2.6%) and pupillary capture requiring repositioning of the IOL (1.3%). Foldable IOLs are associated with a high rate of decentration or dislocation. Decentration/dislocation was responsible for 21% of explanted 3-piece hydrophobic acrylic IOLs in a 2001 survey. In our series clinically significant decentration requiring surgical intervention was noted exclusively in eyes with sulcus fixated foldable IOLs (28.6% - 4/14). Perhaps the rigidity of the poly(methyl methacrylate) (PMMA) IOLs previously used helped to avoid decentration. All of the decentrations were in an inferior direction in male eyes. Perhaps this is due to a higher incidence of trauma among males. Another possible reason is that male eyes have been noted to have longer axial lengths than female eyes (Trivedi et al. AL and K in eyes with pediatric cataract. Poster presented at ASCRS, 2003). We hypothesized that longer eyes may also have a "wider" anterior segment and this wider sulcus-to-sulcus distance may promote IOL decentration. Eyes with an AL of >23 mm were 4-times more likely to develop decentration if implanted with a sulcus-fixated foldable IOL when compare to eyes measuring <23 mm. Another recent study has reported decentration in 6% of eyes after secondary placement of a foldable AcrySof® IOLs in the ciliary sulcus. Jacobi and associates noted decentration of a scleral fixation of a secondary foldable monofocal or multifocal IOL implant in 19.2% of children and young adult eyes. Until the recent past we used heparin surface modified PMMA IOLs for sulcus fixation. However, these IOLs are now no longer available in the US. We now use three-piece AcrySof® IOLs for sulcus fixation in microphthalmic eye and uncoated PMMA lenses for eyes with a longer axial length.

Some reports in the adult literature present a higher incidence of endophthalmitis in secondary IOL patients compared to primary cataract surgery with IOL placement. We have witnessed one patient who was operated for bilateral secondary IOL implantation, who developed unilateral endophthalmitis. A case report of bilateral uveitis (possibly sympathetic ophthalmia) resulting in blindness of a child following secondary IOL implantation for unilateral, congenital cataract has been reported.

We have noted significant improvement in visual acuity outcome after implantation of a secondary IOL in children. In a 1984 series, Hiles reported that 10% of infantile cataract patients achieved best postoperative visual acuities of 20/40 or better. Twelve years later another series reported that 27% of infantile cataract patients achieved visual acuity of 20/40 or better. Another series in 1998 reported that 42% of the patients implanted with an IOL secondarily, had a BCVA of 20/40 or better.

In the Absence of Sufficient Capsular Support

Sharpe and colleagues report their experience with scleral fixation of IOLs in children. Seven IOLs were sutured in the ciliary sulcus of children who could not wear contact lenses but the eye was lacking sufficient capsular support. Six of seven patients had improved visual acuity, with an average improvement of 4 lines. Complications related to scleral fixation included exposure of the scleral fixation suture in one eye, lens decentration in one eye, and lens tilt in one eye after an average follow up of 26 months.

Buckley reported the short-term results and complications of unilateral scleral fixated posterior chamber IOLs in the pediatric population. All patients with scleral fixated IOLs younger than 16 years of age were retrospectively reviewed. Nine patients aged 12 months to 15 years underwent unilateral scleral-fixated IOL implantation using buried polypropylene fixation sutures. Postoperative visual acuity improved in all patients after an average follow up of 2-years. Refractive goals were achieved in all but 1 patient. Complications included elevated intraocular pressure controlled with medications, anterior uveitis, and mild IOL decentration (1 eye each). The author recommended caution when considering this procedure for pediatric patients because the long-term risks are unknown. The authors further noted that the real uncertainty is the issue of the long-term safety of an IOL, which is only supported by a single polypropylene suture. Careful follow-up of these patients will be necessary to determine the stability of the IOL over time and the appropriateness of this procedure for a child.

Zetterstrom and associates evaluated long-term follow-up in eyes of children who had transscleral suture fixation of a sulcus IOL without capsular support. The IOL implantation was primary in 16 eyes and secondary in 5 eyes. An IOL with fixation holes in the haptics was sutured in the ciliary sulcus, with the knots buried in the scleral bed. No complications occurred during surgery. In all cases after IOL implantation, BCVA was equal to or better than their preoperative acuity. After a maximum follow-up of 33-months, posterior synechia formation occurred in 4 eyes, and 4 had cells on the IOL surface. In 2 eyes the IOL optic subluxated into the AC, but both were successfully treated with pilocarpine 4%. The authors concluded that ciliary sulcus placement with scleral fixation of an IOL without capsular support is an option to correct aphakia in children.

Epley and associates reported their experience with pediatric secondary IOL implantation in the absence of capsular support. Postoperative review is presented of 18 eyes with posterior chamber IOLs trans-sclerally sutured into the ciliary sulcus and 10 eyes implanted with AC IOLs. In their series, eyes that became aphakic after the critical period of visual development (>9 years) achieved better overall final visual acuity than the eyes that became aphakic during the critical period. The most common complication with AC IOLs was pigment and protein deposits on the surface of the lenses, none of which were considered to be visually significant. Two patients had visually insignificant corectopia after insertion of the AC- IOL. Progressive migration of the IOL haptic over a period of 6 months with extrusion at the original scleral incision prompted IOL removal in one eye. In the sutured-IOL group, one eye had a small, confined, vitreous hemorrhage near the ciliary body that resolved spontaneously and did not interfere with vision. Two other eyes had visually insignificant corectopia after insertion of a sutured IOL. None of the eyes in any group had evidence of endothelial decompensation, cystoid macular edema, or chronic AC inflammation upon examination. According to the authors, secondary implantation with transsclerally sutured posterior chamber IOLs should be considered in complicated cases when more conservative options have been exhausted.

Vote and colleagues recently reported long-term outcome of scleral-fixated sutured IOL implantation. The most common late complication was breakage of polypropylene sutures, which occurred in 16 of 61 eyes (26.2%). Some eyes had multiple breakages (breakage after resuturing). Multivariate analysis also showed that longer follow-up was significantly associated with suture breakage (P = .014), with the mean time to breakage approximately 4-years after surgery. Younger patients were more likely to suffer the breakage of suture. Age maintained significance (P = .009) even when this variable was corrected for gender, lens status before scleral fixation of PC-IOL, and duration of follow-up. Although this series doesn't include many young patients (age range: 12-80 years), it is important to remember that pediatric eyes may be at higher risk of suture breakage.

We have noted two of six AC-IOL implanted eyes in our series, that required a secondary surgical intervention – one for corectopia and another for traumatic dislocation.

Guell and colleagues report the outcome of Artisan-Verisyse aphakic IOL (Ophthec BV) implanted in adults. The authors noted that the mean endothelial cell loss was 10.9% after 36 months postoperatively. The authors further noted that they are now using the Artiflex lens, a foldable iris fixated IOL that can be implanted through a 2.75 to 3.2 mm incision.

Summary

If sufficient capsular support is available, the most desirable position for the IOL is between the anterior and posterior capsules or "in-the-bag" fixation. However, occasionally, fibrosis and scarring make the anterior and posterior capsule inseparable and this option may not be feasible. Ciliary-sulcus fixation is the best second alternative site for fixation of the IOL. If capsular support is absent, the IOL implantation options are more controversial. In the absence of available capsular support – a sutured IOL, an AC-IOL or an iris claw IOL can be used depending on the surgeon preference, the ocular environment and IOL availability. We prefer to wait for long-term follow-up before commenting on the superiority of one placement preference over the other.

Chapter 7

Management of Pediatric Cataract and Novel Surgery Procedures

Bojan Pajic, Jörg Müller (Switzerland)

Introduction

The management of cataracts in children is a more complex process than treating an adult patient who has previously developed presumably good visual acuity and has it diminished by opacification of the lens. In children, the visual system is in a process of development and will be incompletely developed until age 8 years. Amblyopia may be a determining factor in the final visual outcome in young children. The aim of cataract surgery in children is twofold: first, clear the visual axis to achieve the best possible visual acuity and secondly, to promote development of binocular visual function.

Anatomy of the Child's Eye

Children's eyes are different from adult eyes in several respects. First, they are smaller; at birth the average axial length of the eye is 16.8 mm. The length will increase to the adult length of 23.6 mm by age 16. Most growth occurs during the first two years of childhood and by the end of the second year, the eye will have a mean axial length of 22 mm. The second difference is the steepness of the corneal curvature. During development, the curvature of the cornea will change. At birth, very steep corneal topography readings are common, and will usually measure 47.00 to 51.00 D. The steep configuration decreases to adult readings of 43.50 D. A third consideration is the size of the lens. The horizontal diameter of the lens in an infant is 6.0 mm. This increases to 8.4 mm by 21 months and the lens diameter reaches an adult size, 9.3 mm, by 16 years. The lens capsule in very young children does not lend itself to the current capsulorhexis techniques. The lens substance in children is soft and the lens material or cataract is easily aspirated. The child's eye has a more elastic sclera. Large incisions tend to make the eye collapse during surgery.

The vitreous is more viscous and formed and there may be a persistent attachment between the anterior hyaloid face and the posterior lens capsule. Remnants of the tunica vasculosa lentis may persist to some degree. Frequently, developmental anomalies may coexist with a cataract. These defects may be ocular such as microphthalmia, foveal hypoplasia, optic nerve abnormalities, and persistence of the primary vitreous (PHPV) and of the tunica vasculosa lends. Other defects will be systemic and include: heart, renal, or metabolic conditions which may cause cataracts and also increase risk for administration of general anesthesia.

The visual system in children younger than 8 years is in a process of development. In adults, cataract surgery is associated with vision restoration. In children, the visual system is undergoing development and this needs to be facilitated. This proceeds rapidly during the first 3 or 4 months of life. The rate, and plasticity of development then progress at a slower rate up until the eighth year of life. During this period, amblyopia, deprivation, refractive, and strabismic, must be tested for and treated. Complications such as nystagmus, strabismus, or glaucoma may interfere with a good visual outcome. There are other unique issues that are not experienced in the adult population. For example, children

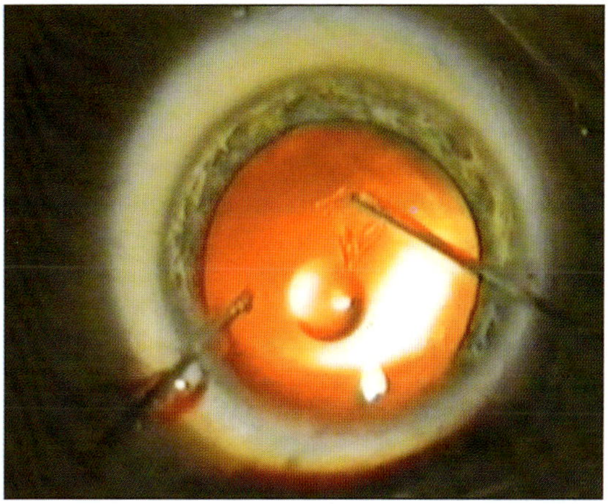

Figure 1: Opening the capsule anterior with a insulin needle to perform a capsulorhexis

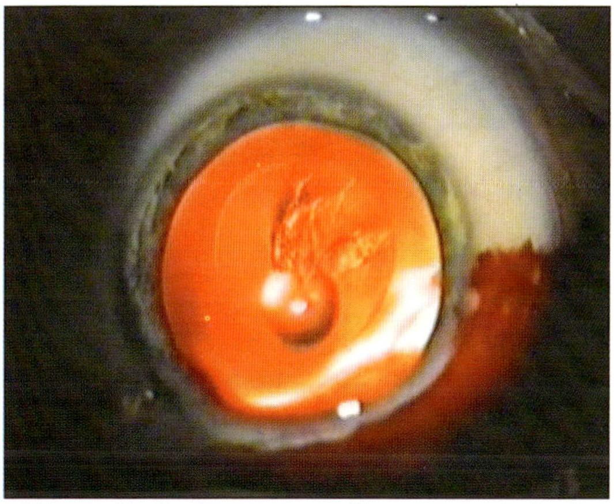

Figure 2: Continuous curvilinear capsulorhexis

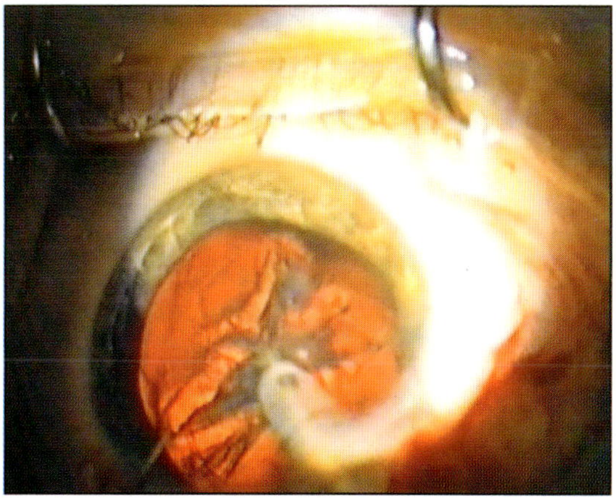

Figure 3: Removing the anterior lens cortex and the lens nucleus with ultrasound

who have a cataract that involves only one eye, are going to be more difficult to achieve a high level of visual acuity because of the resistance of the child, and perhaps the parents, to occlude the good, normally functioning eye. The onset of children's cataracts will vary. Cataracts may be congenital and present at birth or develop later during childhood. Often children have a propensity to develop a cataract as a result of a metabolic condition such as galactosemia. Other cataracts may be acquired following ocular trauma, radiation, inflammation or following administration of corticosteroids. Some partial cataracts will progress to complete lens opacities as is often the case with posterior lenticonus. Successful management of cataracts in children requires a thorough understanding of the complex interplay between all of above issues. Additionally, the surgeon must have the facilities to provide safe general anesthesia for the child. If intraocular lens (IOL) rehabilitation is considered in a young or uncooperative child, equipment should be available in the operating room to perform keratometry and axial length measurements for lens power calculation.

Diagnosis of Cataracts in Children

Children almost never express symptoms related to cataracts. The ophthalmologist must rely upon signs to raise suspicion of the diagnosis. The parent may notice a whitish area in the pupil or the pediatrician may have difficulty examining the fundus during the newborn examination. When the cataracts involve both eyes and are complete, a very noticeable visual deprivation form of nystagmus will occur after 3 months of age. Once this low amplitude, low frequency form of pendular nystagmus ensues, attaining high levels of visual acuity (0.4 or better) is less likely. Some lens defects may be present early in life (posterior lenticonus and PHPV) and the lens remains clear but may later develop opacification of the posterior lens capsule. The same is true for metabolic conditions such as diabetes and galactosemia. Some early lens changes related to metabolic cataracts may be reversible with dietary alteration.

Inheritance

Cataracts may be inherited either as an autosomal dominant, autosomal recessive or with an X-linked pattern. Some genetically transmitted cataracts will occur as a result of inheriting a cataract producing metabolic or chromosomal disorder. Examination of other family members will help to clarify the inheritance pattern.

Classification of Cataracts

Cataracts may be classified by laterality, age of onset, extent, size-density, and by progression.

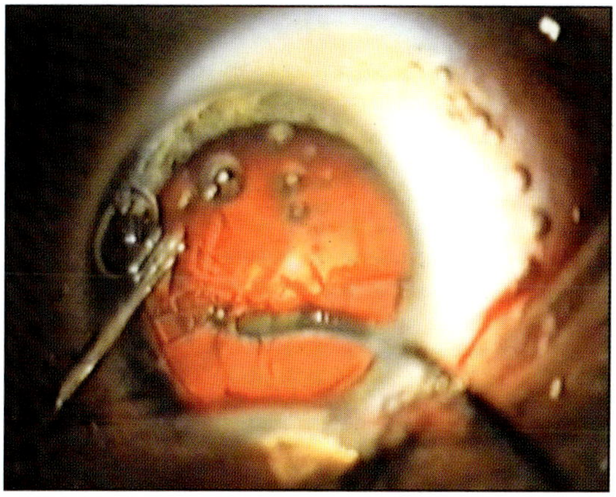

Figure 4: Lens cortex is removed from the fornices of the lens with an I/A Tipp

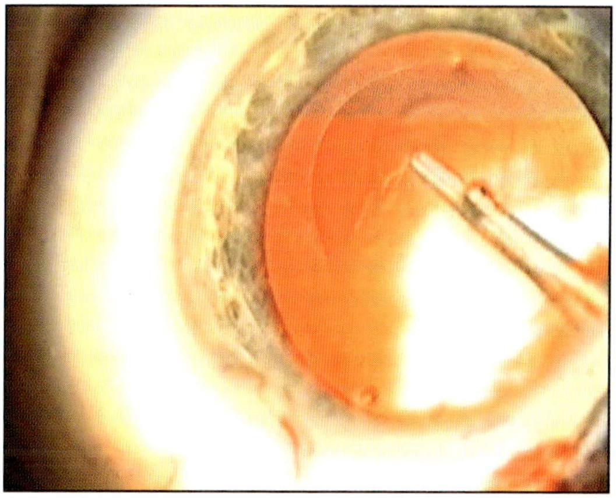

Figure 5: Posterior capsulotomy

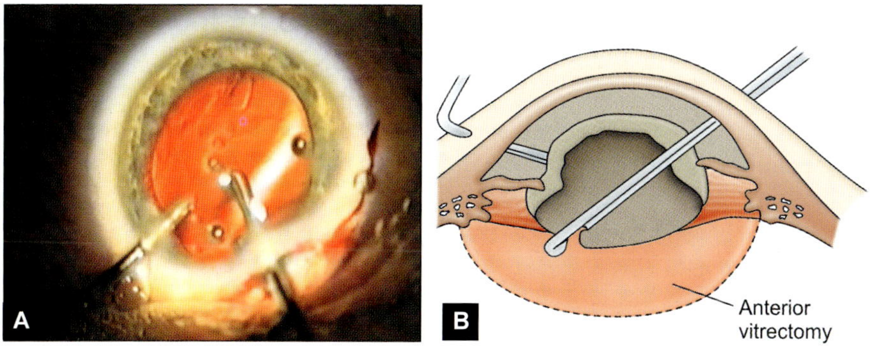

Figures 6A and B: Anterior vitrectomy

Laterality

Cataracts can be classified as unilateral or bilateral. This classification is important because children with unilateral cataracts frequently have a delay in the detection of the cataract and for reasons already mentioned, the visual outcome may be less promising. Visual acuity in patients with bilateral congenital cataracts may be excellent if the cataracts are treated within the critical period of visual development or before the onset of nystagmus.

Age of Onset

Cataracts may be described as congenital if they are present at birth or infantile if they are noticed in the perinatal period. Other cataracts may be acquired later in the child's life as a result of radiation, corticosteroid use, uveitis, or trauma. The term juvenile or adolescent are sometimes used to describe the cataract depending on the age the defect is noted.

The Extent and Location of Cataract

Partial cataracts may be capsular, zonular, cortical, nuclear or a combination of these. Cataracts may be pinpoint and involve only a small portion of the anterior lens capsule. These anterior polar cataracts will usually not show progression and a good visual outcome can be anticipated. Cataracts involving the posterior capsule will usually progress and have a greater impact in the measured visual acuity. Complete cataracts are those which obstruct the visual axis, even when viewed through a dilated pupil.

Some lenses may be clear but on retinoscopy will exhibit a double or distorted refracting system. Examples of these optical defects are seen with dislocated lenses, oil droplet cataracts, or posterior lenticonus or other defects in the posterior capsule of the lens. All of these share the same optical problem. They prevent a clearly focused form image from falling on the retina. When this occurs, development of visual acuity may be impeded and lens surgery should be considered.

Cataract Size and Density

The size of the cataract will have some influence on the level of visual acuity that is attainable. Opacities in the lens that are smaller than 2 mm can usually be observed with frequent monitoring of the vision. Cataracts 2.5 mm or larger will usually require surgery in order to clear the visual axis. Some partial opacities are flake or powderlike and others are opaque but small. Visual acuity may be surprisingly good in some children with partial cataracts. Lamellar cataracts may look "bad" but may not alter VA too much.

Progression

Cataracts may progress in their size or density with time or, in other unusual cases, cataracts may regress with dietary modification. Cataracts related to neonatal tetany and galactosemia may regress with correction of the metabolic

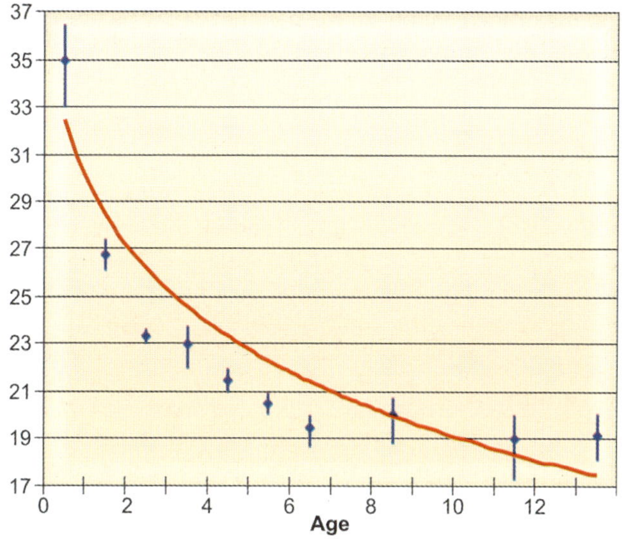

Figure 7: Lens power attitude correlated with age

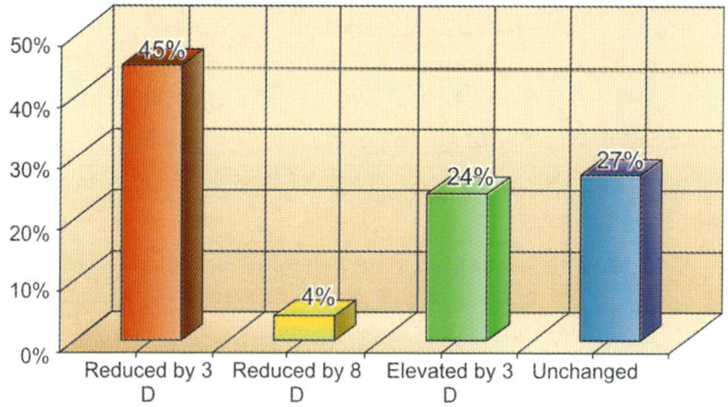

Figure 8: Correlations error after 2 years of age

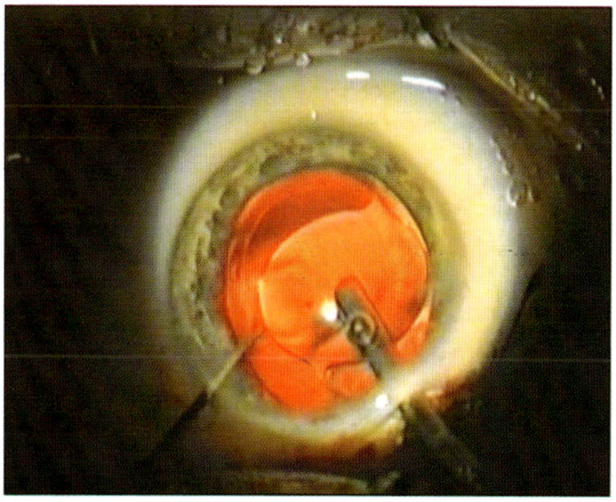

Figure 9: IOL Insertion in the capsule bag after a posterior capsulorhexis and anterior vitrectomy

defect through diet or medication. A transient haze may be present in the lens of premature infants during the early perinatal period. These "cataracts" will frequently regress without treatment.

Evaluation of the Child

Selected patients should be evaluated for cause of the cataract. The decision to proceed with an evaluation will be determined by the character of the cataract, its location, family history, type, and density of the opacity. With this information and the findings on the physical examination to detect systemic problems, a focused laboratory investigation can be planned.

Associated Ocular Defects

Associated defects should be investigated. Some of these defects will modify the procedure and instrumentation that will be used. Other defects may preclude cataract surgery. Eyes that have microphthalmia, as defined by a corneal diameter less than 9 mm, may not be good candidates for lens implantation. Microphthalmia may cause additional problems with instrumentation. Instruments designed for adult cataract surgery may be large and difficult to maneuver in small eyes. Eyes with extensive defects such as posterior staphylomas, optic nerve colobomas, and microphthalmia with cyst may not require cataract surgery because of the expected poor visual prognosis and the risk of loosing the eye as a result of surgery.

Nonsurgical Treatment

Not all pediatric cataracts require surgical treatment. Cataracts that are small and those which are partial and have areas where clear undistorted retinoscopy may require observation only. Frequent monitoring of the visual acuity by assessing the fixation response, watching for sensory strabismus, or measurement acuity using the LEO Visual Acuity Cards are helpful for estimating acuity in nonverbal children. Caution must be exercised in interpreting the results because grating acuity will tend to underestimated amblyopia.

Surgical Treatment

A visual acuity of 0.32 or less would suggest that cataract surgery is indicated. The decrease may be due to the cataract, amblyopia or a combination of these. The onset of strabismus or nystagmus related to visual deprivation is another indication for surgery. Some children who are very young or delayed developmentally may never subjectively provide a measured visual acuity. In these cases, the ophthalmologist's clinical Judgment following assessment of the size, laterality of the cataract, will indicate if and when cataract surgery should be performed.

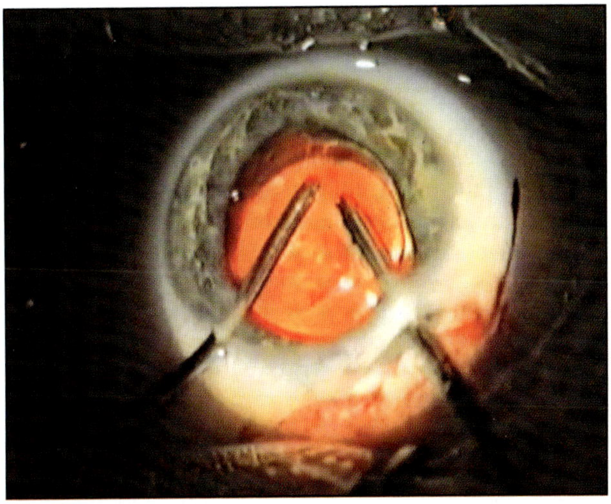

Figure 10: Viscoelastic evacuation with the vitrectome suction unit

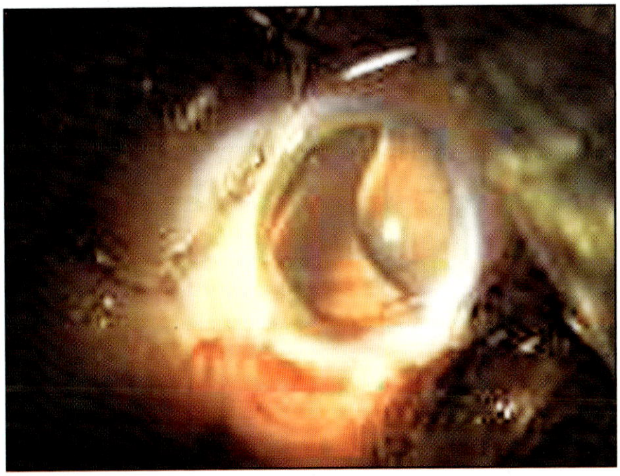

Figure 11: Lens subluxation preoperative

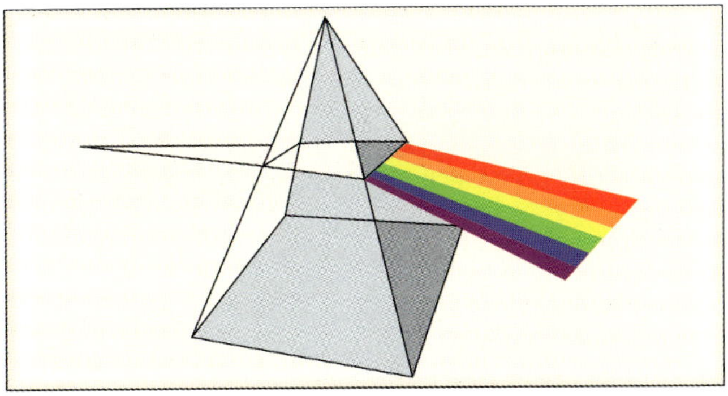

Figure 12: Induction of aberration

Congenital Cataracts

Children with a complete monocular congenital cataract should have surgery performed before 3 months of life. Although there was emphasis at one time on operating and rehabilitating children immediately after birth it is now considered prudent to wait a week or two for the infant to become stable medically, to initiate diagnostic evaluations, and to have sufficient time to initiate appropriate pediatric and anesthesiology consultations to ensure the safety of the administration of general anesthesia. If cataracts involve both eyes, surgery should be performed on the eye with the denser opacity. Once this eye has recovered, (usually 2 to 3 weeks), cataract surgery should be performed on the fellow eye.

Optical Rehabilitation

Once a decision has been made to perform cataract surgery, the next consideration is selection of the method of optical rehabilitation that will be used. For patients with monocular cataracts, aphakic spectacles are not practical. Before 1 year of age, use of contact lens rehabilitation is suggested. After 1 year, an intraocular lens could be considered. In patients with bilateral cataracts, contact lens rehabilitation is recommended before 1 or 2 years. The unpredictable response and growth of an eye in a child younger than 1 year may preclude selection of an intraocular lens as a primary procedure in children.

Table 1: Indications for Use of an IOL in Children

Unilateral Cataract

- Age 1-8 years old with a unilateral congenital cataract, expected or proven contact lens failure
- Age 1-17 years old with an acquired cataract with previously known adequate vision
- Unilateral developmental cataract age 1-17 years old
- Unilateral traumatic cataract

Bilateral Cataracts

- Patient older than 3 or 4 years of age
- Radiation induced cataracts
- Dry eyes
- Large amplitude nystagmus
- Eyelid scars

Table 2: Relative Contraindications for Pediatric IOL Implantation

Age less than 1 year
Microphthalmia
Microcornea (<9.0 mm cornea)
Glaucoma
Inflammation
Aniridia
Dislocated lens

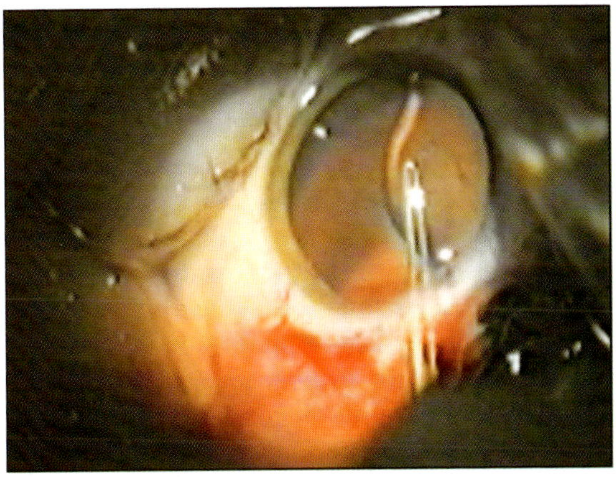

Figure 13: Capsulorhexis

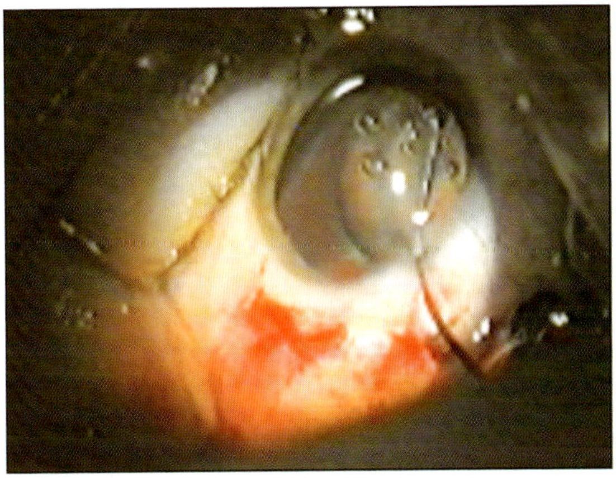

Figure 14: Hydrodissection

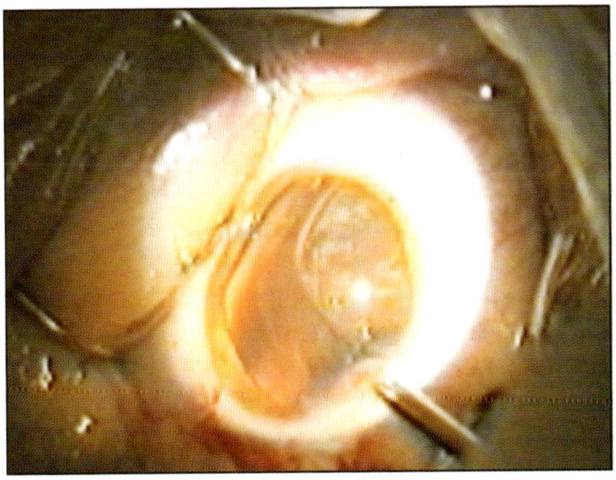

Figure 15: Capsular ring

Complete cataracts diagnosed at birth should be treated with cataract removal using a technique that preserves remnants of the anterior and posterior lens capsule leaflets. In most cases a primary posterior capsulotomy combined with an anterior vitrectomy should be performed. The eye should be rehabilitated with a contact lens. If the child becomes contact lens intolerant or when the child becomes mature, a secondary implant can be placed. Placement of an implant in a child younger than 1 year is technically difficult to perform and the response of a child's eye is unpredictable and in some situations, may be unfavorable to an implanted lens. Infants who have bilateral complete, congenital cataracts should have cataract surgery performed and receive contact lens or spectacle rehabilitation. Once the eye becomes mature or the child becomes resistant to contact lenses or glasses, secondary implants can be considered. Placement of an intraocular lens in a patient with bilateral acquired cataracts below the age of 2 to 4 years is considered by some authors to be unwise. This is due to our uncertainty about long-term effect and safety of implants as well as an incomplete understanding of the effect that an IOL has on the refractive error and growth of the eye over time. Children with a monocular cataract warrant the same concerns but the margin for safety and good vision is greater because of the presence of a sound fellow eye.

The Cataract Procedure

Pupil Dilatation

Children younger than 6 months have their pupils dilated with 0.5 cyclopentolate (Cyclogyl) and 2.5 phenylephrine (Neosynephrine) drops applied twice, 5 minutes apart a half hour prior to coming to the operating room. Use of stronger concentrations of phenylephrine in children may cause elevated blood pressure and irritability of the myocardium. Older children will accept stronger concentrations of these mydriatic agents.

Patient Preparation

Once anesthesia has been administered, axial length determinations can be performed using an A scan probe. If the lens is opaque, a standardized B scan can be performed. The corneal curvature is measured using one of several intraoperative handheld keratometers. If an IOL is going to be used, the pseudophakic lens power calculation can be made while the patient is being propped.

Glaucoma is a problem that occurs in 25 to 31% of children who have a congenital cataract. Presurgical and frequent postsurgical measurements of the intraocular pressure should be made with similar instrumentation, as Perkins applanation tonometer, Tonopen or Schiotz tonometer, so that valid comparison of the pressure can be made.

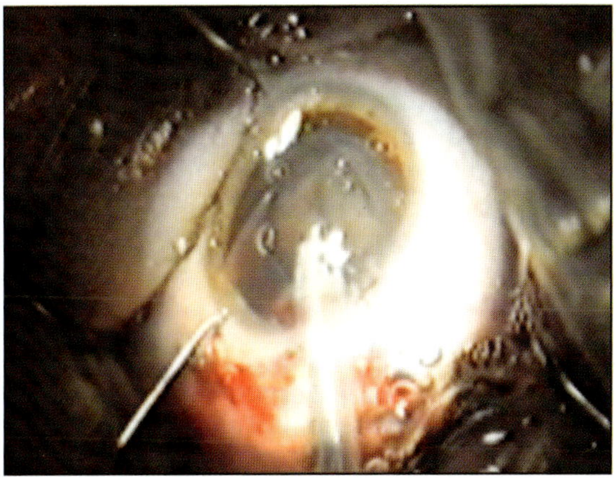

Figure 16: Phacoemulsification

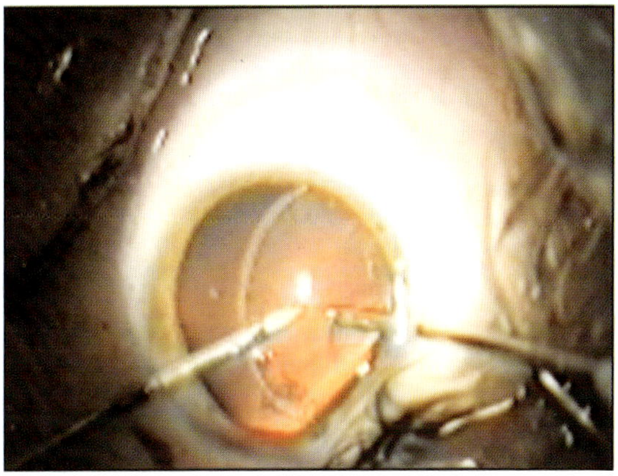

Figure 17: Irrigation / Aspiration

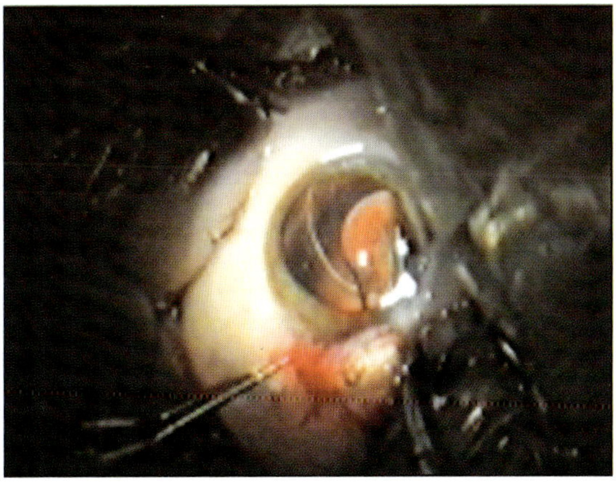

Figure 18: IOL Implantation

Cataract Surgery, Without Placement of an Intraocular Lens

The pars plana or pars plicata incision offers the advantage of having increased ability to remove the lens and to perform an anterior vitrectomy through a single incision. However, there is a risk for hemorrhage, disinsertion of the ciliary body or the vitreous base, and to some degree there is some risk associated with blind passage of instruments behind the iris. Because of these potential problems, we prefer to use a limbal incision. We initially used a scleral frown incision. The advantage of a self-sealing, no stitch incision in a child is not a consideration since most surgeons will suture all wounds for safety. Children will often rub their eyes following surgery.

A small peritomy or fornix based conjunctival flap is opened with a Vannas scissors. Entry is made into the anterior chamber using a 2.8 mm keratome for performing frown incision. Viscoelastic is introduced into the anterior chamber with an at tempt to make the lens-iris diaphragm bow posterior and become somewhat concave. Care should be exercised not to exaggerate this since an increase in the ocular pressure can occur and the vascular supply to the retina could be compromised. A needle with a bent tip is used to engage and tear the central portion of the anterior capsule. With frequent regrasping of the flap and tearing toward the center of the lens while watching for radial tears, a continuous curvilinear capsulorhexis is attempted. This is a very difficult procedure to accomplish in patients younger than 4 years. If there is evidence of extension of the tear radially and it threatens to go to the equator of the lens, this procedure should be abandoned and the remainder of the capsule should be removed with a high frequency capsulotomy device. The lens substance in children is soft and hydrodissection and hydrodelineation are in some cases not performed. The suction part of ultrasound device can be to remove the anterior lens cortex and the lens nucleus. Ultrasound is rarely necessary. Once the nucleus has been aspirated, the peripheral lens cortex is removed from the fornices of the lens with an I/A Tipp. It is best to have linear control of the suction pressure so that remnants of lens cortex can be engaged and then teased from the lens capsule without tearing the capsule. If the child is older than 5 or 6 years and will cooperate for a Nd:YAG laser capsulotomy, the posterior lens capsule, if it is clear, is left intact. However, if the child is too young or problems are anticipated with a Nd:YAG laser capsulotomy, a posterior capsulectomy and anterior vitrectomy should be performed using a suction cutting instrument. Attention to the size and location of the capsular opening is important. Care should be taken to make the anterior lens capsule opening slightly larger than the posterior lens capsule opening. The capsule leaflets will later fuse and form a baffle or a ring of support that may be important for stability of an IOL, if a secondary implant is required later. The pupil should be dilated frequently and kept moving to prevent iris-lens capsule adhesions from forming. The anterior chamber is reestablished with balanced solution saline (BSS) and an iridectomy may be considered. If the child is at low risk for developing glaucoma or the iris is vascular, the surgeon may elect not to perform an iridotomy or an iridectomy. However, in patients with uveitis and in some patients with traumatic cataracts, performing an iridotomy or iridectomy may be prudent. The incision may be

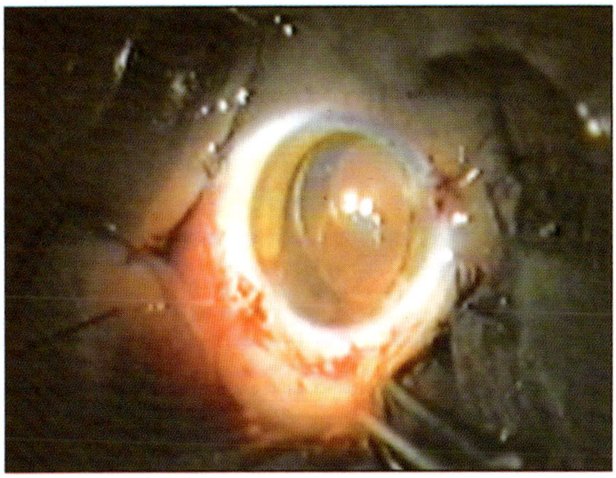

Figure 19: Insufficient centration

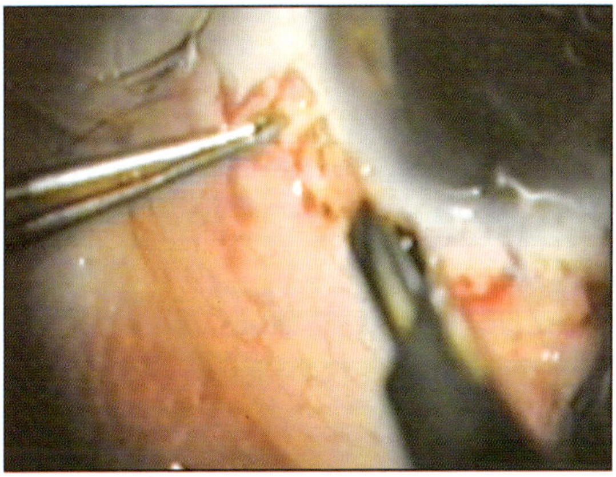

Figure 20: Sclerapocket preparation

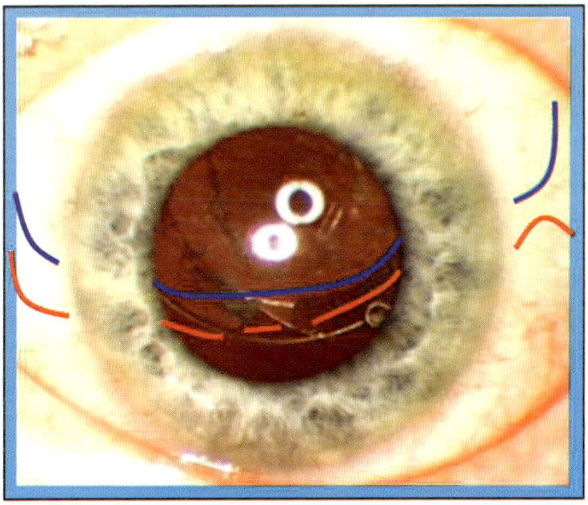

Figure 21: Target suture area

self-sealing by design but it is safer to close all wounds in children with a 10-0 suture.

Postoperative care consists of drops and a shield. I prefer not to use a bandage dressing. Atropine 0.5% is used in children younger than 6 months of age and 1% atropine drops are used twice a day in eyes of children older than 6 months. An antibiotic steroid combination such as Tobradex may be used or Ocufloxacin combined with a steroid such as Prednisolone acetate can be used during the postoperative period. The eye is shielded for 3 days and the patient is usually seen within 48 hours following surgery. Topical medications are discontinued when inflammation has subsided. This is usually 2 or 3 weeks following surgery. Refraction is performed at this time and repeated frequently. Once the refraction is stable, contact lens or spectacle correction is prescribed.

Contact Lens Correction for Aphakic and Pseudophakic Eyes

Optical Supply of an Aphake Eye

The refraction management of children's or baby's aphakic eyes could be done with glasses or contact lenses. The advantage of contact lenses is the better optical quality of retina image and better wearing compliance than with glasses. We prefer soft contact lenses as first choice for aphakic eyes. If corneal irregularities or high astigmatism are detected then we use rigid contact lenses. It's helpful and important to perform a skiaskopy for investigating the final refraction.

Soft Contactlenses – Rigid Contact lenses

We change the soft contact lenses each 30 days. Usually we use the lunelle aphake contact lens with a UV blocker. With this type of contact lenses it is aloud to adjust every parameter as basecurve, dioptrie and diameter.

Monthly Contact lenses are limited by the different parameters. Often the dioptres ends at +6.0dpt. Regarding the hydrations we observe similar problems with new silicon hydrogel material as with Lunelle ES. The clinical outcome and handling with Lunelle material is up to now known for more than twenty years. Usually the contact lenses will be changed every 6 months. Monthly the contact lenses will be cleaned with a tensed, enzymatic cleaner and a consecutive desinfection with peroxyd system. After the enzymatic cleaning, preservative free peroxyd desinfecting system is used again

The target correction is an over correction of 2 up to 3 dpt, what permits a good nearsight for the child. It is quite important because the child's world is within 20 to 50 centimeters.

At age of 0 to 2 years, a visual acuities control is done with preferencial looking tests. The advantage of LEA test is the independence of distance and the knowledge of any letters or numbers.

A soon as possible the stereopsys is inverstigated generally with the Lang Test. The age of the child allows we are checking the stereopsys.

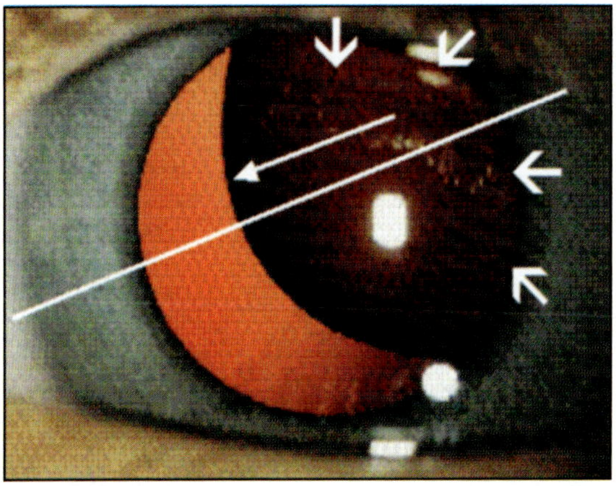

Figure 22: Target zone vector calculation

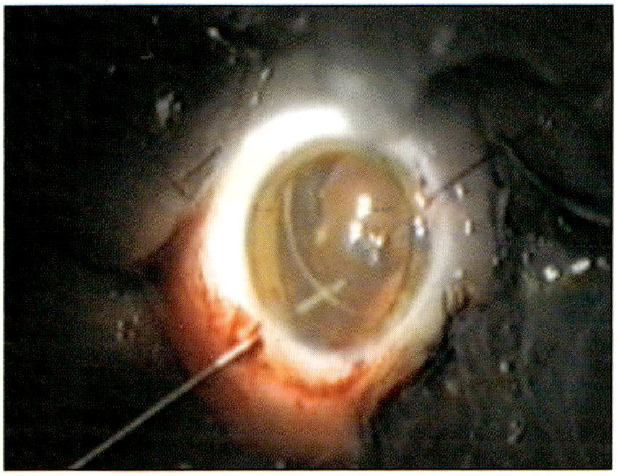

Figure 23: Suture placing

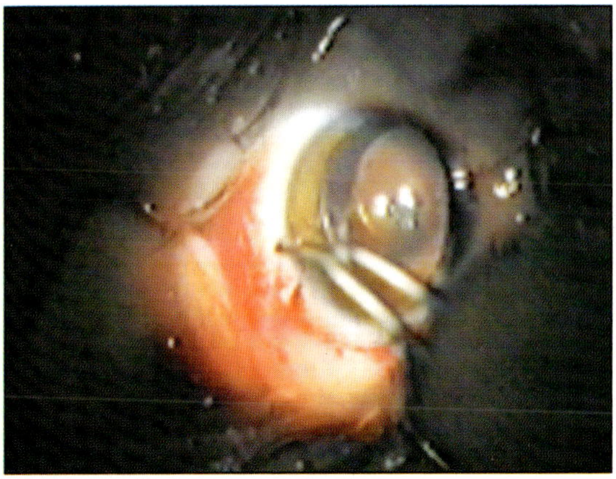

Figure 24: Suture fixation

Every check contains at least the follow points:

- Lids and margins
- Conjunctiva
- Position and movement of the contactlenses on eye
- Cornea
- Tears quality
- Sciascopy / Refraction
- Visual acuities
- Quality control of the contactlenses
- Compliance

The instruction of the parents in handling with the contactlenses is very important for ever regarding save wearing. During the night we recommend to remove rigid contactlenses. After the second birthday the fare vision becomes more important. One good solution is to fit bifocal - or progressive lenses. The results with progressive lenses are good, forever because they are better accept by parents!

Cataract Surgery with Lens Implantation

Patient Selection

Patients with monocular cataracts who are older than 2 year or those who are contact lens resistant or those with inadequate family support to provide reliable and consistent application and removal of contact lenses are candidates for an IOL.

Lens Style and Power

The lens style should be biconvex and have a 6 to 6.5 mm optic diameter optic that has a UV coating. The haptics are angulated and should be between 12 and 13.5 mm in diameter with soft C or J loop configuration. Usually PMMA or acrylic IOL are used as lens material.

The acrylic lens is able to be folded and inserted through a smaller incision in the case if we apply clear corneal technique. We have used the 6 mm optic size for implantation in children. We choose this relatively large optic size because the lens capsule may frequently contract and displace the lens, even when the lens is within the capsular bag. The 6.0 mm optic provides a larger area of optical correction to provide an extra margin area if the lens is displaced within the capsular bag. Stager, et al. have been pleased with the performance of this lens in children. Long-term studies regarding the safety and tolerance of pediatric eyes to this lens are lacking.

Lens Power

Measures should be taken to select a lens of appropriate power for the age of the child. Replacement of an IOL that has been placed in the eye of a child is difficult. Adhesions between the IOL and the lens capsule will be fibrotic and replacement or explanation of the lens will be difficult and hazardous. If possible

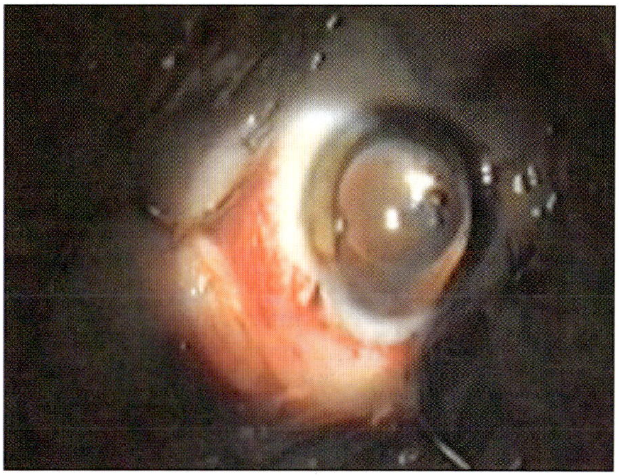

Figure 25: Perfect centration

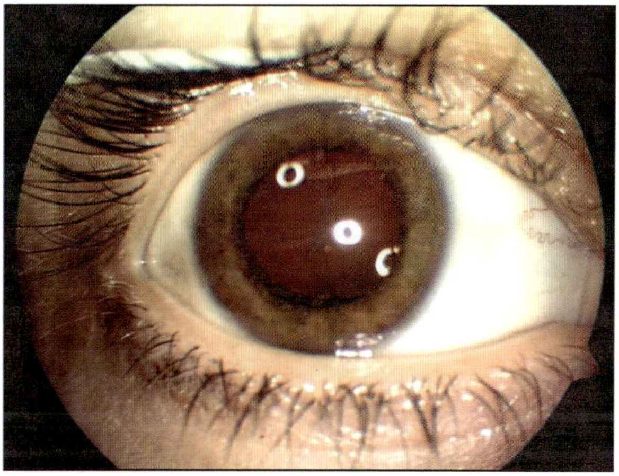

Figure 26: Result after one year

the power selection should be one that is appropriate for a lifetime. The surgeon should attempt to anticipate the refractive error at maturity. Some of the considerations in selecting a lens power are the age of the child, the refractive error of the fellow eye, and the refractive error of the parents. The lens power is calculate for the eye to achieve emmetropia. Biometric readings may be difficult to obtain in children. If the child has not had axial length determination or is uncooperative for preoperative studies, the axial length determination and keratometry are performed in the operating room after the child has been anesthetized. Lens power calculations are performed while the patient is being propped and draped and the surgical microscope is being positioned. There are a few studies that have evaluated the growth of the eye of primates and humans following cataract surgery with and without an IOL. The studies issue conflicting information on the growth patterns of the eye. In children with dense lens opacities, the eye may have a longer than expected axial length. Other studies have shown that growth of the eye is reduced following implantation of a lens. Other studies have shown that the aphakic eye continues to elongate axially so that the correction of aphakia reduces with time even until age 20. We set as our goal to achieve a refractive error in adulthood that produces 1.50 D or less of anisometropia. In children younger than 2 years of age, the power selected should provide a final power that is close to the power that the fellow eye is expected to achieve. For example, if the fellow eye in a 2-year-old has a piano refractive error and the child has a traumatic cataract, it would be assumed that the power of the sound eye would eventually develop a myopic refractive error of about -2.00 D. If we calculated a lens power of+20.00 to achieve a piano refractive error in the injured eye, we would reduce the lens calculated power by -2.00 D and implant a +18.00 lens. Between 2 and 8 years of age, the lens power would be reduced by 1.50 D. In children older than 8 years of age, the refractive error is calculated to match the fellow eye.

Implantation of an Intraocular Lens

The technique used to implant an IOL is a modification of the procedure used to remove a cataract without an IOL. Style and power of the lens are selected and confirmed by the surgeon. This will facilitate maneuvering instruments in the anterior chamber. When implanting a PMMA 6.5 mm optic lens, a fornix based conjunctival perimetry is made. A frown incision is constructed at the mid-limbal position and entry is made into the anterior chamber with a keratome. Viscoelastic is introduced to partially fill the anterior chamber. A bent needle is used to puncture the anterior lens capsule and a capsulorhexis is performed with a needle or capsulorhexis forceps. The lens material is removed as described in the previous section. After all cortical remnants are removed the posterior lens capsule is polished. A posterior capsulectomy combined with a small anterior vitrectomy using a vitrecome or similar suction cutting instrument is performed. If one desires, the sleeve can be removed and a separate irrigation cannula can be placed through a stab incision in the peripheral cornea. Viscoelastic is introduced into the anterior chamber. Viscoelastic is used to separate the lens capsule leaflets. The lens is irrigated with a balanced salt solution and the inferior haptic is inserted into the capsular bag under direct visualization. The superior haptic is grasped with a nontooth forceps and, with gentle pressure, is inserted into the superior lens capsular bag. The lens is then dialed into position with a Sinsky hook so the lens is centered and the haptics are positioned with a 3 and 9 o'clock orientation. If the lens capsule has a radial tear that precludes lens placement within the capsular bag, the haptics may be alternatively placed in the ciliary sulcus. The haptics must both be either in the capsular bag or both in the ciliary sulcus. One in each position will cause decentration and possible iris capture. The frown incision is adapted for security with one or two 10-0 sutures. Viscoelastic is aspirated with the vitrectome suction unit from the anterior chamber. An iridotomy may be performed at this time. If the surgery has been uneventful and the patient is at low risk for developing glaucoma, an iridotomy or iridectomy is not performed. When the posterior lens capsule is clear and the patient of 6 age or more with a good cooperation of the child, we will leave it intact. We are fortunate to have access to the microruptor three Nd:YAG laser to treat capsular opacification. Alternative methods to "manage" the posterior capsule are to complete the lens implantation and then make a separate pars plana or a pars plicata incision. An irrigation cannula is inserted into the anterior chamber and an vitrectome or similar suction cutting device is placed through the pars plana incision to perform a posterior capsulotomy and removal of the anterior vitreous. We use a capsulorhexis technique to open the posterior capsule with a consecutive anterior vitrectomy. The anterior capsule leaflet is reflected and a Utrata forceps is inserted behind the lens but above the surface of the posterior capsule to perform a posterior capsule capsulorhexis. A further modification is to prolapse the lens optic through the posterior capsule opening in effort to block lens epithelial cell migration in an effort to reduce the formation of secondary membranes. These maneuvers are technically difficult to perform and there is an increased risk for creating a radial tear in the capsule which may cause the lens to decenter.

Surgical Technique of Congenital Lens Subluxation

The aim of the novel surgical technique is to preserve the capsule with implanting the IOL in the bag.

In figure the preoperative situation of a congenital lens subluxation can be seen. The lens edge of the subluxated lens induces an aberration of higher order, which is heavily to correct with glases or contact lenses. The Capsulorhexis we perform with a needle or/and forceps. After the hydrodissection a capsular ring have to be implanted in the capsular bag. With low energy of phacoemulsification the lens content can be take away following irrigation and aspiration. The IOL implantation in the bag leeds to a better centration, but it is still not sufficient. The suture is fixed anterior and posterior the IOL haptic, capsular ring and lens capsule in the direction of the calculated optimal, main mathematical vector. The next step is to prepare a sclerapocket 1 mm from the limbus. With a insulin needle the suture is placed in the area of the scleralpocket. A consecutive suture fixation can be done using a perfect centration can be stated after surgery, even after 1 year later. The advantage of the novel surgery method is a long-term fixation and centering of chamber posterior IOL at the physiological space. The capsule is adherent with the ciliary body after months. The known disadvantages of the aphakia and chamber anterior IOL could be avoid. The surgical treatment of a congenital lens subluxation is sophisticated surgery method which shows excellent results.

Secondary IOL Implantation in Children

Secondary IOL implantation in children is common because many children will have congenital complete cataracts that require removal at an age where implantation of a lens is not commonly performed. When there is sufficient residual lens capsule to support a sulcus fixated IOL, fixation with a suture is not necessary. The technique for implanting a secondary IOL is similar for PMMA or the foldable lens. Viscoelastic is used to hydraulically separate the fused capsular leaflets from the iris. The cannula for the viscoelastic may be introduced through a peripheral iridotomy or iridectomy. The firm adhesions between the iris and lens capsule can be separated with a Barraquer spatula. The cataract wound is extended with frow incision technique and a 6.5 mm optic all PMMA lens is inserted. The haptics are placed in the ciliary sulcus. Alternatively, the wound can be enlarged with a 3.5 mm keratome and a foldable acrylic lens may be inserted into the ciliary sulcus. The implants are dialed into position to be sure they are well centered and wound closure is similar for the other procedures.

Secondary Intraocular Lens, Placement Without Capsular Support

In the previous decade, there was great concern about the formation of secondary membranes and their effect on treating amblyopia in children. Several surgeons advocated removal of the posterior lens capsule soon after the suction cutting instruments became available. Some surgeons zealously removed the entire lens using a pars plana approach. When these children refuse to wear a contact lens or spectacles, placement of an IOL is difficult because of lack of capsular material to provide stabilization of an IOL.

Most surgeons feel uncomfortable about the placement of an anterior chamber IOL in a child. The long-term apposition of the lens haptic to the filtration angle and potential for loss of corneal endothelium and dislocation are valid concerns. We have placed a few secondary implants with suture fixation in children and young adults who have refused to wear contact lenses and have inadequate capsular support. This procedure is hazardous and the long-term outcome remains unclear. However, observing these implants, the eyes seem to tolerate the suture fixated implants well. The potential for endophthalmitis related to suture erosion is reduced by placing the 10-0 monofilament sutures that anchor the lens at the 3 and 9 o'clock position underneath a prepared half thickness scleral flap. Lens tilt, dislocation, erosion of the suture or haptic and a risk for endophthalmitis are all valid concerns. However, suture placement is a reasonable alternative in these patients who are functionally aphakic. A technique with frown incision allowed to fixate the IOL at 6 and 12 o'clock at the level of the frown tunnel. That is a very safe and fast procedure. A lens tilt is not seen at this procedure.

Follow-up Care

Following cataract surgery and optical rehabilitation with either contact lens or implant, amblyopia must be addressed. Over-correction of the eye with spectacle lenses must be continuously updated to ensure that clear, focused images are placed on the retina during times when occlusion therapy is used. All children will opacity the posterior capsule. There is no way to prevent this. The posterior capsule will opacity in approximately 2 to 3 years if the capsule is not opened at the initial surgical procedure. Children who have had extensive posterior capsulotomies with anterior vitrectomies may still have sufficient growth of lens epithelium to require, in some cases, removal of secondary membranes using vitrectome or a Nd:YAG laser. Repeat capsulotomies are common in children.

Following cataract surgery in children, it is common to require more than 10 office visits over the first year to monitor the clarity of the visual axis, the refractive error, and for those patients with contact lenses, to replace, adjust power, and fit of the contact. Later, the children need a 3 months follow-up visits to detect glaucoma, strabismus, and to continue to treat amblyopia.

Conclusion

Early identification and prompt surgical treatment of pediatric cataracts followed by prescription of accurate optical correction and amblyopia treatment will ensure the best visual result. Pre-existing eye conditions, absence of the fovea, undetected retinal problems, late onset glaucoma, secondary membrane formation, and difficulties in treatment of amblyopia are concerns to the treating ophthalmologist. Progress has been made in the management of children with cataracts. Three decades ago, cataract surgery for children with unilateral complete cataracts was not a consideration. Results that are reported now frequently yield visual acuities better than 0.5 and in some patients, high levels of binocular function are being reported.

Chapter 8

Bag-in-the-Lens in Babies and Infants

MJ Tassignon, I De Veuster,
D Godts, L Gobin (Belgium)

Introduction

The concept of the Bag-in-the-lens (BIL) has been patented by the US Patent Office in February 2000 and by the European Patent Office in 2004 As shown, the concept of this new IOL consists in putting the anterior and posterior capsule, after having performed a capsulorhexis of the same size in both capsules, within a peripheral groove and defined by an anterior and posterior haptic.

In the theory first major advantage of this IOL is the quasi absence of contact between the biomaterial and the lens capsule reducing by this the inflammatory reaction related to the biomaterial. In the theory second major advantage of this implantation technique is the entrapment of the LECs within the peripheral capsule reducing the risk of transformation of the LECs into fibroblasts or myofibroblasts as triggered by inflammatory mediators released by the stress due to the surgery. Because the LECs remain in their physiological condition within the lens capsule, we hypothesized that this would favor transparency, flexibility and growth of the lens capsule postoperatively. The in theory third advantage of the BIL is the absolute avoidance of anterior vitrectomy. We will further study whether these theoretical advantages of the BIL are confirmed in clinical practice.

The BIL has been implanted in 37 eyes of 22 children. All 37 eyes had a posterior capsulorhexis but none of these eyes had anterior vitrectomy except in four eyes presenting Persistant Fetal Vasculature (PFV). In this last condition, vitrectomy is necessary for obvious reasons.

DVD 1 shows the surgical technique in a child with congenital cataract. DVD 2 shows the surgical technique in a child with congenital cataract associated with PFV.

The implantation of the BIL in the first eyes of babies and infants showed excellent results and motivated the department of paediatric ophthalmology to start immediately postoperative visual training programmes, especially in children with unilateral cataract.

In Table 1 the age at surgery, the number of eyes operated and the underlying cause of the cataract are listed. Congenital cataract without PFV was present in 30 eyes and PFV was concomitantly present in 4 eyes. One child presented a cataract after orbital radiotherapy. Bilateral cataract was present in 15 patients and unilateral cataract was present in 7 patients.

The postoperative follow-up of these 37 eyes ranged between 68 months for the longest follow-up and 6 months for the shortest (17.49 months ± 18.50 months).

Pre- and postoperative visual acuity is listed. The bilateral cataract clearly result in better postoperative results compared to the unilateral cataract. Postoperative refractive results are listed in Table 2.

The mean postoperative spherical equivalent is –0.2 D ± 1.7 D for a mean aimed refraction of –0.12 D ± 0.06 D and a mean follow-up of 17.49 ± 18.50 months. This means that the A-constant used is correct, which is 118.2.

Within this follow-up period the number of secondary surgical procedures was reduced to two: one eye presented a dropped IOL one week after surgery

Table 1: Preoperative age and postoperative follow-up

Patient	*Operated eye*	*Pathology*	*Age at surgery (years/months)*	*Postoperative follow-up (months)*
1	OD	congenital cataract	4 years	68,8
	OS	" "	4 years	63,8
2	OD	congenital cataract	5 years	41,5
	OS	" "	5 years	41,1
3	OD	congenital cataract	1 year	
	OS	" "	1 year	42,3
4	OD	congenital cataract + PFV	7 months	29,1
5	OD	congenital cataract	3 years	31,8
	OS	" "	3 years	32,0
6	OD	congenital cataract	7 years	8,7
7	OD	congenital cataract + PFV	15 months	13,8
8	OD	congenital cataract	8 years	30,1
	OS	" "	9 years	20,4
9	OD	congenital cataract	12 years	8,5
	OS	" "	not yet operated	
10	OD	congenital cataract	12 years	14,0
	OS	" "	12 years	13,9
11	OD	congenital cataract	13 years	2,7
	OS	" "	13 years	1,0
12	OS	congenital cataract	2 years	14,7
13	OD	congenital cataract	14 years	2,1
	OS	" "	14 years	3,5
14	OD	congenital cataract	13 years	5,5
	OS	" "	13 years	5,8
15	OS	radiotherapy-induced cataract	7 years	4,0
16	OD	congenital cataract + PFV *	5 months	4,5
17	OD	congenital cataract + PFV	4 years	5,0
18	OD	congenital cataract + trisomia 21	not yet operated	
	OS	" " "	6 years	1,0
19	OD	spherophakia + dysgenesis AC **	3 years	6,2
	OS	" " "	3 years	5,9
20	OD	congenital cataract*** + dysgenesis AC	5 months	2,3
	OS	" " " "	5 months	2,5
21	OD	congenital cataract*	2 months	5,0
	OS	" "	2 months	5,0
22	OD	congenital cataract	10 years	1
	OS	" "	10 years	1

Table 2: Refractive results (mean spherical equivalent refraction: –0.2 ± 1.7 D; mean follow-up: 17.48 ± 18.50 months; mean aimed refraction: –0.12 ± 0.06 D). Pre- and postoperative visual acuity. Mean accommodation: 5.2 ± 2.3 D measured with the RAF test.

Patient	Operated eye	Preoperative BCVA	Axial length (mm)	Preoperative keratometry (D)	Preoperative corneal astigmatism (D)	Postoperative UCVA	Postoperative BCVA	Postoperative spherical equivalent (D)	Postoperative corneal astigmatism (D)	Intraocular pressure (mmHg)	Accommodation RAF (D)
1	OD	0,4	21,5	43,0	0,4	0,4	1,0	2,5	–1,0	15	4,0
	OS	0,4	21,0	42,0	0,4	0,4	1,0	3,5	–0,5	15	4,0
2	OD	0,2	22,6	43,7	1,8	0,4	0,8	–0,9	–1,3	19	5,0
	OS	0,2	22,4	43,8	2,1	0,3	0,5	–1,8	–2,0	19	5,0
3	OS		19,5								
4	OD					0,07		–2,6	–3,3		
5	OD	0,2	19,9	47,9	3,4		1,2	0,4	–2,3	19	
	OS	0,1	18,6	47,6	4,1		0,8	1,5	–3,0	19	5,0
6	OD	0,1	22,5	41,2	1,3	0,07		–0,9	–0,8	16	
7	OD		19,9				0,1			15	4,0
8	OD	0,1	24,2	44,1	1,0	0,2	1,0	–4,5	0,0	17	3,5
	OS	0,1	23,9	44,3	0,2	0,5	1,0	–2,5	0,0	16	3,0
9	OD	0,3	23,0	44,8	1,6	0,2	1,2	–1,5	–2,0	13	3,0
10	OD	0,2	20,7	43,9	0,5	0,8	1,0	–0,8	0,0	19	3,0
	OS	0,3	20,9	44,1	0,7	0,8	1,0	–0,5	–1,0	19	3,0
11	OD	0,2	25,0	41,6	1,7	0,6	1,0	–1,0	–2,0	17	
	OS	0,3	25,0	42,0	2,2	0,7	1,0	–1,0	–2,0	17	
12	OS		21,5							18	6,0
13	OD	0,2	24,1	42,9	1,4	0,8	0,8	0,0	0,0	21	3,0
	OS	0,1	24,4	43,4	1,7	0,9	0,9	0,0	0,0	14	12,0
14	OD	0,3	22,6	47,9	3,1	0,7	0,8	–1,0	–1,0	16	
	OS	0,3	22,0	48,4	2,8	0,7		0,0	0,0	17	
15	OS	0,4	23,4	40,4	0,6		0,8	0,0	0,0	11	2,5
16	OD		20,5	46,0	0,0			1,3	–2,0	16	
17	OD	0,1	20,0	46,4	2,4		0,3			11	
18	OS		22,2	45,8	0,0						
19	OD	0,2	21,8	43,4	2,5		0,5	5,0		20	
	OS	0,2	21,7	43,2	2,9		0,5	3,5		30	
20	OD		18,4	41,2	1,9			+6	–3	19	
	OS		18,4	41,2	2,1			+3	–2,75	13	
21	OD		18,5	44,4	1,4						
	OS		18,0	44,8	1,5						
22	OD	0,15	21,52	47,4	1,8	0,4	0,7	–1,25	–1,50	15	
	OS	0,15	21,58	47,5	2,65	0,8	0,8	0	0	15	

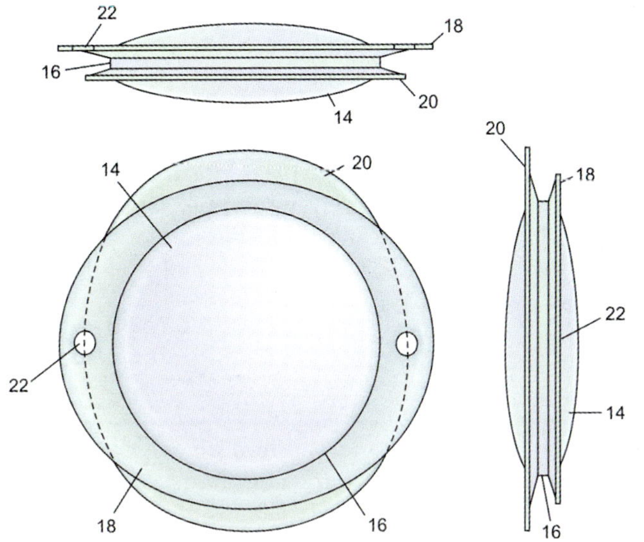

Figure 1: Top: Schematic drawing of the BIL showing the main circular central optic surrounded by the haptic. The two haptics are oriented perpendicularly to each other to ensure optimal lens stability. The side view shows the characteristic groove in which both lens capsules will be positioned. (1 = optic; 2 = groove; 3 = oval-shaped posterior haptic; 4 = oval-shaped anterior haptic; 5 = positioning holes, optional)

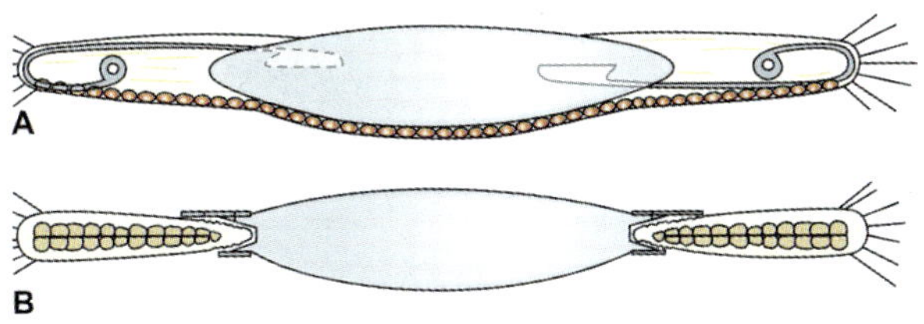

Figure 2: (A) Schematic drawing of the lens-in-the-bag implantation. (B) Schematic drawing of the bag-in-the-lens implantation

because of an oversized anterior and posterior rhexis (before the introduction of the ring caliper to calibrate the rhexis diameter). One child presented an ocular trauma one week after surgery with IOL luxation into the anterior chamber as a result. This IOL could be repositioned surgically.

None of these eyes needed a surgical intervention for glaucoma. None of the children presented visual axis reproliferation (VAR) during this follow-up period (17.49 ± 18.50 months), which is a unique result compared to the literature.

Postoperative images are all alike: a clear optical zone, no vitreous reaction and a quiet anterior chamber. One of the pleasant surprises of the implantation of the BIL in children is the relatively large postoperative accommodation capacity of these children. The mean postoperative accommodation measured with the RAF test was 5.2 D ± 2.3 D, which allows most of the children to read without spectacles.

Conclusion

The BIL implantation in babies and children gives very promising results. Although this lens may show some difficulties to implant in very small babies and in eyes presenting congenital malformations, it is however worthwhile to afine the technique for these very challenging cases.

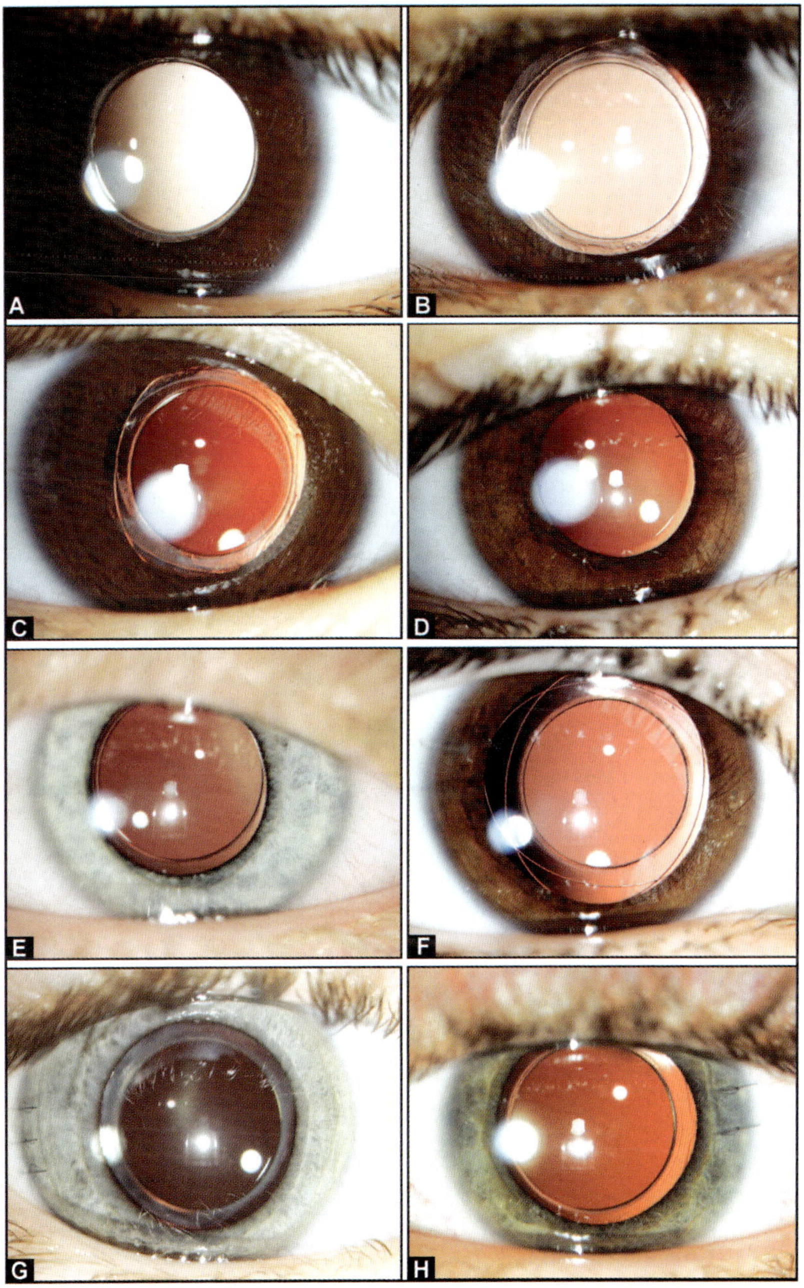

Figure 3: Postoperative results after BIL implantation

A. 64 months follow-up
B. 41 months follow-up
C. 29 months follow-up
D. 18 months follow-up
E. 14 months follow-up
F. 8 months follow-up
G. 3 months follow-up
H. 1 month follow-up

Chapter 9

Pediatric Aphakia

Ewa Oleszczynska Prost (Poland)

Introduction

Congenital cataracts continue to be a major cause of decreased vision and blindness in children, despite dramatic improvements in the surgery treatment of infantile cataracts.

Good vision and binocularity may be attained nowadays, in great percentage of children following the removal of congenital unilateral and bilateral cataracts. The best outcomes after surgery depend on several variables. This includes:

- The extend of cataract
- Associated ocular abnormalities
- Associated systemic abnormalities
- Early diagnosis
- Early treatment
- Surgical techniques of cataract removal
- Optimum optical correction
- Visual rehabilitation for years

Amblyopia associated with congenital and infantile cataract is the major cause of poor vision. It is important to start the treatment in early critical period of visual development, in the first few months of life when the visual areas in the brain are developing rapidly in response to the visual stimuli from the eyes.

There are two solutions of pediatric aphakia correction:

1. Primary lens implantation technique
2. Postoperative aphakia correction

Clinical Findings

- Monocular or binocular, post cataract surgery, lack of lenses
- Microphthalmos especially in unilateral cases
- Often irregularity of pupil
- Opacified peripheral capsular ring
- Sometimes heterochromia of iris
- Esodeviation or exodeviation
- Hyperphoria on the aphakic eye
- DVD or oblique dysfunction
- Nystagmus horizontal, vertical or rotation, also monocular
- Torticollis ocularis

Investigation

- Patient's history
- Keratorefraction by hand-held autokeratorefractometer (Retinomax)
- Eye examination on slit lamp
- Fundus examination
- Ultrasonic axial length measurements

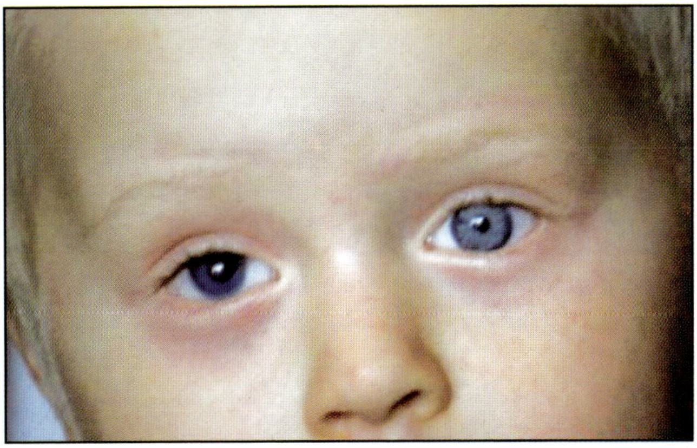

Figure 1: Lack of lenses post monocular cataract surgery

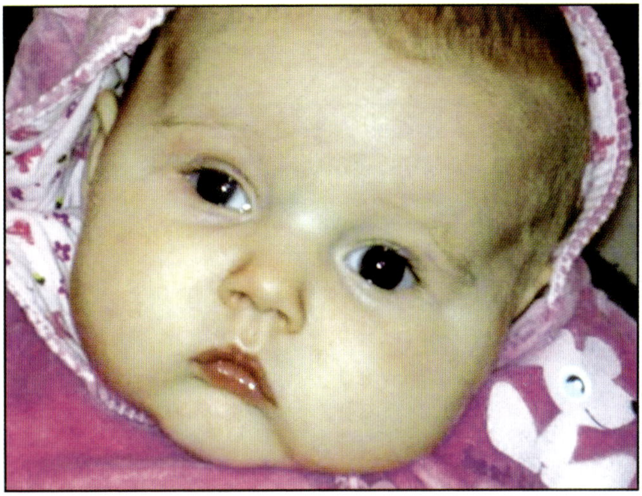

Figure 2: Microphthalmic right eye in unilateral aphakia

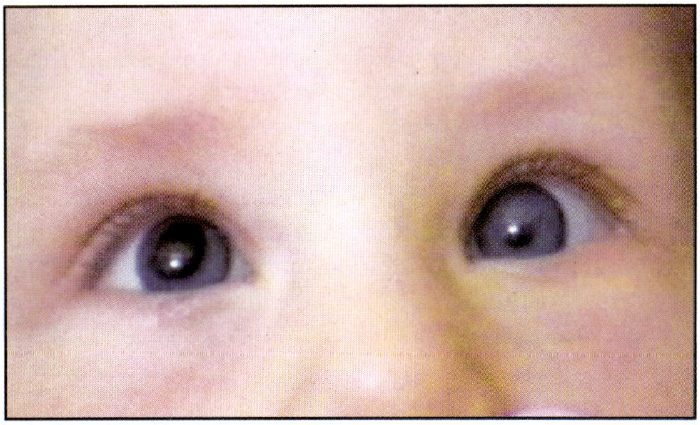

Figure 3: Irregularity of pupil in the aphakic right eye

- Hirschberg light reflex test
- Krimsky's prismatic test
- Eye movements examination in 9 cardinal position of gaze
- Cover-uncover test
- Evaluation of vision acuity
- Fixation testing for amblyopia

Differential Diagnosis

- Lens coloboma
- Congenital lens dislocation
- Congenital esotropia
- Nystagmus
- Anisometropia

Treatment

- Contact lens performed as soon as possible after surgery
- Aggressive occlusion therapy in unilateral aphakia
- Pleoptic treatment
- Penalization method treatment
- Prismatic correction of strabismus
- Localization method treatment with exercises in hypercorrection prismatic glasses
- Orthoptic exercises
- BTA injections
- Strabismus or nystagmus surgery

Prognosis

Monocular Aphakia

- The amount of patching required visual development of the aphakic eye depends on the age when the retinal image was cleared.
- If surgery and optical correction (contact lenses) is provided in early critical period of visual development, especially by 2 months of age, monocular congenital cataracts have a relatively good prognosis (visual acuity range 20/200 to 20/25)with motor and bifoveal fusion after a part time patching.
- Patients with relatively late cataract surgery (by 17 weeks of age), received full-time occlusion therapy to achieve their good visual results with developed strabismus

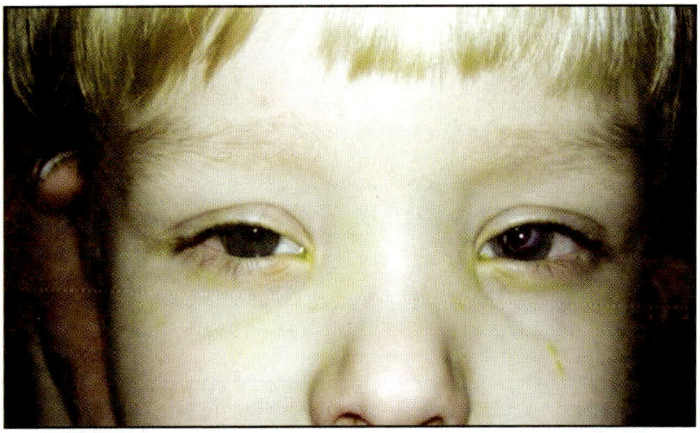

Figure 4: The child with binocular aphakia. The opacified peripheral capsular ring seen in the left pupil

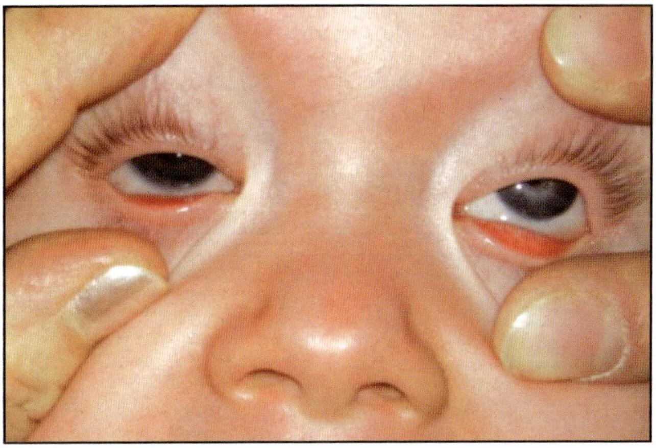

Figure 5: Heterochromia of iris after congenital cataract surgery

Binocular Aphakia

- If surgery and exact optical correction (contact lenses) is provided in early critical period of visual development, especially by 2 months of age, binocular congenital cataracts have a good prognosis (visual acuity range 20/100 to 20/30) with full fusion and stereopsis.
- Patients who developed nystagmus or strabismus required often visual rehabilitation (optical correction and orthoptic treatment) after surgery or BTA injection.

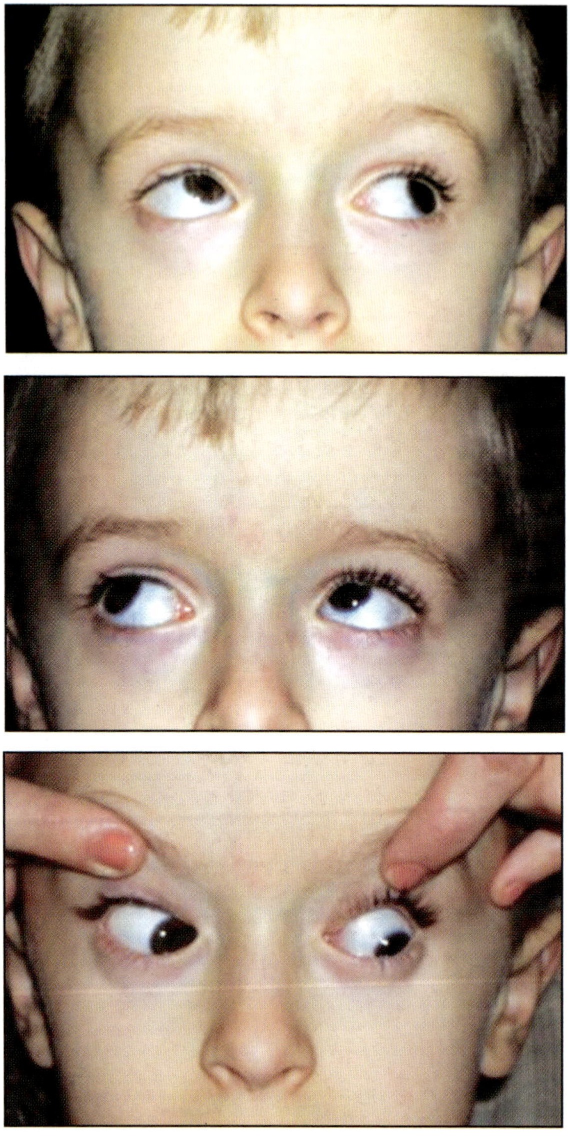

Figure 6: Inferior oblique dysfunction on the right sound eye. See aphakia in the left eye

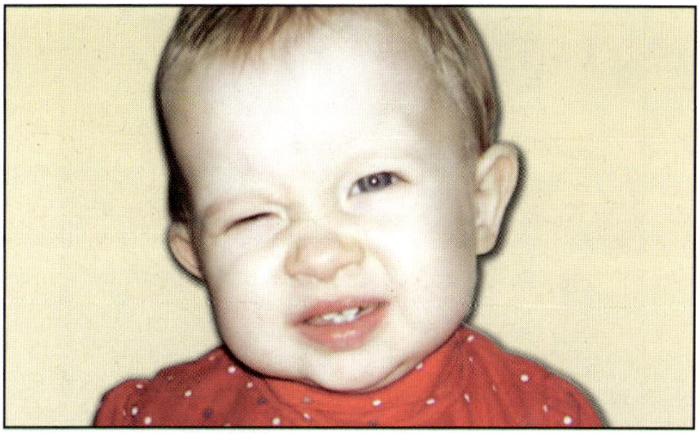

Figure 7: Torticollis ocularis

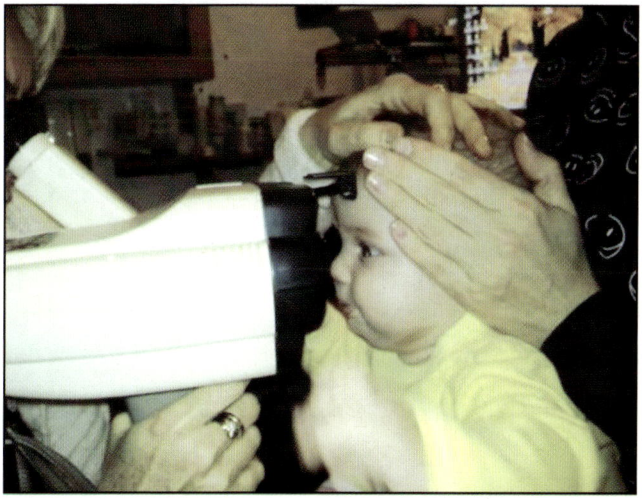

Figure 8: Evaluation of refraction in very young children by use hand-held autokeratorefractometer (Retinomax)

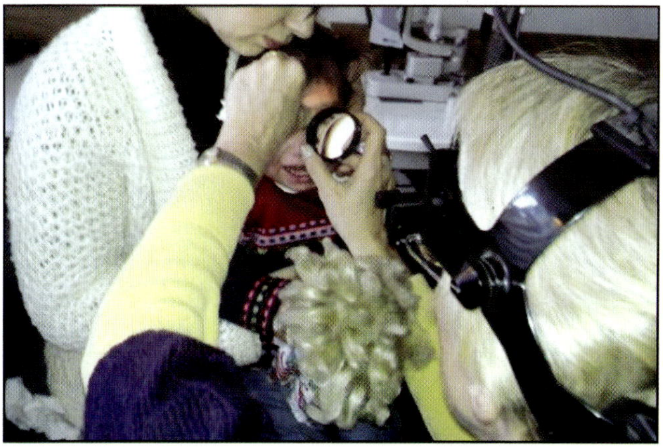

Figure 9: Fundus examination

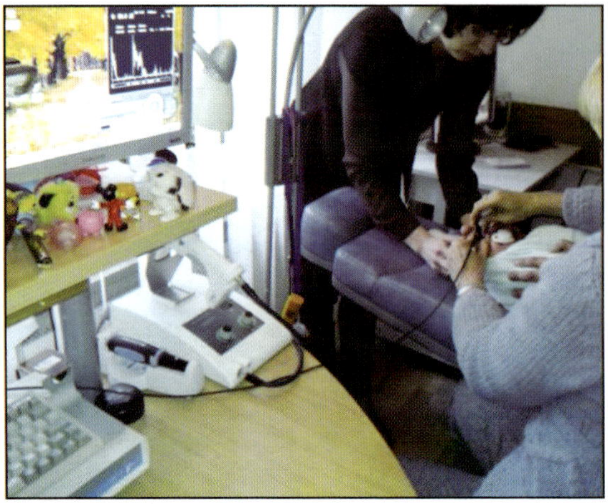

Figure 10: The ultrasonic axial length measurements in 3 year old child

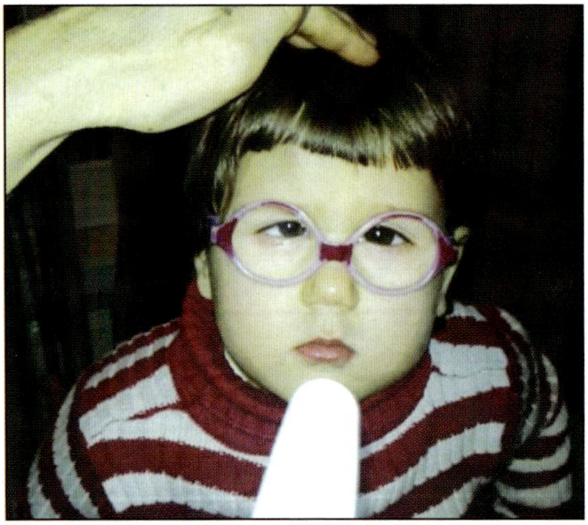

Figure 11: Hirschberg light reflex test

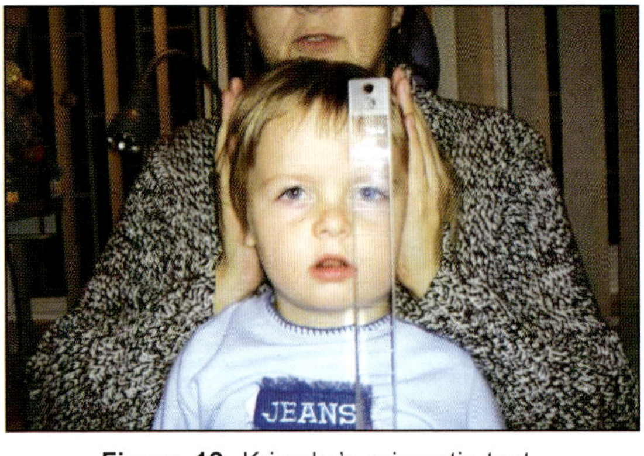

Figure 12: Krimsky's prismatic test

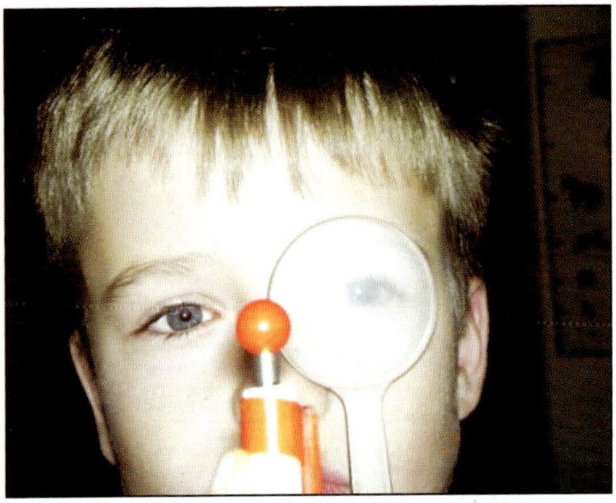

Figure 13: Cover-uncover test

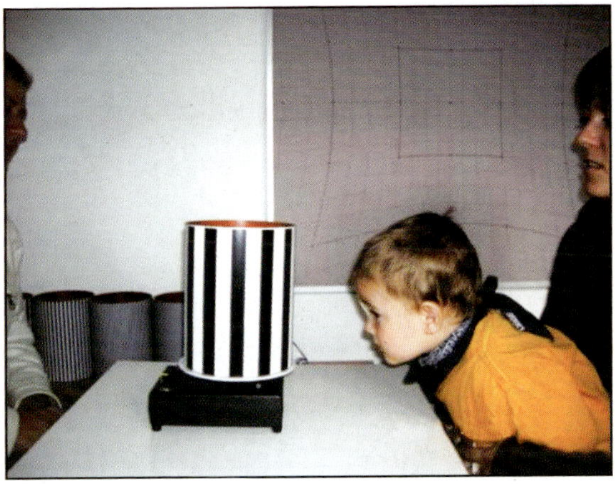

Figure 14: Evaluation of vision acuity with using OKN

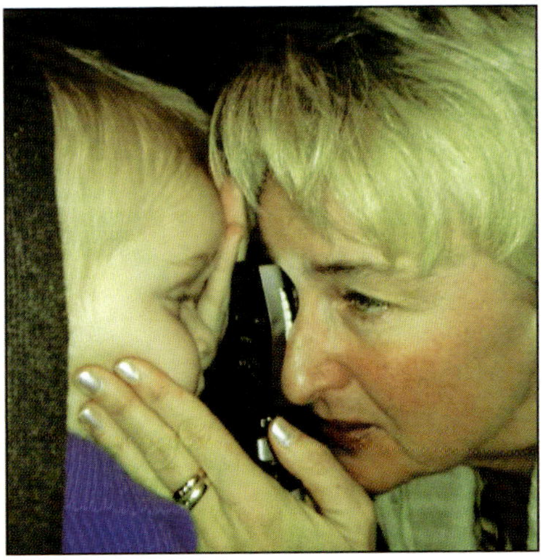

Figure 15: Fixation testing for amblyopia

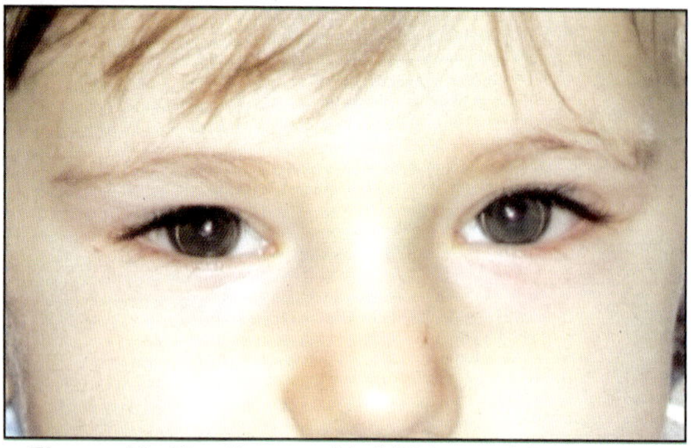

Figure 16: The 2-year-old child treated for binocular aphakia by using contact lenses

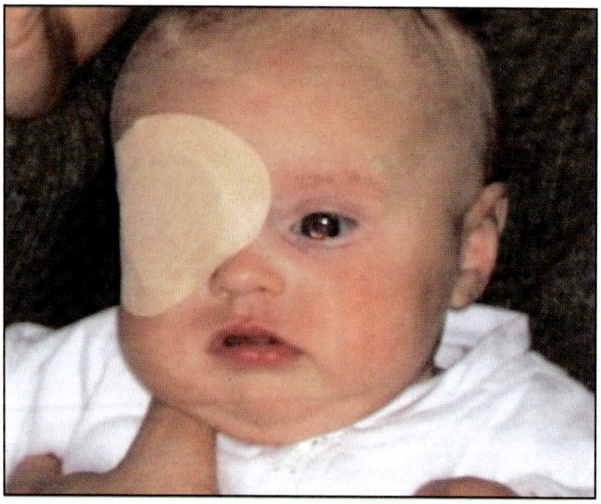

Figure 17: Aggressive occlusion therapy in unilateral aphakia

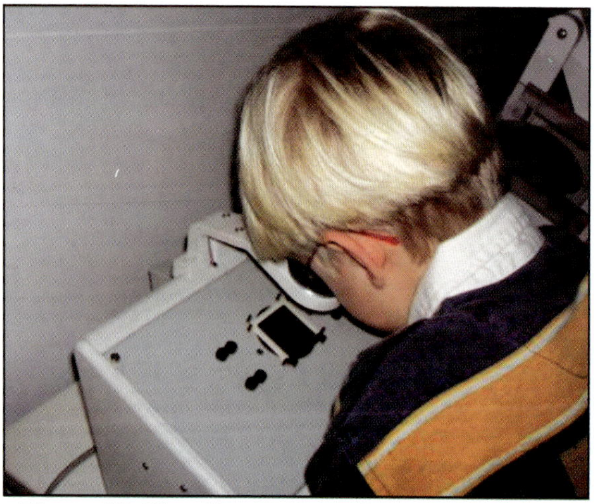

Figure 18: Pleoptic treatment of aphakic amblyopia

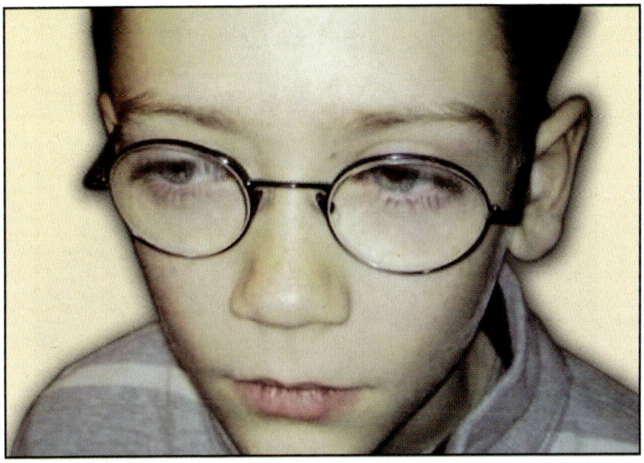

Figure 19: Prismatic glasses for correction of strabismus

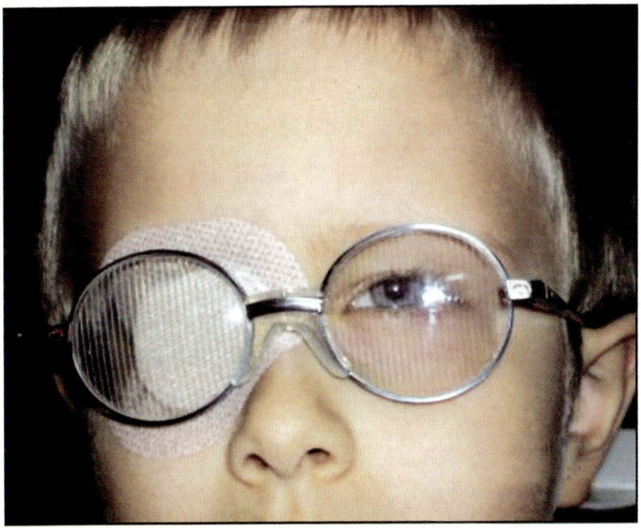

Figure 20: Localization method treatment with exercises in hypercorrection prismatic glasses

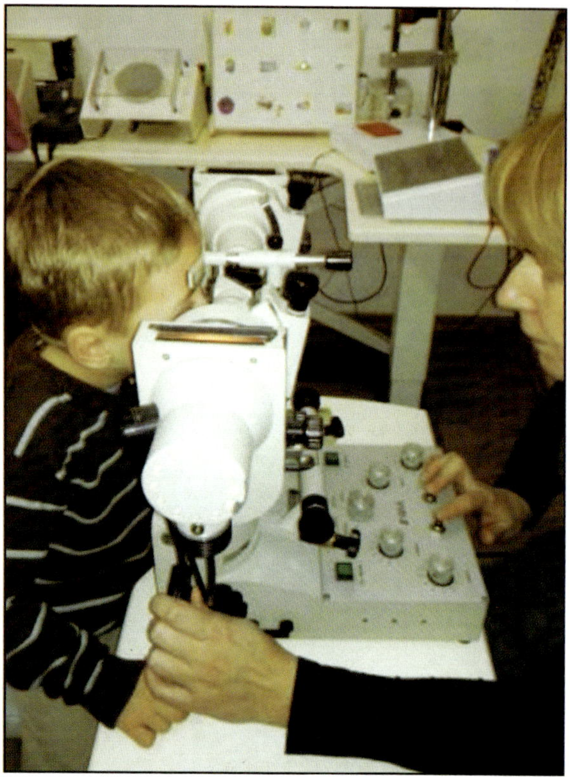

Figure 21: Orthoptic treatment –exercises on synoptophore

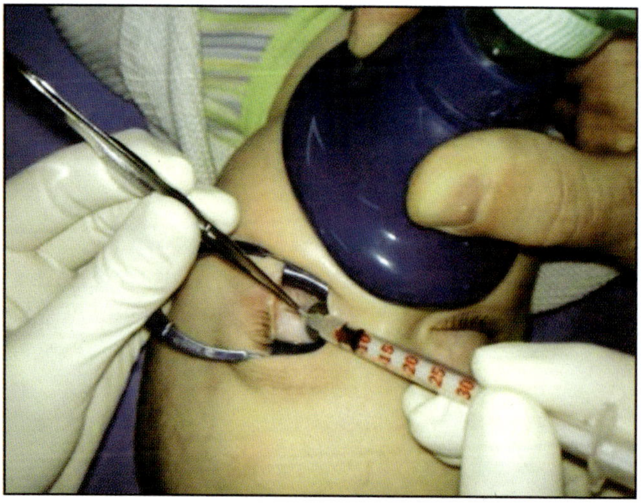

Figure 22: BTA injection in 5 years old

Chapter 10

Removable Piggyback IOL in Managing Cataract in Infants

Keiki R Mehta, Cyres K Mehta (India)

Introduction

Mananging to give an accurate power to a child, operated in its infancy, following a cataract, is at best a probem. There are many alternatives available but none of them really measure up.

Children's eyes are continuously growing, and as the body grows quickest in infancy and slows down later, so do the eyes.

The constant size of the adult eye ensures that the refraction of an adult pseudophakic eye is stable. However ocular growth has gross effects on refraction, having a tendency to produce a large myopic shift.

In essence, we would like the child to have a good visual acuity when he grows up with as low a power as is possible. To achieve this goal however a large number of factors need to be considered.

Calculating the Intraocular Lens Power Calculation for Children.

Biometry

Perhaps the most important factor to consider. As is routine, we need to consider the axial length (AL) and corneal power (K). In addition we need to consider, corneal diameter, intraocular pressure (lOP), and corneal thickness.

Recording any measurements in a child is, at best, difficult though after the age of 6 or 7 with a little reassurance the child will cooperate adequately to let that happen. Alternatively. these measurements can be done quite easily in the operating room while the child is asleep. A-Scan ultrasound can be done using either contact or immersion methods. Care must be taken that the scan is directed toward the macula and that the tip does not indent the relatively soft cornea. We routinely use immersion biometry with the Alcon unit and are quite satisfied with it.

Recording the curvature we place an autokeratometer at the side of the bed and simply tilt the childs face. The readings need to be transposed by 90 degrees but otherwise are perfectly easy to do. Portable autokeratometers are also available.

Glaucoma is a frequent occurrence in aphakic and pseudophakic children's eyes, and the IOP should also be measured at the initiation of anesthesia whenever a child has cataract-related surgery and at subsequent examinations under anesthesia. An hand held applanation tonometry is fairly accurate can be significantly affected by cornea thickness and thus pachymetry should also be carried out the first time the child is examined.

IOL Formulas

It is interesting to consider the optics of an aphakic eye. For all practical purposes, the refraction depends on Axial Length and corneal power alone.However a pseudophakic eye has two additional factors to consider: the IOL power and its position in the eye. Most formulae will work well. The only variable is the

Age	*Sag length*	*Corneal dia*	*IOL power*
Term	16.8-17.3	8.8-9.9	34.4-38 D
6 months	17.8-18.2	8.9-10.4	31.3-34.7D
12 months	20.6-21.4	10.1-11.5	28.2-31.6D
1 year	22.2-23.5	10.8-12.1	21.6-23.8D

Data from Jeanty P et al: Radiology 143:513,1982; Swan K.C Wilkins JH: J. Pediatr Ophthal Strab 21:44,1984:Agarwal. J; J All India Ophthal Soc 49:873.1986

Figure 1: Physical ocular characteristics

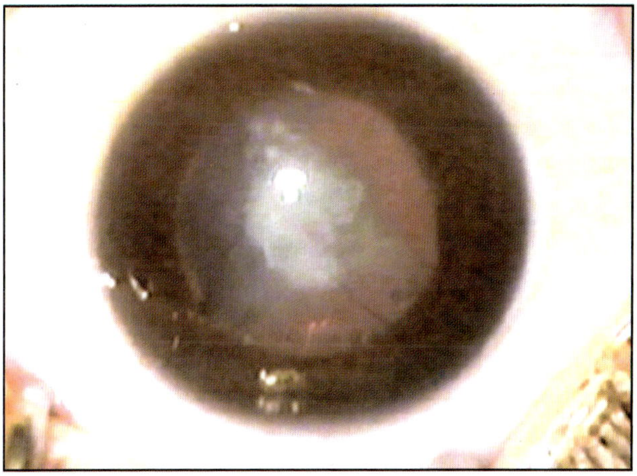

Figure 2: 9 month child with gradual fall in vision

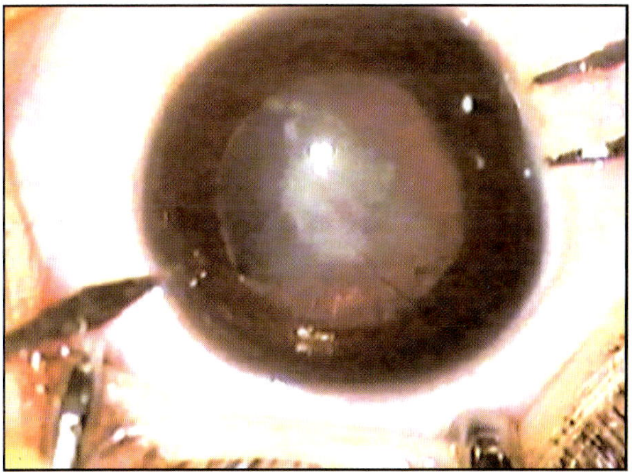

Figure 3: Side port with MVR blade, supporting from the opposite side

growing differences in children's anterior segment anatomy which affect the position of the IOL immediately after surgery, thus slightly changing the initial postoperative refraction.

The formulas used for calculation of IOL powers are designed to take into account the final position of the IOL in the eye. Depending on the type of the implant, its relative final position in the bag will be different. An IOL that is relatively anterior in the eye will have a greater refractive effect than one that is relatively posterior.

One of the first IOL calculation formulas was the SRK formula, an empiric, linear formula that made calculations by hand and calculator quite simple. This formula worked well for most eyes but gave incorrect calculations for eyes that were short or long or had an unusual anterior segment anatomy.

In an effort to compensate for variance in anterior segment anatomy on IOL calculation a host of newer generations of IOL formulas are available. Modern theoretic formulas, such as the SRK- T, Holladay I and II, Hoffer Q, and Haigis, take these factors into account. In adults, the theoretic formulas are more accurate than the SRK I or SRK II formulas, and in published series they show a mean absolute error of <±0.6 D (diopter). However the studies in children have shown larger errors in IOL formula predictions than are found in adults.

Andreo et al studied 47 consecutive pseudophakic pediatric patients, age 3 months to 16 years. They compared the actual initial postoperative pseudophakic refractions to those predicted by four formulas (SRK-II, SRK-T, Holladay, and Hoffer Q). They found no significant difference in accuracy between the formulas: the average initial postoperative refractive error was between 1.2 and 1.4 D in all formulas. Another study found that the mean difference between the predicted and the actual postoperative refractions was slightly more accurate using theoretic formulas (1.06 D, vs. 1.22 D with regression formulas). Which IOL formula should be used for children? Because of the relatively large IOL formula errors demonstrated in pediatric studies, it is not clear that any formula can be considered accurate for all children. Although no formula has been proven to have an advantage it is recommended (McClatchy & Hofmesiter) to use the theoretic formulas because they are generally more accurate for small eyes, and may be more accurate in general.

The Growth of the Eye

The growth of the eye (McClatchy & Hofmesiter) follows a logarithmic curve. The greatest change is in early childhood, but there is no sharp cutoff: the refractive growth continues up to age 20 years. This growth has profound effects on the refraction of aphakic and pseudophakic eyes.

In normal children, the growth of the eye affects both the AL and the cornea curvature. Most of the growth occurs in the first 2 years of life, but there is a smoothly changing curve, with some growth until adulthood. The AL increases from an average of 16.8 mm at birth to 23.6 mm in adulthood, while K decreases from an average power of 51.2 to 43.5 D. Aphakic children's eyes become less

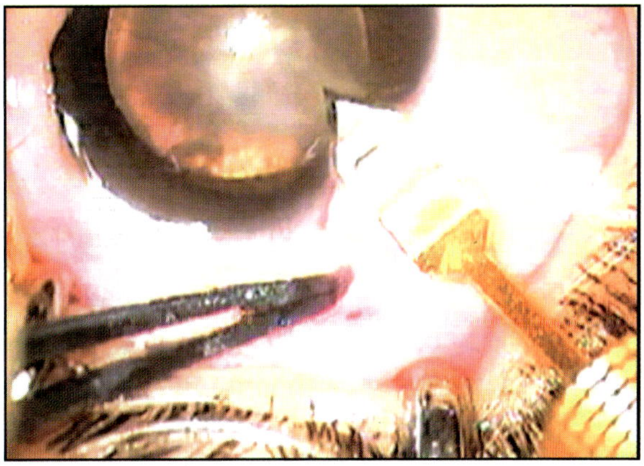

Figure 4: Diamond knife tunnel corneal incision. Care to make a deep tunnel

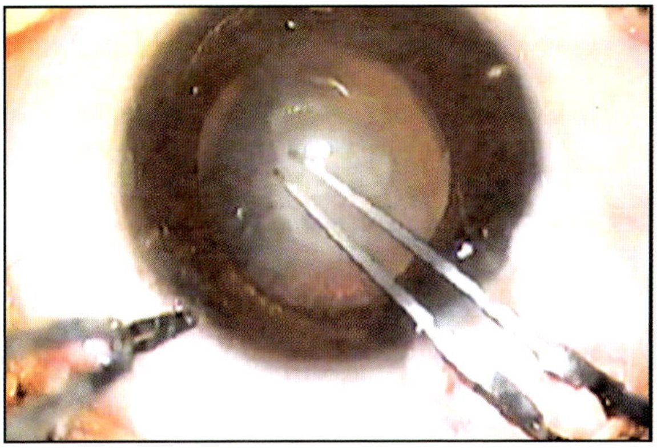

Figure 5: Rhexis commenced with sharp pointed utrata forceps

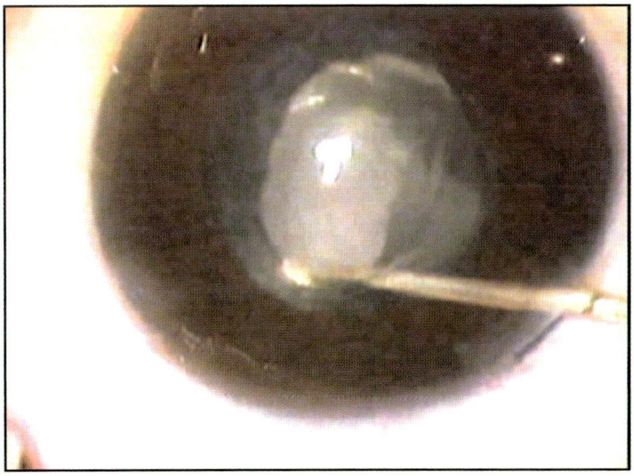

Figure 6: Hydrodissection with blunt cannula

hyperopic with time: they have an average myopic shift of 10 D from infancy to adulthood. In contrast, the refraction of normal eyes changes much less, approximately -0.9 D.

In an effort to understand this variance, Gordon and Donzis performed a biometric study of normal children of various ages and found that the natural lens power decreases dramatically as the eye grows. Indeed, this must be true for the optical system of the eye to focus on the retina at all ages: as long as all parts of the eye grow proportionally from infancy, the focus will remain unchanged. As the natural lens is scaled up in size with the growth of the eye, the surfaces of the lens have greater radii of curvature. This causes the lens to have a longer focal length (lower power) and thus focus well onto the more distant retina. If a child has a lens removed, the eye is left hyperopic in relation to the power of the lens that was removed. Thus, the quantity of hyperopia of a child's aphakic growing eye decreases with time, just as the power of the natural lens decreases with time.

The slope of the line was originally given the name "rate of myopic shift" when it applied only to aphakic children. The slope in the logarithmic model can be calculated for pseudophakic eyes by mathematically removing the optical effect of the IOL. The slope in this case is not a direct measure of myopic shift, so it was renamed "rate of refractive growth" (RRG), because it is analogous to other rates and is a measure of the refractive change due to the growth of the eye.

For this model to be extended to pseudophakic eyes, we must know the effect of IOL implantation on the growth of the eye. The largest long-term studies of refractive growth in aphakic and pseudophakic children show that the eyes of aphakic and pseudophakic children have a similar growth curve, with a slightly lower rate of refractive growth in pseudophakic eyes. Most of the refractive change occurs in the first few years of life, with a gradually decreasing rate of myopic shift (reduction in hyperopia). RRG is lower in children <6 months of age at surgery.

Cataract surgery after 6 months of age has little effect on the growth of the eye, with or without IOL implantation.

Extending the Refractive Growth Model to Early Pregnancy

Evaluation of children who have surgery at between 3 and 6 months of age have a lower RRG. A study of children who had surgery at between 3 and 6 months of age found an RRG lower than that seen in older children.

The cutoff age is not inherently obvious, but by inspection of the refraction graphs, the age of 3 months was chosen. Therefore, a different model must be used for ages <3 months where the rate changes fairly significantly.

Another important variable which has to be considered is that as the pseudophakic eye grows, the distance from the IOL to the retina increases. This effectively moves the focal point of the IOL anterior in the eye. This refractive change is analogous to the refractive difference between contacts and spectacles:

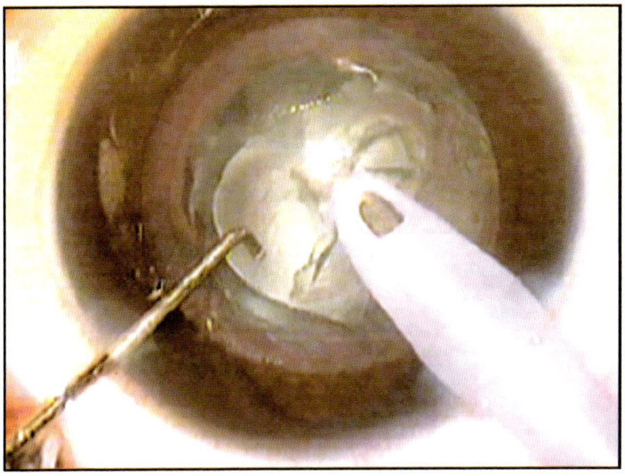

Figure 7: Phaco with high aspiration, occasional pulse

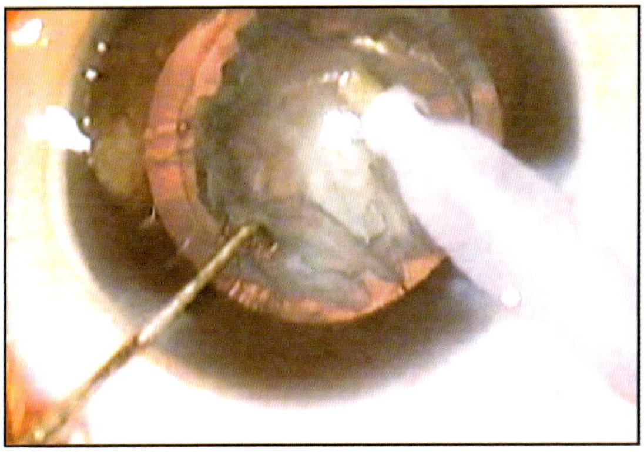

Figure 8: Fragments aspirated out carefully. Note edge of rhexis

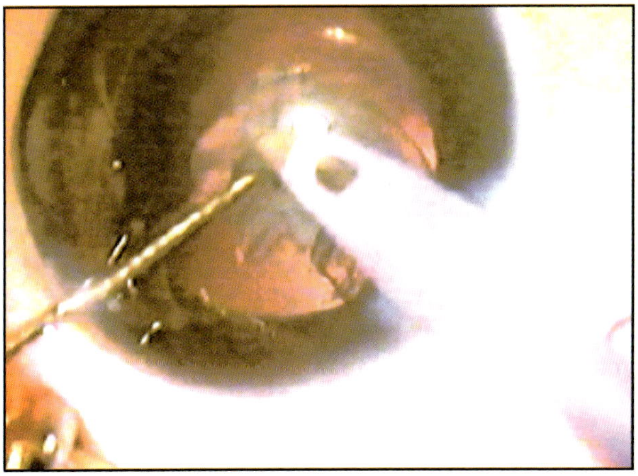

Figure 9: Final fragments aspirated out

the optical effect of vertex distance for a high-power correction is significant. For example, an aphakic patient who is corrected with a + 12.00-D spectacle lens at a vertex distance of 12 mm would require a contact lens power of + 14.0 D. The need for increased power in the contact lens is caused by the optical effect of vertex distance.

The higher the power of the lens, the greater the effect. For example, a patient who required a +20.00-D spectacle lens would require a contact lens power of +26.3 D.

Practical Considerations in IOL Power Choice

We think it is useful to start with the goal in mind. Ideally, we would like the child to grow up to have good visual acuity and emmetropia in adulthood. The IOL power choice is only one step in the path to this goal, which also includes amblyopia management and refractive correction with glasses or contact lenses. Ultimately a refractive surgery such as photo refractive keratectomy can eliminate any significant refractive error in adulthood. Of course, not all young children with cataracts will end up with this ideal, because of coexisting ocular abnormalities,

What then are the Options?

Surgeons have taken four approaches to IOL power choice. At first, when biometry was difficult, some surgeons chose to use an IOL with a typical adult power. With biometry readily available, surgeons can now choose an initial postoperative refractive goal. Some choose hyperopia, with the expectation of myopic shift with time; others choose emmetropia or myopia to help with amblyopia management. Each of these approaches has advantages and disadvantages. There is no study showing a visual advantage of one approach over the other.

Many surgeons prefer to leave the eye moderately hyperopic, using a logical approach based on knowledge of how the refraction is likely to change with age. They also customize the choice of initial postoperative refraction based on the child, accounting for the refraction of the opposite eye and whether the surgery is unilateral or bilateral, among other factors.

In infants and in very small eyes, refractive correction may require more than a single IOL. The surgeon may choose to leave the pseudophakic eye strongly hyperopic and to correct the hyperopia with a contact lens or spectacles. Another option is to place piggyback IOLs, with a high-power IOL in the bag and a second, lower-power IOL in the sUlcuS. Piggyback IOLs offer unique advantages and challenges in this situation, and long-term studies in children have not yet been published. As the eye grows, the refraction may become dramatically less hyperopic; in this case the piggyback IOL can be easily removed. On the other hand, some eyes have little refractive growth with age, and the two lenses could be left in place indefinitely.

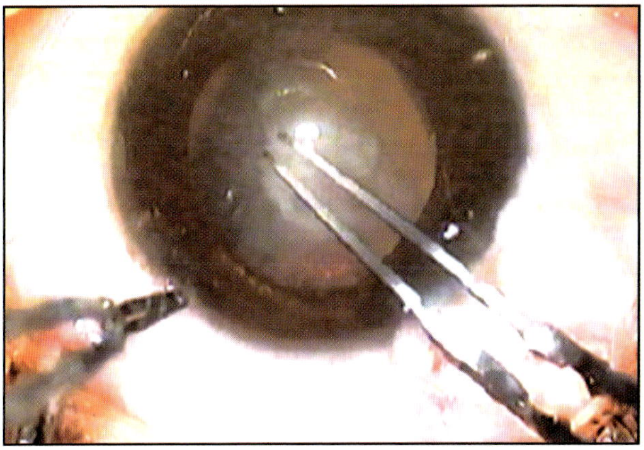

Figure 10: Posterior rhexis with the utrata forceps

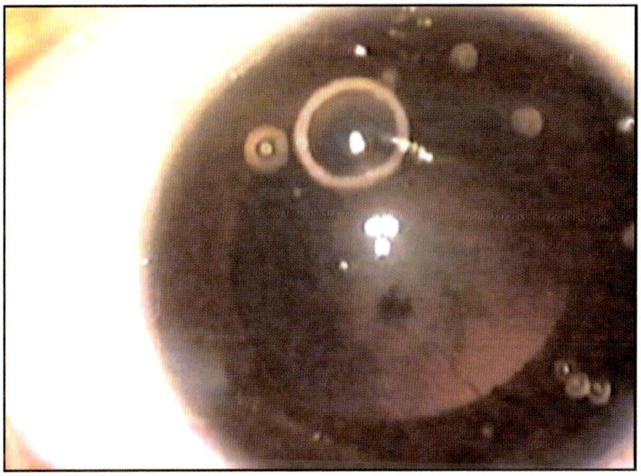

Figure 11: Posterior rhexis with the utrata forceps

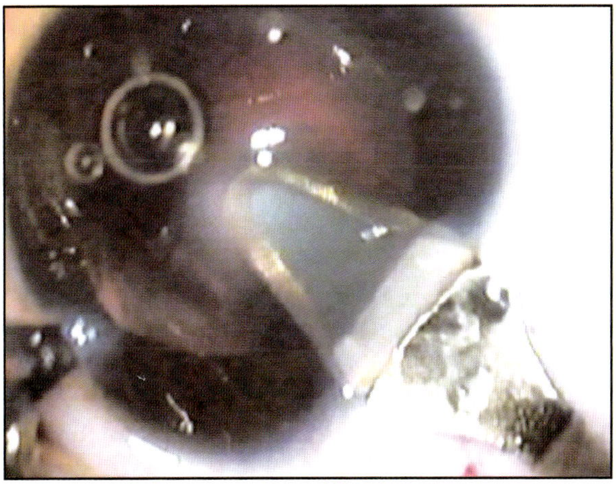

Figure 12: Incision widened to 3.8 mm using a keratome. Note width of tunnel

If piggyback IOLs are placed, it is imperative that that care should be taken to remove as many of the lens epithelial cells as possible. The space between the two IOLs can provide a scaffold for the rapidly growing lens cells, resulting in obscuration of the visual pathway.

Calculation of predicted refractions of pseudophakic children as they grow can be done in several ways, including spreadsheets and commercial IOL programs. To date, the authors are not aware of a commercial program that uses the logarithmic model. The surgeon should keep in mind that the goal postoperative refraction may be different for children with bilateral cataracts than for those with unilateral cataracts, and account may need to be taken for difficult social circumstances or other factors.

This chapter will consider the implications of the piggy back removable system which seems to work well and can be fine tuned to deliver the accuracy desired.

Two Surgical Approaches

Two different surgical approaches have been proposed to avoid complications with piggyback IOLs:

- In the first, both IOLs are implanted in the capsular bag with a larger diameter capsulorhexis, The cut edge of the capsulorhexis may fuse with the posterior capsule, which should help sequester the retained/ proliferative equatorial lens epithelial cells within the equatorial fornix and prevent cell migration toward the interlenticular space.
- In the second approach, the posterior IOL is implanted in the capsular bag with the cut edge of a small-diameter capsulorhexis resting on its anterior optical surface, Dr. Werner reported. The anterior IOL is placed with the haptics in the ciliary sulcus, anterior to the capsulorhexis. Retained/ proliferative lens epithelial cells are confined to the compartment of the capsular bag around the rear IOL, but the interlenticular space in front of the capsulorhexis is also sequestered.

In addition, careful cortical cleanup to remove most remaining cells from the equatorial lens bow can help prevent complications, To do this, aspirate the lens epithelial cells, even off the undersurface of the anterior capsule, in addition to using 12 hydrodissection waves, one for each clock hour. The availability of the new Alcon AquaLase which uses pulses of warmed water leaves extremely clear capsules and is highly recommended for children.

Which Lens?

Most available IOL optic materials, including PMMA, silicone and hydrophobic acrylic materials, have been used for piggyback implantation.

The longest experience has been with PMMA lenses, but they require a larger incision. "That is why people went to the foldable AcrySof. However, interlenticular opacification seems to be more common with the AcrySof lens, and so it is preferred not to use two AcrySof lenses in the bag for piggybacking."

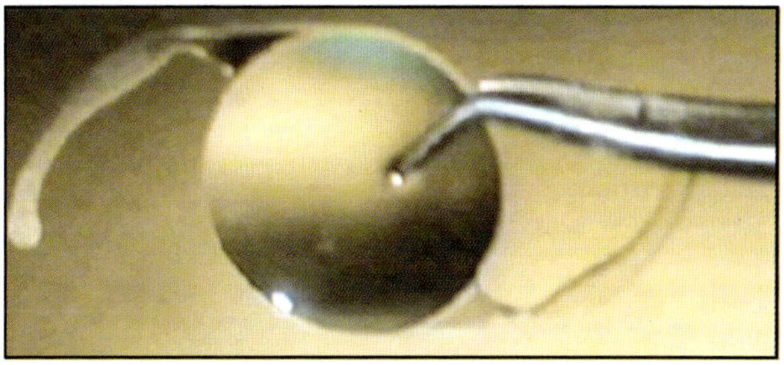

Figure 13: Acrysof lens prepared for injection insertion

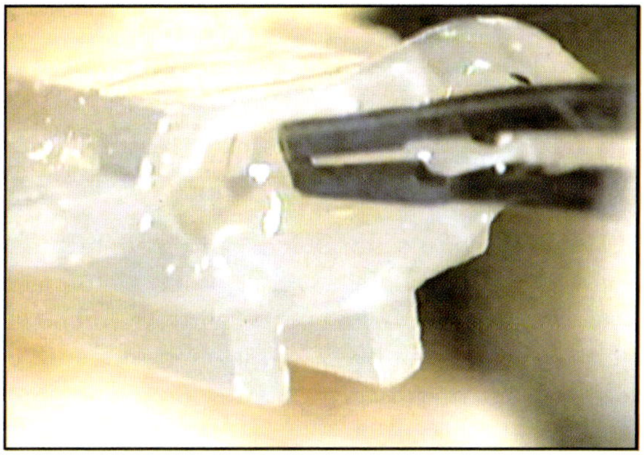

Figure 14: Loading lens in the monarch injector cartridge

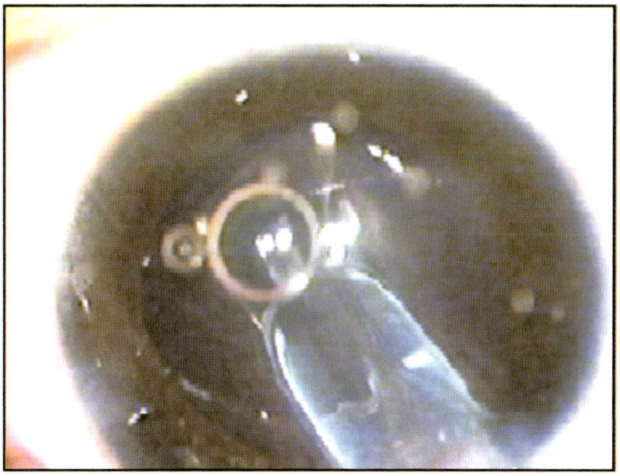

Figure 15: Acrysof lens being injected into the posterior chamber

In search of the ideal for primary piggybacking, we tried different lens combinations. The ideal answer is to use a Acrysof as the "permanent" IOL and to use a pure Hema Disc IOL as the "removable" IOL.

The advantage of the Hema IOL is that it induces no adherence at all and is placed in the ciliary sulcus

Piggy Backing

The most functional concept

Advantages

1. Easy to compute
2. Better stimulus for amblyopic prevention
3. Easy to calculate the appropriate time for removal
4. In case of gross inaccuracy, another permanent piggy back can be replaced later

Disadvantages

1. Difficult to do surgery with multiple IOL with tendency to optic capture
2. Virtually impossible with the present crop of lenses to place both in bag
3. Interface debris (red-rock) problems especially when both PMMA
4. Removal requires transection of IOL and is often more difficult due to deep adhesions. If both bagged, difficulty still more.

Answer

1. Use the permanent lens of the most tried and tested material. Acrysof (Alcon)
2. Use the IOL to be removed of a pure HEMA material. HEMA induces no adhesions and hence can be removed easily.
3. Make the Hema lens in the shape of an inverted dome, so it can be bagged easily.

Material of the Hema Domed Implant

Wohlk (German) soft contact lens material, Hexa methyl meth-acrylate with cross polymers and EGDA

Refractive Index	1.44
Elasticity at break	1.40
Oxygen permeability	4.43×10^{-9}

Hema Intraocular Domed IOL

Hydration

Saline content	38.8 %
Water uptake	62.3 %
Saline uptake	63.6 %

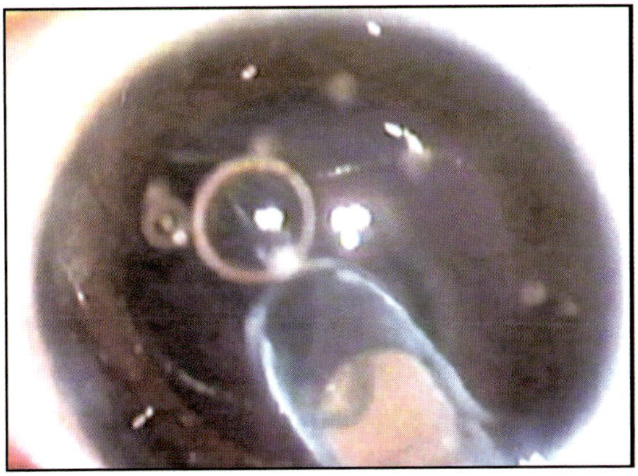

Figure 16: Note Acrysof lens going below the rhexis, into the bag. Care to be taken that it does not snag on the edge of the posterior rhexis

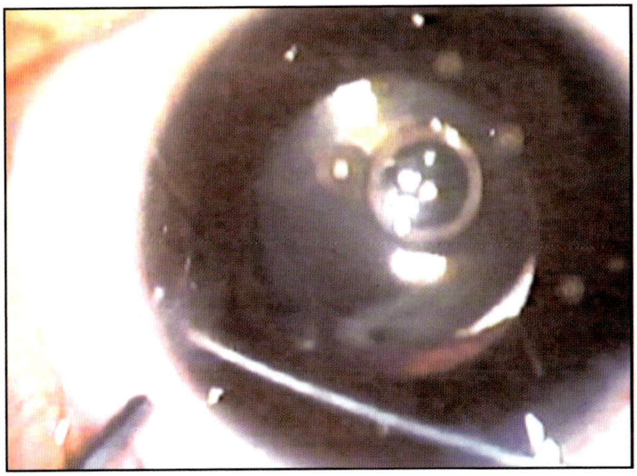

Figure 17: Acrysof lens in place

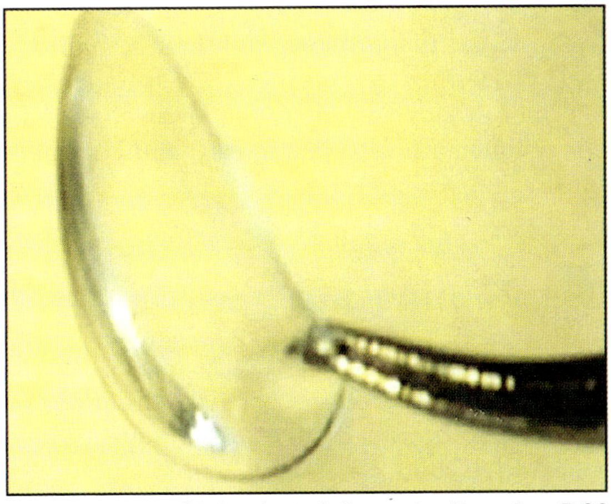

Figure 18: Hema domed IOL implant. 9.5 mm in diameter, 5.00 mm optics, periphery very thin. Note bevel on edge to permit easy insertion.

Temperature resistance: No change in parameters after boiling for 24 hours
Light Transmission 400-800 nM: Ash Content. .0.1 mg in 3.00 gm ashed

Specification of the Domed IOL

Made by IOL Tech India Ltd: An WHO certified, ISO 9001 company. Now FDA approved.

9.5 mm in diameter, 5.00mm optics, with the optic on the external convex side, with a base curve of 6.8 mm, with an bevel on the external aspect permitting easier bag entry.

Can be easily folded or rolled over and entry and removal via a minimum 2.8 mm incision

Criteria for Selection of IOL

1. Under anesthesia, measure corneal curvature with auto keratometer on table. Take axial length reading with A- Scan, using SRK –T formula, calculate IOL power.
2. Extrapolate to age of two years based on reading (a baby at 3 months, with an IOL power of 28 –30 D will be 23 D at 2 years).
3. Place the anticipated IOL power as Acrysof in the bag first, place the residual power as the Hema lens over it.

Criteria for Removal of IOL

1. When anticipated IOL refraction reaches –4.00, remove IOL. Example. Baby placed IOL at 3 months of 31 D, 23.00D as Acrysof, + 6 D as Hema (under correcting by 20%). Will reach –4.00 at age of 18 months when IOL removed.
2. We use the rule of 4 as a variation of 4 dioptres from emmetropia rarely induces significant amblyopia.

Anesthesia Requirements

Satisfactory anesthesia for the pediatric ophthalmic patient presents many special challenges. These include control of the intraocular pressure (IOP), awareness of the oculocardiac reflex, thorough knowledge of drug interactions, smooth anesthetic maintenance and emergence, and control or prevention of postoperative nausea and vomiting (PONV).

Perioperative Routine and Selection of Anesthetic Agents

There is no need to separate children and parent as this is a very trying time for both. Too early an separation leads to aa distraught mother and a crying unhappy non cooperative child.

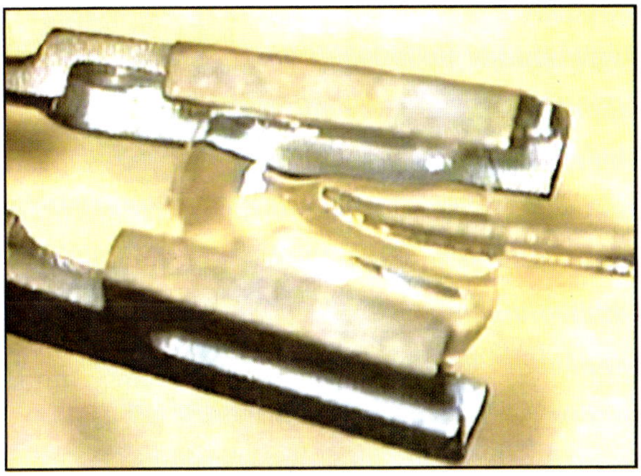

Figure 19: Lens placed in the folder to permit easy holding. The lens is folded on itself like a roll in the folder

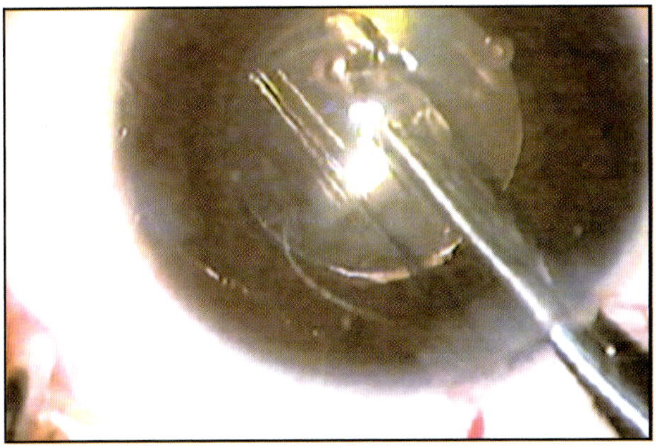

Figure 20: Hema IOL inserted into the chamber, note its rolled state

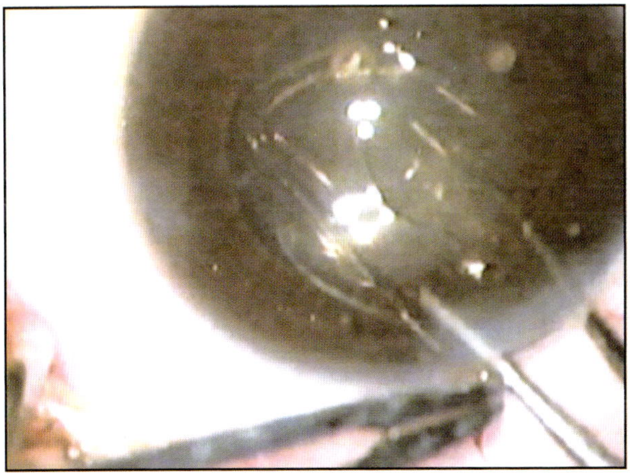

Figure 21: Hema lens opening up. Care must be taken to insert the rim under the iris edge and under the rhexis

Ideally children may receive clear liquids 2 to 3 hr before surgery without increasing the risk of aspiration.! Adequate preoperative hydration decreases the incidence of intraoperative hypoglycemia and hypovolemia and postoperative nausea and vomiting.

Though many institutions routinely use premedication for young children (between 18 months and 5 years of age) before ophthalmic procedures we have never found it necessary.

Both inhalational and intravenous general anesthetic techniques have been used successfully for pediatric cataract surgery. However, with the exception a history or a family history of malignant hyperthermia, most general anesthesia in young children undergoing cataract surgery is done with an inhalational agent. Isoflurane has widely replaced halothane as the induction agent of choice in children. It possesses a less offensive odor than other volatile agents, is less stimulating to the airway, and lacks the arrhythmogenic properties of halothane.

Nitrous oxide, traditionally used with volatile anesthetics, may increase postoperative nausea and vomiting. The cause-and-effect relationship between nausea/vomiting and nitrous oxide remains controversial.

Propofol is the intravenous induction agent of choice for cataract surgery in older pediatric patients and those with preoperative intravenous access. Propofol is an isopropyl phenol that has a rapid onset and offset of action. It is used for the induction and maintenance of anesthesia or sedation. Intravenous injection of a therapeutic dose of propofol produces hypnosis rapidly with minimal excitation. Propofol is also believed to have antiemetic properties. It effectively produces hypnosis of short duration with minimal "hangover."

We usually combine it with ketamine hydrochloride, a dissociative anesthetic that can be used for the induction and maintenance of anesthesia. However ketamine hydrochloride does causes an increase in IOP, which should be kept in mind when following patients with glaucoma.

During anesthesia, even in patients whose IOP is usually normal, an increase in pressure can produce catastrophic effects. And may lead to prolapse of the iris and lens and loss of vitreous. Therefore, proper control of IOP is critical. We usually supplement the anesthesia with a1.5 cc sub Tenon block and let the eye soften for 3 minutes which obviates much of the risk of inhalation or injectable anesthesia.

Bell's phenomenon is a useful indicator an can be seen at any time during anesthesia when the patient's depth of anesthesia has changed. It manifests as upward (or sometime downward) movement of the eye. It is usually a sign of being light, although the patient is not awake. It is an indicator that the anesthesiologist should be prepared to "deepen" the anesthesia to facilitate surgery.

Oculocardiac Reflex

The oculocardiac reflex is stimulated by pressure on the globe and/or by traction on the extraocular muscles, the conjunctiva, or the orbital structures. The afferent

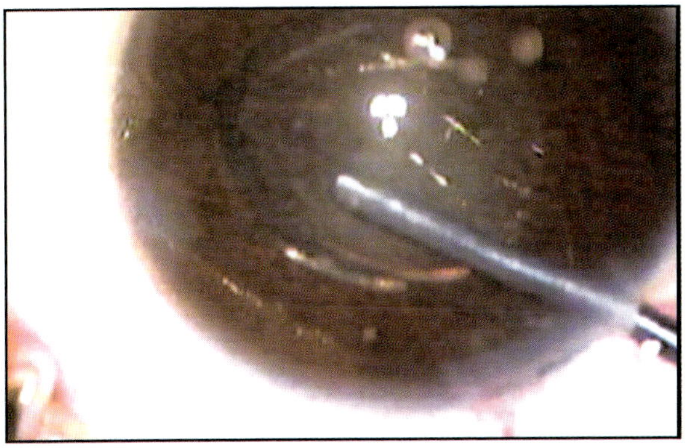

Figure 22: Lens is tyre ironed under the rhexis rim and gradually worked into the position. It goes in surprisingly easily due to the edge bevel

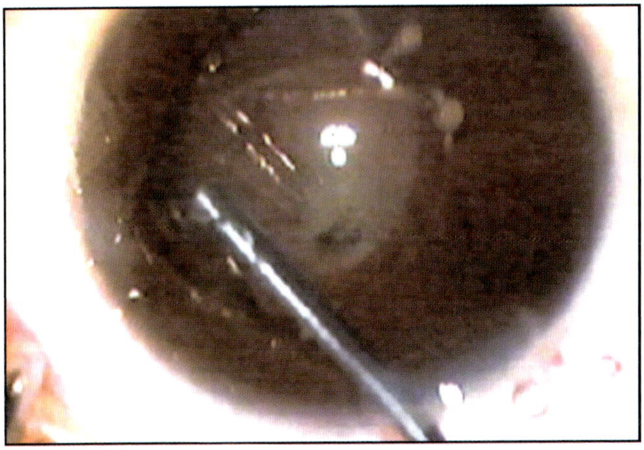

Figure 23: Final edge is slipped in

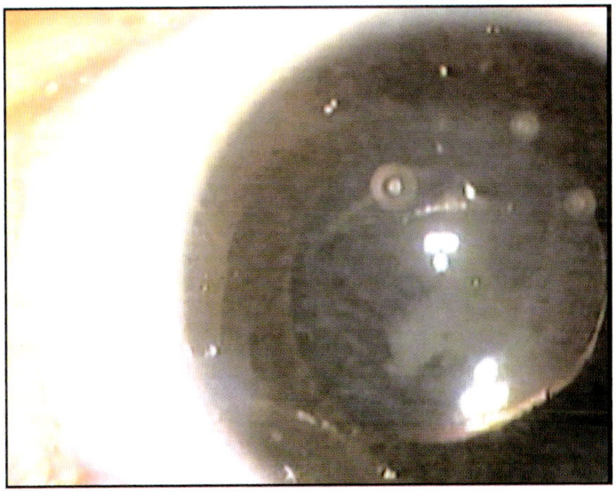

Figure 24: It is a very easy procedure. Both IOLs are stable. Thanks to the beveled edge of the IOL, insertion under the rhexis is easy

limb is trigeminal and the efferent limb is vagal. Although the oculocardiac reflex is commonly associated with bradycardia, virtually any dysrhythmia, including ventricular tachycardia and asystole, may be seen.

It must be remembered that Children have increased vagal tone and, therefore, are more likely to present with the reflex.. If a dysrhythmia appears, the surgeon to cease the manipulation. Check that the depth of anesthesia and ventilatory status are adequate.

Usually, the heart rate and rhythm return to baseline within 20 sec.. If the reflex becomes a problem, atropine should be given intravenously.

Surgical Technique

A well made surgical tunnel is mandatory for babies and young children.. It is important that the tunnels be made well. The first step is to make two 0.8 mm tunnels at 9.00 o'clock and 2.00 o'clock. The tunnels are made by applanating the scleral surface so that the tunnels are longer than they are broad. The next step is to fill the eye with an OVD (Ophthalmic Viscosurgical device). The best in the opinion of the authors is Viscoat (Alcon). The next best is Healon 5. The most economical is methylcellulose which unfortunately runs out freely. If Methylcellulose is to be utilized it should be frozen (kept under the freezer). Methylcellulose increases its viscosity by a factor of 3 if frozen and does not run out at all. However once it warms up it runs again freely.

The next step is to carefully 'construct' the corneal incision. Refill OVD. Once again taking a 2.8 mm diamond blade (ideal for children) applanated it to the sclera and then advance. Only enter the tunnel after the length is more than the breadth. BE CAREFUL WHEN REMOVING THE BLADE NOT TO INCISE THE SIDES OF THE TUNNEL.

Rhexis in young children is best commenced with a sharp bent 27 G needle cystitome as the capsule is tough and does not give way easily and then continue the rhexis with a capsule forceps refilling the OVD at regular intervals. Do remember in children that the tendency is for the rhexis to increase.. So plan for a 5 mm rhexis, and it invariably becomes bigger. If the eye is soft, after a block, rhexis is far easier. To do a rhexis in a tight eye is foolish as it will run away.

Hydrodissection under the rhexis is done with a blunt tipped side ported 24 G cannula. That way accidental injury to the capsule is avoided if the chamber suddenly shallows. The Hydrodissection is started at ther 7.00 o'clock position and fluid injected slowly in all the clock hours. Usually the nucleus will tumble out if the cataract is soft.

The authors use the Alcon AquaLase which uses bursts of warmed water as a routine in children. It has a polymer blunt tip which protects the capsule. It is essential not to increase the suction too much. Usually all the cortex can be easily removed with the AquaLase but if any is left behind it can be easily removed with an I/A bimanual system.

AquaLase polishing if the capsule is essential. It leaves a very clean capsule. If not available than manual polishing of the capsule is compulsory.

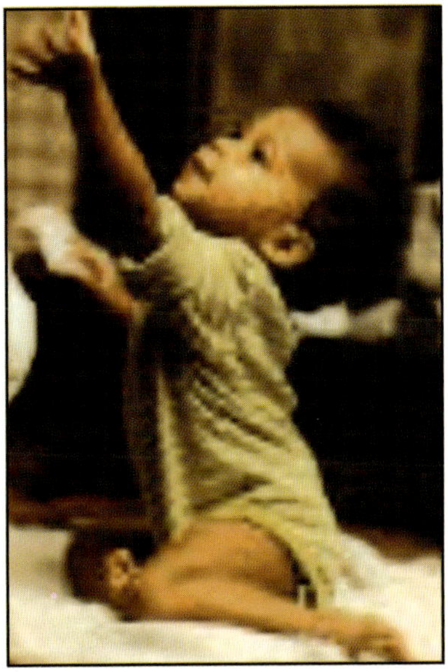

Children	Number Unilateral	Percentage	Number Bilateral	Percentage
16	5	31.25%	11	68.75%

Figure 25: Unilateral or bilateral cataract

Age at Implantation	*Number*	*Males*	*Females*
2 months	5	4	1
3 months	3	1	2
5 months	4	3	1
7 months	5	3	2
8 months	5	1	4
10 months	3	3	0
13 months	1	0	1
15 months	1	1	0
Total	27	16	11

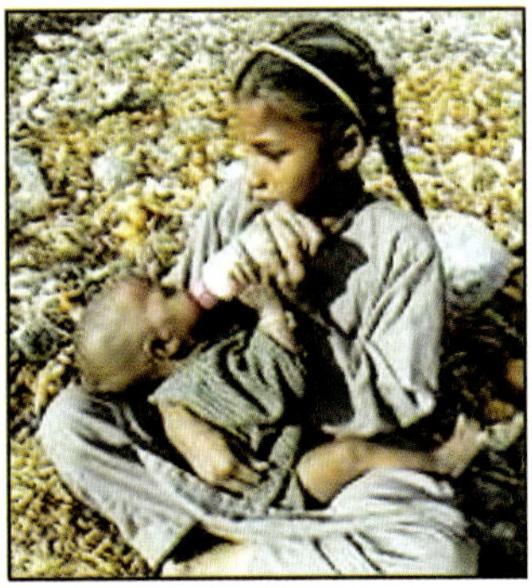

Figure 26: Age at Implantation

Refill the chamber with the OVD of your choice and inject in the IOL. Our personal preference for the permanent IOL remains the AcrySof 60AT with the Monarch II injector. Once the IOL is perfect centered. The Hema domed IOL of the appropriate power is taken. It is inserted after being folded twice (both the sides are folded to meet in the middle. The entire IOL is then taken and placed in the Rayner injector and simply injected in the eye. The Hema IOL is allowed to open outside on the anterior capsule.

The next step is to insert it under the edge of the rhexis. Lens is tyre- ironed under the rhexis rim and gradually worked into the position. It goes in surprisingly easily due to the edge bevel. Unlike PMMA or other IOL which are placed in the sulcus (sulcus fixated, the Hema IOL is placed in the bag. Hema induces no reaction and lies stable. The reason for placing it under the edge of the bag is that otherwise Hema being very soft tends to ruck.

The pupil is narrowed with a miotic (Intracameral pilocarpine 1% with no preservative works well.) The pupil must be brought down to less than 4 mm prior leaving the case as in a child any sudden pressure will lead to the domed Hema IOL being captured in the iris.

We have stopped doing a posterior rhexis as following the AquaLase polishing the capsules are very clear and even after a posterior rhexis, unless vitrectomy is done the capsule closes again.

The chamber should reform, and stay formed on the table. If the chamber immediately flattens, it is prudent to take a single 10/0 Vicryl buried stitch at the site of the corneal incision.

Postoperative treatment is fairly simple. We do not permit the mother to handle a babies eyes under any circumstance. The mother is taught to place the drops in the inner corner of the eye and simply pat the child on the abdomen gently and wait. The moment the eye opens the drops go in. The child lids are very tight and very closely apposed to the eye. Any forcible effort only leads to the drops being literally "wipered" off. Previously we used to use Tobramycin, now replaced by Moxifloxacin eye drops t.i.d with Prednisolone eye drops t.i.d.

It is coupled with oral steroids. Oral drops of Betamethasone, 10 drops, bid for children under 3 years of age, tid for upto 5 years of age and qid for over that for a month. This usually takes care of any inflammation. We do not use mydriatics, but prefer to use a drop of 1% pilocar once a day for a month. In this regime, we never get lens capture, get perfectly centered pupils and do not have any inflammation.

Criteria for Selection of IOL

Under anesthesia, measure corneal curvature with auto keratometer on table. Take axial length reading with A- Scan, using SRK –T formula, calculate IOL power. Extrapolate to age of two years based on reading (a baby at 3 months, with an IOL power of 28 –30 D will be 23 D at 2 years).Place the anticipated IOL power as Acrysof in the bag first, place the residue as Hema over it.

Age at Hema Explantation	*Number*	*Precentage*
18 months	3	11.1
22 months	4	14.8
25 months	6	22.2
28 months	14	51.9
Total	27	100

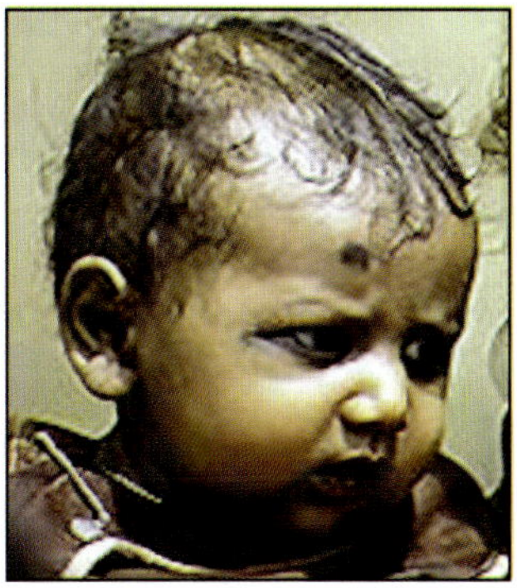

Figure 27: Age at Explantation of the Hema IOL

Residual ametropia	*No*	*Precentage*
+/- 0.50	3	9.7
+/- 1.00	4	12.9
+/- 1.50	6	19.4
+/- 2.00	0	00.0
+/- 2.50	3	9.7
+/- 3.00	5	16.1
+/- 3.50	4	12.9
+/- 4.00	1	3.2
+/- 4.50	3	9.7
- 5.50	1	3.2
- 7.00	1	3.2

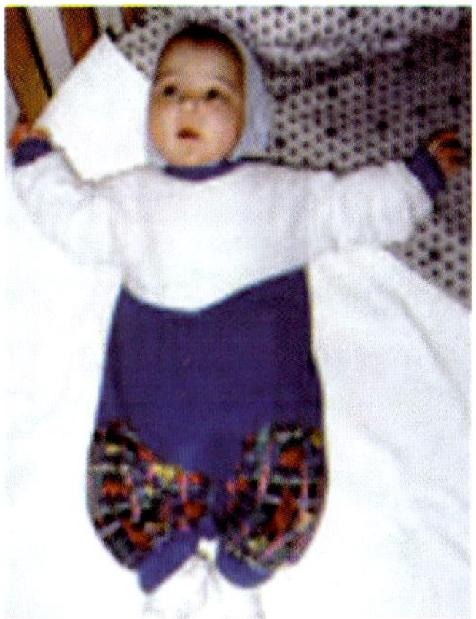

Figure 28: Residual ametropia after removal of Hema IOL

Complications	*Number*	*Percentage*
Corneal abrasion	2	7.4
Shallow A/C	9	33.3
Iritis	6	22.2
Hema IOL Pupil capture	2	7.4
Raised IOP : Temporary	7	25.9
Raised IOP : Needed Surgery	3	11.1
Hyphema	5	18.5

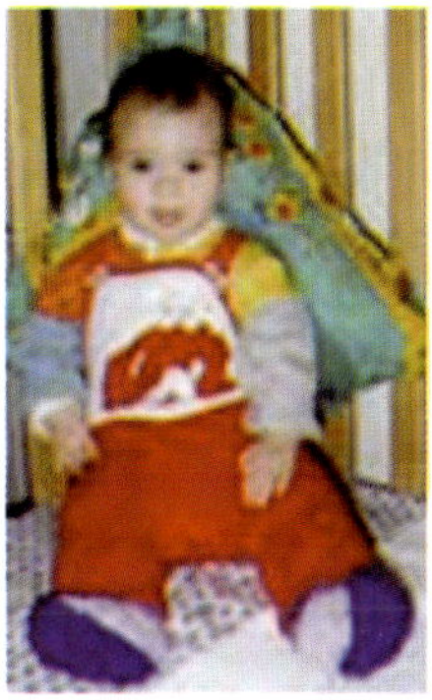

Figure 29: Complications n = 27

Criteria for Removal of IOL

When anticipated IOL refraction reaches –4.00, remove IOL. Example. Baby placed IOL at 3 months of 31 D, 23.00D as Acrysof, + 6 D as Hema (under correcting by 20%). Will reach –4.00 at age of 18 months when IOL removed. We use the rule of 4 as a variation of 4 dioptres from emmetropia rarely induces significant amblyopia.

Chapter 11

Management of Postoperative Complications after Pediatric Cataract Surgery

Rupal H Trivedi
M Edward Wilson (USA)

Introduction

Cataract surgery in children is the first stepping-stone in the long way to visual rehabilitation. The cataract surgery is not the end of the journey; it is the beginning. Surgery is only one component of the *treatment package* for a child with cataract. The main immediate goals are to remove the cataract and to correct residual refractive error. The main long-term goals are to diagnose and to treat postoperative complications as soon as possible. Maintenance of a clear visual axis and correction of changing residual refractive errors are the two most important aspects while following the children after cataract surgery. Pediatric cataract surgery is a complex issue best left to expert hands that are familiar with the long-term complications and the lengthy follow-up. The best outcome can be achieved by a *"team approach"* – a team consisting of an ophthalmologist, a pediatrician, an anesthesiologist, and most importantly the child's primary caretakers.

Methods of cataract surgery with intraocular lens (IOL) implantation in children have undergone dramatic changes during the last several years because of advances in surgical technique and technology. Still, postoperative complications associated with pediatric cataract-IOL surgery continue to be a major concern. The risk of postoperative complications is higher due to a greater inflammatory response after pediatric intraocular surgery. Close follow-up to detect and treat the complications early is mandatory. In this chapter, we discuss postoperative complications of pediatric cataract surgery, and address their management.

Visual Axis Opacification

Visual axis opacification (VAO) remains the most frequent complication of pediatric cataract surgery. *Note that we prefer the term "visual axis opacification" for children since a primary posterior capsulectomy has often been performed. VAO is distinguish from posterior capsule opacification (PCO), which is a term we avoid using in eyes after a primary posterior capsulectomy has been performed.*

VAO interferes with the main goals of the operation and is a potential cause for amblyopia. It should be prevented or treated promptly. Since children may be unable to report decreased vision, early VAO may go unnoticed and lead to amblyopia. VAO is almost inevitable after pediatric cataract surgery if the posterior capsule is left intact. It may occur as a result of proliferation, metaplasia and migration of equatorial lens epithelial cells on the posterior capsule. Despite removal of the posterior capsule, secondary membranes and media opacity may still develop. An intact hyaloid face can serve as a scaffold for migration of lens epithelial cells and their subsequent proliferation and transformation.

The most critical factor influencing the occurrence of VAO is age. While opacification of an intact posterior capsule is nearly universal in infantile eyes, the incidence decreases with increasing age. Besides age, the incidence and severity of VAO also depends on the type of cataract (congenital, developmental, or traumatic), associated ocular abnormalities (e.g. uveitis, persistent fetal

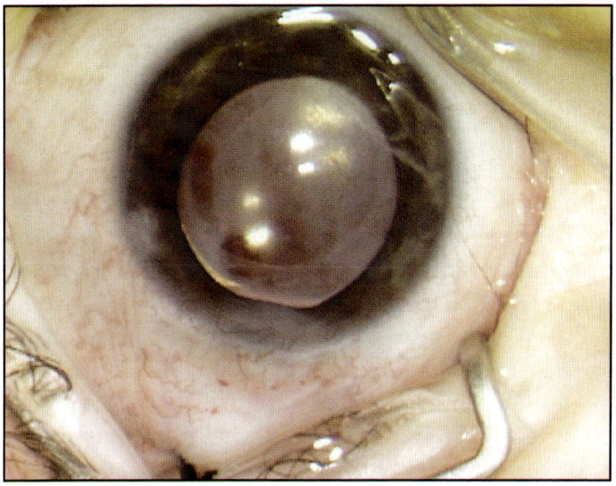

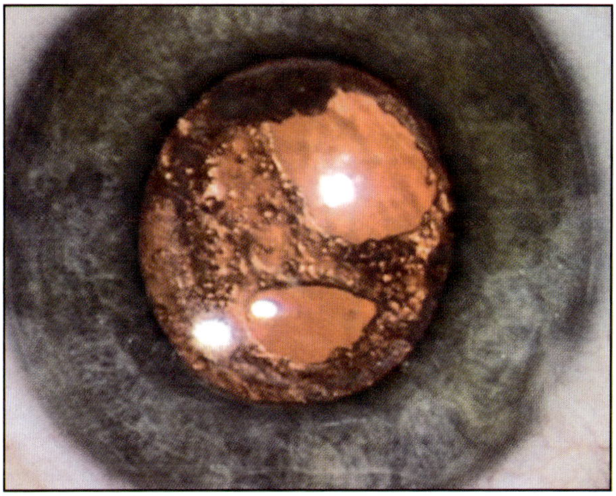

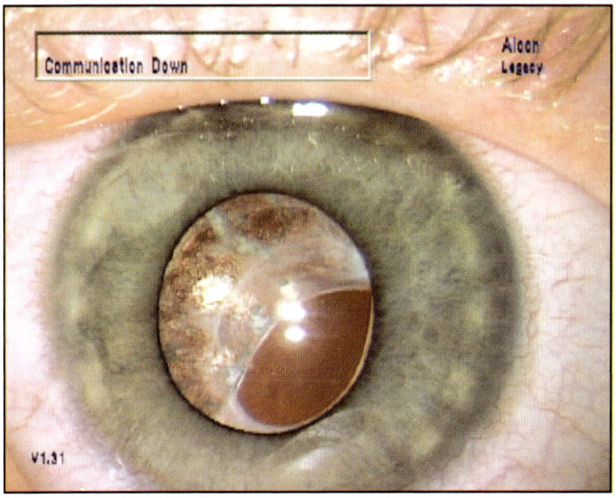

Figures 1 to 3: Visual axis opacification after pediatric cataract surgery

vasculature), aphakia versus pseudophakia, type of IOL, and ciliary sulcus versus capsular bag fixation. Additionally, the duration of follow-up affects the incidence of VAO. The longer the follow-up, the more VAO becomes manifest.

Prevention

Primary posterior capsulectomy and vitrectomy are effective in preventing VAO in children beyond their first birthday. Primary posterior capsulectomy is often can be performed up-to age 5-8 years. In children at 5-8 years of age when posterior capsule is left intact, VAO (in this case it is PCO) occurs generally after 18-24 months. If child cooperates for slit-lamp examination during preoperative assessment for cataract, it may be assumed that the child will cooperate for YAG laser capsulotomy after 18-24 months if needed. The posterior capsule can be left intact in such children. However, posterior capsulectomy and vitrectomy is advisable under certain circumstances even in older children. Eyes with pre-existing posterior capsule defects and dense posterior capsule plaques require primary posterior capsulectomy and vitrectomy. Patients where follow-up is questionable, patients with multi-system disorders where cooperation with YAG is questionable, and where facilities for YAG is not available are benefited by primary posterior capsulectomy and vitrectomy even at older ages within childhood. Eyes with traumatic cataract develop VAO more rapidly and severely. Thus, in eyes with traumatic cataract, primary posterior capsulectomy is often can be performed even in older children. Gimbel and colleagues calculated the cumulative incidence of need for capsulotomy to be 41% for congenital or developmental cataracts and 66% for traumatic cataracts over 2 years. The apparently increased need of secondary capsulotomy in traumatic cataracts may be due to more severe inflammation in the traumatized eye and less possibility of in-the-bag IOL implantation.

To prevent VAO, the recent literature has also reported the use of "bag-in-the-lens" IOL (or twin-capsulorhexis IOL) which seems promising in reducing or eliminating VAO. Here, the insertion of anterior and posterior capsules are in a peripheral groove of the IOL optic. Also, the sealed capsule irrigation device has potential clinical usefulness for reducing the incidence of VAO. This device needs further testing in pediatric eyes.

Treatment

Despite posterior capsulectomy and anterior vitrectomy, secondary VAO may occur. Predisposing factors for recurrent opacification include the following: small-sized capsulectomy (< 4 mm), young age, type of cataract, ciliary sulcus fixation of the IOL, reaction to IOL material and associated ocular or systemic inflammatory conditions.

VAO can be amblyogenic if it occurs in younger children. In cases of dense, thick VAO surgical posterior capsulectomy combined with anterior vitrectomy is required to clear the visual axis. Secondary posterior capsulectomy can be performed through the limbal route, however most eyes require a pars plicata approach. Fibrous opacification is better to remove early after detection, not

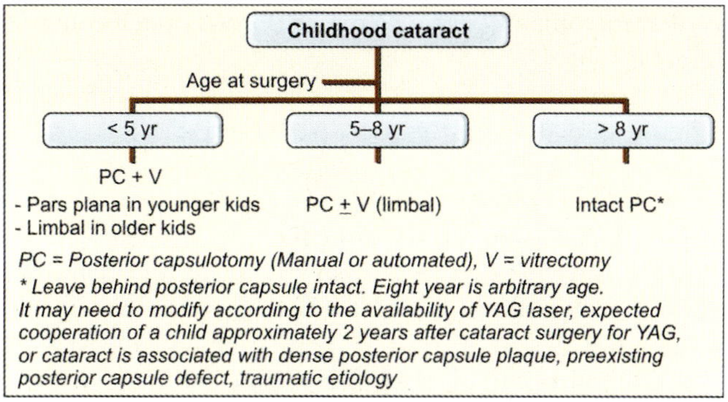

Figure 4: Management of posterior capsule and anterior vitreous at the time of pediatric cataract surgery

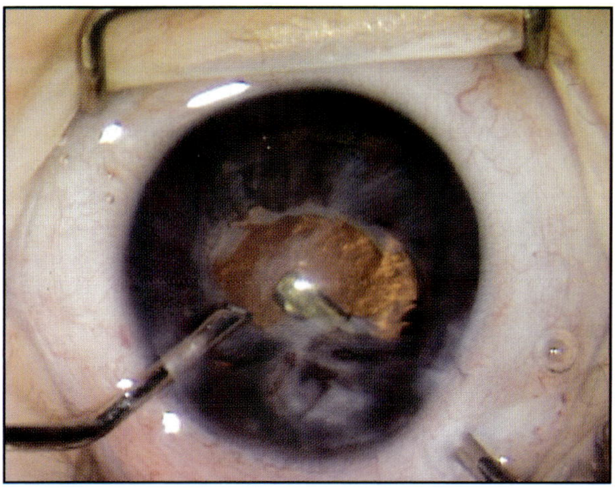

Figure 5: Surgical removal of visual axis opacification

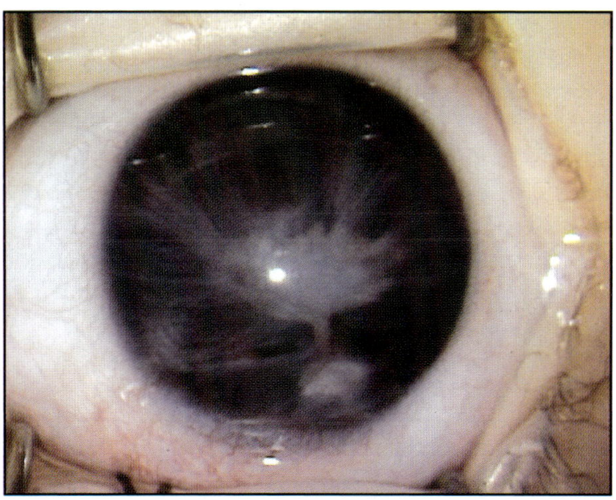

Figure 6: Glaucoma developed in a child operated at 2-month of age

only to prevent amblyopia but because dense fibrous opacification is also more difficult to remove.

Nd:YAG laser can also be used to perform posterior capsulectomy when VAO is not dense and the child can cooperate for YAG laser capsulotomy. However, reopacification of YAG-laser openings have been reported in pediatric eyes. Hutcheson and colleagues reported 57% (13/23) reopacification after YAG laser in pediatric eyes. Four eyes (17%) in the YAG treated group required a third treatment for opacification in this series. Stager and colleagues reported that 60% of the eyes developed recurrent opacification following Nd-YAG laser treatment in the younger age group (< 4 years), which suggested that surgical posterior capsulectomy and vitrectomy rather than YAG laser posterior capsulectomy may be more beneficial in younger kids.

IOL Opacification

Visual axis opacification can occur as a result of IOL opacification. Postoperative opacification of the foldable hydrophilic acrylic lens designs is a major concern among surgeons and manufacturers. Three major hydrophilic acrylic lenses, explanted due to varying degrees of IOL opacification, secondary to different patterns of dystrophic calcification, include the Bausch and Lomb Hydroview™, Medical Developmental Research- SC60B-OUV™ and Ophthalmic Innovations International, Aqua-Sense™. A recent report describes the opacification of hydrophilic acrylic IOLs in children (Kleinmann G, Werner L, Pandey SK et al. Opacification of surface of hydrophilic acrylic intraocular lenses in children, Presented at ASCRS Symposium on Cataract, IOL, and Refractive Surgery, San Diego, CA, May 2004). An IOL explantation/exchange is currently the only available treatment.

Intraocular Pressure Spike due to Residual Ophthalmic Viscosurgical Devices

As in adults, retained ophthalmic viscosurgical devices (OVDs) can cause marked postoperative intraocular pressure (IOP) elevation after surgery for childhood cataracts. Englert and Wilson, have suggested the need for more meticulous removal of OVDs. The cohesive OVDs, while responsible for most IOP spikes, are easier to remove than dispersive OVDs. OVDs can be removed with irrigation/aspiration using a small bimanual hand-piece or the vitrector hand-piece.

Postoperative Glaucoma

The incidence of glaucoma after surgery for a congenital cataract varies from 3% to 41%. Eyes with a cataract diagnosed and treated at an early age are at high-risk for development of glaucoma. Ophthalmologists must be vigilant about assessing for postoperative glaucoma in children left aphakic or pseudophakic.

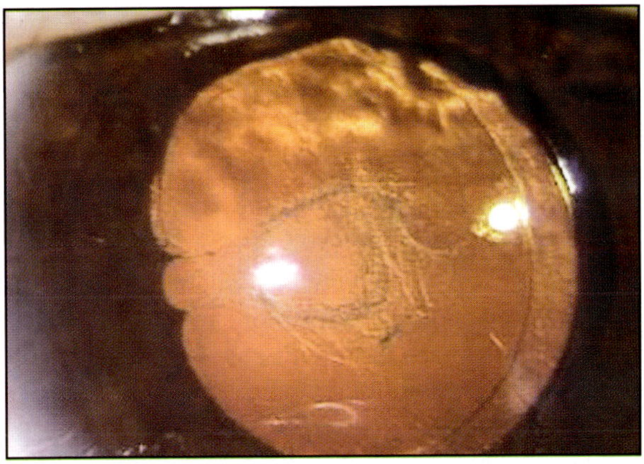

Figure 7: Early postoperative uveitis

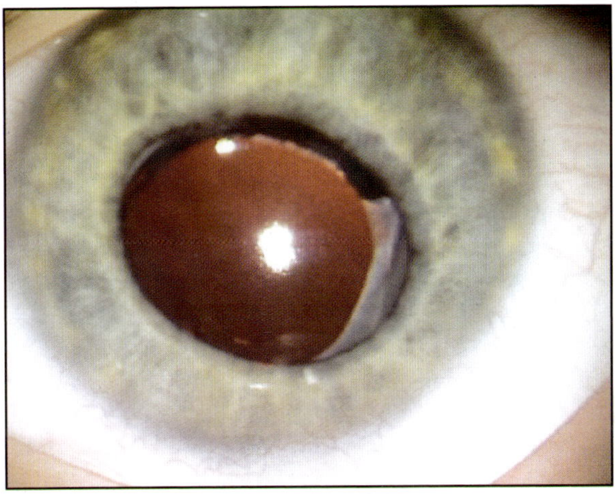

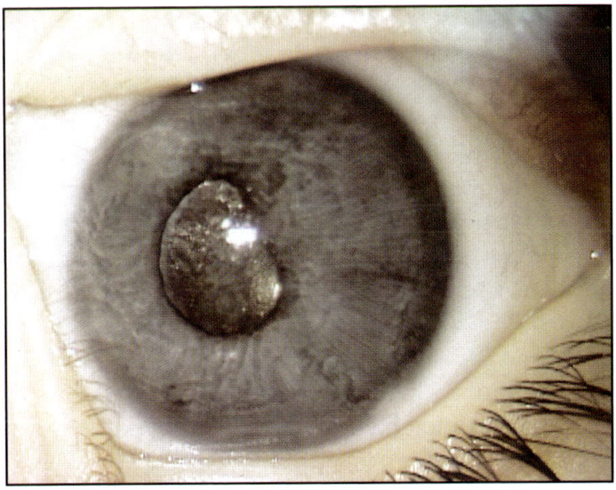

Figures 8 and 9: Synechiae after cataract surgery in children

It is vital to examine the patients on a regular basis after uneventful infantile cataract surgery with or without IOL implantation. Examinations under anesthesia can be scheduled when clinic examinations with IOP measurements or refractions are technically impossible.

Treatment

Pupillary block was once the leading cause of postoperative aphakic glaucoma. Acute angle closure rarely occurs in aphakic patients after recent advancement in surgery, open angle glaucoma occurs more frequently. A surgical or laser peripheral iridectomy is standard treatment once pupillary block is recognized.

Medical management is often initiated after aphakic glaucoma is diagnosed. One retrospective study of 64 eyes of 38 patients with glaucoma reported medications alone controlled IOP in 63.6% (21/33 eyes) of patients, almost all of whom had open-angle glaucoma. When medical management fails, realistic surgical options include seton implantation, trabeculectomy or cyclo-destructive procedures. Aphakia has been previously reported as a significant risk factor for failure of trabeculectomy with mitomycin-C (TMMC) in not only adult patients, but also in pediatric patients; the latter studies are discussed below.

Freedman et al retrospectively evaluated results of 17 consecutive children (21 eyes) under 17 years of age (median age 2.6 years) who had failed maximum medical therapy, prior angle or filtration surgery (goniotomy, trabeculotomy, trabeculectomy), or both. TMMC with or without postoperative 5-Fluorouracil (5-FU) or laser suture lysis or both were performed. Aphakic eyes performed worse than phakic, whether TMMC was performed before or after one year of age. Success was poor in all patients less than a year of age, whether phakic (3/8 eyes) or aphakic (0/2 eyes). Success rates were higher in patients one year of age or older, both for phakic (6/6 eyes) and aphakic (2/5) groups. The authors concluded that laser-suture lysis or 5-FU augmentation of TMMC did not improve success in younger, aphakic children and may have increased the complication rate. The study is limited by the small number of patients in each subgroup and limited (median 23 months) follow-up of successful cases.

Beck and colleagues provide another report of failure of TMMC in aphakic patients less than a year of age. Records of 49 patients (60 eyes) 17 years of age or younger (mean age 7.6 years) who had undergone TMMC for various etiologies were retrospectively reviewed. Success (IOP $\leq$ 22 without glaucoma progression or visually devastating complications) rates were 67% at one year and 59% at two years. Young age ($\leq$ 1 year) and aphakic status were statistically significant risk factors in multivariate analysis. Failure occurred in 60% of 20 aphakic eyes and in 24% of 29 phakic eyes. Failure occurred in seven of eight eyes of children less than 1 year old and in 29% of 41 eyes of patients one to 17 years of age. Late onset, bleb-related endophthalmitis occurred in five of 60 (8%) eyes. Although TMMC demonstrated considerable efficacy in phakic patients greater than one year old in this and other reports, the authors express concern about the 'substantial' risk of infection with TMMC in aphakic infants.

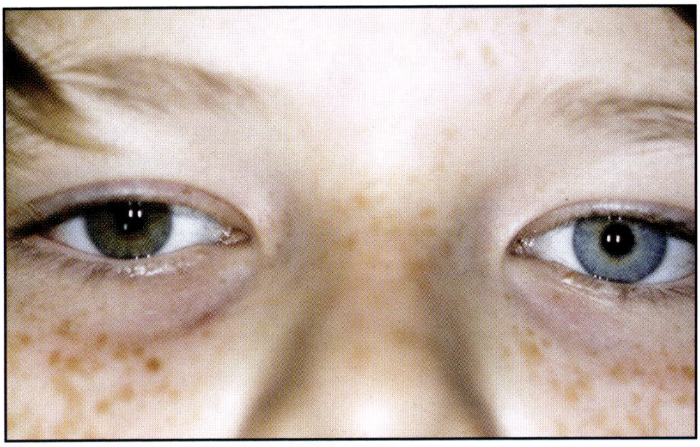

Figure 10: Heterochromia irides

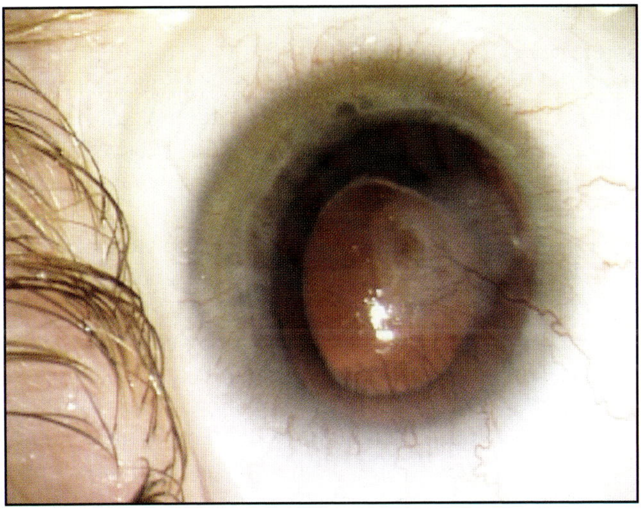

Figure 11: A healed cornea ulcer in an aphakic eye after prolonged use of contact lens

Age less than one year and aphakia are risk factors for failure of TMMC in the two aforementioned retrospective studies. How do aqueous shunt devices (ASD) compare? For children two years and younger, Beck and colleagues report greater efficacy of aqueous shunt devices over TMMC. Only the minority of these patients studied were aphakic or pseudophakic. In this retrospective, age-matched comparison of ASD and TMMC, Beck and colleagues determined the likelihood of maintaining an IOP of less than 23 mmHg in 46 eyes of 32 patients under two years of age. According to the authors, pressure below this level provides clinical stability in very young patients with glaucoma. For the 46 eyes receiving ASD, 16 eyes (34.8%) were aphakic or pseudophakic compared to three of 24 eyes (12.5%) in the TMMC group. Beck and colleagues employed Baerveldt implants for 32 eyes and Ahmed valves for 14 eyes. After the aforementioned procedures, success achieved at one and three years was 87% and 53% in the ASD group, respectively, compared to 36% and 19% with the TMMC group at the same intervals. Interestingly, although the seton implantation group was comprised of more high-risk patients (16/46 (34.8%) eyes aphakic or pseudophakic) than the TMMC group (3/24 (12.5%) eyes), the seton group overall (no separate success rates were reported for aphakic and pseudophakic patients) fared better (72% success versus 21% success in TMMC group) and had no infections (versus 8.3% in TMMC group.

The poor success rates and potential for infection with TMMC for young, aphakic patients in the retrospective studies previously discussed corroborate the results of Beck's work discussed above. For the first surgical procedure for aphakic or pseudophakic patients on maximal medical therapy, seton implantation appears more likely to succeed in controlling IOP than TMMC, especially in infants.

Seton implantation size and type are additional surgical considerations. Higher success rates can be obtained with Ahmed glaucoma valve implants, Baerveldt implants, and double-plate Molteno implants than single-plate Molteno implants. An attractive feature of Ahmed valve implants is the immediate pressure lowering effect delivered to the glaucomatous eye without a high risking of hypotomy. The non-valved Baerveldt implants have a limited pressure lowering effect until the temporary tube occluder is removed at least one month after the original surgery. Without this temporary tube occlusion, the Baerveldt implant would produce marked early hypotony. Rapid IOP reduction may be less crucial in aphakic glaucoma than in patients with congenital glaucoma who fail angle surgery — these latter patients depend upon rapid clearing of the visual axis from lower pressure. Patients with aphakic glaucoma typically have clear corneas. It is easier to implant an Ahmed glaucoma valve than a Baerveldt in an infant due to eye and orbit size, but aphakic glaucoma is most commonly diagnosed four to five years after the cataract surgery. The valve in the Ahmed implant may fail, and there is a greater probability of having a hypertensive phase in an Ahmed valve than in a Baerveldt in pediatric patients. The hypertensive phase tends to peak at a month and resolve by six months after Ahmed implantation in adults. Since all types of glaucoma implants will demonstrate a decline in success rates over time, the ideal seton implant for the aphakic or pseudophakic child with glaucoma is not currently agreed upon.

Cycloablative techniques have been generally reserved for refractory cases of glaucoma in children. The success rate is low if these techniques are used as the initial surgical option. Cyclocryotherapy and laser cyclophotocoagulation in children may result in severe complications in some patients. Retinal detachment, sympathetic ophthalmia, and phthisis can occur. Surgical revision or addition of a second tube implant can also be associated with high rates of complications such as new corneal edema. Supplemental transscleral laser photocoagulation is a viable alternative for children suffering tube failure. Several laser treatments may be required to achieve long-term control. Endocyclophotocoagulation is a relatively recently applied technique which has demonstrated some promise in treating refractory glaucoma in children and adults. Neely and Plager reported on 51 endoscopic diode laser cyclophotocoagulation procedures performed on 36 eyes of 29 pediatric patients. Cumulative success rates after all procedures at a mean of 19 months of follow-up was 43%. Severe visual complication rates were lowest with endocyclophotocoagulation. The authors noted that only 1/123 diode endolaser treated eyes progressed to phthisis. Nonetheless, for aphakic patients especially, Neely and Plager report that endocyclophotocoagulation is not undertaken without risk, as retinal detachment, hypotony, and decreased vision all have occurred. Long-term results are not available, so this procedure should still be used with caution in children with refractory aphakic glaucoma.

Astigmatism

Postoperative astigmatism is of greater importance in children than in adults because of the adverse effect it has on visual development and the risk of amblyopia. Children, however, show regression of astigmatism during the initial postoperative period. Astigmatism of 3.1 ±2.8 D and 2.1 ±1.7 D at 1 week postoperative period (in scleral tunnel and corneal tunnel group respectively) decreases to 1.1 ±1.2 and 0.9 ±1.0 D at 5 months postoperatively. Bradfield and colleagues report mean postoperative retinoscopic cylinder of 0.63 D (range 0.0 to 4.50 D) at 1 month, 0.40 D (range 0.0 to 1.75 D) at 6 months, and 0.51 D (range 0.0 to 2.50 D) at 1 year. The authors reported less astigmatism in children having surgery before they were 36 months old.

Postoperative Anterior Uveitis

Postoperative anterior uveitis is more frequent in children as compared with adults due to increased tissue reactivity in children. No-iris- touch surgery and in-the-bag fixation helps to reduce the postoperative anterior uveitis.

Prevention

Frequent topical steroids and even systemic steroids may be needed in selected cases to reduce postoperative inflammation. Brady and colleague recommend five units of intravenous heparin in 500 ml of irrigating solution. Rumelt and colleagues report using 40 mg of Enoxaparin (low molecular weight heparin) in 500 ml of BSS.

Treatment

Fibrinous exudates can be dissolved with intraocular streptokinase (500-1000 IU) and recombinant tissue plasminogen activator (rt-PA).

IOL Deposits and Synechiae

The deposits on IOL optic are often seen during the early postoperative period. They are usually not visually significant. They occur much more commonly in children with a dark iris, with a ciliary-sulcus fixated IOL, and when compliance with postoperative medications has been poor. Synechiae formation to the IOL optic occur more frequently in eyes implanted at younger age and in eyes with incomplete capsulorhexis. Neither deposits nor synechiae require any treatment in general.

Heterochromia Iridis

In some children, cataract surgery is associated with a darkening of the iris color in the operated eye. Authors hypothesized that the darkening may results from an exuberant prostaglandin release stimulated by the cataract surgery and may occur through the same or a similar mechanism by which Latanoprost causes the darkening of iris color.

Pupillary Capture

Pupillary capture of an IOL occurs more frequently when an IOL is placed in the ciliary sulcus and when the anterior capsulorhexis is large. Placing the IOL in the capsular bag with an anterior capsulotomy smaller than the IOL optic helps to prevent pupillary capture. When it occurs, pupillary capture can be left untreated if it is not associated with decreased visual acuity, IOL malposition or glaucoma. However, surgical repair recreates a more round pupil shape and IOL centration and reduces the risk of an ongoing mild uveitis.

Corneal Complication

Corneal edema may be caused by irrigation fluids, toxic substances, excessive intraocular manipulations or IOL touch during implantation. Long-term use of contact lens can lead to corneal problems. Use of ophthalmic viscosurgical devices have helped to avoid corneal endothelial problems. Basti and colleagues reported that endothelial cell loss is within acceptable limits. Long-term effect of pediatric cataract surgery on endothelium is yet to be established.

Endophthalmitis

Endophthalmitis does occur as a rare complication of pediatric cataract extraction. Techniques to avoid endophthalmitis remain controversial in all cataract procedures. Some surgeons advise the use of topical antibiotic ophthalmic solutions applied to the cataractous eye for 24 hours preoperatively. However, it is unclear whether this decreases the incidence of infectious complications. Other authorities emphasize the need to use an undiluted povidone-iodine (Betadine™) solution not only applied to the skin but also instilled in the eye at the time of the operation to reduce the bacterial flora in the operative field.

Identifying endophthalmitis in the young child is often much more difficult than in the adult patient. Careful slit-lamp examination may not be possible, even with a hand-held device. The most likely time for endophthalmitis to become clinically apparent in the postoperative period is between 48 and 96 hours postoperatively. Postoperative schedules for evaluating these patients should be drafted with this fact in mind in this era of ambulatory surgical therapy.

IOL Malposition

Decentration of an IOL can occur because of traumatic zonular loss and/or inadequate capsular support. Sharma and colleagues report IOL decentration in 33.3% of eye. Asymmetric IOL fixation, with one haptic in the capsular bag and the other in the ciliary sulcus can also lead to decentration and should be avoided. Complete IOL dislocation can occur after trauma. Posterior capture of the IOL optic also results in better centration of the implanted IOL. Explantation or repositioning of the IOL may be necessary in some cases presenting with significant decentration/dislocation.

Retinal Detachment

The incidence of retinal detachment (RD) following pediatric cataract surgery is approximately 1 to 1.5%. The incidence appears to be decreasing as surgical techniques advance and evolve. The use of modern high-speed vitreous cutter reduces the traction on the retina. Most cases have a history of multiple reoperations performed in the years prior to the introduction of automated lensectomy and vitrectomy. A long-term follow-up is critical in children as the RD can occur many years after the cataract surgery. This is especially important for those eyes at a higher risk for RD by virtue of a long axial length for age, PFV or multiple surgeries.

Treatment

The goal is to identify and close all the retinal breaks. Several techniques, as they pertain to repair of RD can be employed, based on the type and location of the hole/tear. The surgical management often involves a scleral buckle with or without vitrectomy. An encircling band is often used in aphakic or pseudophakic detachments. The band helps to close retinal holes near the vitreous base and can relieve vitreous traction that might lead to new break formation. Vitrectomy may be an ideal procedure for these cases as vitreoretinal traction may be relieved in an efficient manner without regard to potential damage to the lens by scleral depression. Fluid-air exchanges in pseudophakic eyes with an open capsule may pose a problem. Fluid condensation on the surface of the IOL may impair the visibility of the retina, making completion of the fluid-air exchange challenging. Pars plana vitrectomy, an encircling band, internal drainage, and intraocular tamponade are effective and efficient methods of repairing primary pseudophakic RDs.

Cystoid Macular Edema

The retention of the posterior capsule during cataract surgery has a protective effect on the occurrence of postoperative CME. However, while managing pediatric cataracts, posterior capsulectomy and vitrectomy are necessary surgical steps to maintain a clear visual axis long-term. Despite this, current studies appear to indicate that with present techniques of cataract surgery and IOL implantation, this complication is quite rare in children. Although the reasons for this are not clear, it may be due to a healthier vasculature, a general lack of systemic vascular disease, possible differences in prostaglandin physiologic structure, and differences in operative techniques in children. Assessment of CME in children can be complicated by poor cooperation of young children for slit-lamp biomicroscopy. Inaccuracies in visual acuity estimation in the early postoperative period in these young children, many of whom also have amblyopia, would reduce the effectiveness of clinical CME assessment. Because of the difficulty of performing fluorescein angiography in young patients, surgeons seldom evaluate children for this complication. Ahmadieh et al evaluated 45 eyes of 31 children undergoing cataract surgery and IOL implantation, using intravenous fluorescein and fundus fluorescein angiography. CME was not detected in any eye at 6 weeks after surgery. Rao et al performed evaluation four to six weeks after surgery, using oral fluorescein and angioscopy, in 25 eyes of children and did not detect CME in any of them. The incidence of CME may be higher in children with uveitis.

Prevention

The use of topical non-steroidal eye drops prior to cataract surgery can decrease the occurrence of intraoperative miosis and also reduce the incidence of postoperative CME. There is as yet no evidence of the effectiveness of this approach in pediatric cataract surgery. In patients with uveitis, surgery is best performed after clinical resolution of ocular inflammation. Such eyes can be treated with a sub-tenon injection of triamcinolone 20 mg, 3 days prior to surgery, and topical steroids and cycloplegics for 3 days prior to surgery. A better understanding of the mechanisms of post-cataract surgery intraocular inflammation, and the availability of newer pharmacological agents like the non-steroidal anti-inflammatory drugs, has improved the postoperative care of the pediatric eye. Diclofenac 0.1% eye drops can be used to prevent CME. Indomethacin 1.0% eye drops and ketorolac 0.5% eye drops can also be effective in the treatment of CME. These studies report outcomes in adults, but the use of these medications is efficacious in pediatric cataract surgery as well.

Treatment

In the event of persistent CME following surgery, traditional methods of treatment include the use of topical and oral steroids, topical and oral non-steroidal agents and the use of carbonic anhydrase inhibitors.

Hemorrhagic Retinopathy

This complication may occur following infantile cataract surgery in up to one-third of eyes as reported by Mets and Del Monte. Hemorrhagic retinopathy presents with flame-shaped retinal hemorrhages and may be associated with concurrent vitreous hemorrhage. The hemorrhages develop during the first 24 hours following surgery, are non-progressive and resolve within few weeks. The occurrence of this complication may be higher. However, these eyes do not undergo examination frequently during early postoperative period and thus may have been underestimated.

Myopic Shift of Refraction

The surgeon who performs pediatric cataract surgery must be prepared for a wide variation in long-term myopic shift. Both the magnitude of and the variance in this myopic shift are likely to be greater among children who undergo cataract surgery in the first few years of life. Much of the myopic shift can be attributed to normal eye growth; however other causes including age at surgery, visual input, presence or absence of an IOL, and laterality also play a role in this process.

As time passes, more and more children will be presenting for treatment with significant pseudophakic myopia. For aphakic eyes, treatment choices include secondary IOL implantation (if enough capsule support exists), and corneal refractive surgery. For pseudophakic eyes, choices include IOL exchange, implantation of a piggyback IOL, or corneal refractive surgery. Each of the currently available procedures has advantages and disadvantages when pediatric use is expected. LASIK allows faster visual rehabilitation and needs a shorter course of postoperative medications. The corneal flap, however, may be vulnerable to childhood trauma. PRK would hold up much better to trauma, but has a slower healing and needs a longer course of postoperative medications. LASEK (laser assisted sub-epithelial keratectomy) has also been used in children as a variation in the PRK procedure. Each of these procedures could be used for the moderate degree of myopia that will develop in most pseudophakic children and young adults. If high myopia develops, an IOL exchange would likely be chosen over laser refractive surgery. After cataract surgery, children will most likely need laser refractive surgery at the end of their growing years. At that age, predictability and stability may approach that found in adults.

Strabismus

Although not a complication of cataract surgery itself, strabismus is frequently seen in aphakic and pseudophakic eyes and are thus included here. Strabismus occurs more frequently in pseudophakic pediatric patients than in the general pediatric population. Strabismus was reported in 39% (37/94) of pediatric pseudophakic eyes. Exotropia (46%) was more common than esotropia (41%). Earlier onset unilateral cataracts have the highest risk for strabismus and late-onset bilateral cataracts have the least risk. Also, as a general rule, the patients with partial cataracts and relatively good preoperative visual acuity have less strabismus. Long delays in detection and treatment of visually significant cataracts increase the risk of strabismus, even when the cataracts are incomplete. Strabismus at presentation is often an indication that the cataract is long-standing and that significant amblyopia is likely to be present. In review of the literature since 1980 we found that strabismus was present in 33.3% of patients preoperatively, and in 78.1% of patients postoperatively. The higher incidence of strabismus after treatment than before may reflect the intensity of the occlusion prescribed, the ongoing susceptibility of the infantile eye to amblyopia due to an uncorrected refractive error, or the easier detection of strabismus in older children. Strabismus surgery is often delayed until after the initial amblyopia treatment has improved the visual acuity somewhat. Occasionally, an intermittent strabismus will resolve as the visual acuity improves. However, this is the exception rather than the rule. Strabismus associated with cataracts in children usually needs surgery. If the strabismus angle and pattern are stable, correction is planned at an elective time such as during a scheduled examination under anesthesia where intraocular pressure, retinal examination and serial axial length measurements are planned.

Stability of alignment after strabismus surgery in aphakic or pseudophakic children is difficult to predict. Generally, children with better visual outcomes and better binocularity have better stability of ocular alignment. Dense deprivation amblyopia lessens the chance of long-term correction of strabismus but despite this, a cosmetically acceptable alignment if often maintained for many years. Overall, the success of strabismus surgery is higher for strabismus that develops after the cataract surgery as compared to strabismus that is present preoperatively, at initial presentation. Although occlusion therapy for amblyopia must usually be continued after surgical realignment of the eyes, full-time occlusion is not recommended since it carries a higher risk for recurrence of strabismus.

Summary

Postoperative complications may develop in the early postoperative period or after many years. Therefore, it is crucial to follow children closely on a long-term basis after pediatric cataract surgery. If child is not cooperative for routine examination we recommend yearly examination under anesthesia.

Chapter 12

PCO in Childhood: Prevention and Management

Frederic Hehn (France)

Introduction

Posterior capsule opacification (PCO) results from the proliferation of the lens epithelial cells (LEC) that remain in the lens bag, especially in the equatorial region. Albert Galand developed in 1996 the concept of a systematic posterior continuous curvilinear capsulorhexis (PCCC), but there is some risks of retinal detachment, and the learning curve of this technique is hard. Marie-josé Tassignon developed the concept of 'the bag in the lens to avoid the PCO, but the stability of the lens and the realization of this difficult technique are in concern. The square edge IOL design provides a lower rate of PCO, but does not eradicate it. Depending on the length of the follow-up, the PCO occurs and has been reported in up to 80% of eyes having a cataract extraction with an IOL Implantation.

But in childhood PCO is systematic and occurs faster and harder. Today the consensus still remains PCCC and anterior vitrectomy or not in prevention of PCO.

MICS (microincision cataract surgery) and frequently implantation of a soft IOL in the bag even in pediatric eye can modified our strategy of prevention and treatment of PCO in childhood.

The main question is the possibility or not to conserve the integrity of posterior capsule, to respect the vitreous body and decrease the rate of vitreo-retinal complications.

Characteristics of Cataract Surgery in Childhood

The first specific point concern the crystalline capsule: Capsular thickness is approximately 10 µm in anterior part, only 5 µm in post-part and get the more width in equatorial region 15 µm. But the major parameter in childhood is the more elasticity of the capsule. This extend of elasticity give some difficulties to perform ant and post-capsulorhexis. To well control capsulorhexis, we must begin smaller, to avoid zonular tears.

The second concern is about the extreme inflammatory reaction after pediatric cataract surgery: Increasing the rate of uveitis, cystoid macular edema, glaucoma, capsular bag retraction and opacification. With difficulties of management of the both recurrent PCO and high level of capsular shrinkage, with volting and possibilities of IOL displacement.

Modern Cataract Surgery in Childhood

Before 3 years old is not recommended to realize an IOL implantation, because the bag is too small, and the evolution of refraction too unforeseeable (often steep keratometry and small axial length). Contact lens remains a good option to fight against amblyopia due to ametropia of aphakia. Then before 3 years old the only solution still remains PCCC and anterior vitrectomy, without implantation in prevention of PCO. In this case to let a good anterior capsular ring is useful to permit a later in sulcus implantation when the growth of the eye and refraction become more stable.

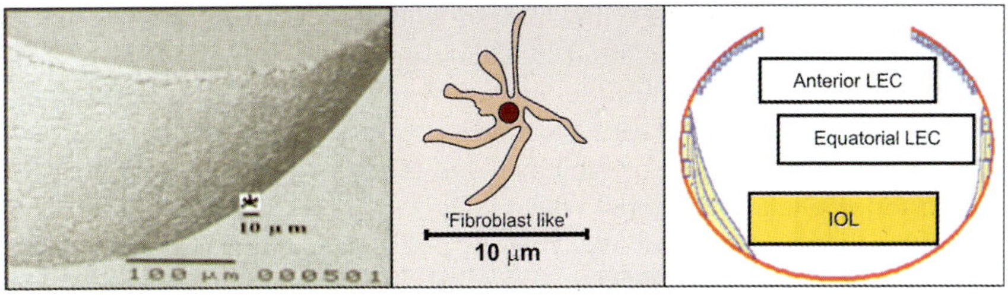

Figure 1: Cellular scale (Escobar-Gomez) a SEM (scanning electron micrograph) of the SA30AL at the scale of 100 µm. On this figure a virtual 'fibroblast like' wide of 10 µm has been drawn by the author

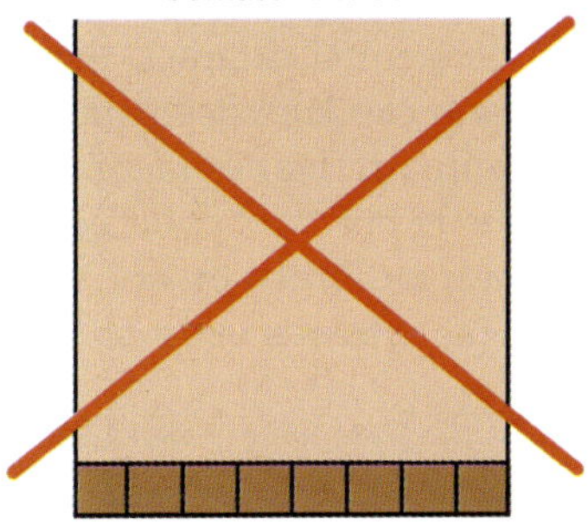

Figure 2: Contact inhibition. At the scale of 10 µm the IOL optic material, seems to be porous and rough, and the SE sharp of the IOL becomes a very academic point of view

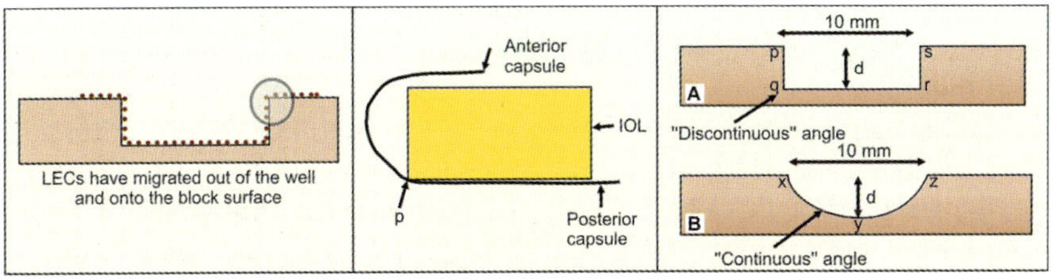

Figure 3: Boyce and Al experience: LEC are not inhibited by the square egde itself

Then we considered that with children who are more than 3 years old, the PCO management looks like adult PCO management.

If possible, anterior technique, microincision, and phacoemulsification is the best way of pediatric cataract, for a better control of total nucleus and cortex ablation, decrease of induce astigmatism and safety of implantation rather than by a posterior phako-vitrectomy way.

Different kind of IOL are available for pediatric cataract surgery, after the classical one piece hard PMMA, some others like soft hydrophobic even hydrophilic IOL are used in this surgery. Of course, the soft IOL, is also useful for a later exchange is necessary due the modification of refraction. Sure the both design and material of the IOL can influence PCO formation.

With MICS, bimanual technique consisting in separate irrigation and aspiration; It allows micro-incision of 1.5 mm width for entirely procedure from corneal incision until IOL implantation. But in regard of PCO the problem is the same that it was in conventional 3.2 incision cataract surgery.

The problem is that even in case of PCCC and anterior vitrectomy, PCO can be sometimes recurrent in congenital cataract, then multiple Nd yag capsulotomy, or iterative pars plana capsulovitrectomy increase the rate of great complications: Endophthalmitis, retinal detachment, glaucoma, uveitis, iris atrophia. Then this consensus is not the “panacea”.

The main question is the possibility or not to conserve the integrity of posterior capsule, to respect the vitreous body and decrease the rate of vitreo-retinal complications.

Preventing Factors of PCO

The well known preventing factors of a PCO are: No IOL decentration, a 360° IOL overlapping of capsulorhexis, an ablation of visco-elastic behind the optic, a reduction of the retro-optical space, no folds on posterior capsule, the speed of the capsular bend formation, the adhesion between the optic and posterior capsule by fibronectin, IOL materials, and of course Square Edge IOL design. But only a total cleaning of anterior and equatorial LEC could be efficient to avoid the PCO.

The LEC give always anterior or posterior capsular bag opacification in the shape of fibrosis or pearls and sometimes shrinkage with IOL displacement.

The problem of PCO is not only the cost and the morbidity of Nd:yag capsulotomy, but the real challenge is to keep a soft capsular bag . With a soft capsular bag, LEC free, it will be possible to restore accommodation in pseudophakic eyes with the “phacoersatz” and avoid practice anterior vitrectomy and PCCC in children’s cataract surgery.

There are only two ways to avoid PCO, Block LEC migration, or kill the LEC. Until we will be not able to take off or kill entirely the equatorial LEC, PCO occurs irreversibly from month to month after cataract surgery.

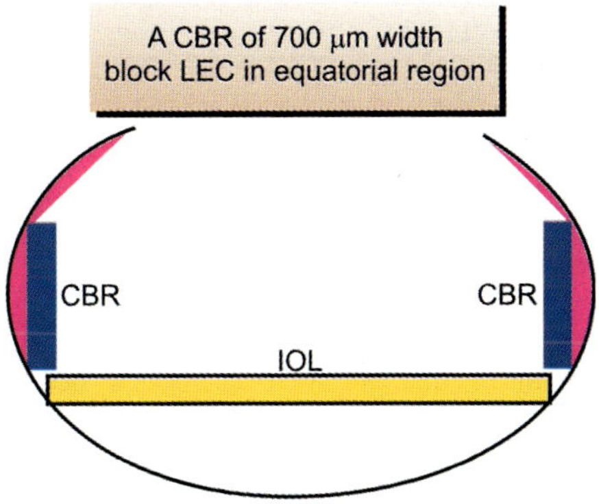

Figure 4: Effect of CBR in the bag: It block the LEC in equatorial region

Hydrophobic	Without CTR	n = 41	12, 19%(5)	With CTR	n = 96	5,20%(5)	p < 0.01
Hydrophilic	Without CTR	n = 33	21, 21%(7)	With CTR	n = 106	10,37%(11)	p < 0.001
Silicone	Without CTR	n = 31	19, 35%(6)	With CTR	n = 108	9,25%(10)	p < 0.01

Figure 5: Rate % of Nd:yag for PCO at 24 months follow-up

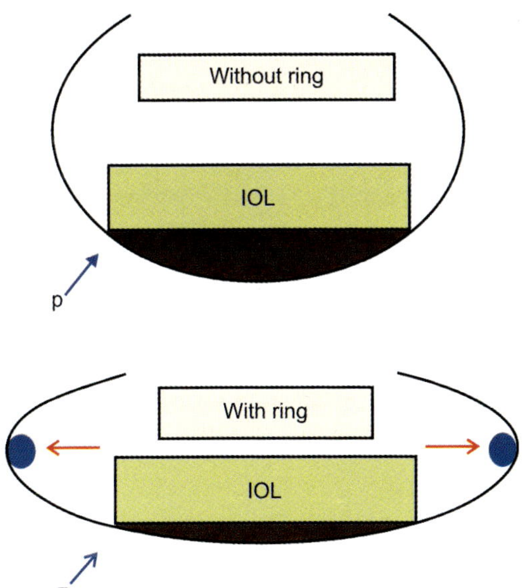

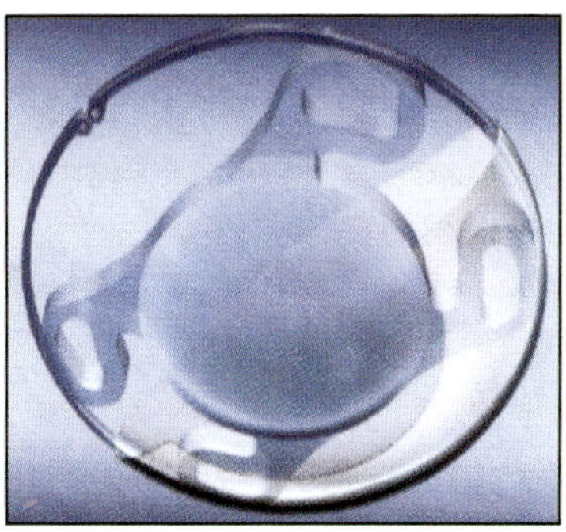

Figures 6 and 7: IOL and CTR = immediate capsular bag tension, preventing LEC migration

Block LEC Migration

There are two possibilities to block cell migration; the first is to block them by IOL shape "the square edge", the second is to block LEC in equatorial region with a capsular tension ring.

Square Edge

What are we speaking about? We are speaking about cell. At first the LEC are not cubic in the equatorial region. Secondly, they are modified cells and become 'fibroblast like' from 10 µm diameter << IOL' optic diameter (800 µ or more).

'Fibroblasts like' have got *'arms and legs and hands and feet'* and they try to conquer the retro-optical space. Be sure that 'Fibroblast like' are not afraid of a SE IOL design and that they can pass it round. Obviously the square edge shape concept does not exist at the cellular scale. Because the fibroblast like cells are not at all cubic, and they have got three-dimensional coordinates. Secondly, the IOL itself at the cellular scale of 1 to 10 µm is not smooth at all and it is not perfectly polished but rough and porous.

But is there nothing right at all about a SE IOL design effect? Some studies show there is a SE effect on the PCO regardless of the type of IOL material. Other studies show that the difference in terms of PCO rate is due to the IOL material, and not statistically due to the SE effect. Obviously both factors, SE IOL design and type of IOL's material, influence the PCO rate. We now know that, of course, there is a SE effect but it is not a contact cellular inhibition, but it is a mechanical tension effect. **Boyce, Bhermi and Spalton** have shown, by a mathematical model, that in fact a SE IOL design exerts twice more pressure than a round edge at the point p . This 'p' point is the contact between the corner of the edge and the posterior capsule. This high pressure blocks the LEC migration.

Capsular Rings: CBR and CTR Respective Actions Against PCO

Many other systems failed to completely clean the capsular bag without any risk for the zonula, the endothelium or the posterior capsule. Only a ring is able to go to the equatorial region, to try to mechanically block the LEC, or to block it by a disposable drug delivery system like 5FU and so on...

There are two methods with rings; the first is to block LEC in equatorial region by a CBR: Capsular bending ring which is large enough 700 µm, that the study of NISHI, but with this technique, because the CBR is large it avoid the collapse and adhesion between anterior and posterior capsule (which increase the risk of LEC migration).

CBR

HEMA IOL HM60 STORZ + 13 mm CTR PMMA square edge not polished 0.7 mm width and 0.2 mm thickness ONE EYE IOL + CTR SECOND EYE ONLY IOL

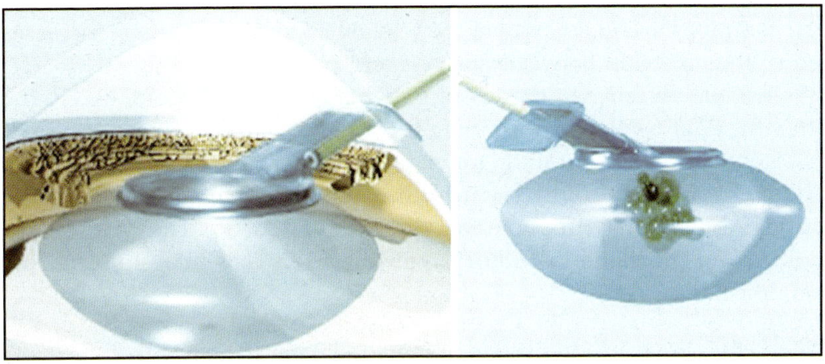

Figure 8: Perfect capsule

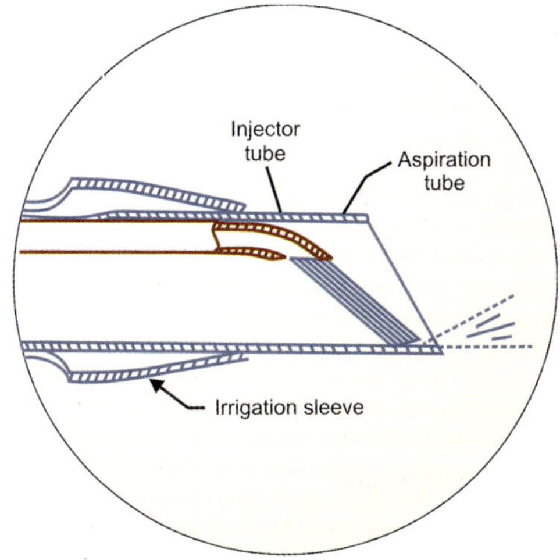

Figure 9 : Aqualase

2 YEARS FOLLOW-UP 84 eyes of 42 patients EPCO computer image analysis

Rate of Nd:yag capsulotomy	**5% (4/84) ring**	**20% (17/84) without**
Folds post-cap	0% with ring	25 % without ring

CTR

At the contrary Dr HEHN explore the way of classical CTR which increases the speed of the adhesion between anterior and post-capsule.

We have analyzed two groups of patients with and without a CTR, during the months after a cataract surgery and we have compared the rate of Nd yag capsulotomy and EPCO grading for evaluate the PCO. We have got 3 groups of 3 kinds of IOL's materials. Hydrophilic acrylic (Stabibag Ioltech), silicone (Clariflex AMO) and hydrophobic acrylic (SA60AT Alcon). The CTR was simply a choice from the same laboratory than the IOL: Tensiobag Ioltech, Reform Alcon, Injectoring AMO.

When the ring is inside the bag, it exerts a tangential tension of the posterior capsule all around 360°. Therefore a CTR increases the pressure at the 'p' point and then the SE tension effect of IOL, to mechanically block the LEC migration. That is the most fundamental effect of a CTR against the PCO but it is not the only one.

Previous research, by Rupert **Menapace** suggested that capsular tension rings prevent the PCO through more than one mechanism. First, the ring causes posterior capsule stretching, which reduces the IOL capsule distance. The well tension of the capsular bag reduces the retro-optical space: The CTR increases the 'no space no cell ' theory.

The immediate well tension of the bag with the ring (before the natural retraction of the capsular bag), increases the speed of the capsular bend formation, before the LEC get enough time to conquer the retro-optical space: The CTR increases the CBI (Capsular bending index), which is fundamental, to avoid the LEC migration. The instantaneous tension of the bag by the ring facilitates the capsular adhesion between the posterior capsule and the IOL optic by fibronectin, laminin or collagen type IV, which are present on capsular or on LEC surface, and so on, are free to absorb the IOL surface after the break of the blood aqueous barrier: The CTR increases the 'sandwich' theory.

I expect so that a CTR would probably increase the LEC destruction by a direct cell compression. Other well known properties of the ring can be combined to reduce the PCO rate, like the better long-terms centration for all lens with a CTR. CTR facilitates the equatorial LEC removal by an IOL rotation inside the capsular bag without any risk for the zonula, it facilitates the retro-optical viscoelastic ablation too, according to the 'no space no cell' theory, it facilitates the anterior capsular bag cleaning to prevent capsular shrinkage. Eventually, a CTR decreases capsular fold of posterior capsule and then it avoids the LEC migration along the folds.

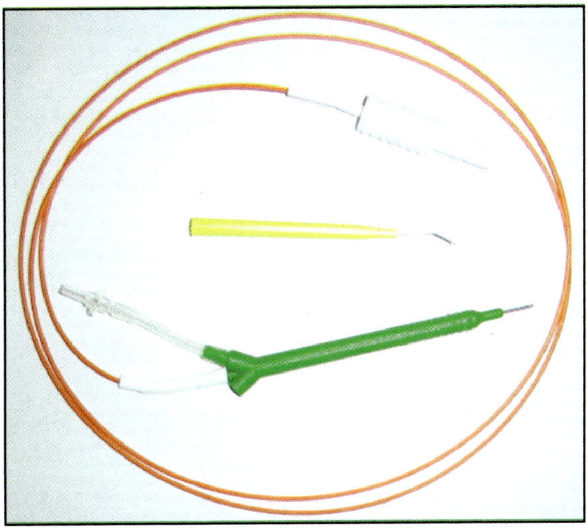

Figure 10: Phacolaser

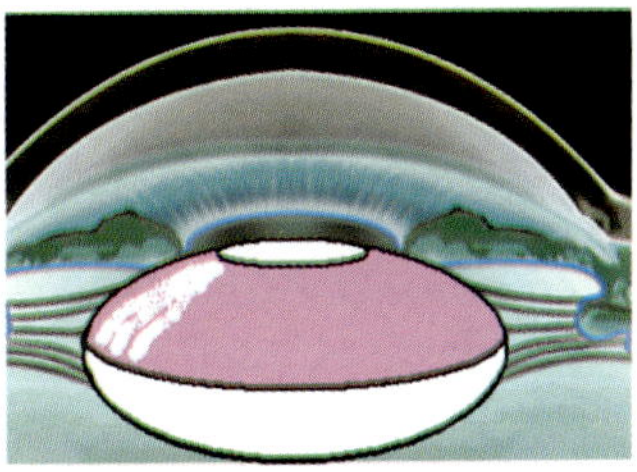

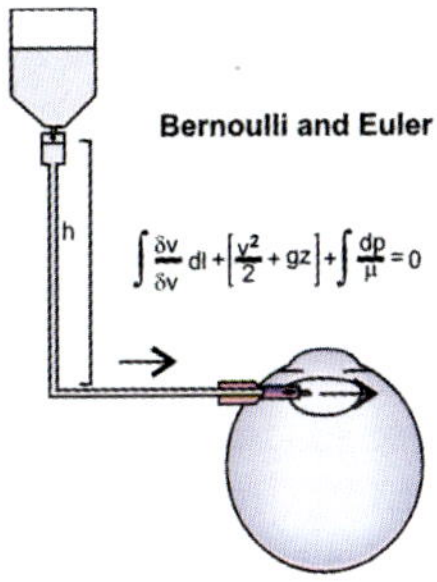

Figure 11: CBJ principle

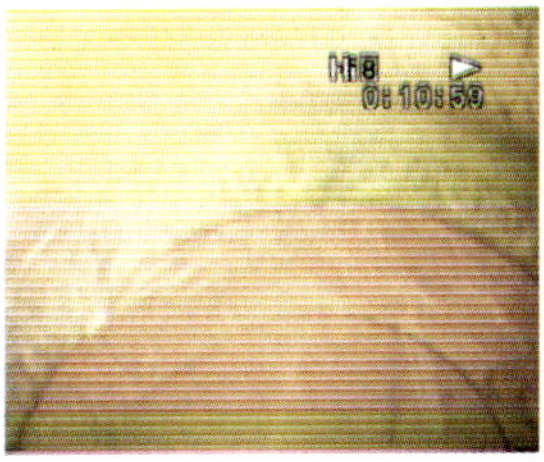

Figure 12: CBJ human surgical view

Properties to Prevent PCO

We can say that there are ten specific CTR preventing PCO factors, which are summed up in the schema just below:

01. The CTR increases the pressure at the 'p' point and then the SE IOL design tension effect.
02. The CTR reduces the retro-optical space too, according to the 'no space, no cell ' theory.
03. The CTR increases the speed of the capsular bend formation.
04. The CRT facilitates the adhesion between the capsule and the IOL according to the 'sandwich' theory.
05. The CTR probably makes some equatorial LEC destruction by direct cell compression.
06. The CTR prevents IOL decentration, deformation and tilting with soft IOL.
07. The CTR facilitates the equatorial LEC removal by an IOL rotation inside the capsular bag.
08. The CTR facilitates the retro-optical viscoelastic ablation too, according to the 'no space no cell' theory.
09. The CTR facilitates the anterior capsular bag cleaning to prevent capsular shrinkage.
10. The CTR decreases the capsular folds of posterior capsule.

Pediatric Example of Cataract Surgery with Acrylic IOL and CTR

It is a world wide acceptance that in case of a pediatric cataract, surgeons are obliged to practice both PCCC and anterior vitrectomy, otherwise, early, strong and recurrent PCO occurs.

But unfortunately, every pediatric cataract surgeon knows that even with the PCCC and anterior vitrectomy, a PCO can often occur and repeat itself. Some surgeons suggest that the bag should be cleaned by aspiration with the 'cap vac' phaco-mode in case of Elschnig pearls; then with the current tendency which consists in changing PMMA IOL in congenital cataract for a soft acrylic IOL, especially hydrophobic; and thirdly with the excellent preliminary results of our own study: We decided to treat a child with the same bi-implantation technique by IOL and CTR.

The goal was to respect the anatomy of his eye as long as possible and to avoid complications of initial vitrectomy (retinal detachment, glaucoma and uveitis). This bi-implantation technique has been performed on only one patient with a congenital cataract. This case is about a 5 years old boy. A bilateral cataract surgery with a hydrophilic acrylic stabibag and a CTR tensiobag 10.00 PMMA diameter from ioltech, were implanted in October 2001. For children with a PMMA CTR, we can give the rigidity of a PMMA IOL and benefit from a soft lens implantation by a micro-corneal incision. Neither posterior continuous capsular capsulorhexis, nor anterior vitrectomy has been performed. After 18 months of follow-up no Nd yag capsulotomy was necessary. The right eye +1.50 (180°-2.50) BCVA 4/20 J3 before the implantation and +1.00(10°-1.00) BCVA 14/20 J2 before the implantation. The left eye, amblyopia –6.00 (175°-

5.00) BCVA 4/20 J5 before and +3.00 (180°-1.75) 5/20 J4 18 months after the implantation.

We perfectly know that a CTR is not the final solution to prevent PCO in childhood or in adulthood, but it is certainly good to use all the techniques that can delay PCO as long as possible. Especially in this case, it will be better to practice Nd: yag at 7 or 8 years old rather than a PCCC and anterior vitrectomy at 5 years old. This very interesting result will be analyzed with EPCO software for a next publication.

Kill the LEC

Perfect Capsule™

That's perfect capsule system, which is able to kill the LEC by hypo-osmolarity, but there is some risk for endothelium if the succion leaks. Actually perfect casule device is not available for MICS because it needs a 5.0 mm width cornea insision.

Aqualase®

An hot hydrojet, able to lyse the nucleus of the crystalline, is there any possibilities to lyse the LEC in equatorial region? Actually aqualase is compatible with bimanual technique, but not with MICS because the needle of aqualase handpiece needs of 3.2 incision, the next generation of aqualase certainly will be compatible with MICS.

Phaco-laser

Phaco-laser (the Dodick photolysis) is compatible with MICS, recently at ARVO 2004 meeting, it has been shown the possibility of direct LEC destruction by Nd yag laser on anterior capsule.

CBJ: Cleanbagjet®

It is a new phaco handpiece, which produce a micro-hydrojet able to clean the LEC even in equatorial region, developed by Ioltech laboratories, first clinical results are attempted in ASCRS 2005.

Conclusion

PCO remains the really final frontier in cataract surgery, especially in pediatric cataract surgery.

Before three years old implantation is not recommended, and the classical technique with anterior and posterior CCC and anterior vitrectomy is still the consensus for congenital cataract management. But in this case, to let a good anterior capsule ring seems to be useful for a later IOL in the sulcus implantation.

After 3 years old, generally pediatric catatract can benefit of all refinement of MICS technique; some new device like CTR, aqualase, phacolaser, perfect capsule and clean bag jet seem to be useful to decrease or delay PCO. We hope that soon without PCO, it will be possible to treat accommodation in pseudophakic eye and perform cataract surgery as easily in children than in adult without anterior vitrectomy nor PCCC.

Chapter 13

Early Onset Developmental Glaucoma (Primary Congenital Glaucoma)

Ahmad K Khalil (Egypt)

Introduction

Developmental glaucoma is a glaucoma caused by maldevelopment of the eye's aqueous outflow system. Depending on the severity of this maldevelopment the resultant elevated intraocular pressure may occur at birth or anytime thereafter. Most cases present at birth (congenital) or within the first year of life (infantile), and on these entities, we refer as early onset developmental glaucoma (EODG). Due to the elastic nature of the embryonic tissues, the eye ball stretches and enlarges in congenital cases, with subsequent Descemet's membrane ruptures, corneal edema and cloudiness. Pressure on the elastic optic nerve head and *lamina cribrosa* leads to early (distension) cupping, but eventually functional loss and glaucomatous optic atrophy ensue.

The disease is bilateral in 75% of the cases, males more commonly affected (65%). There is sporadic occurrence in 90% of the cases, the remainder; autosomal recessive with variable penetrance. Its incidence is 1:10,000 births in the West and 1:2500 births in the Middle East. More than 80% present before 1 year.

Genetically, EODG appears to be a genetically heterogeneous disorder in that there is an unequal sex distribution and fewer numbers of affected siblings. To date, 2 loci have been found for EODG: GLC3A (chromosome 2p21) and GLC3B (chromosome 1p36).

Clinical Signs and Symptoms

Epiphora, photophobia and blepharospasm are often the first symptoms to alarm the parents. Any of these symptoms warrants careful examination with glaucoma in mind. I have seen infants with a moderate degree of glaucoma who were referred because of persistent epiphora after nasolacrimal probing.

Grayish discoloration (cloudiness of the cornea) is usually the presenting symptom of more advanced cases.

Corneal enlargement without cloudiness is a less often presenting symptom, as it is often thought by parents as a beauty sign, rather than an abnormal alerting sign.

Examination

The normal IOP in the newborn well falls in the 1 digit mmHg readings. The disc has almost no cup. The cornea is clear, its horizontal diameter in a full-term newborn is 10 to 10.5 mm and increases to the adult diameter of approximately 11.5 to 12 mm by 2 years of age.

IOP

Examination is ideally done under general anesthesia, where it would be possible to make a full examination at no haste. This is at least necessary for a first full examination for decision-making and a couple of follow-up examinations as thought necessary. Follow-up examinations can then

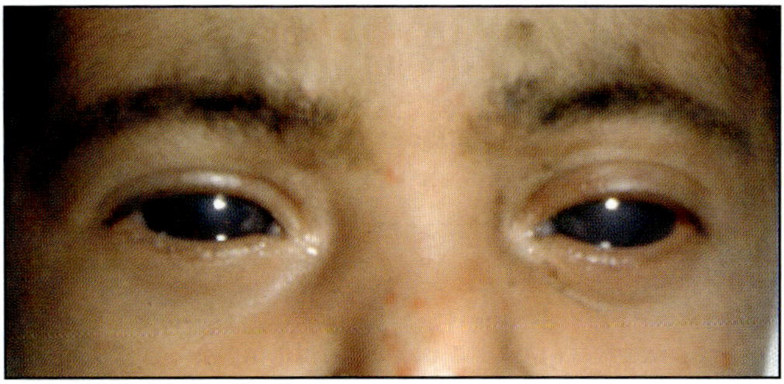

Figure 1: Classically described EODG with photophobia, epiphora, corneal enlargement and cloudiness

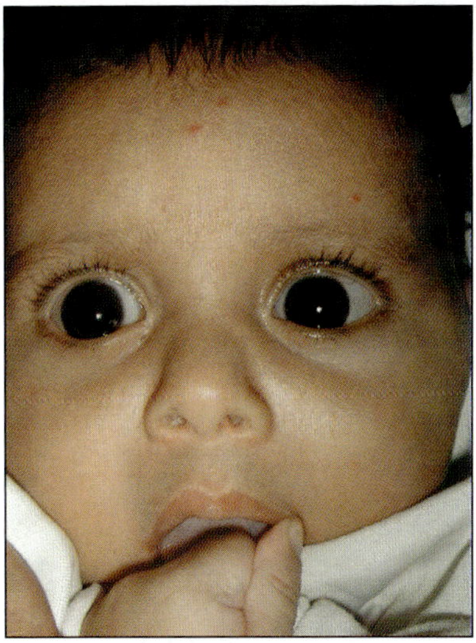

Figure 2: Parents are often peaceful with larger corneas of their infants seeing it as a sign of beauty, and often overlooking the mild corneal cloudiness seen in the right eye of this infant

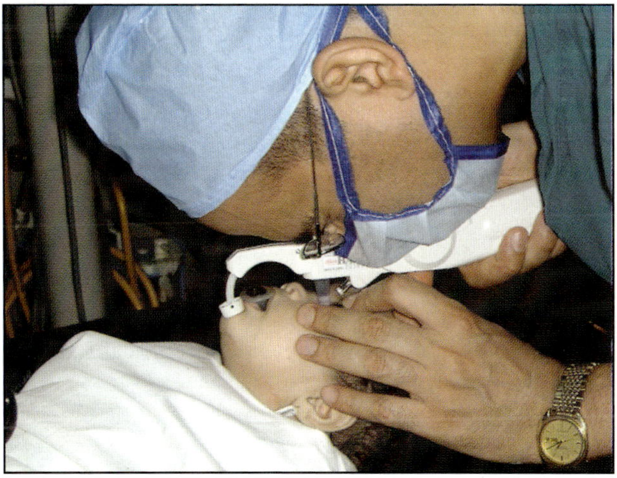

Figure 3: Measuring the IOP under general anesthesia using the Perkins tonometer in the operation theater. For follow-up examinations, a mask anesthesia with an oral airway is usually adequate

adequately be made with sedation (chloral hydrate), and with proper training afterwards, without sedation as early as the second year of life.

Most general anesthetics tend to lower IOP readings, and a knowledge of the anesthetic used and its behavior is needed. A hand-held applannation tonometer, is a good device in this regard. Lid and canthal pressure can lead to false high IOP readings with forceful opening of the eye lids.

Cornea

Using the surgical microscope or a portable slit lamp, early corneal edema or more pronounced clouding and breaks in Descemet's membrane should be looked for. A diameter greater than 12 mm in an infant is highly suggestive of EODG. Developmental anomalies of the cornea and iris must be noted because they may alter diagnosis and treatment. Corneal clouding is usually reversible after IOP control.

Rupture lines of Descemet's membrane (Haab's striae) with associated localized areas of edema can be seen in moderate to severe untreated cases. Glassy lines can be seen long after glaucoma control, and might be the only indication of self-limited IOP rise episodes in infancy.

The Optic Nerve Head

A cup/disc ratios greater than 0.3 in an infant is suggestive of glaucoma. Changes in the optic disc occur readily with changes in IOP in infants due to increased tissue elasticity which translates IOP increase into mechanical distortion in the disc supporting elements. Globe enlargement further magnifies this mechanical cupping. This cupping is easily reversible typically within 4-6 weeks after normalization of IOP. The younger the child, the faster the reversibility. If left untreated, neuronal loss eventually ensues, with irreversible damage. Together with regression of photophobia, reversibility of optic disc cupping is one of the best criteria for surgical success in most cases.

Gonioscopy

Gonioscopy is performed by use of a gonioprism, a Koeppe or a barkan operating lens (a truncated koeppe lens) and binocular microscope for the evaluation of goniodysgenesis.

Axial Length Measurements

Measuring the axial length was proposed as a diagnostic and follow-up procedure. It is generally thought, however that corneal diameter is a more sensitive tool in this context.

Differential Diagnosis

Mild to moderate cases can easily be confused by entities which increase corneal diameter (megalocornea), cases with corneal cloudiness (sclerocornea,

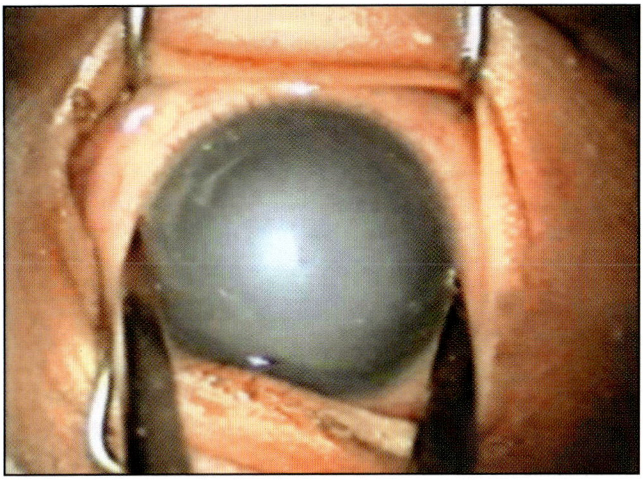

Figure 4: Measuring of the white to white corneal diameter

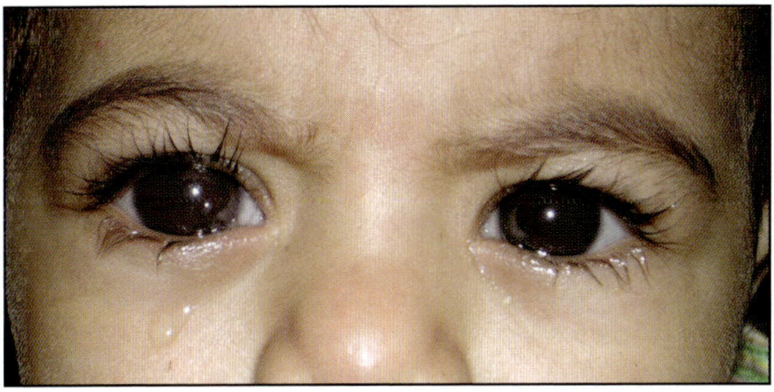

Figure 5: Corneal cloudiness clearing in the left eye 5 days after surgery as compared to the right still cloudy non-operated eye (watering is caused by child crying rather than epiphora)

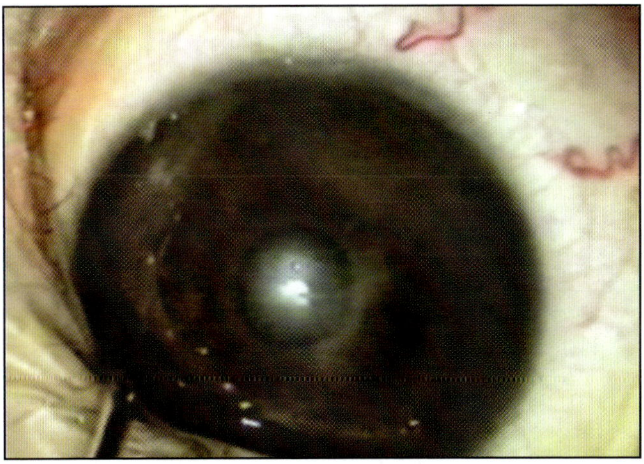

Figure 6: Rupture lines of Descemet's membrane (Haab's striae) with associated localized areas of edema

dystrophies like Meesman's and Reis-Buckler), or other causes of epiphora (NLD obstruction).

Management

Surgery is the first line of therapy for EODG for the following reasons: (1) Since this type of glaucoma results from abnormal anatomical development of the anterior chamber angle, anatomical or surgical correction is recommended. (2) Accumulated experience shows the effectiveness of surgery. (3) It is difficult to determine the effectiveness of medical therapy in infants and children because the procedure is complicated and may require anesthesia. The long-term effectiveness and complications of different anti-glaucoma drugs have not been well studied.

Surgical Management

Trabeculotomy and Goniotomy

Trabeculotomy and goniotomy remain the first line surgical procedures for EODG. They directly attack the faulty site with minimal surgical trauma, as compared with trabeculectomy, hence inviting much less tissue reaction and fibrosis which very often compromise the surgical outcome. The absence of external aqueous filtration precludes delayed filtering bleb-related complications, such as infection, hypotony, and leaks.

Trabeculotomy and goniotomy seem to be in some ways equivalent, and both are particularly successful in previously unoperated cases of EODG. Goniotomy, however, does not have a good success rate when done below 1 month or over 2 years of age. It is usually associated with a relatively high rate of recurrence, and multiple goniotomies are needed to achieve a success rate similar to that of trabeculotomy. Trabeculotomy is probably a more demanding technique with which it may be more difficult to achieve a technically perfect procedure than it is with goniotomy, but it is the preferred choice of the author of this chapter, with a 5-year cumulative success rate of 92%.

Goniotomy

Goniotomy involves the creation of a superficial incision into uveal TM, allowing the iris root to move posteriorly and presumably relieving the mechanical obstruction to aqueous outflow. This procedure is performed under direct visualization through a gonioscopic contact lens and the operating microscope.

Trabeculotomy

Trabeculotomy is my first choice for surgery in all cases of EODG, regardless any previous surgery, as long as there is a sound non-scarred 120 degrees of limbic circumference. A properly performed trabeculotomy gives good results in most of these eyes. Bad prognostic signs include; eyes with corneal diameter

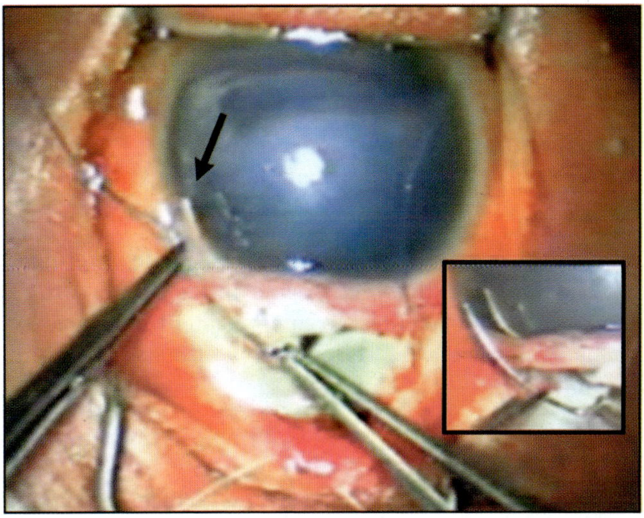

Figure 7: The second trabeculotomy probe is being rotated into the AC

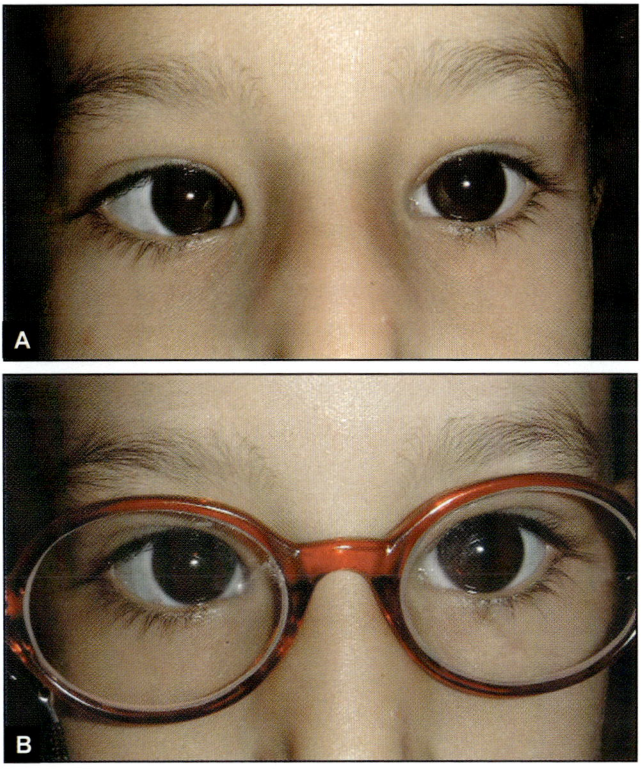

Figures 8A and B: 3 years after bilateral successful trabeculotomy for EODG, this case presented with anisometropia (one eye myopic, the other low hyperopic) and strabismus. Glasses correction and amblyopia management could achieve a bilateral 0.8 visual acuity

14.5 or more, advanced congenital cases, and multiple previous surgeries. It involves creating a superficial sclera flap and then making a limbal radial incision to reach and incise open the Canal of Schlemm, which is then probed on either side by specially designed probes. When these are rotated into the AC, they sever the malformed trabecular/angle tissue.

Trabeculectomy

The decision to perform this procedure must be made carefully because in infants and children, filtering bleb formation may be difficult despite intraoperative use of antimetabolites. Even after filtering blebs are successfully formed, the patients may be exposed to the risk of post-surgical infections for the rest of their life.

Deep Sclerectomy

No much role as it leaves the trabecular beams, which are the main site for resistance to outflow in EODG, untouched.

Aqueous Shunt Implantation

The enhanced success with aqueous shunt devices is associated with a higher likelihood of postoperative complications. They can probably used as a last resort in refractory cases with multiple previous surgeries and compromised angle structures.

Medical Treatment

Because of poor efficacy, a greater potential for adverse systemic side effects, medical treatment is used as an auxiliary means to temporarily control IOP till surgery is performed or in the rare instance when repeated surgeries fail to control IOP. **Brimonidine** should be used with caution in young children because of the potential for CNS depression.

Prognosis

Even after successful surgery with IOP control and regression/stabilization of optic disc cupping, regular follow-up and rehabilitation measures will be necessary to achieve a favorable outcome and prognosis. It is near meaningless to save an eye from sight threatening glaucoma, and lose it.

Chapter 14

Late (Adult) Onset Developmental Glaucoma

Ahmad K Khalil (Egypt)

Introduction

This is an evolving entity which would include in older literature entities like juvenile glaucoma and many cases of primary open angle glaucoma (POAG). This type of glaucoma results from maldevelopment of the eye's aqueous outflow system, but as the extent of such morphological anomalies is slight; the age of onset is delayed until late teens, twenties, or even later.

Clinical Signs and Symptoms

Accidental discovery of a moderately high IOP or optic disc cupping in a late teen who is known not to be glaucomatous in previous examinations is not uncommon. Onset and diagnosis can be even delayed to the age of fourties or fifties. Less frequently, patients presents by visual complaint caused by advanced visual loss and cupping.

IOP rise ranges between low twenties to mid fourties. Sudden IOP rise can occur which brings the patient complaining of headache. Cupping can be seen in these subacute cases, and I have seen a patient in his mid-fourties presenting with high IOP, and optic disc cupping of 0.6 which was reversed on IOP control to 0.3. This denotes the rapid onset as well as the residual elasticity of optic nerve head structures up to this adult age.

The hallmark of LODG is the typical angle changes. **Mal-development of the angle (gonio-dysgenesis)** with anterior insertion of the iris root into the trabecular area and/or embryonic iris processes reaching to Schwalbe's line and the corneal periphery. **Corneal diameter** is typically within the normal adult size. Finding of a larger corneal diameter or endothelial (Haab's) striae/lines denote an infantile onset of a milder glaucoma. LODG should be considered when evaluating cases with pre-senile cataracts, as it can be the inciting factor.

Regular glaucoma tests including diurnal variations, visual field testing, and nerve fiber layer analysis, should be pursued in all cases. Most structural tests do not still have a normative database for younger individuals, but even though; such tests can still be done for future comparison and potential progression evaluation with evolving newer technology.

Differential Diagnosis

When encountering glaucoma with developmental angle changes in an adult, the differentiation should be made whether this is a late onset developmental glaucoma or a self-limited mild glaucoma developed in infancy and passed unnoticed, whether this is a newly developed glaucoma or a newly discovered glaucoma! This becomes particulary important in cases with borderline findings like a 20 mmHg IOP, a 0.6 C/D ratio. This can be a self-aborting case of EODG which does not require more than follow-up, and can be an evolving case of LODG which requires immediate attention and management. As mentioned above, the presence of corneal enlargement and/or Haab's striae denotes an

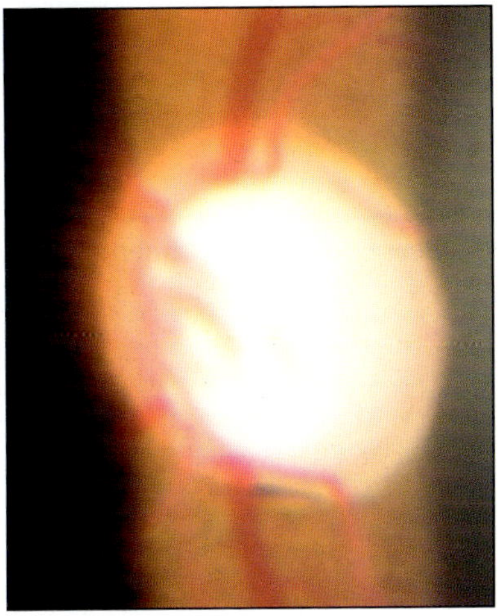

Figure 1: Advance cupping in a recently diagnosed case of LODG, female age 19 years

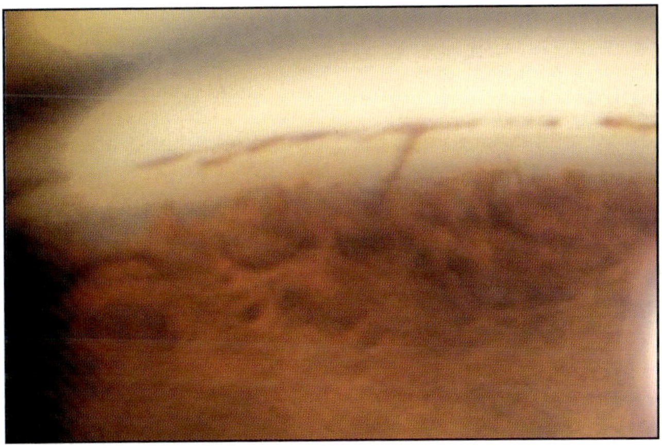

Figure 2: Gonio-dysgenesis; anterior insertion of iris root into anterior trabecular area

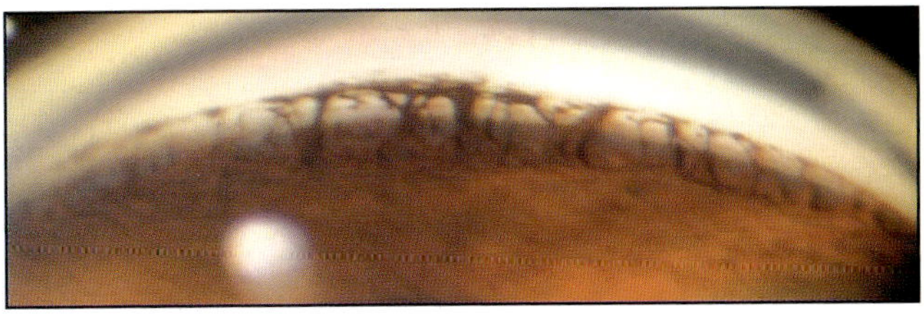

Figure 3: Gonio-dysgenesis; embryonic iris processes bridging and covering most of the angle structures and reaching to the corneal periphery

earlier onset. When uncertain, closer follow-up is advised for IOP fluctuations and visual field changes.

Treatment

Similar to EODG but to a lesser extent, treatment is mainly surgical. Medical treatment, however, has a wider place here and is more effective than that very limited role in EODG.

Surgical Options

Trabeculotomy

Similar to EODG as the main pathology is in the trabecular area, trabeculotomy remains the preferred surgical option regardless the age of the patient. Different from trabeculotomy in the newborn, Schlemm's canal should be sought more anteriorly in the limbus area, as there is less ocular stretch. For the same reason, the canal is also deeper and narrower. After probing both cut ends of the canal simultaneously with trabeculotomy probes, they are rotated into the AC severing the faulty trabecular tissue.

Trabeculectomy

Trabeculectomy can have a role in this population when trabeculotomy can not be performed. The addition of antimetabolites is more warranted in younger age populations.

Prognosis

When detected at an early stage, the prognosis is favorable, as it usually responds well to medical and surgical management. The major negative prognostic factor in cases with LODG, however, is that it inflicts an age range, for which, more often than not, IOP measurement is skipped even during professional ophthalmological examination, and cases can be diagnosed when one eye has an almost total visual field loss, and the other has an advanced loss.

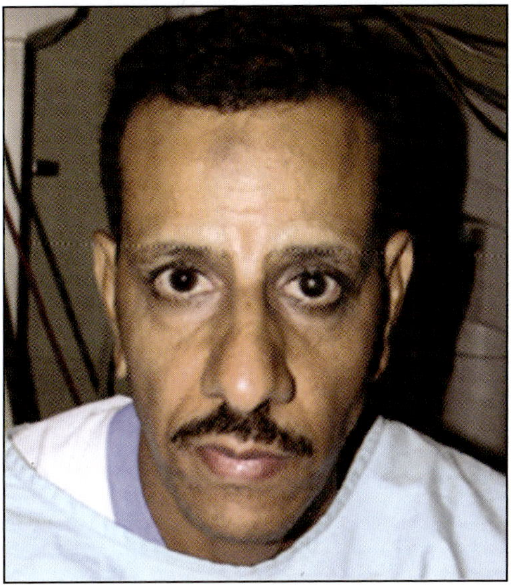

Figure 4: A case presenting with left pre-senile cataract, gonio-dysgenesis and a pressure in the mid 40s were found

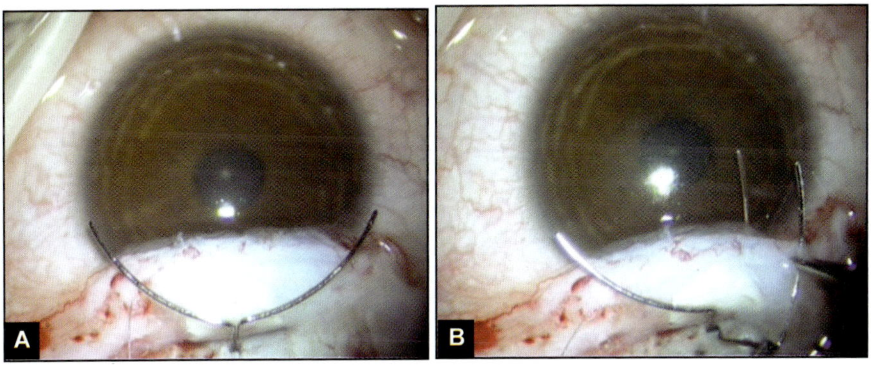

Figures 5 A and B: Trabeculotomy in an adult eye; (A) Both trabeculotomes in place, a limb inside Schlemm's canal and the outer guiding limb conforming with the limbal circumference. (B) The first trabeculotome is rotated into the AC

Chapter 15

Primary Infantile Glaucoma

Maria Da Luz Freitas (Portugal)

Introduction

The term *Developmental Glaucoma* includes primary congenital glaucoma and glaucoma associated with other developmental anomalies, either ocular or systemic. Glaucoma associated with other anomalies, either ocular or systemic may be inherited or acquired. *Primary Congenital or Infantile Glaucoma* is evident either at birth or within the first few years of life. This condition is believed to be caused by dysplasia of the anterior chamber angle without other ocular or systemic abnormalities. *Secondary infantile glaucoma* is associated with inflammatory, neoplastic, hamartomatous, metabolic, or other congenital abnormalities of the eye.

Developmental glaucoma occurs in about 1 in 10.000 live births and *Primary Congenital or Infantile Glaucoma* is believed to occur 1 in 30.000 births; 60% are diagnosed by the age of 6 months and 80% within the first year of the life. Approximately 65% of patients are male, and the involvement is bilateral in 70% of cases. Most cases occur sporadically.

Various classifications of the *Development Glaucoma* have been used. Hoskins *et al* have suggested an anatomic classification. Clinically identifiable anatomic defects of the eye were chosen as the basis for this system because they are readily apparent on examination and do not require supplemental information. The goniodysgenesis that leads to glaucoma occurs in a variety of ways and may involve one or more of the three angle structures: the trabecular meshwork, the iris and the cornea, so the extent of maldevelopment is indicated by the presence or absence and degree of trabeculodysgenesis, iridodysgenesis and corneodysgenesis. These defects occur in a variety of combinations with attributes that have therapeutic and prognostic significance.

Table 1: Hoskins's anatomic classification of developmental glaucomas

I. Isolated trabeculodysgenesis (malformation of trabecular meshwork in the absence of iris or corneal anomalies)		
	A Flat iris insertion	1. Anterior insertion
		2. Posterior insertion
		3. Mixed insertion
II. Iridotrabeculodysgenesis (trabeculodysgenesis with iris anomalies)		
	A Anterior stromal defects	1. Hypoplasia
		2. Hyperplasia
	B. Anomalous iris vessels	1. Persistence of tunica vasculosa lentis
		2. Anomalous superficial vesssels
	C. Structural anomalies	1. Holes
		2. Colobomata
		3. Aniridia
III. Corneotrabeculodysgenesis (usually has associated iris anomalies)		
	A. Peripheral	
	B. Midperipheral	
	C. Central	
	D. Cornea size	

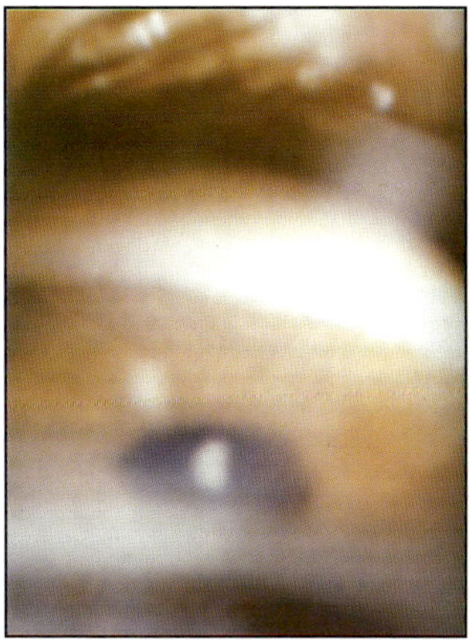

Figure 1: Anterior insertion

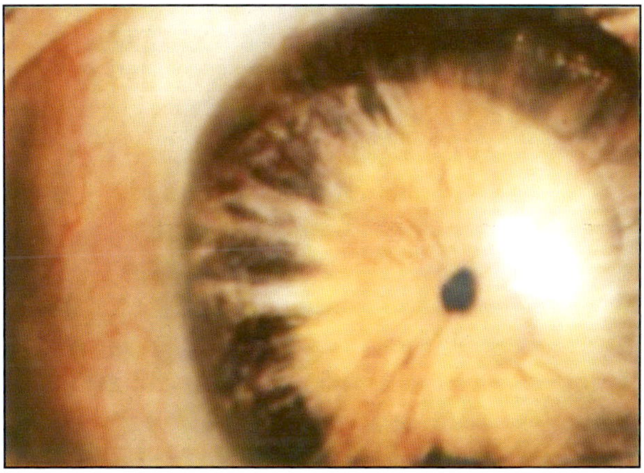

Figure 2: Hypoplasia iris

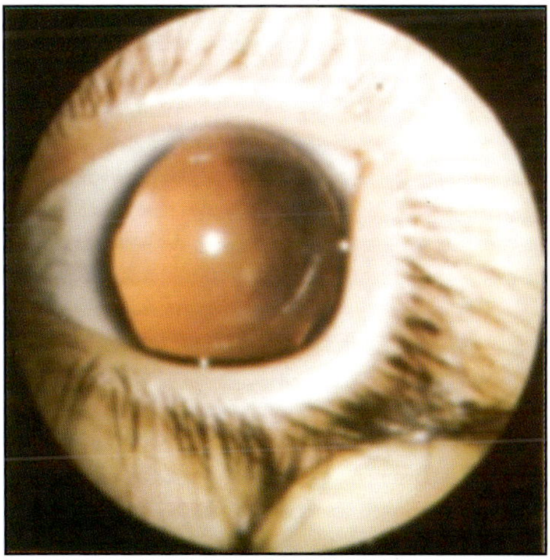

Figure 3: Aniridia congenita

Pathophysiology

Although the exact mechanism of *Primary Infantile Glaucoma* remains unproven, it is generally related to an iridocorneal angle malformation, with an obstacle to aqueous humor outflow. Some investigators have suggested that a cellular or membranous abnormality in the trabecular meshwork is the primary pathologic mechanism. This abnormality is described as either an anomalous impermeable trabecular meshwork or a Barkan membrane covering the trabecular meshwork. Other investigators have emphasized a more widespread anterior segment anomaly, including abnormal insertion of the ciliary muscle. Many of these features suggest a development arrest in the late embryonic period.

Clinical Features

Diagnosis of *Infantile Glaucoma* depends on careful clinical evaluation, including IOP measurement, measurement of corneal diameter, gonioscopy, measurement of axial length by ultrasonography and retinoscopy, and ophthalmoscopy.

Table 2: Diagnosis of Infantile Glaucoma

Name:		
Birthday:		
	Right eye	Left eye
Corneal		
edema		
Horizontal diameter		
Vertical diameter		
Gonioscopy		
Iris		
Lens		
IOP (type of tonometer)		
Ultrasonography		
AC		
Axial length		
Paquimetry		
Ophthalmoscopy		

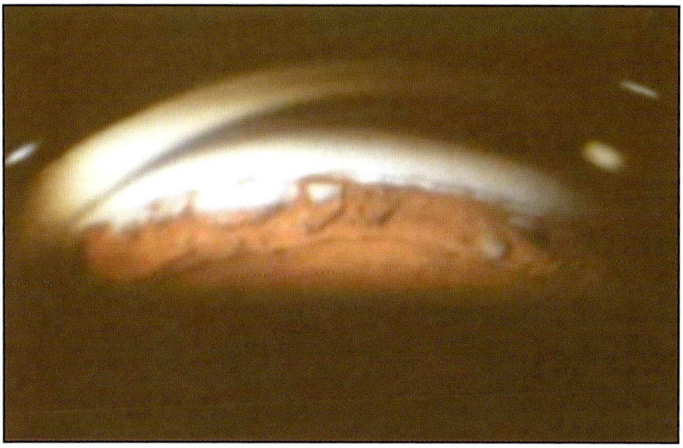

Figure 4: Axenfeld syndrome

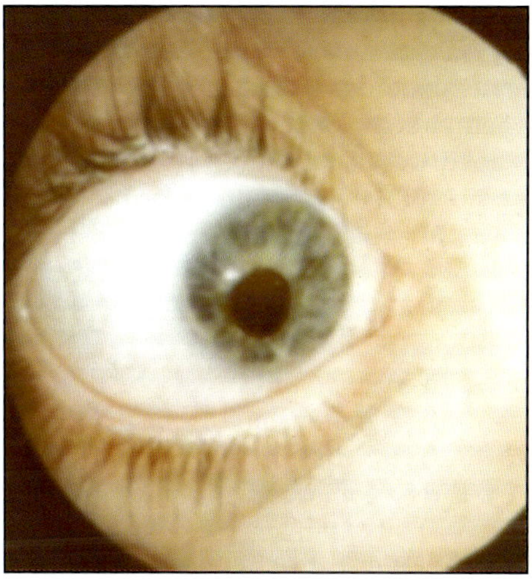

Figure 5: Axenfeld-Rieger syndrome

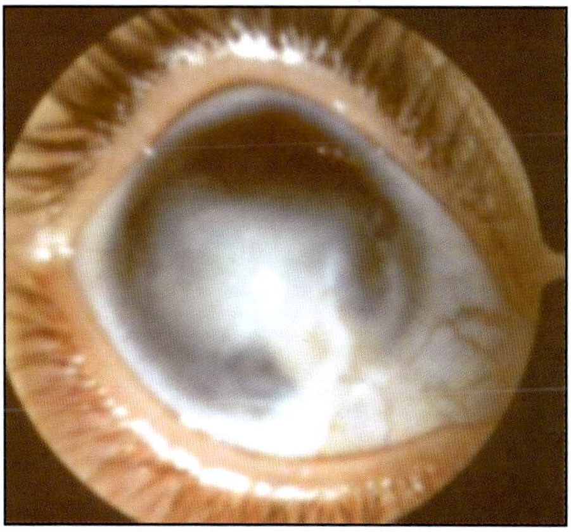

Figure 6: Peters anomaly

Characteristic findings of *Infantile Glaucoma* include the classic triad of presenting symptoms in the newborn: *epiphora, photophobia and blepharospasm.* External eye examination may reveal *buphthalmos* with corneal enlargement greater than 12 mm in diameter during the first year of life (the normal horizontal corneal diameter is 9.5-10.5 mm in the full-term newborns and smaller in premature newborns). Corneal edema may range from mild haze to dense opacification of the corneal stroma because of elevated IOP (corneal edema is present in 25% of affected infants at birth and in more than 60% by the sixth month). Tears in Descemet's membrane called *Haab's striae* may occur acutely as a result of corneal stretching.

Critical evaluation of infants requires an examination under anesthesia. Most general anesthesic agents and sedatives lower IOP, so the normal IOP in an infant under anesthesia may range form 10 to 15 mm Hg, depending on the tonometer. Measurement of corneal diameter with a caliper, gonioscopy, measurement of axial length by ultrasonography and ophthalmoscopy under anesthesia is recommended.

In *Primary Infantile Glaucoma*, the anterior chamber is characteristically deep with normal iris structure. Findings include a high and flat iris insertion, absence of angle recess, peripheral iris hypoplasia, tenting of the peripheral iris pigment epithelium and thickened uveal trabecular meshwork. The angle is typically open, with a high insertion of the iris root that forms a scalloped line as a result of abnormal tissue with a shagreened, glistening appearance. This tissue holds the peripheral iris anteriorly. The angle is usually avascular, but loops of vessels from the major arterial circle may be seen above the iris root. The normal anterior chamber angle in childhood is different from the adult angle. Many of the findings just listed are nonspecific, and it may be difficult to distinguish the gonioscopic findings in infantile glaucoma from a normal infant angle.

Visualization of the optic disk may be facilitated by using a direct ophthalmoscope and a direct gonioscopic or fundus lens on the cornea. The optic nerve head of a normal infant is pink with a small physiologic cup. Glaucomatous cupping in childhood resembles the cupping in adulthood, with preferential loss of neural tissue in the superior and inferior poles. In childhood, the scleral canal enlarges in response to the elevated IOP, causing enlargement of the cup. Cupping may be reversible if IOP is lowered, and progressive cupping indicates poor control of IOP.

Medications have limited long-term value for *Infantile Glaucoma* in most cases, and the preferred therapy is surgical.

If there are high suspect of glaucoma, the parents must be inform and the surgical procedure must be done immediately after the first examination under anesthesia.

Surgical Treatment

Introduction

Surgery is preferred for several reasons, including problems with compliance with medications, lack of knowledge about the systemic effects of medications

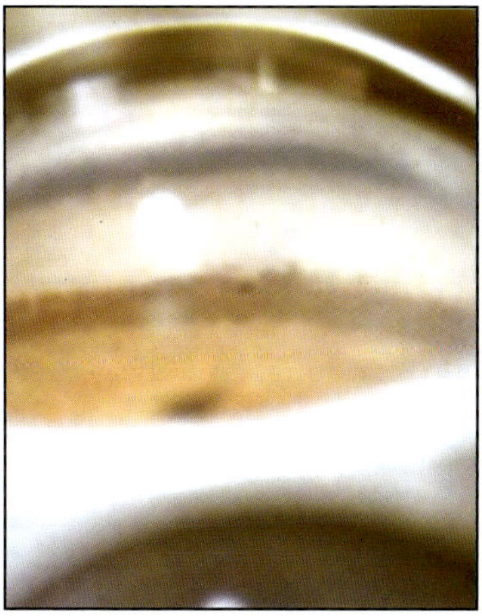

Figure 7: Abnormal angle

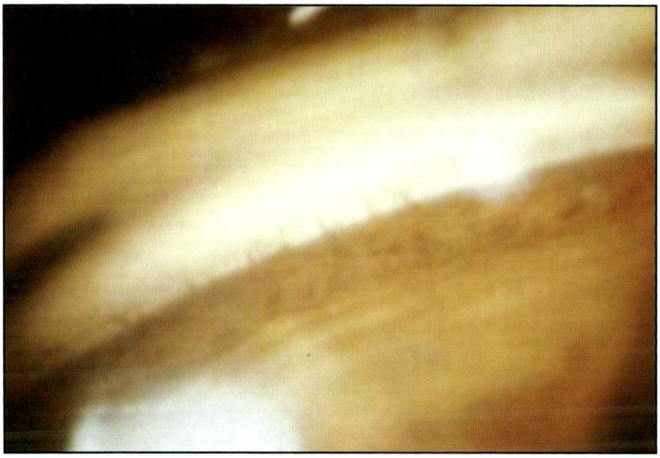

Figure 8: Iris process

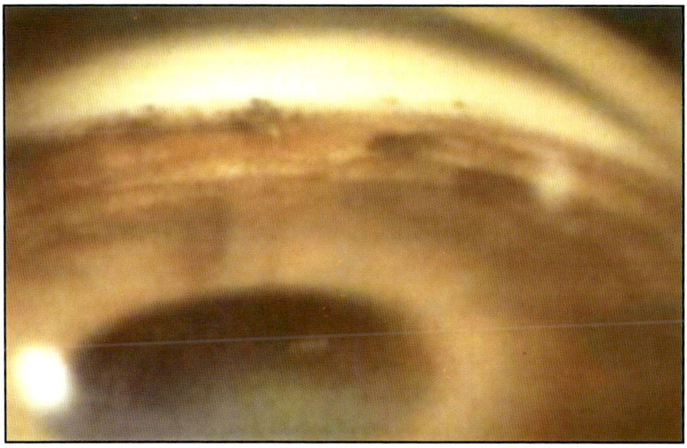

Figure 9: Pigmented angle

in the infant and infants' generally poor response to medications. Most important, surgery has a high success rate (however, success rates vary markedly among the anatomic forms of infantile glaucoma) and a low incidence of complications.

In children under 2 to 3 years of age goniotomy or trabeculotomy are recommended. Trabeculotomy is recommended for children over 2 to 3 years of age and for all children in whom corneal clouding prevents adequate visualization of the angle. Combined trabeculotomy — trabeculectomy is recommended in the group of iridotrabeculodysgenesis or failed previous angle surgery (2 or < goniotomies and/or trabeculotomies). Drainage implant surgery is done after failed trabeculectomy with intraoperative mitomycin C and when there is reasonable visual potential or high-risk for complications with filtraction surgery (e.g., Sturge-Weber syndrome). Transscleral cyclophotocoagulation is recommended in failed angle surgery and minimal visual potential, failed trabeculectomy and/or implant with poor central vision, IOP too high after glaucoma implant with encapsulation but not blockage and high-risk for complications with filtraction surgery (e.g., Sturge-Weber syndrome).

Preoperative Management

Some time medications play an auxiliary role before the surgery. Oral carbonic anhydrase inhibitors, primary acetazolamide, have effectively reduced elevated IOP. When administered orally with food or milk three or four times dairy (total dose 10 to 20 mg/kg/day), acetazolamide is fairly well tolerated. Topical dorzolamide together with apraclonidine 0.5% could be used in select cases. In goniotomy and trabeculotomy, to obtain miosis, pilocarpine 1% should be placed onto the eye to be operated upon just before surgery to protect the crystalline lens from injury during surgery.

Angle Surgery

The introduction of angle surgery made a revolution in infantile glaucoma procedures. In fact, the poor prognosis of infantile glaucoma changed dramatically with the introduction of goniotomy by Otta Bakan in 1938 (Gk. *gonio*, "angle", and *tomein*, "to cut"). Although the instrumentation has since been refined and the operating microscope now permits more precise visualization of the angle structures, the operation has remained essentially unchanged.

A further advance in management came in the 1960s with the introduction of trabeculotomy by Allen and Burian and Smith , which was popularized by Harms and Dannheim .

Both goniotomy and trabeculotomy have their staunch advocates. Trabeculotomy is our preferred operation for the following reasons :

- Trabeculotomy has a documented higher success than goniotomy. The latter controls intraocular pressure is about 74% of the eyes having glaucoma of all degrees of severity, although control may be as high as 85% if eyes with corneal clouding are excluded.

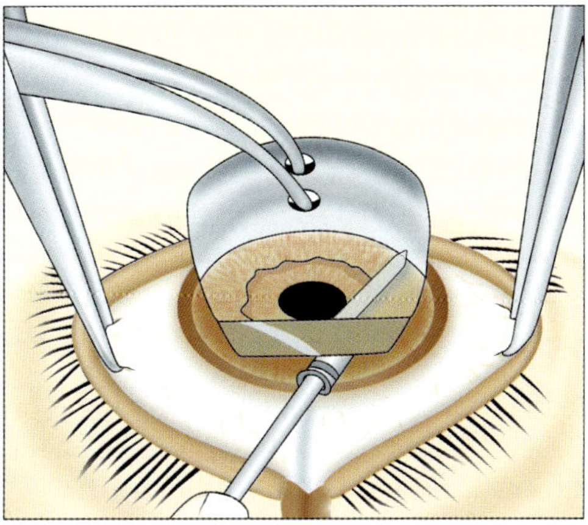

Figure 10: Goniotomy using a Barkan lens and Swan goniotomy knife

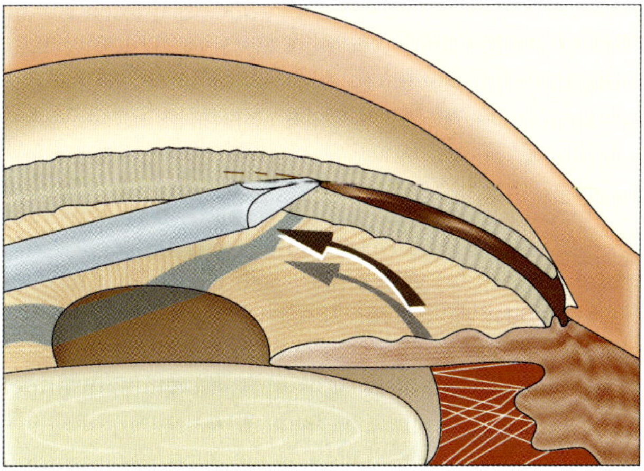

Figure 11: Correct location and depth of the goniotomy incision

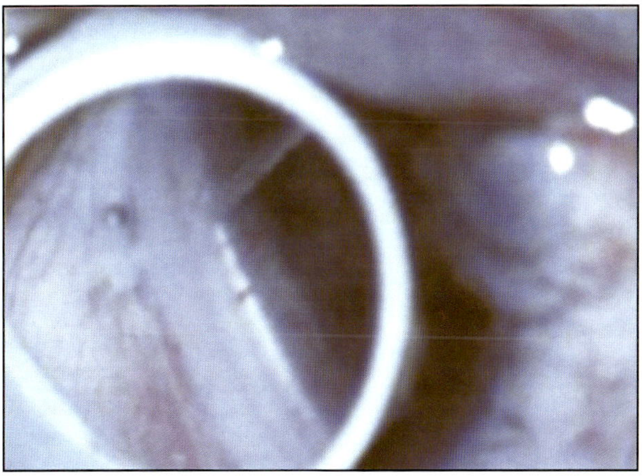

Figure 12: Goniotomy using a Swan-Jacob lens

- Trabeculotomy is technically easier for a well-trained microsurgeon because it does not require the introduction of sharp instruments across the anterior chamber, which increases the risk of damage to other ocular tissues. It can be performed with the same accuracy in advanced cases in which the cornea is edematous or scarred and there is poor visibility in the anterior chamber.
- There no need for the surgeon to adapt to the visual distortion produced by the operating gonioprism.
- A trabeculotomy is anatomically more precise in creating an opening between the anterior chamber and Schlemm's canal, and there is the advantage to associate a viscocanulostomy.
- The success of trabeculotomy depends only on the type of angle anomaly and not dependent on the severity of the glaucoma, the size of the cornea, or the presence of corneal edema, as the goniotomy does.

Goniotomy

The aim of goniotomy is to open a route for aqueous humor to exist the anterior chamber into Schlemm's canal by removing obstructing tissue and it is performed using a surgical goniolens and a goniotomy knife. There are several available goniolenses, in addition to the round-domed Barkan goniolens, including the Lister modification, which includes irrigation, or the Swan-Jacob's lens, which incorporates a handle and facilitates use of a microscope, or Worst lens. Numerous modifications of Barkan's goniotomy knife have been described, including attached fiber optics for intraocular illumination . A non-tapered Swan knife enters the anterior chamber easily and cuts in either direction. Alternatively, a disposable 23- or 25-gauge needle attached to a syringe containing viscoelastic may used in place of a knife, allowing the anterior chamber to be deepened before incision and to be maintained upon instrument removal. The perform goniotomy safely and effectively, corneal clarity must be sufficient to allow an adequate view of the angle structures. The surgeon usually sits opposite the portion of the angle to be operated, with the patient's head slightly rotated away from the surgeon. Viscoelastic may placed onto the central cornea just before placing the operating goniolens. The goniolens may be stabilized with a nontoothed fine forceps in the positioning holes of the lens, or it may be modified to include a handle. The goniotomy knife or needle is placed through peripheral clear cornea 1 mm from the limbus, opposite the midpoint of the intended goniotomy, in a plane parallel to the iris. It is guided over the iris tissue to engage trabecular meshwork in its anterior third, just posterior to Schwalbe's line. A circumferential incision is then made for about 4 to 5 clock hours. The incision must be superficial. Postoperative treatment includes the use of topical antibiotic, steroid, and miotic.

Mild to moderate hyphemas commonly occur after goniotomy, but they almost always clear rapidly without sequelae over several days. Other complications following goniotomy are rare and include iridodialysis, cyclodialysis, small peripheral anterior synechiae in the incised angle, damage to the crystalline lens.

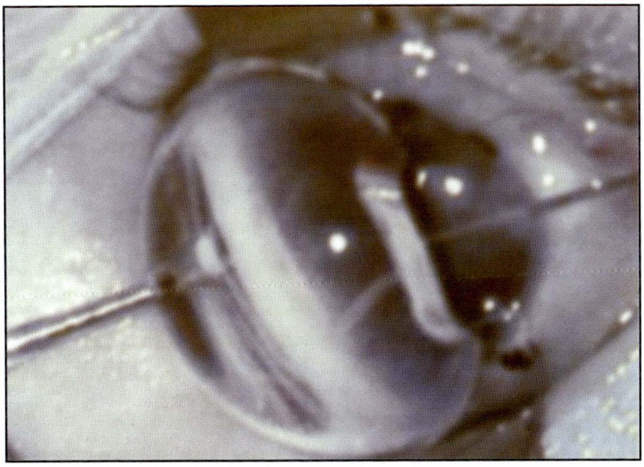

Figure 13: Goniotomy using a Worst lens

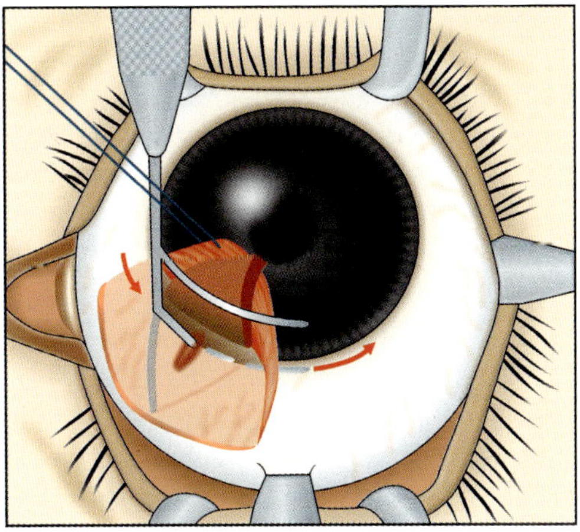

Figure 14: Trabeculotomy under a limbus-based conjunctival and partial-thickness scleral flap

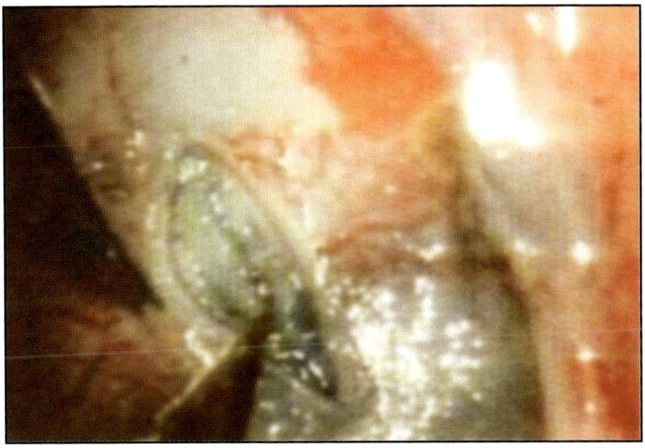

Figure 15: Radial incision of the Schlemm's canal

The results of goniotomy should be evaluated weekly in the immediate postoperative period. Gonioscopy after successful goniotomy often reveal a widened angle in the previous incision site, with improved visibility of the ciliary band and scleral spur. Because 4 to 5 clock hours of angle tissue are incised with single goniotomy, repeat procedures in untreated portions of the angle may enhance pressure control in selected cases. Goniotomy may fail to control infantile glaucoma in some instances because of improper placement and depth of the angle incision, or the obliteration of the incision by peripheral synechiae.

The success of goniotomy in controlling glaucoma varies with the etiology of the glaucoma. The best results – 80% to more than 90% success after one or two procedures – are achieved in infants with primary infantile glaucoma presenting between 3 months and 1 year of age . Success rates are much lower for cases of primary infantile glaucoma presenting either at birth or after 12 months of age (about 30 to 50%) . The success of goniotomy depends also on the size of the cornea, or the presence of corneal edema .

The need to use a multiple lens system (operating microscope, goniotomy lens, lens-cornea-fluid meniscus and cornea) to visualize the angle, as well as the above changes in the cornea that reduce visualization, combine to make goniotomy a difficult and hazardous procedure. To improve visualization the corneal epithelium may be removed. Use of prismatic lenses to view the angle also usually requires tilting of the operating microscope, further reducing its resolution power.

Trabeculotomy

The surgical technique of trabeculotomy is performed by cannulating Schlemm's canal from external approach and then tearing through the trabecular meshwork into the anterior chamber. This procedure thus creates a direct communication between the anterior chamber and Schlemm's canal.

In the surgical technique described by McPherson , a limbal based conjunctival flap and a partial-thickness triangular or rectangular scleral flap are created as for standard trabeculectomy.

Alternatively, the procedure may be easier to perform under a small fornix-based conjunctival peritomy. After partial-thickness scleral flap has been created, a radial scratch incision is made in the bed of the scleral flap across the sclerolimbal junction (2.5 to 3 mm posteriorly the surgical limbus). This scratch incision is gradually deepened under high magnification until Schlemm's canal is identified just anterior to the circumferential fibers of the scleral spur (near the posterior aspect of the limbal "gray zone").

Often a small amount of blood or aqueous humor refluxes through the cut ends of Schlemm's canal, and the internal wall of the canal appear slightly pigmented. To confirm the identity of the canal, a Grieshaber cannula should threat easily to both the left and right sides of the radial incision. If resistance is met, the radial incision must be deepened, or a second parallel radial incision must be done. Once the canal has been located, I like to do viscocanalostomy

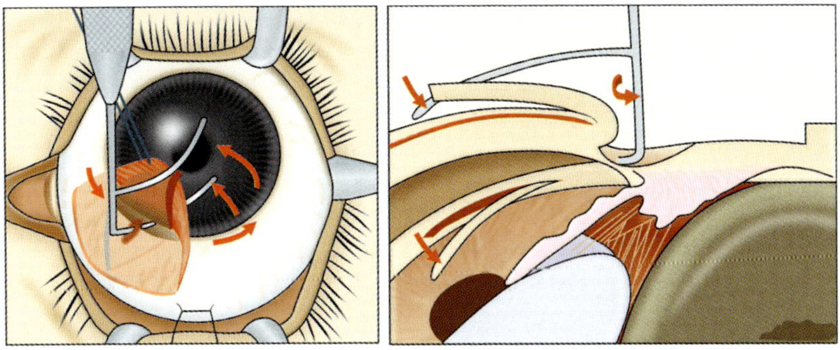

Figure 16: Rotation of the trabeculotome into the anterior chamber

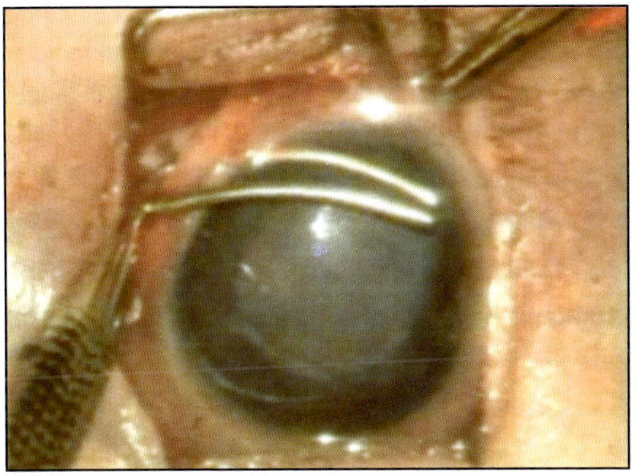

Figure 17: Trabeculotomy

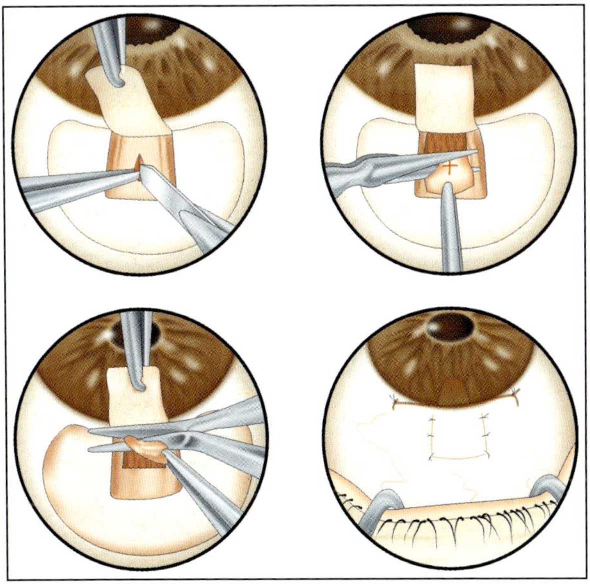

Figure 18: Technique for combined trabeculotomy—trabeculectomy

with Grieshaber cannula with and sodium hyaluronate at 1.4%. This procedure turns the introduction of the trabeculotome easier, enlarging the Schlemm's canal and destroying any bands. After this, the internal arms of the trabeculotome should be passed gently into the canal as far as possible without meeting resistance, and using the parallel external arm as a guide. The internal arm is then gently rotated into the anterior chamber, with care to avoid entry into the peripheral cornea or beneath the iris plate. Rotation of the trabeculotome into the anterior chamber tears through the intervening trabecular meshwork and requires very little force. Rotation should be halted once about 75 to 80% of the internal arm of the trabeculotome is visible in the anterior chamber. The trabeculotome is removed from the eye along its path. In similar fashion, the trabeculotome should be placed into the other side of the radial incision and the procedure repeated. The scleral flap and the conjunctive are then sutured with 8-00 polyglactin. Subconjunctival antibiotic and steroid may be given at the end of surgery.

Postoperatively, patients are treated with topical antibiotics and steroids. While small hyphema occurs commonly after trabeculotomy, rarer complications include inadvertent filtering blebs, choroidal detachment, iridotomy, damage of the lens, false passages into the anterior chamber or suprachoroidal space, and infection .

The effects of trabeculotomy should be determined 3 to 4 weeks after surgery. This procedure may be repeated in the different portion of the angle if the effect is inadequate following the first procedure.

Success rates varying from 73 to 100% have been reported for trabeculotomy in infantile glaucoma . In a series of 71 patients (most with primary infantile glaucoma), Akimoto and colleagues reported total success probabilities of one or more trabeculotomies of 92.5% and 76.5% at 5 and 10 years, respectively .

Combined Trabeculotomy—Trabeculectomy

If Schlemm's canal has not been successfully cannulated or if previous similar trabeculotomy procedures have failed to control intraocular pressure, the trabeculotomy can be combined with a trabeculectomy by removal of a full-thickness block of limbal tissue in the bed of the scleral flap, followed by peripheral iridectomy as in the standard trabeculectomy.

Penetration into the anterior chamber is made slowed. The anterior chamber is entered at one corner through a small opening by careful dissection through Descemet's membrane, allowing aqueous humor to seep slowly out until the eye becomes soft, but without losing the anterior chamber. In buphthalmic eyes, the zonules may be stretched and, with penetration into the anterior chamber, vitreous can prolapse through the chamber. The risk of this complication can be reduced by slowly reducing intraocular pressure before completing the trabeculectomy. After the eye has softened, air or balanced salt solution is injected into the anterior chamber to maintain a moderate depth. The iridecotmy should be made carefully because vitreous may prolapse through a stretched and ruptured zonule and erupt through the iridectomy. If this occurs, a limited

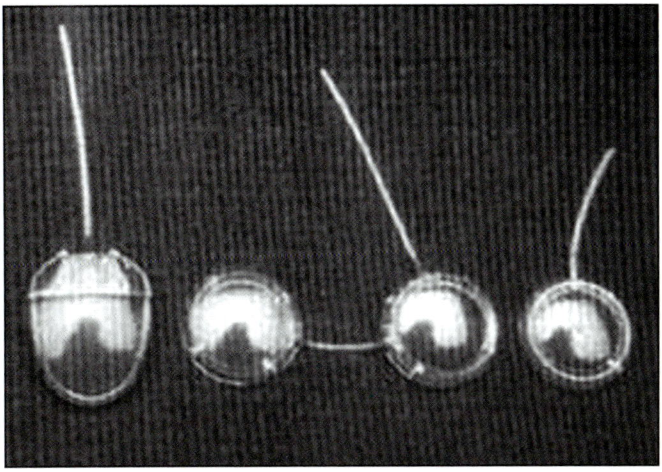

Figure 19: Ahmed valve Implant, double-plate and single-plate Molteno Implant

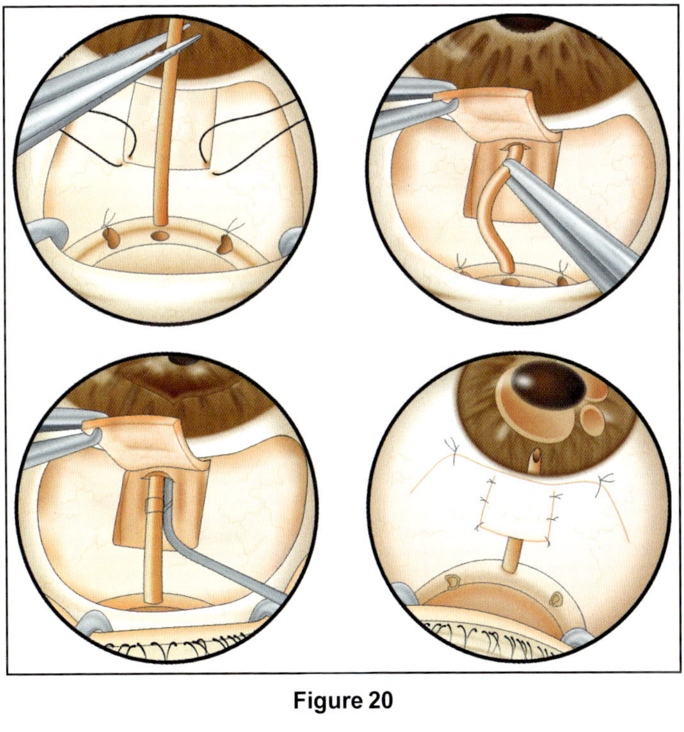

Figure 20

vitrectomy must be performed, removing all vitreous from the iridectomy and the immediately surrounding iris surface. This is best accomplished using sponges and Vannas scissors. The scleral flap and the conjunctiva are then sutured with 8-00 polyglactin. Subconjunctival antibiotic and steroid may be given at the end of surgery. If antimetabolites are used, I prefer limbus-based conjunctiva-Tenon's capsula flap, and is closed with continuous suture.

The postoperative management for the trabeculotomy, combined trabeculotomy—trabeculectomy or isolated trabeculectomy is the same. Intraocular pressure is checked in the office or by examination under anesthesia within 6 weeks of the surgical procedure. A cycloplegic is used in combined trabeculotomy—trabeculectomy or isolated trabeculectomy if there is a significant postoperative inflammation.

Some surgeons advocate combined trabeculotomy—trabeculectomy as the first surgery for infantile glaucoma.

Trabeculectomy

Filtering surgery is usually done when goniotomy and trabeculotomy either failed or are unlike to succeed. Poor outcome from trabeculectomy is most likely multifactorial, but several authors have reported much higher rates of success using primary trabeculectomy in children with glaucoma, mostly in infantile cases . Although subconjunctival 5-fluorouracil has been administered postoperatively in children after trabeculectomy, resulting in successful filtration, its administration usually requires multiple sequential anesthesias and is limited by corneal epithelial toxicity, as in the adults . The intraoperative use of mitomycin C has greatly enhanced the success of trabeculectomy in controlling glaucoma, presumable by limiting postoperative scaring by Tenon's capsula and scleral fibroblasts. The success of mitomycin C augmented trabeculectomy in chidren is much higher in those who are older and phakic. Hence several authors independently found young age and aphakia to be negative predictors of success . I do not use mitomycin C in a very young children, because the response is extremely variable, with some patients scarring rapidly despite antifibrotic therapy and others developing hypotony with large avascular filtraction blebs .

Synthetic Drainage Implants

Drainage implant surgery is done when it is a children whom failed trabeculectomy with intraoperative mitomycin C and reasonable visual potential or high-risk for complications with filtration surgery (e.g. Sturge-Weber syndrome). All modern drainage implant devices have the same basic design, which typically consist of a silicone tube that extends from the anterior chamber to a plate, disk, or encircling element beneath conjunctiva and Tenon's capsule. The edge of the external plate has a ridge, through which the distal end of the tube inserts onto the upper surface of the plate. The ridge decreases the risk of obstruction of the posterior opening of the tube with the surrounding tissue and fibrous capsule. The plates of the glaucoma drainage devices have large

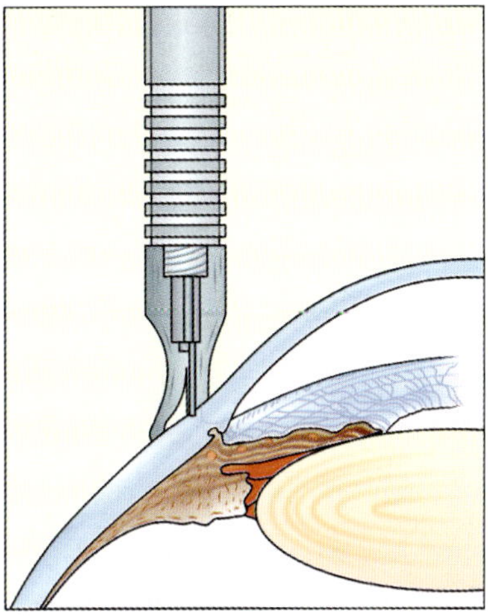

Figure 21: G-Probe

surface areas and promote the formation of the filtering bleb posteriorly, near the equator.

Performance of similar drainage devices can vary significantly, depending on the size, shape, and materials from which the external component and tube are constructed. One of the most fundamental design differences is the way the device has an open, unobstructed drainage tube or one that contains a pressure-regulating valve. Baerveldt, Molteno, and Schocket implants are the examples of open tube implants. Ahmed and Krupin implants are designed to have a flow-restricting valve mechanism.

Molteno Implant is the prototype drainage implant device and has had the longest and most extensive clinical experience since it was introduced by Molteno in 1969.

Ahmed glaucoma valve implant has a mechanism to decrease early postoperative hypotony by providing resistance to the flow and therefore regulating the pressure within a desired range. In this valved drainage implant design, a silicone tube is connected to a silicone sheet valve, which is held in a polypropylene body. The valve mechanism consists of two thin silicone elastomer membranes, which allows one-way regulation of the flow with a goal of keeping the IOP between 8 and 10 mm Hg in the early postoperative period. The inlet cross section of the chamber is wider than the outlet, which offers a theoretical small pressure differential between the anterior chamber and subconjunctival space, which is claimed to enable the valve to remain open even when only a small difference in pressure exist.

Only Molteno and Ahmed glaucoma valve implants are usually used in children eyes. Although certain variations of surgical techniques are required for implantation of the different implants, the basic surgical principles apply in general to all drainage implant devices.

Adequate surgical expose is dependent on proper placement of a traction suture. A 6-0 polyglactin or silk traction suture on a spatulated needle is placed through superficial cornea near the superior limbus and attached to the drape beneath the eye. A fornix-based conjunctive-Tenon's capsule flap is created, usually in the superotemporal quadrant, to expose the scleral bed. The initial conjunctival incision may be made approximately 2-3 mm from the limbus, to create a limbal based flap and to permit easier closed suture. The flap is slightly elevated to allow for blunt dissection between Tenon's and episclera with blunt Westcott scissors. Because it is necessary to have surgical exposure to or beyond the equador of the globe, radial relaxing incisions should be placed on one or both sides of the conjunctival flap. A muscle hook is then used to isolate the two rectus muscles on either side of the surgical site. With Ahmed valve implant it is necessary to irrigate balanced salt solution though the tube using 27-gauge cannula, before the insertion into the anterior chamber, to ensure that the valve opens properly. The external plate is then tucked posteriorly into sub-Tenon's space one sutured to sclera with 8-00 nylon sutures through the anterior positional holes of the plate. The anterior, border depending on the size of the globe, must be 6 to 8 mm posterior the limbus. After the plate been sutured a lamellar scleral flap must been dissected with 6 × 4 mm. Preplaced sutures at the corners of the flap will be looped out of the way. The tube of the flap is trimmed to size at its anterior end (2 to 3 mm into the anterior chamber). The anterior end of the tube is inserted into the anterior chamber via the needle track using a nontoothed forceps and is secured to the sclera with a loose nylon suture. The scleral falp is sutured back in place. The conjunctiva is then sutured back its original position using polyglactin sutures. Subconjuntival steroids and antibiotic are injected.

With Molteno implant, restriction of aqueous flow to avoid severe early postopearative hypotony can be achieved by using a two-stage implantation technique, in which the external plate is placed in the subconjunctival space without inserting the tube into the anterior chamber. The tube is inserted 6 to 8 weeks later, after the fibrous capsule has formed around the external plate. A more popular technique is to occlude the tube, this provides the advantage over the two-stage technique of avoiding a second operation. The tube can be occluded in different ways: a ligature of 6-0, 7-0, or 8-0 polyglactin before inserting it into the anterior chamber; an adjustable suture could be done.

Complications of drainage implantation in children include tube malposition, flat anterior chamber, tube obstruction by iris or vitreous, cataract, cornea-tube touch, choroidal detachment, corneal edema and corneal abrasion.

Cyclodestructive Procedures

The surgical procedures previously described all share the goal of increasing aqueous outflow from the eye. Cyclodestructive procedures reduce the rate of aqueous production by injuring the ciliary processes.

Indications for cyclodestructive procedures is usually reserved for situations in which repeated filtraction surgery are failure and when there is severely buphthalmic eye with extensive optic nerve pathology and a poor visual prognosis.

The success of the cyclodestrutive procedures is also modest (about 50%), results are often unpredictable, but with lower reported incidence of phthisis bulbi and hypotony. The cyclodestructive procedures used are cyclocryotherapy and transscleral cyclophotocoagulation.

Cyclocryotherapy presumably destroys the ability of ciliary processes to produce aqueous humor by the biphasic mechanism of intracellular ice crystal formation and ischemic necrosis.

The mechanism by which transscleral cyclophotocoagulation lowers IOP is not fully understood. The prevailing theory is that it reduces aqueous production by damaging the pars plicata, although it is not clear whether this due to direct destruction of the ciliary epithelium or reduced vascular perfusion. In ours days it is available the *neodymium:YAG* and the *semiconductor diode* lasers. Advantages of these laser techniques over cyclocriotherapy include less transient IOP rise, a less exuberant uveitic response, and less pain postoperative.

Cyclocryotherapy

Cyclocryotherapy has been used as therapy for infantile glaucomas for many years, and is applied with a similar technique to that used in adults. In children, cryotherapy should be applied to a maximum of 180 degrees of the circumference of the eye at one session, using six or seven freezes (60 seconds each at – 80 degrees Celsius) with the anterior edge of a 2.5 mm diameter cryoprobe placed 1 to 1.5 mm from the limbus, in a nonbuphthalmic eye, and placed 1.5 to 2 mm from the limbus in a buphthalmic eye. Placement of the probe directly over the 3 and 9 o' clock positions should be avoided to prevent damage to the long posterior ciliary vessels. In addition to limited success rates, the risk includes not only hypotony or phthisis, but also uveitis, cataract formation, and attendant visual loss. Al Faran et al. reported 30% success after one or more treatments in a large series of children with advanced infantile glaucoma .

Trans-scleral Cyclophotocoagulation

Neodymium:YAG Lasers

Neodymium:yttrium aluminum garnet (Nd:YAG) lasers, with a wavelength of 1,064 nm, are useful for transscleral cyclophotocoagulation because they transverse the sclera with relatively low absorption and scatter. They may be operated in a continuous-wave mode, and be delivered by a contact probe, fiberoptic system.

Continuous-wave mode: The SLT CL60 (Surgical Laser Technologies) provides contact probe delivery in a continuous-wave of 0.1 to 10 seconds. A 2.2 mm Sappire-tipped, handheld probe, which is focused at 1.5 to 2 mm in air, is coupled to a fiberoptic delivery system. The unit can provide powers in excess of 10 W. the SLT is the unit on which most of the early experience with contact, continuous-wave Nd:YAG transscleral cyclophotocoagulation is based. A subsequent instrument, the Microruptor 3 (MR3) also provides continuous-wave Nd:YAG laser energy, which can be delivered by either a 600 μm, flat tip, quartz fiber probe or a slit-lamp.

This technique has been performed primary with the SLT, using exposure times of 0.5 to 0.7 seconds. The laser focus is fixed by the design of the probe tip, which is held perpendicular to the surface of the conjunctiva with the anterior edge of the probe 0.5 to 1.5 mm behind the limbus; 32 to 40 applications of 7 to 9 W for 0.5 to 0.7 seconds are applied for 360 degrees, often sparing the 3 and 9 o′ clock positions. Limited experience with Nd:YAG contact transscleral cyclophotocoagulation in young children with advanced, uncontrolled glaucoma suggest effective pressure reduction in approximately 40% after a single 360 degrees treatment.

Semiconductor Diode Lasers

Although semiconductor diode lasers, with a range of wavelengths between 750 and 850 nm, do not transverse the sclera as efficiently as Nd:YAG lasers, they have the advantage of greater absorption by uveal melanin. In addition, they have the advantage of solid-state construction with compact size, lower maintenance requirements, and no special requirement for electric outlet or water cooling. The Oculight SLx (Iris Medical Instruments) is a continuous-wave, contact delivery diode laser with a wavelength of 810 nm, a maximum power output of 2.5 to 3.0 W, and a maximum duration of 9.9 seconds. The probe (G-Probe) consists of a 600 μm quartz fiberoptic, protruding 0.7 mm from a handpiece, which is fabricated to center the fiberoptic 1.2 mm behind the surgical limbus and parallel to the visual axis. The back of the G-Probe pushes the limbus away from the surgical site, and the sides can be used to aide in spacing the laser applications. Initial settings are 1,750 mW and 2 seconds. If a popping sound is heard with the initial application, the power is reduced by increments of 250 mW until no pop is heard. If no pop is heard with the initial application, the power is increased by the increments until the sound is heard and then reduced by one increment. The laser applications are spaced circumferentially by placing the side of the G-probe footplate adjacent to the indentation mark of the previous fiberoptic placement. The original protocol involved 18 applications for 270 degrees, avoiding the 3 and 9 o'clock positions because this reduce the chances of occluding the long posterior ciliary vessels and thus reduce the chance of anterior segment ischemia. The rate success of this technique is of 30 to 75% after one or more treatments.

Postoperative inflammation can be a significant problem, requiring special prophylactic measures. One approach is to give a subconjunctival injection of a short acting steroid at the end of the procedure and to prescribe topical atropine and steroid for approximately 10 days. Postoperative pain also tends to be mild, with many patients requiring no analgesic. The most significant complication associated with transscleral cyclophotocoagulation is loss of visual acuity. The precise mechanisms are not fully understood, but likely causes include macular edema associated with the inflammatory. Maximum pressure reduction is typically achieved in 1 month, and it is usually desirable to wit at least this long before retreating.

Long-term Follow-up

Patients with infantile glaucoma require follow-up examinations for life.

Long-term medical therapy in children can be difficult because of side effects and compliance problems. Medical therapy is used primary in difficult cases that have not responded well to surgical intervention.

Prognostic Factors

It appears that the surgical prognosis for patients with infantile glaucoma is best when the onset of the disease occurs between the first and the twenty-fourth month of life. The reasons for this are unclear. Earlier cases with onset at birth may represent a more severe developmental disorder. Later, possibly changes of trabecular tissues or apposition and compression of the wall of Schlemm's canal or impermeability of the canal's inner wall play a role.

Various factors, such as the age of onset, may affect the prognosis . On the other hand, surgery is generally more successful when performed as early as possible. It is generally accepted that the success of goniotomy is not as good in eyes with significant buphthalmos.

The appearance of the anterior chamber angle is of great prognostic significance. In the group of isolated trabeculodysgenesis, the angle anomaly may be result of incomplete development of tissue derived from neural crest cells. These patients have the best prognosis for either goniotomy or trabeculotomy, over 90% achieving intraocular pressure control. In the group of iridotrabeculodysgenesis, the anomaly involves the peripheral iris and the trabecular meshwork and is the result of a cicatricial process in the periphery of the anterior chamber angle. These patients have a far poorer prognosis with surgery, particularly goniotomy or trabeculotomy, which have success rates approximately 30%. Patients undergoing trabeculectomy, combined trabeculotomy—trabeculectomy have success rate of approximately 50%. When filtration surgery fails, a glaucoma drainage implant or cyclodestructive procedure would be indicated. Some surgeons consider drainage implants as the primary procedure in these patients. In the group of corneotrabeculodysgenesis (Axenfeld-Rieger syndrome and Peters' anomaly, for example) the prognosis is also poor with trabeculotomy or goniotomy and better with trabeculectomy, but many of these patiens also finally require a drainage implant or cyclodestrutive procedure. However, even with the use of a drainage implant, the prognosis for successful surgery in groups 2 and 3 probably not exceed 60%.

Chapter 16

Pediatric Glaucoma

Nicola Freeman (South Africa)

Introduction

The pediatric glaucomas are a heterogeneous group of conditions. Primary maldevelopment of the aqueous outflow system may be named ***primary congenital glaucoma*** when presenting at birth, ***primary infantile glaucoma*** when presenting at birth to three years of age or ***primary juvenile glaucoma*** when presenting at three to sixteen years old. The secondary pediatric glaucomas include the ***secondary developmental glaucomas***, e.g. aniridia, Sturge-Weber/ periorbital port wine stain, neurofibromatosis, hyperplastic primary vitreous, Peter's anomaly and the ***secondary pediatric glaucomas***, e.g. aphakic, uveitic, traumatic, cicatricial ROP, ectopia lentis, intraocular neoplasm and steroid induced glaucomas.

Clinical Presentation

Primary Congenital Glaucoma (PCG) and Primary Infantile Glaucoma (PIG)

- Epiphora, photophobia, blepharospasm = clinical triad of PCG
- Corneal clouding, corneal enlargement, corneal edema
- Haab's striae (curvilinear breaks in Descemet's membrane)
- Optic disk cupping (stretching of optic canal in young patients; may be reversible)
- Raised intraocular pressure on tonometry (Tonopen, Perkins or Goldman tonometry).

Secondary Developmental Glaucomas and Secondary Pediatric Glaucomas

- Seldom present with the above mentioned symptoms
- Diligent follow-up and IOP monitoring essential in conditions such as aphakia, uveitis, trauma, ROP, intraocular neoplasm, aniridia, periorbital port wine stain, neurofibromatosis, hyperplastic primary vitreous and Peter's anomaly.
- Up to 1/3 of pediatric aphakic and pseudophakic eyes develop glaucoma. There are usually no clinical symptoms and long-term vigilance is necessary to make the diagnosis early.

Differential Diagnosis

1. Of epiphora:
    - Nasolacrimal duct obstruction
    - Conjunctivitis
    - Corneal epithelial defect or abrasion
    - Ocular inflammation.

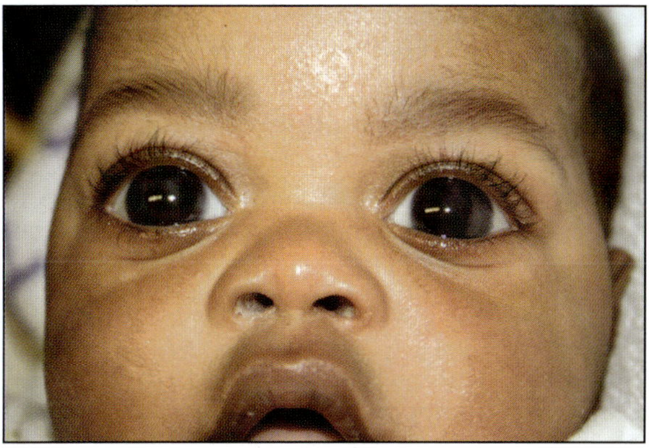

Figure 1: Bilateral buphthalmos with corneal enlargement and scarring

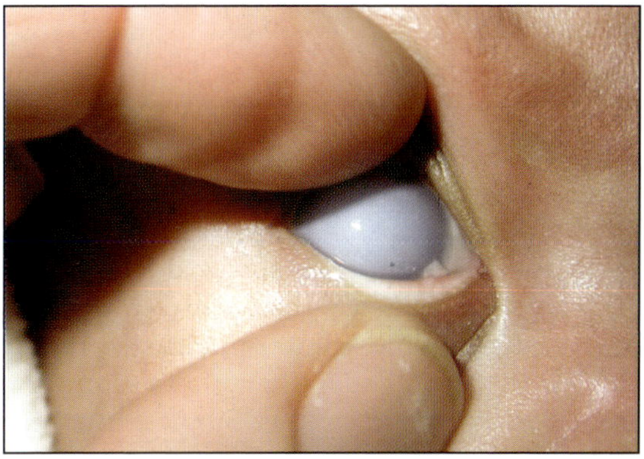

Figure 2: Differential diagnosis: The cloudy cornea of Rubella keratitis

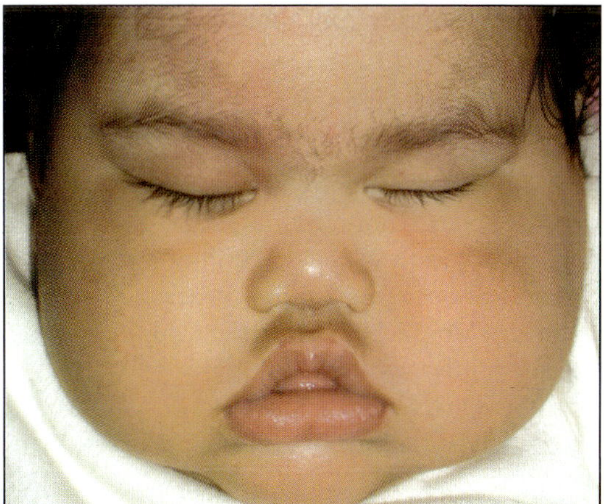

Figure 3: Right periorbital port wine stain or cutaneous hemangioma in Sturge Weber can be subtle in infancy. This child was born with right buphthalmos and had a diffuse choroidal hemangioma of the right eye with leptomeningeal changes on CT scan

2. Of corneal edema or opacification:
   - Rubella keratitis – Rubella also causes microphthalmos and congenital glaucoma
   - Birth trauma – forceps delivery causing Descemet's tear
   - Congenital anomalies – Sclerocornea, Peter's anomaly
   - Storage diseases – Mucopolysaccharidoses, cystinosis
   - Corneal dystrophies – congenital hereditary endothelial and posterior polymorphous dystrophy.
3. Of enlarged cornea:
   - Megalocornea
   - Axial myopia.
4. Of enlarged optic nerve cupping:
   - Optic nerve coloboma or malformations
   - Optic nerve hypoplasia or atrophy.

Management

General Management

- Examination under anesthesia (EUA): Ketamine hydrochloride IVI using local anesthetic patch. Atropine and midazolam pre-med. NB Inhalation anesthetics all decrease IOP unpredictably and substantially.
- Examination: IOP, corneal diameters and corneal changes, corneal thickness, anterior segment, angle gonioscopy, optic disks, retina and vitreous, refraction, axial lengths and AC depth with ultrasound if possible.
- *Primary congenital and infantile glaucomas*: Surgical intervention—treatment of choice with medical used preoperatively and as adjunct to surgery.
- *Secondary developmental and secondary pediatric glaucomas*: Medical treatment first-line. Surgical intervention only when medical fails.

Surgical Intervention Options

- *Goniotomy:* corneal clarity required, angle surgery under direct visualization with goniotomy lens and goniotomy blade
- *Trabeculotomy:* corneal clarity not required, trabeculotome inserted into canal of Schlemm and swept into anterior chamber rupturing the trabecular meshwork. A temporal approach spares superior conjunctiva
- *Trabeculectomy:* antimetabolite modification usually necessary
- Combined trabeculectomy and trabeculotomy
- *Artificial drainage shunts:* refractory cases
- *Cyclodiode laser:* usually in last resort refractory cases.

Medical Treatment Options

- Punctal occlusion for 5 minutes reduces systemic effects.
- Topical beta-blocker: Betaxolol 0.25% (Betoptic S), Timolol 0.25% (Timoptic XE) (Beware asthma and cardiac problems)

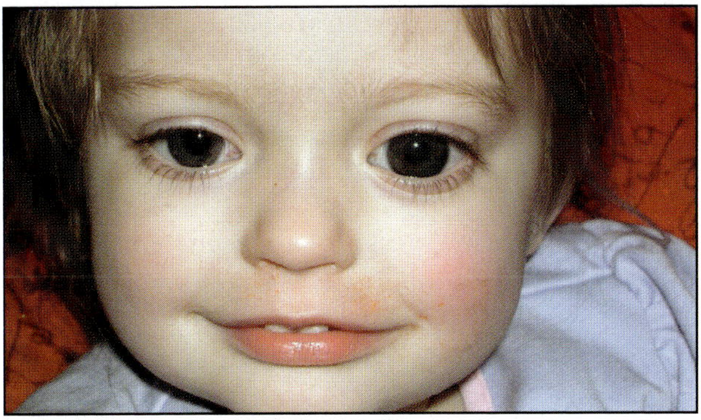

Figure 4: Left buphthalmos. The right eye is receiving atropine penalization for amblyopia management

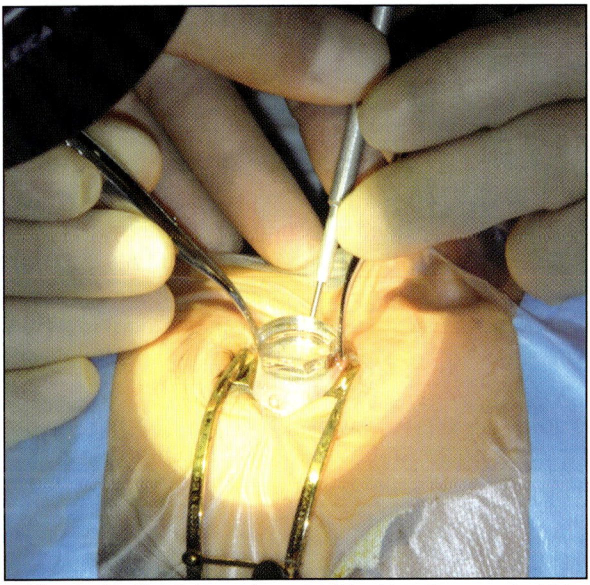

Figure 5: Goniotomy lens and locking forceps held by assistant in goniotomy procedure

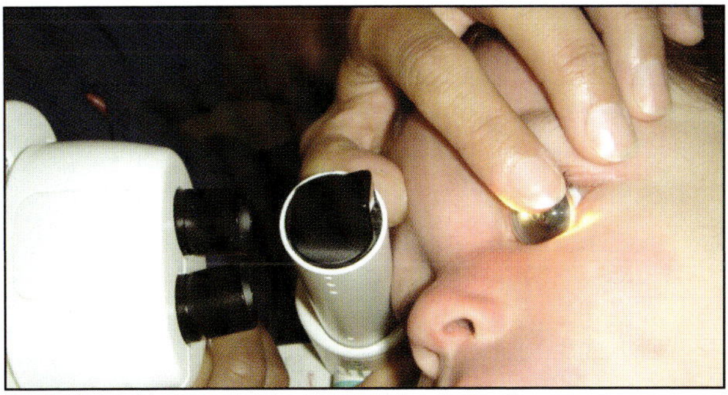

Figure 6: Slit-lamp examination with the Koeppe lens in a child with Sturge-Weber glaucoma

- *Topical carbonic anhydrase inhibitors:* Dorzolamide (Trusopt), Brinzolomide (Azopt)
- *Prostaglandin derivatives:* Travaprost (Travatan), Bimatoprost (Lumigan), (Latanoprost (Xalatan)
- *Oral carbonic anhydrase inhibitors:* Acetazolamide (Diamox) 10-30 mg/kg/day; qid
  (Beware metabolic acidosis. Use short-term preoperatively only)
- A*lphaagonists:* may cause apnea, bradycardia, hypotension.

Follow-up

- Regular EUAs required when uncooperative age
- Monitor IOP, Corneal diameters, axial lengths, refraction
- Early detection and treatment of amblyopia.

Prognosis

Visual loss in childhood glaucoma is multifactorial. It may result from corneal scarring, optic nerve damage or amblyopia secondary to myopia, astigmatism or anisometropia.

Onset at birth, corneal diameter >14 mm and failed angle surgery are all poor prognostic indicators for *Primary congenital and primary infantile glaucoma.*

The poor prognostic indicators for Aphakic and pseudophakic glaucomas are younger age at cataract surgery and pre-existing ocular abnormalities. The role of preservation of the vitreous face at surgery and IOL placement is still uncertain.

Even in poor prognosis eyes, all attempts at IOP control should be continued. Any amount of vision preservation in a growing child is important for neural integration development.

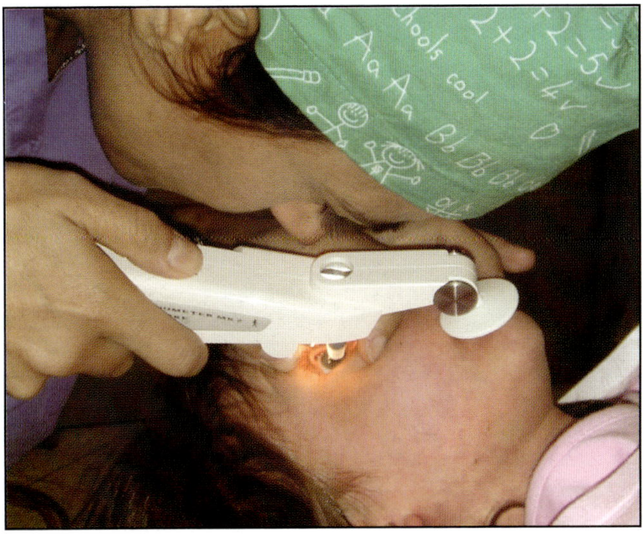

Figure 7: Perkins tonometer used in the examination under anesthesia

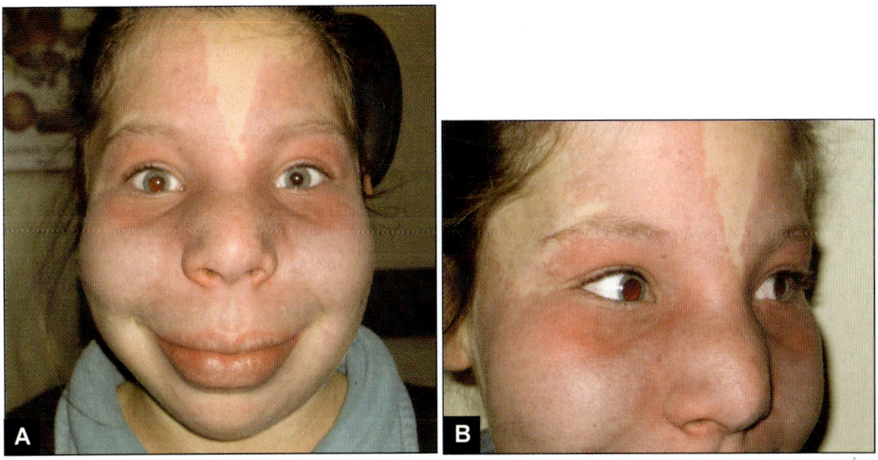

Figures 8A and B: Bilateral Sturge-Weber syndrome

Chapter 17

Glaucoma Implants in the Treatment of Pediatric Glaucoma

Peter WT de Waard (Netherlands)

Introduction

Management of primary congenital glaucomas is primarily surgical. Goniotomy or trabeculotomy each have success rates of 40-90% in the management of primary congenital glaucoma. In case of secondary glaucoma's associated with, e.g. aphakia, aniridia, anterior segment dysgenesis and Sturge-Weber syndrome, goniotomy or trabeculotomy success rates are low. When goniotomy or trabeculotomy fail or are inappropriate to control intraocular pressure (IOP) in pediatric patients, alternatives include filtering surgery or drainage implants.

Beck found that aqueous shunt implantation (Ahmed or Baerveldt) offers a significantly greater chance of successful IOP control compared with trabeculectomy with Mitomycine-C in infants up to 24 months of age. They found cumulative probabilities of success at 12 months of 87% for the aqueous shunt group and 36% in the trabeculectomy group. In pediatric patients in whom goniotomy, and/or trabeculectomy with or without antimetabolites have failed, success rates of 56-95% have been reported with these glaucoma implants.

Choice of Implant

As the normal IOP in children is the same as in adults, we may assume that the aqueous production at least equals that of adults. Studies showed that glaucoma implants with a large surface, like the Baerveldt 350 (mm^2), have higher success rates then the ones with smaller surfaces, like the Baerveldt 250 (mm^2) and the Ahmed (184 and 96 mm^2). So it seems justified to implant the Baerveldt 350 in children without a compromized aqueous production. The latter can be found in uveitic glaucoma or after cyclodestructive procedures. In these cases one should choose a smaller implant to reduce the risk of hypotony. In case one needs immediate lowering of the IOP, e.g. very high IOP unresponsive to maximal tolerable medical therapy, the valved Ahmed implant is the best choice.

Operation Technique of Baerveldt Implant

The sclera in the superior temporal quadrant is exposed with a limbus-based conjunctival flap, and the superior and lateral rectus muscles are identified and isolated with muscle hooks. The wings of the implant are positioned under the insertions of the muscles. The plate is secured 1-2 mm posterior to the insertions with 2 interrupted 9-0 nylon sutures. The tube is trimmed so that it would extend 1-2 mm beyond the posterior surgical limbus with the bevel toward the corneal endothelium. A stent (3-0 prolene), 1-2 mm in length, is passed into and down the tube and positioned ± 7 mm behind the limbus. The tube is ligated with 7-0 vicryl around the stent. This stent is used for easy constriction of the tube and ensures a watertight closure, preventing early postoperative hypotony. The stent itself hardly affects the flow through the tube (personal measurements with donor eyes). The tube will opened after 5-7 weeks. A paracentesis track through the cornea into the anterior chamber is made to

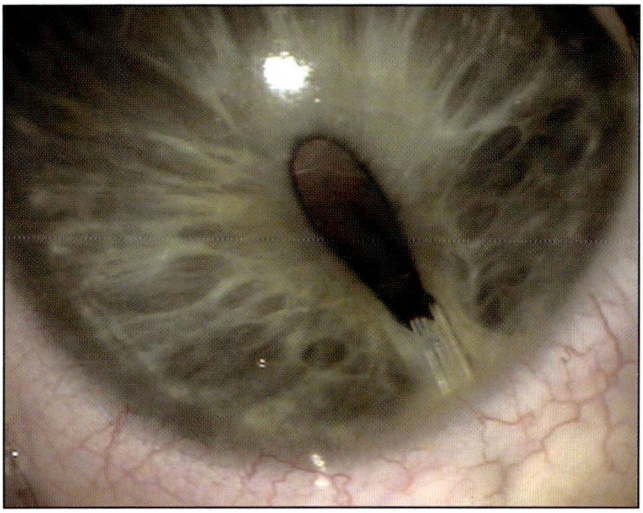

Figure 1: Dyscoria in buphthalmic eye with BGI

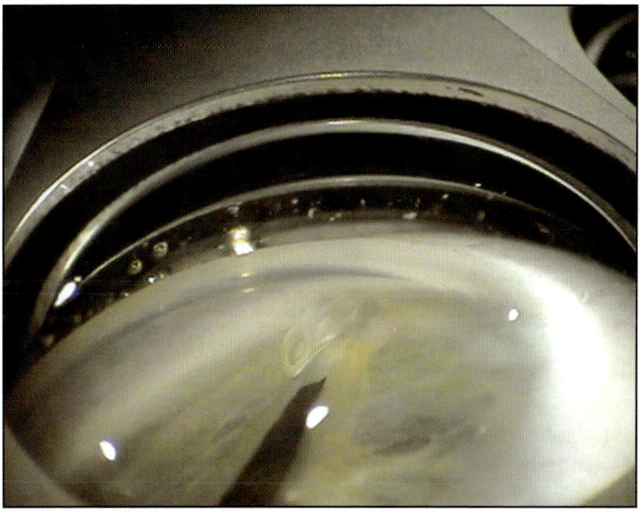

Figure 2: Gonioscopic view of dyscoria of Figure 1. Entrapment of peripheral iris in tube-track can be seen

control the IOP and the anterior chamber depth intraoperatively. A 23-gauge needle is used to create an opening for insertion of the tube into the anterior chamber. Glycerin-preserved donor sclera is used to cover the tube near the limbus and secured with interrupted 9-0 vicryl sutures. Finally tenon and conjunctiva are reapposed with running 9-0 vicryl sutures. A subconjunctival injection of corticosteroids is administered before the eye is patched. Postoperatively, topical steroids are tapered slowly and glaucoma medications are removed or added as IOP and clinical status requires. Many but not all steps apply to the other glaucoma implants as well.

Preoperative and postoperative examinations must include slit-lamp examination, ophthalmoscopy, IOP measurement with a pneumatonometer (Model 30 classic, Mentor O and O, Norwell, MA, USA), and measurement of axial length by ultrasound A-scan (A-5500 A-scan system, Sonomed, Lake Success, NY, USA). Most examinations are performed under general anesthesia in patients younger than 6 years. Older patients may be able to undergo examinations in the office.

Complications

Early postoperative high IOP can be medically treated. Early postoperative hypotony does not require treatment as long as the anterior chamber (AC) is not flat. Logically, IOP lowering medication can be stopped. This hypotony can be caused by a little flow of aqueous through the needle-track round the tube or more serious by inadequate closure of the tube. The latter will very often lead to a flat anterior chamber needing reclosure of the tube with 7-0 vicryl under general anaesthesia as soon as possible.

The tube will open 5-7 weeks postoperatively. A relatively large volume of aqueous will flow through the tube from the anterior chamber to the filtration bleb formed around the plate of the BGI. Consequently, a transient shallow anterior chamber and hypotony can be seen until the bleb is filled with aqueous and an equilibrium is reached between the IOP and the counterpressure in the bleb.

After opening of the tube the IOP depends on the diffusion of aqueous through the wall of the bleb. In its turn, this diffusion depends on the surface and the thickness of the blebwall. The surface is controlled by the choice of platesize (e.g. Baerveldt 350 or 250 mm^2). The thickness depends on the reaction of Tenon´s to the silicon implant before and to aqueous humor after opening of the tube. As the active reaction to aqueous continues for life, slow changes in the thickness of the blebwall will lead to IOP changes. In this way, late hypotony can not only be caused by compromized aqueous production but also by thinning of the blebwall due to inhibition of the mitotic activity of fibroblasts (e.g. methotrexate in the treatment of juvenile idiopathic arthritis). The latter cause of hypotony can be treated by temporary occlusion of the tube (vicryl 7.0) and injection of autologous blood in the bleb to increase the thickness of the blebwall. Antimetabolites should be reduced or stopped if possible.

In case the blebwall becomes to thick and the resulting high IOP can not be medically controlled, a second glaucoma implant should be placed because the thickness of the blebwall can only be controlled (thinning) with a, probably nonacceptable, longlasting treatment with antimetabolites.

The most frequent complication of the BGI is tube related, varying from mild dyscoria to tube exposure. Studies reported 6.5-39.1% tube related complications. The variability in the published incidence of tube related complications after BGI, may be partly due to inclusion of differing proportions of buphthalmic eyes in these studies. The thin elastic sclera in buphthalmic eyes gives little support to the implanted tube and predisposes these eyes to changes in size and shape when the IOP is reduced, leading in turn to tube related complications.

In our study dyscoria was observed, only in buphthalmic eyes, shortly after opening of the tube caused by entrapment of a tuft of peripheral iris tissue in the needle-track. The entrapment could be a result of a shallow anterior chamber during the period of hypotony after opening of the tube, in combination with movement of the tube in the needle-track creating space next to the tube due to thin elastic sclera. It seems likely that movement of the tube is induced by movement of the eyelids over a hypotonous eye. In combination with the dycoria we often see an anterior movement of the tube, eroding through the thin sclera, frequently coming in close contact with the cornea endothelium. These eyes need to be reoperated by opening the conjunctiva/tenon at the limbus, removing the tube from the anterior chamber, closing the tube-track and replacing the tube in the AC through a new track. The latter must be made as long as possible, the sclera giving more support to the tube. Future adjustments to the tube and avoiding the hypotonous period with valves could diminish or even prevent these tube related problems.

In case of tube exposure immediate recovering of the tube with donor sclera, tenon and conjunctiva is required because of the high-risk of endophthalmitis.

Tube retraction asks for extension of the tube. This is best performed in the fornix near the connection of tube and plate. The tenon and conjunctiva overlying the tube is opened (± 6 mm) and the soft fibrous capsule encircling the tube is incised. The exposed tube is cut (± 5 mm proximal to the connection of tube and plate) and the extension is placed between the two ends. Because the silicon tube slides through the encircling capsule very easily, the long proximal part of the tube can be advanced into the AC. Sometimes the conjunctiva/tenon has to be opened at the limbus to assist the (re)entrance of the tube into the AC.

In case the tube in the AC becomes too long, the diameter of the bulbus becoming smaller after lowering of the IOP, the AC can be filled with viscoelastics and the tube can be shortened intraocularly with fine vitreous scissors. The cut end is removed by vitreous forceps through the same paracentesis.

Studies of pediatric patients with glaucoma implants report motility disturbances in 0-16% after implantation. Similar findings (0-10%) were noted after implantation of an Ahmed or Molteno implant in pediatric patients. Motility problems are believed to be secondary to a mass effect from the equatorial filtering bleb, a Faden or posterior fixation effect induced by scarring under the rectus muscle, or fat adherence syndrome. In our study we found mild motility disturbances postoperatively in 7.3% of the patients. Strabismus surgery was necessary in only one patient, the motility disturbances in the other patients being transient after 4-6 months.

Conclusion

Glaucoma implants are effective and safe in the management of pediatric glaucoma, despite its propensity for tube related postoperative complications. One must be prepared to follow these patients a life time and deal with many possible complications, especially the tube related problems.

Chapter 18

Sclerothalamotomy ab Interno: A Minimally Invasive Surgical Option for Glaucoma

Bojan Pajic (Switzerland)

Introduction

The ongoing devote on recent developments in glaucoma surgery reflects that an ideal solution is not available which would promise long-term IOP reduction and eliminate the necessity of supplementary pressure-reducing medication at low complication rates. Trabeculectomy, first described in the sixties, is probably the most widespread approach in glaucoma surgery presently. The intention of trabeculectomy is to bypass the resistance of trabecular meshwork by channelling aqueous humor directly to the Schlemm's canal. In literature the success rate of trabeculectomy ranges between 32–96%. On the other hand, postoperative complications like hypotony and choroidal detachment are reported up to 24%. Variation of success rates may be explained by different criteria of surgical indications, selection of cases, various diagnoses, the various degrees of surgical experience and variations in postoperative medical treatment. Failure of pressure regulations is associated with the assence of a filtering bleb and depends on the duration of follow-up involved. It has become evident that successful reduction in IOP following trabeculectomy is clearly related to the presence of a filtering bleb.

The more recent method of non-penetrating deep sclerectomy, was first described by Fjodorov in the eighties. This techniques tries to achieves an improved uveoscleral outflow and therefore is not depending on the presence of a filtering bleb. Koslov expanded this method by introducing a collagen implant. Literature on non-penetrating deep sclerectomy indicates a success rate of 58 to 74% without collagen implant and 74 to 90% with collagen implantation.

In 1976, Benedikt described that the exposure of the ciliary body (i.e. a form of penetrating sclerectomy) was leading to successful long-term IOP regulation in 27 of 38 cases involving hemorrhagic, aphakic and irreversible angle-closure glaucoma after initially failed filtering surgery. This technique was the basis for later development of perforating deep sclerectomy, a method which has been used since 1985 was described previously (as "*sclerothalamectomy*"). Bypassing of the trabecular meshwork is an alternative for aqueous humor outflow from the anterior chamber to the Schlemm canal. It is the principal mechanism for non-penetrating glaucoma surgery, in particular, for deep sclerectomy and viscocanalostomy. These surgical procedures provide effective IOP reduction as well as the elimination of typical filtration bleb complications. So far clinical application of these procedures has been limited by technical difficulties to perform this kind of surgery and a poor predictability of pressure reduction.

The concept of trabecular meshwork bypass as a surgical principle for glaucoma treatment evolved from the discovery that pathologic outflow resistance is caused primarily by the juxtacanicular conjunctive tissue of the trabecular meshwork and, in particular, by the inner wall of the Schlemm canal. A further publication in this area indicates that 35% of the outflow resistance arises distally to the inner wall of the Schlemm canal.

Spiegel et al have described a new surgical technique involving the use of an implanted tube, the so-called trabecular meshwork bypass tube shunt, which

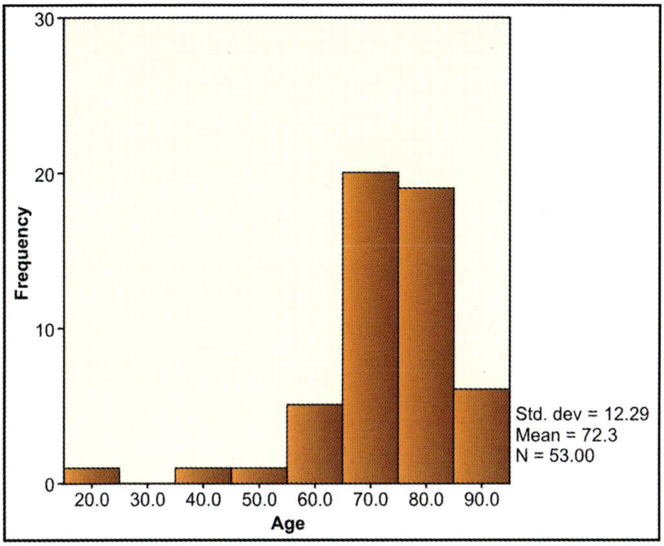

Figure 1: Mean age

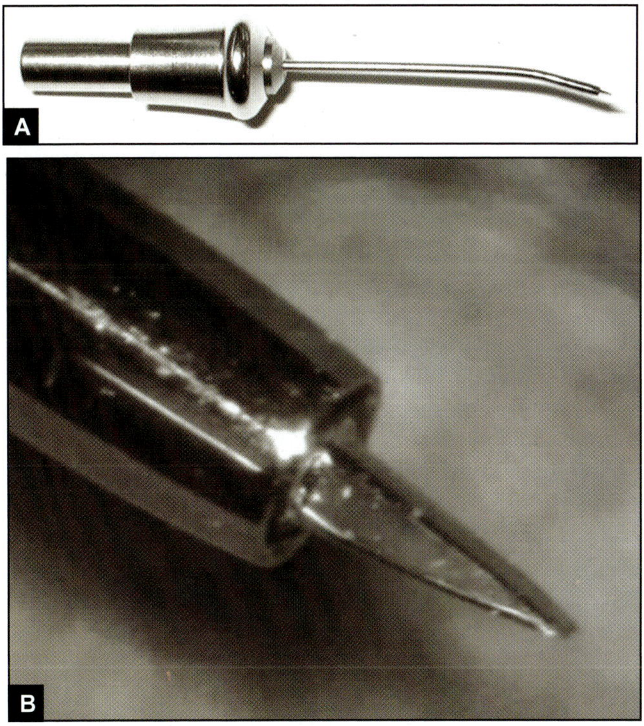

Figures 2A and B: STT glaucoma tip (Oertli Reference VE 201750)

should provide a direct connection between Schlemm's canal and the anterior chamber. This surgical technique avoids technical difficulties of non-penetrating deep sclerectomy, especially the delicate microperforation of the trabecular meshwork in order to ensure the permeability of the Descemet membrane. Furthermore, these techniques avoid the disadvantages of filtration blebs.

All surgical procedures for glaucoma involving the creation of external access may be complicated by the risk of fibroblast proliferation and failure of filtration. The novel procedure published offers a chance to avoid some of the above-mentioned disadvantages. We refer to this technique as *sclerothalamotomy ab interno.*

Patients and Methods

Before beginning the clinical study phase, the tips used for the STT ab interno procedure were developed using a large number of pigs' eyes. The high-frequency diathermic technique was already very well known in the application for capsulorhexis in cataract surgery. It was important to create a design for optimal application of the STT probe in the iridocorneal angle and to evaluate the charcteristic of the achieved deep sclerotomy. By virtue of this results the STT ab interno probe development as describe below.

53 sclerothalamotomies ab interno in 53 patients were carried out in primary open-angle glaucoma between 1 April 2002 and 31 July 2002. Main inclusion criterion into this study was an insufficient response to medical treatment of IOP. Data was documented according to a prospective study protocol. Mean age of patients was 72.3 ± 12.3 years (range: 15-92 years). 17 patients (32%) were female, 36 patients (68%) male. In 25 cases (47.4%) the right eye in 28 cases (52.6%) the left eye was treated. There was no patient who received bilateral surgery. Snellen visual acuity was 0.7 ± 0.3 (range 0.1 to 1.0) preoperatively. In 5 cases a moderate cataract was observed which didn't have influence on the visual acuity.

A complete ophthalmologic status check was carried out in each patient prior to surgery including: uncorrected and best corrected visual acuity, IOP applanation tonometry, biomicroscopy of anterior segment, funduscopy (in particular, stereoscopie evaluation of the optic nerve head) and computerized visual field testing (Octopus 101, program G2).

Complete ophthalmologic follow-up examinations were carried out postoperatively at day 1, 2, 3 and 4, after 1, 2 and 4 weeks, and 2, 3, 6, 12, 15, 18, 21, 24, 27, 30, 33 and 36 months.

In a pilot study with at least of 24 months follow-up, 5 patients with therapy-resistant juvenile glaucoma were treated.

High-frequency Diathermic Probe

The high-frequency diathermic probe consists of an inner platinum electrode which is isolated from the outer coaxial electrode. The platinum probe tip is

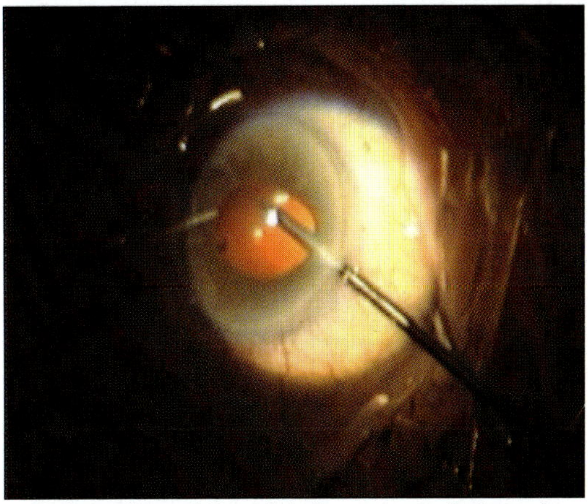

Figure 3: Insertion of the high-frequency diathermic probe (Oertli) through the temporal corneal insertion

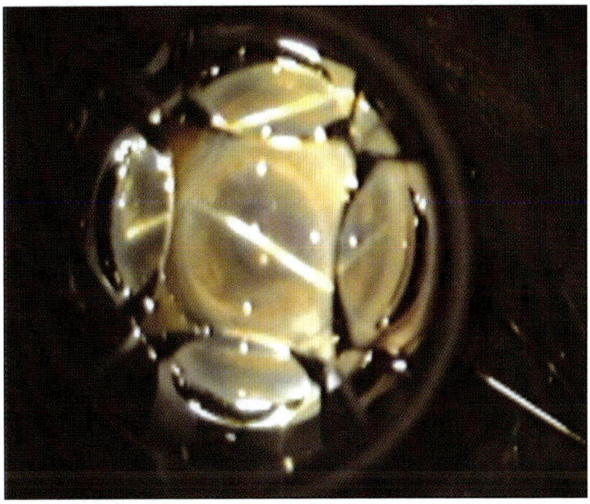

Figure 4: Visual inspection of the target zone (opposite iridocorneal angle) by a 4-mirror gonioscopic lens

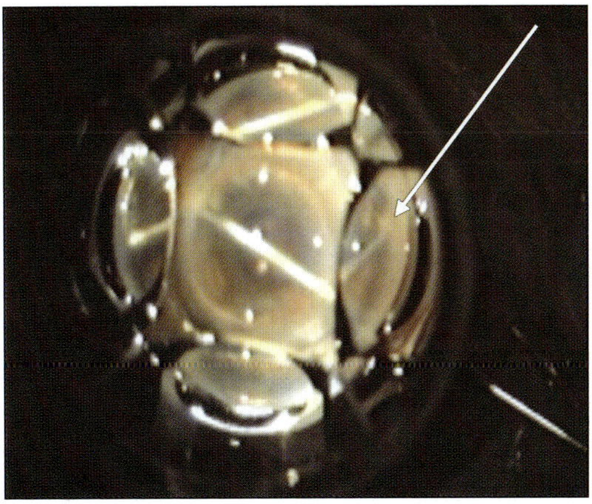

Figure 5: Penetration of the high frequency tip

1 mm in length, 0.3 mm high and 0.6 mm width and is bent posteriorly at an angle of 15°. The external diameter of the probe measures 0.9 mm. Modulated 500 kHz current generates a temperature of approximate 130°C at the tip of the probe. The setup provides high frequency power dissipation in close vicinity of the tip. As a result, heating of tissue is locally very limited and is applied as a rotationed ellipsoid.

Surgical Procedure

A clear cornea incision (1.2 mm wide) was placed in the temporal upper quadrant using a diamond knife. A second corneal incision was performed 120° apart from the first followed by injection of Healon GV. The high-frequency diathermic probe (Oertli) was inserted through the temporal corneal insertion. Visual inspection of the target zone (opposite iridocorneal angle) was observed by a 4-mirror gonioscopic lens. The high-frequency tip penetrates up to 1mm nasal into the sclera through the trabecular meshwork and Schlemm canal, forming a deep sclerotomy (i.e. "thalami") of 0.3 mm high and 0.6 mm width. This procedure was repeated 4 times within one quadrant. Healon GV was evacuated from the anterior chamber with bimanual irrigation/aspiration. Tobramycin/ Dexamethason eye drops were then applied 3x daily for 1 month and Pilocarpin 2% eye drops 3x daily for 10 days.

Evaluation of the Results

Statistical evaluation of results was calculated with SPSS Program Version 10. Two-tailed Student t-test was used for statistical evaluation of parametric data. The unit of significance was set at a critical p value of < 0.05, including Bonferroni correlation for repetitive use of data sets.

Results

Mean preoperative IOP in the study population of 53 patients with primary open-angle glaucoma was 25.6 ± 2.3 mm Hg (range 18 to 48 mm Hg). Average IOP was 17.6 ± 2.7 mm Hg (range 2 to 36 mm Hg) after a follow-up period of 1 day, 14.9 ± 2.4 mm Hg (range 2 to 30 mm Hg) after 2 days, 15.7 ± 2.4 mm Hg (range 4 to 28 mm Hg) after 3 days, 16.0 ± 2.6 mm Hg (range 4 to 36 mm Hg) after 4 days, 19.0 ± 2.6 mm Hg (range 12 to 39 mm Hg) after 7 days, 16.9 ± 2.5 mm Hg (range 9 to 44 mm Hg) after 1 month, 15.1 ± 1.8 mm Hg (range 11 to 20 mm Hg) after 3 months, 14.7 ± 1.7 mm Hg (range 11 to 20 mm Hg) after 6 months, 14.8 ± 1.7 mm Hg (range 10 to 20 mm Hg) after 9 months, 14.7 ± 1.7 mm Hg (range 10 to 20 mm Hg) after 12 months, 15.5 ± 1.7 mm Hg (range 11 to 20 mm Hg) after 15 months, 14.1 ± 1.6 mm Hg (range 11 to 20 mm Hg) after 18 months, 16.5 ± 1.7 mm Hg (range 12 to 22 mm Hg) after 21 months, 15.0 ± 1.6 mm Hg (range 11 to 20 mm Hg) after 24 months, 14.7 ± 1.7 mm Hg (range 11 to 20 mm Hg) after 27

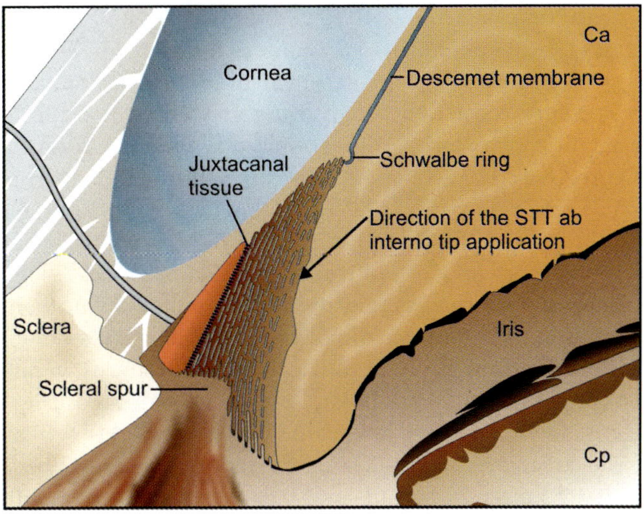

Figure 6: Penetration up to 1 mm nasal into the sclera through the trabecular meshwork and Schlemm canal

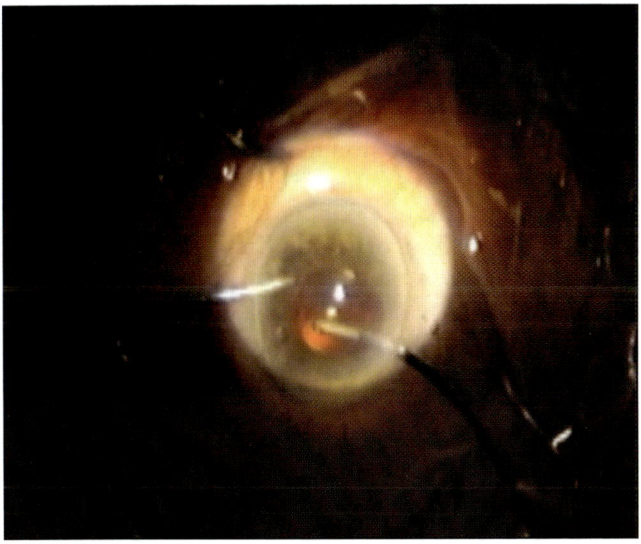

Figure 7: Healon GV was evacuated from the anterior chamber with bimanual irrigation/aspiration

months, 14.7 ± 1.7 mm Hg (range 10 to 20 mm Hg) after 30 months, 15.5 ± 1.7 mm Hg (range 11 to 20 mm Hg) after 33 months and 14.6 ± 1.7 mm Hg (range 10 to 20 mm Hg) after 36 months a result which, at $p < 0.005$, is statistically highly significant. Pressure reduction at any time of standardised follow-up was statistically significant compared to preoperative data at a level of $\alpha < 0.03$ (Bonferroni corrected). For all patients the follow-up was 36 months.

At month 36, 54.7% of patients had an IOP< 15 mm Hg, 77,4% had an IOP< 18 mm Hg and 83% had an IOP< 21 mm Hg. After 36 months, 86.8% achieved > 20% reduction in IOPs and 77% of treated patients achieved > 30% reductions of the IOP. The complete success rate, defined as an IOP lower than 21 mm Hg without medication, was 83% at 36 month. Qualified success rate, defined as an IOP lower than 21 mm Hg with medication, was 100% at 36 months.

The average preoperative administration of pressure-reducing eye agents was 2.6 ± 1.0. Following surgery, this value was decreased to 0.45 ± 0.72 after 1 month, 0.38 ± 0.60 after 3 months 0.38 ± 0.69 after 6 months, 0.19 ± 0.52 after 12 months, 0.21 ± 0.53 after 24 months and 0.50 ± 0.90 after 36 months. After 36 months, it was necessary to administer IOP reducing medication in only 9 eyes, a figure which corresponds to 17% of all cases.

Average visual acuity after treatment was 0.69 ± 0.31 (range 0.05 to 1.0). In 6 eyes (11.3%) moderate cataract development after surgery which was without influence of visual acuity. Another 3 eyes (5.7%) developed cataract with decreased visual acuity of one Snellen line.

There is no significant difference regarding the cup/disk ratio at baseline with 0.65 ± 0.18 and at 36 months with 0.66 ± 0.19 ($p = 0.11$).

There is no significant changes comparing the visual field at baseline with mean defect MD 9.45 ± 2.32, loss variance LV 30.0 ± 5.11 and at 36 months with MD 9.29 ± 2.59, LV 31.4 ± 5.66 ($p = 0.78$ for MD, $p = 0.96$ for LV).

Temporary IOP elevation higher than 21 mm Hg was observed in 12 of 53 eyes (22.6%). These patients responded well to pressure-reducing treatment with one agent and medication could gradually be withdrawn in all of these patients. A single case of hypotension (1.9%) that lasted for 3 days after surgery was observed. Hyphema was present in 6 cases (11.4%) which disappeared within the first 2 weeks after surgery. One eye (1.9%) exhibited transient fibrin formation at pupillary level. Fibrin was cleared within one day after frequent application of topical Dexamethason.

In a pilot study 5 patients with therapy-resistant juvenile glaucoma were treated. We observed an IOP reduction from 41 ± 6.4 mm Hg prior to surgery to 12 ± 2.6 mm Hg after surgery, a result that has remained stable without any additional pressure-reducing therapy for 24 months.

Discussion

This study reports long-term results of a new surgical technique for treating open angle glaucoma. The STT ab interno method intends the creation of a direct channel between the anterior chamber and the Schlemm canal. Persistence

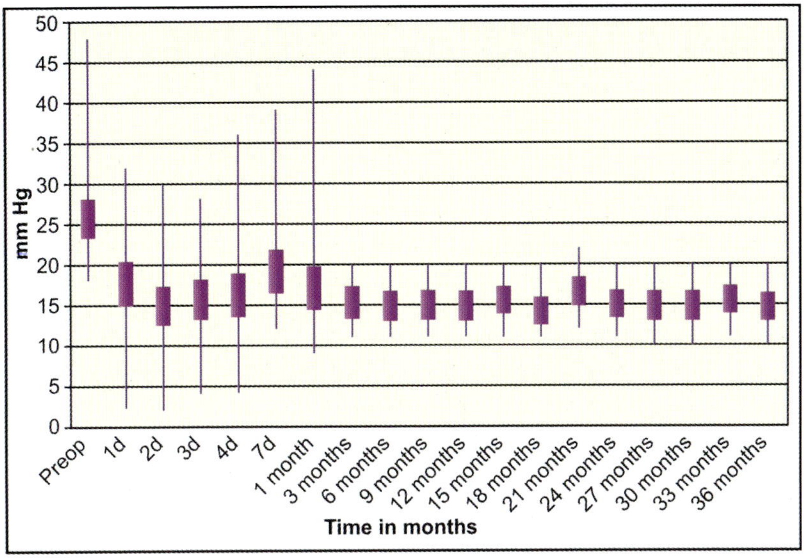

Figure 8: Average level of intraocular pressure (IOP) after Sclerothalamotomy (STT) ab interno surgery for all 53 cases at the time of scheduled examination

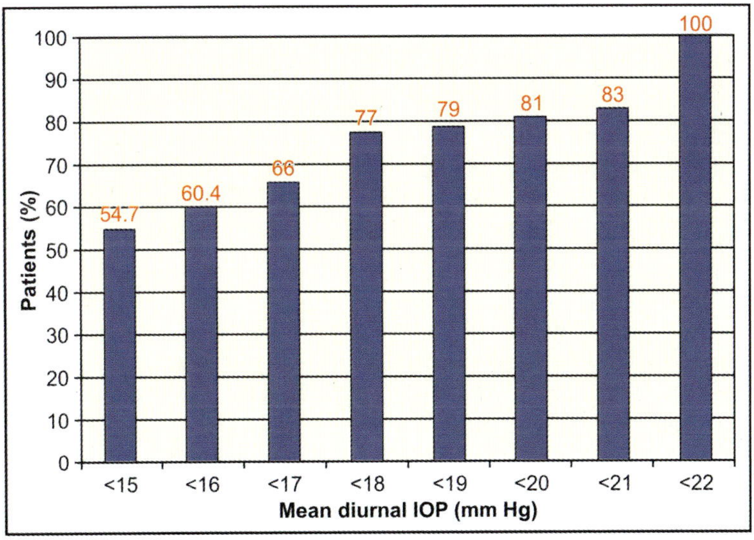

Figure 9: Percentages of patients reaching specified intraocular pressure (IOP) levels

of the sclerotomy can be investigated with a 3-mirror Lens (Goldmann 903). The STT ab interno tip creates a deep sclerotomy with subsequent access of aqueous to the scleral layer. Both aspects may facilitate a bypass effect of aqueous outflow. In light of the fact that about 85% of the aqueous humor drains (in physiological terms) transtrabecularly, we suspect an additional route for aqueous humor absorption in the case of elevated IOP. There is evidence in literature that such bypass effects may be present after surgical intervention which do not lead to the formation of filtering blebs. In a previous study, it was ascertained that eyes without filter bleb exhibited very stable long-term IOP regulation postoperatively. In addition to the bypassing of trabecular outflow resistance caused by STT ab interno treatment, outflow resistance may be further reduced by scleral thinning at the base of the thalamus. In addition to that aqueous humor could perhaps be absorbed by the ciliary body. After early postoperative reduction, the average IOP continued to decline gradually over a period of 6 months before reaching a relatively a constant level . It can be speculated that newly formed blood vessel and lymph vessel close to the surgical site, may contribute to the decrease of IOP level during follow-up.

In literature the success rate range for trabeculectomy ranges between 57% and 96%, for deep sclerectomy without collagen device between 57 % and 74 %, and for deep sclerectomy with collagen device between 58 % and 90 %. The STT ab interno technique with a complete success rate of 90.6% is comparable with other so far published surgery methods.

Advantages of the STT ab interno method, compared with trabeculectomy and perforating and non-perforating deep sclerectomy seem to be a rate of postoperative complications and a constant level of reduced IOP. Hypotension, a frequent finding in trabeculectomy, perforating deep sclerectomy and non-perforating deep sclerectomy, is a relatively rare postoperative complication. The most frequent early complications in trabeculectomy are hyphaema (24.6%), shallow anterior chamber (23.9%), hypotony (24.3%), wound leak (17.8%) and choroidale detachment (14.1%). The most frequent late complications are cataract (20.2%), visual loss (18.8%), iris incarceration (5.1%) and encapsulated bleb (3.4%). After STT ab interno cataract development was seen in 17% with only 5.7% loss of one line of visual acuity after 36 months. Compared with other techniques STT ab interno seems to be a relatively save surgical technique.

Transient IOP elevation after STT ab interno may occur in the first 6 weeks and can be effectively brought under control with the use of a topical medication. In most cases, IOP-reducing therapy could be gradually withdrawn after 3 weeks postsurgery. It was necessary to continue pressure-reducing therapy in 5 of 53 eyes, in all this cases medication was effective in controlling IOP.

Problems of scarring to the Tenon's capsule, fibroblast proliferation and secondary occlusion associated with trabeculectomy which are induced by the surgical procedure itself may the reason behind the practice of antimetabolites applications (Mitomycin C at concentration of 0.2-0.4 mg/ml for 1-5 minutes). Although this practice was conceived to modulate wound healing and thus to counteract scar formation, it often resulted in serious complications, such as scleral necrosis and an increased incidence of avascular filter bleb and their

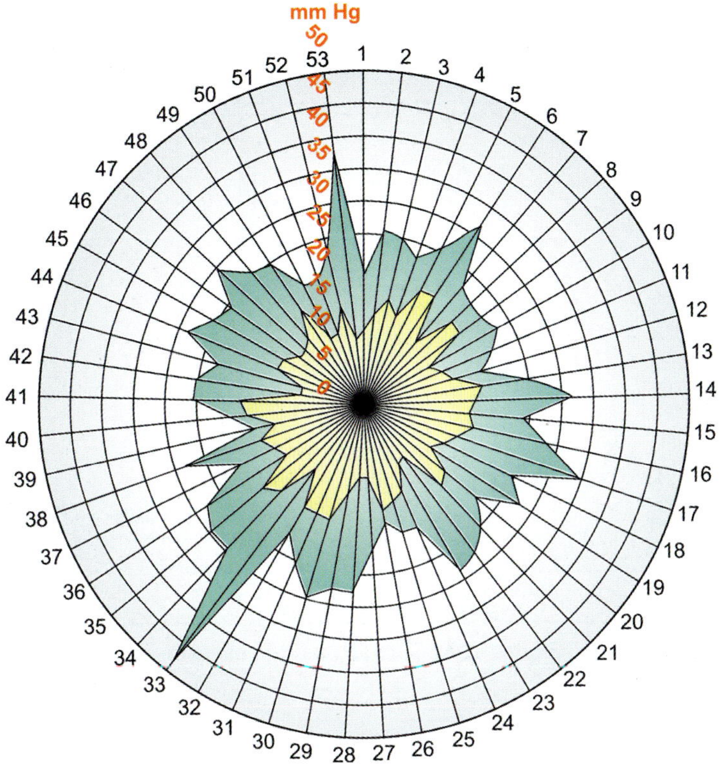

Figure 10: Preoperative and postoperative level of IOP 36 months of follow-up

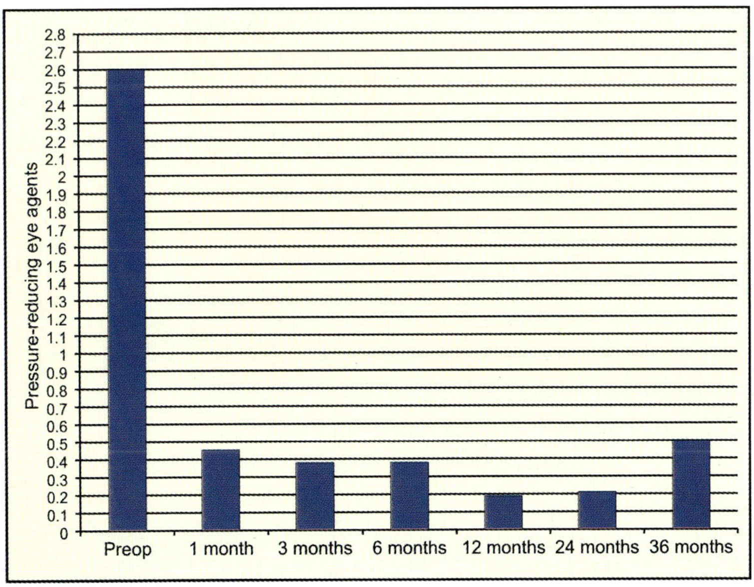

Figure 11: Administration of pressure-reducing eye agents during 36 months

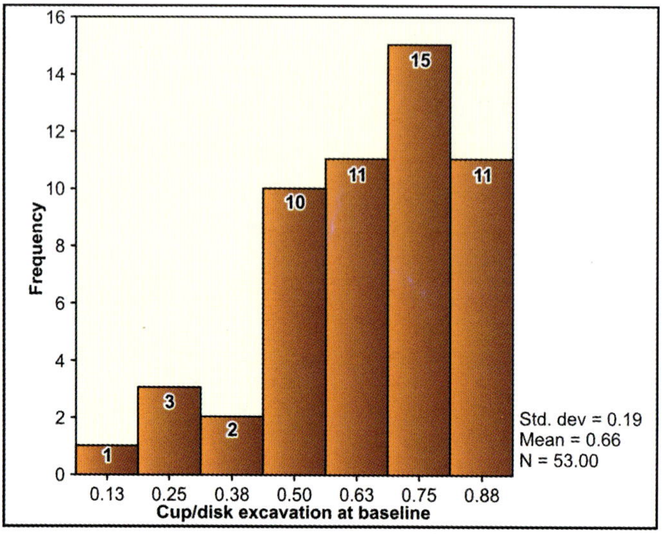

Figure 12A: Cup/disk ratio at baseline

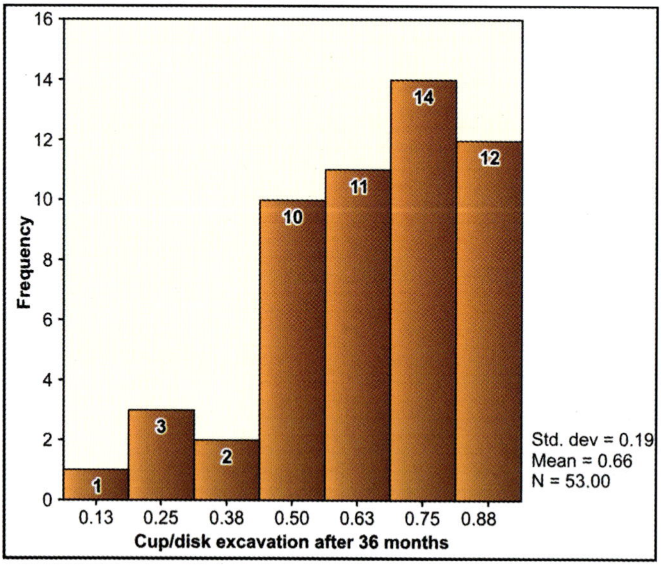

Figure 12B: Cup/disk ratio at 36 months

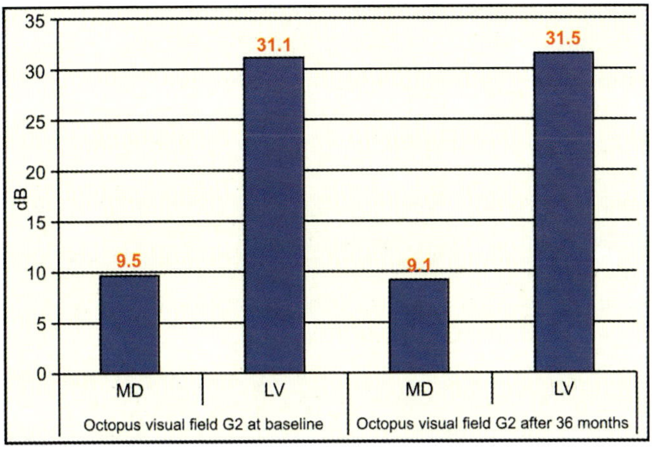

Figure 13: Visual field analysis

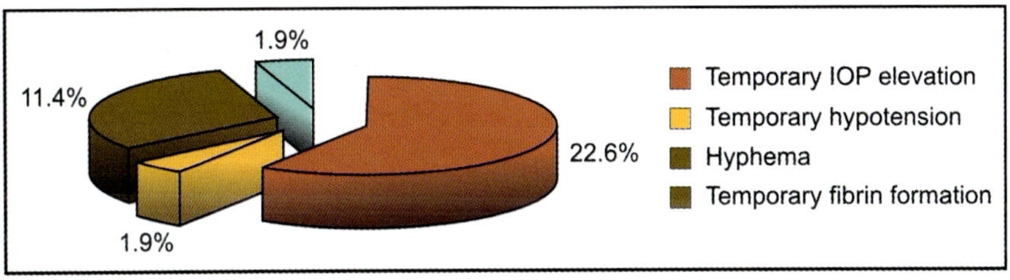

Figure 14: Complications after Sclerothalamotomy (STT) ab interno surgery

late complications. The surgical procedure applied in this study avoids stimulation of episcleral and conjunctival proliferations and may therefore be related with less secondary cell invasion at the filtrating bypass.

Preliminary histological investigations of postmortem human eyes following STT ab interno did not indicate signs of indirect necrosis in cell layers adjacent to the thalamus formed by high-frequency diathermy. It is yet unknown, if the inner surface of the thalamus will be covered by endothelial cells of corneal or trabecular origin, and whether the thalamus and its function will remain intact on a much longer time scale.

Avantages to STT ab interno include the comparative simplicity and quickness of the surgical procedure itself.

This study point out, that the performance of 4 thalami has so far proved sufficient, what corresponds to a resorption surface area of 2.4 mm^2. The number of 4 thalami was defined empirical. Regarding the results of this study the creation of 4 thalami seems to provide a sufficient long-term decrease of IOP as a low rate of postoperative complications. For a further potentiality of IOP decreasing effect we recommend to perform up to 6 thalami.

A randomized multicentre study will be conducted in the future to compare STT ab interno, trabeculectomy, and deep sclerectomy for the surgical treatment of primary open angle glaucoma.

Chapter 19

Congenital Eyelid Anomalies

Roshmi Gupta, Ramesh Murthy
Savari Desai, Santosh G Honavar (India)

Introduction

Congenital lid anomalies are a heterogeneous group of disorders. Broadly they may be classified into malformations and malpositions of the eyelids. Some conditions may be innocuous, while others may have serious visual consequences, and need prompt attention.

Development of Eyelids

The eyelids develop from lid folds that first appear in the surface ectoderm overlying the optic vesicle in the 16 mm stage of the embryo, and grow till the 32 mm stage. Between the 32 to 37 mm stages of the embryo, the upper and lower lid folds fuse together. They begin to separate at the fifth month of gestational age, starting at the nasal side, and the separation is completed by the sixth month.

Cryptophthalmos

Etiology

Partial or complete failure of eye lid fold formation causes cryptophthalmos.

Signs and Symptoms

Cryptophthalmos presents with three grades of severity.

- Complete cryptophthalmos is usually associated with other developmental anomalies, and often bilaterally symmetrical. A smooth skin passes from the forehead to the cheek. Eyebrows and lashes are usually absent.
- Partial cryptophthalmos shows partially formed eyelids and a disorganized anterior segment. The lids are often colobomatous. Facial skin fuses with the medial aspect of the globe.
- Abortive cryptophthalmos has a formed globe, with partial absence of the eyelids in some parts; symblepharon is seen at these areas. Cornea is covered by keratinized and stratified epithelium.

Associated ophthalmic features include microphthalmos, anterior segment anomalies such as small anterior chamber, absent trabecular meshwork, subluxated lens, posterior segment anomalies like uveal coloboma, adnexal abnormalities like dermoids, supernumerary brow and absent lacrimal and accessory glands.

Cryptophthalmos may also have associated nonophthalmic abnormalities, including cleft lip or palate, hernia, aplasia of kidneys, malformed genitalia, meningomyelocele, and mental retardation.

Hereditary transmission of an autosomal recessive nature has been reported.

Differential Diagnosis

Complete cryptophthalmos has a characteristic appearance that is diagnostic. Incomplete cryptophthalmos needs to be differentiated from isolated lid

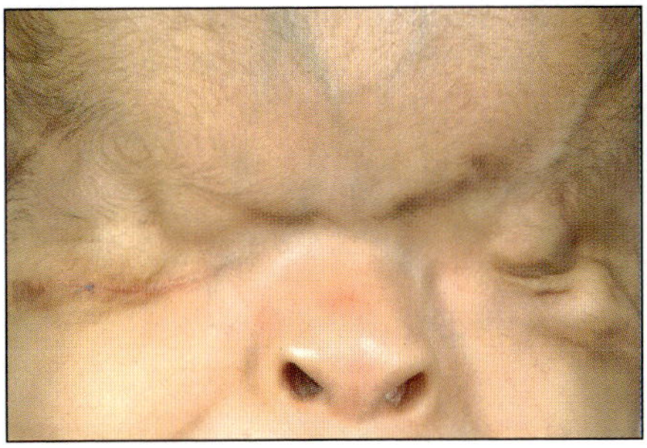

Figure 1A: Clinical photograph of bilateral complete cryptophthalmos

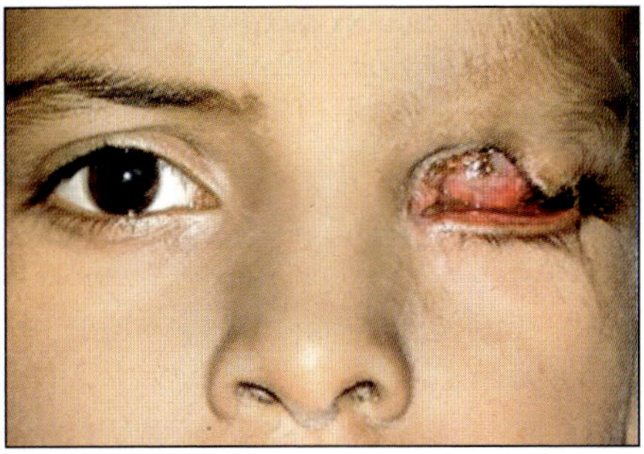

Figure 1B: Partial cryptophthalmos. There is a disorganized anterior segment and partial formation of eyelids

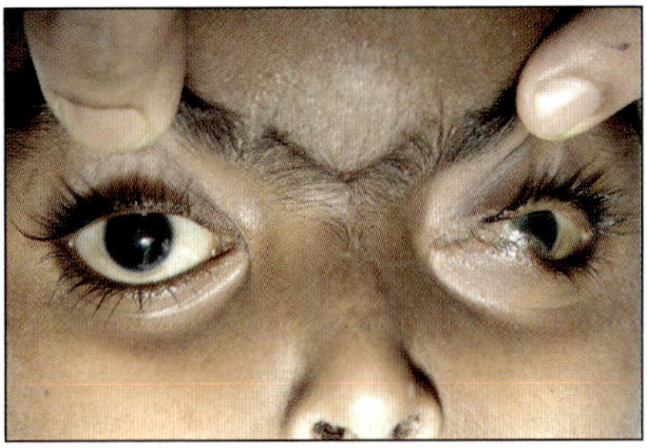

Figure 1C: Abortive cryptophthalmos, with incomplete formation of the nasal end of the eyelids, with symblepharon formation

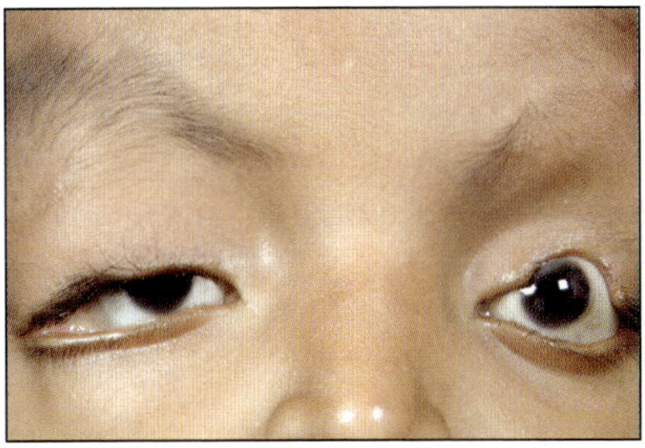

Figure 2A: Clinical photograph of patient with right eye lateral canthal ectopia, congenital ptosis, and left eye upper lid coloboma with corneal scarring due to exposure

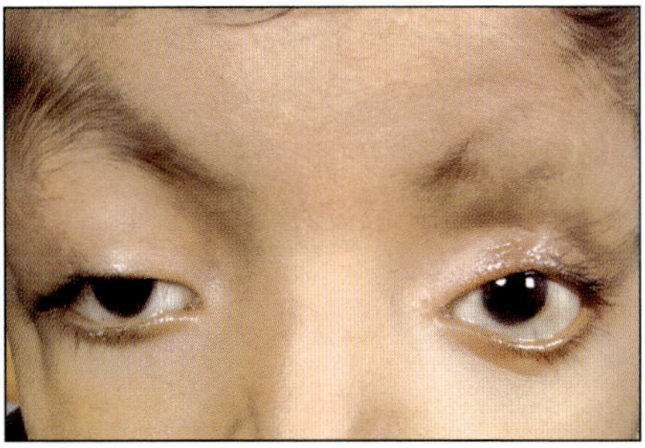

Figure 2B: Postoperative clinical photograph of the same patient, with well-corrected coloboma

colobomas.Causes ofacquired symblepharon are to be differentiated fron abortive cryptophthalmos.

Investigation

Ultrasound B scan and computed tomography may help to assess the condition of the globe.

A thorough systemic evaluation is required to detect any associated anomalies.

Management

The management is surgical, with staged reconstruction of eyelids and the ocular surface. The visual outcome is poor.

Lid Colobomas

Etiology

Lid colobomas form due to delay in fusion of the mesodermal components of the frontonasal and maxillary processes of the face.

Signs and Symptoms

A coloboma is a partial or full thickness absence of the eyelid, which may be triangular, quadrilateral, W-shaped or irregular. The edges are rounded and covered with conjunctiva. The partial thickness coloboma may show the lid margin structures such as lashes. The upper lid colobomas are usually in the middle and the nasal third of the lid. The lower lid colobomas are often situated temporally. If situated at the medial end of the lower lid, they are associated with abnormalities of the lacrimal drainage system.

The cornea may be visible through the coloboma even when the lid is closed, and show exposure keratopathy on slit-lap examination.

Differential Diagnosis

Congenital colobomas need to be differentiated from acquired coloboma caused by trauma.

A coloboma may be isolated, or be a part of the Goldenhar syndrome.

Investigation

The child requires systemic evaluation to rule out other congenital abnoamalities.

Management

The urgency of surgical repair of a coloboma depends on the severity of exposure caused by it. Any coloboma larger than one-third the horizontal extent of the

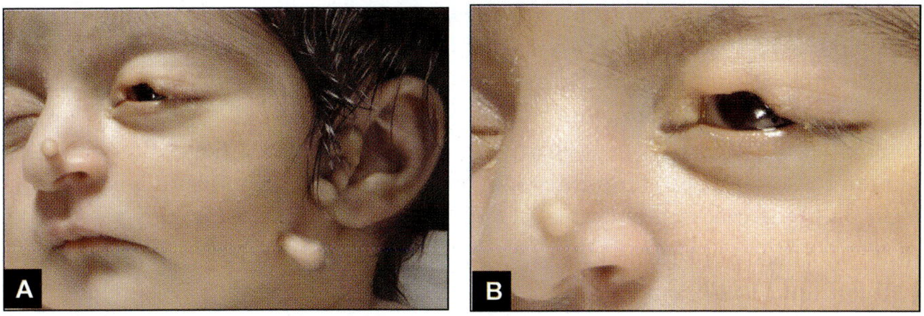

Figures 3A and B: Goldenhar syndrome with left eye upper lid coloboma and preauricular and external nasal skin tags

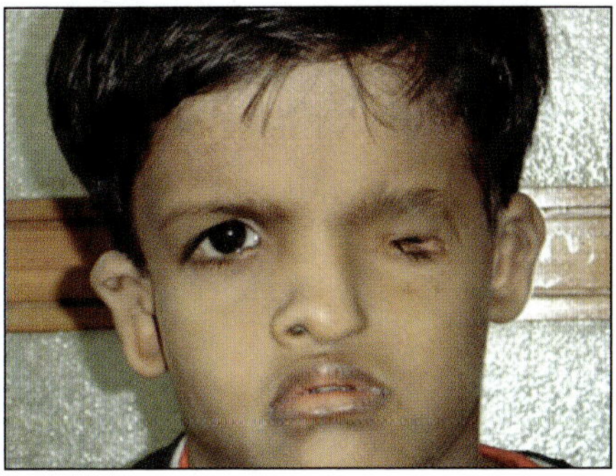

Figure 4: Patient with right eye euryblepharon, left eye clinical anophthalmos with upper and lower lid microblepharon. The eyelids are short vertically as well as horizontally

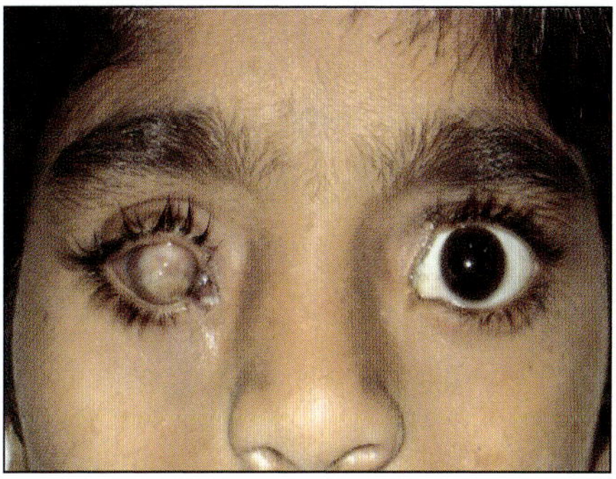

Figure 5: Clinical photograph of patient with right eye corneal dermoid, medial canthal ectopia both eyes and small colobomatous lid notching in left eye. The medial canthus is displaced downwards, and is associated with congenital nasolacrimal duct obstruction. The patient has undergone surgical correction of cleft lip and palate previously

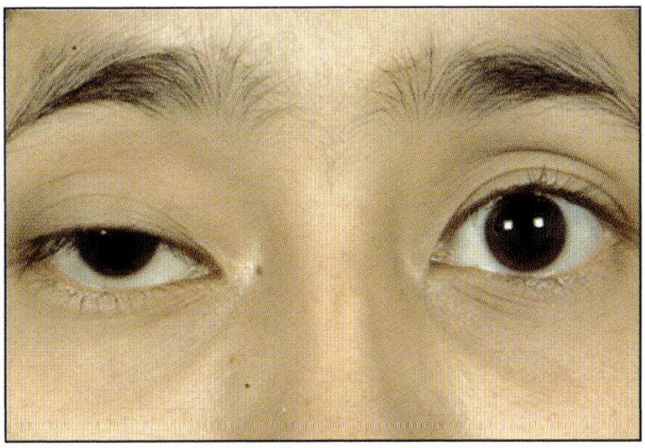

Figure 6A: Patient with right eye congenital ptosis, with epicanthus tarsalis both eyes. A fold of skin extends from the upper lid to the lower lid at the medial canthus

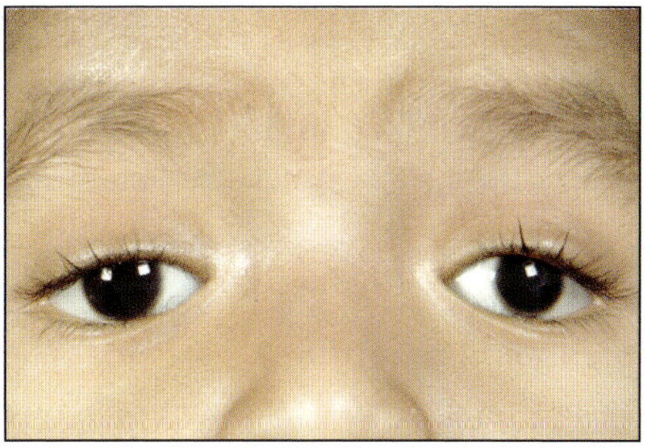

Figure 6B: Patient with bilateral congenital ptosis and bilateral epicanthus inversus. A semilunar fold of skin extends from the upper lid to the lower lid

eyelid poses danger to the cornea, and must have early surgical correction. Any smaller one may undergo elective correction, and have conservative management with lubricants, moist chambers or bandage contact lenses. The edges of the coloboma should be manually pulled together to assess the actual size of the coloboma, to plan appropriate surgery. Smaller ones may have direct closure. Larger ones may need more extensive reconstruction. When using a lid-sharing technique, the risk of amblyopia in a young child should be remembered.

Goldenhar Syndrome

Lid coloboma is a common association with Goldenhar syndrome, in addition to corneal or epibulbar dermoids, and preauricular skin tags and external ear deformities.

Microblepharon and Ablepharon

Introduction, Signs and Symptoms

A microblepharon is a rare vertical foreshortening of the eyelid. The upper lid is more commonly affected. Apparent ablepharon may be a severe microblepharon, and one should look carefully for rudimentary eyelids. It may be associated with clinical anophthalmos. It is associated with lagophthalmos and exposure keratopathy. There may be additional ocular and systemic abnormalities.

Investigation

Evaluation should be performed for addditonal systemic and ocular abnormalities. In a microphthalmic eye, assessment for visual potential is required.

Differential Diagnosis

Microblepharon and ablepharon should be differentiated from lid colobomas.

Management

The surgical management plan depends on the visual potential and the specific features. Correction may require rotation flaps from the cheek, lid sharing procedures, pedicle flaps or skin grafts.

Ankyloblepharon Filiforme Adnatum

Signs and Symptoms

The condition shows fine extensile cords attaching upper and lower lids, which may be single or multiple. The cords decrease the palpebral fissure height and reduce lid excursion. It has been reported n association with trisomy 18.

This may be associated with ectodermal dysplasia and cleft lip or cleft palate – this is the autosomal dominant Hay-Well's syndrome.

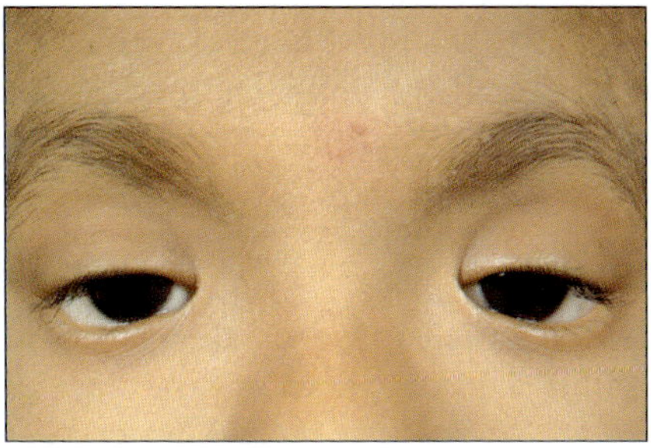

Figure 6C: Epicanthus palpebralis, with a semilunar fold of skin extending on both upper and lower lids. The epicanthal fold obscures the medial canthal structures and gives an appearance of pseudostrabismus

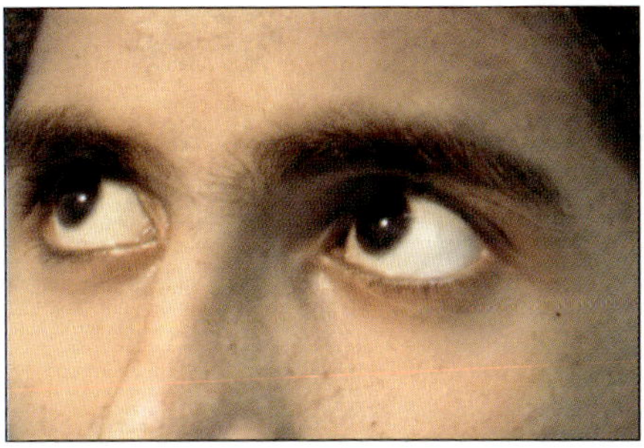

Figure 7: Patient with Centurion syndrome, with sharp medial canthal angles, square eyebrows, and elongated horizontal palpebral aperture. The medial canthal tendon is prominent and attached anteriorly, not allowing proper apposition of the lacrimal punctum to the tear meniscus

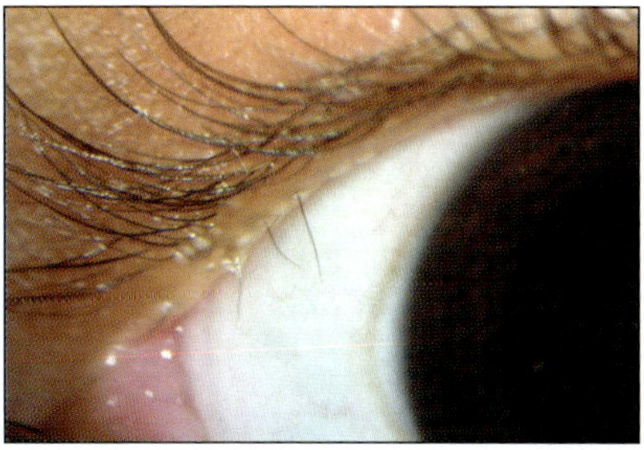

Figure 8: Incomplete row of eyelashes growing on the medial aspect of the upper lid; the lashes are at the sites of meibomian gland orifices

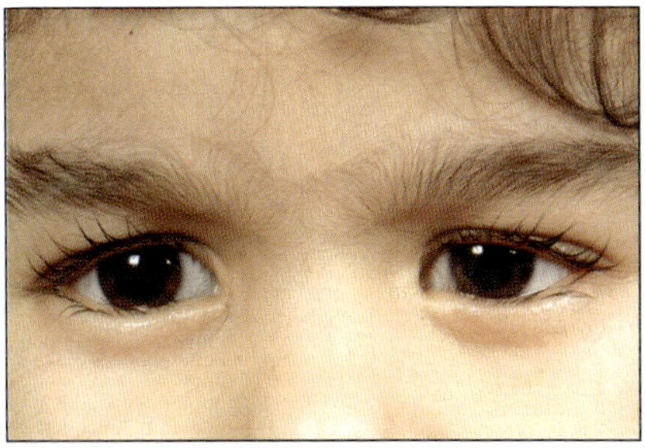

Figure 9A: Patient with bilateral epiblepharon with high tear meniscus

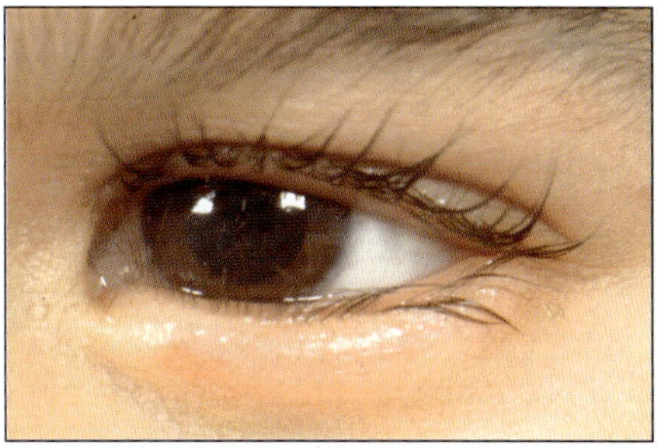

Figure 9B: Clinical photograph showing redundant horizontal fold of lower lid skin and orbicularis, with vertical orientation of eyelashes

Treatment

The cord is simply severed, and the epithelial tags involute.

Congenital Ankyloblepharon

Introduction

Congenital ankyloblepharon is caused by developmental arrest leading to growth aberration at either canthus, inner or outer.

Signs and Symptoms

It is caused by partial fusion of the upper and lower lid, and results in horizontal foreshortening of the palpebral fissure. The commoner external variety is at the lateral canthus, causing an appearance of pseudoexotropia. The internal ankyloblepharon at the inner canthus causes pseudoesotropia.

Differential Diagnosis

Pseudo- eso- or exotropia must be differentiated from true strabismus.

Treatment

Ankyloblepharon requires surgical separation of the eyelids.

Medial Canthal Ectopia

Introduction

Medial canthal ectopia is caused by developmental arrest in the second month of intrauterine life.

Signs and Symptoms

The medial canthal tendon is displaced inferiorly along with surrounding canthal structures. It attaches to the junction of the medial wall of the orbit and the inferior orbital rim. There may be associated nasal cleft deformities and nasolacrimal duct obstruction.

Differential Diagnosis

The condition is to be differentiated from medial canthal dystopia acquired after trauma.

Investigation

The child should be assessed for nasolacrimal duct obstruction.

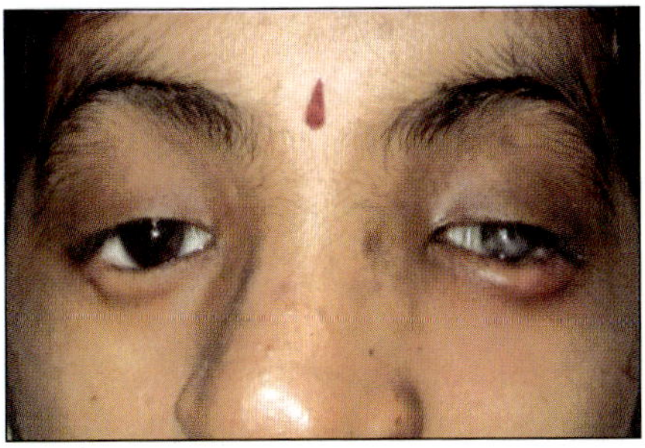

Figure 10: Clinical photograph of patient with bilateral congenital ptosis, with antimongoloid slant of palpebral fissures, with lower lid entropion. Left eye shows a failed corneal graft and lower lid external hordeolum

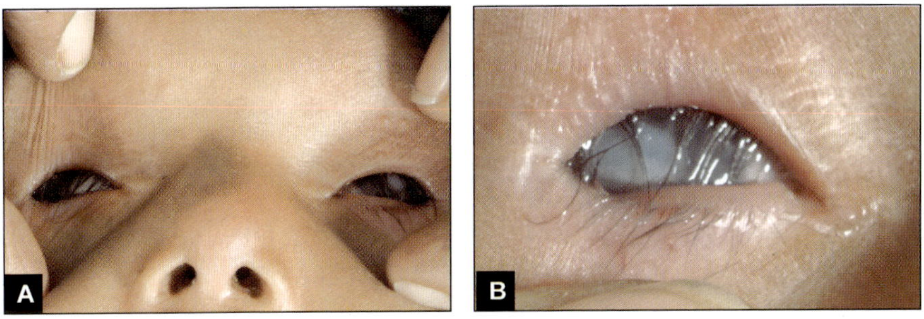

Figures 11A and B: Patient with bilateral tarsal kink and bilateral corneal ulcers. The upper lids show severe entropion, with obscuration of lid margin and absent lid crease

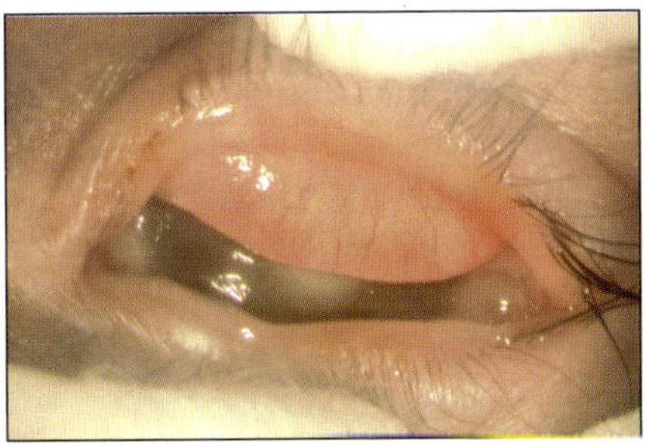

Figure 11C: The everted eyelid shows a crease in the tarsal plate along the entire horizontal length

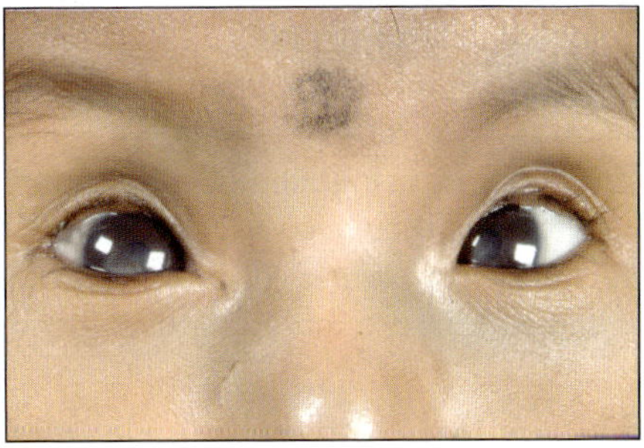

Figure 11D: The clinical photograph of the same patient after surgical correction of the entropion

Treatment

The condition requires surgical supraplacement of the medial canthal tendon: a Z-plasty or a Y-V plasty may be used. The associated nasolacrimal duct obstruction should also be corrected.

Epicanthus

Introduction, Signs and Symptoms

Epicanthus is a semilunar fold of skin at the medial canthus, with its concavity directed outward. The epicanthal fold obscures the view of the medial canthal angle, the caruncle and plica. An epicanthus may be isolated or be an associated feature in a patient with congenital ptosis or Blepharophimosis syndrome. There are several varieties of epicanthus:

- Epicanthus tarsalis extends from the upper lid
- Epicanthus inversus extends from the lower lid (associated with Blepharophimosis-ptosis-epicanthus inversus syndrome - BPES)
- Epicanthus palpebralis extends from the upper lid to the lower lid
- Epicanthus superciliaris extends from below the eyebrow.
  Epicanthus may give an appearance of pseudoesotropia.

Differential Diagnosis

Any epicanthus should be examined to rule out associated BPES.

Treatment

Epicanthus is corrected by Mustarde double Z-plasty, modified Y-V plasty or C-U plasty.

Centurion Syndrome

Introduction, Signs and Symptoms

The patient of centurion syndrome has a history of epiphora since childhood, which worsens at puberty. Syringing of the nasolacrimal duct is patent. The syndrome derives its name from the resemblance of the patients to the Roman centurions in their helmets. The medial canthal tendon is taut and attached anteriorly, causing medial stand-off of the lower lid and punctum. The lacrimal punctum is displaced forward out of the lacrimal lake, causing epiphora. The facial appearance is typical, with a sharp medial canthus, long horizontal palpebral fissure and square eyebrows.

Differential Diagnosis

The condition is to be differentiated from other causes of epiphora.

Investigation

 Lacrimal syringing will be patent, but dye disappearance will be delayed.

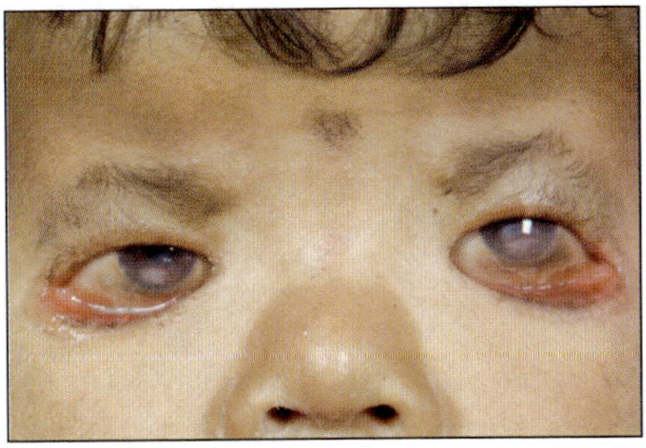

Figure 12A: Clinical photograph of patient with bilateral congenital ptosis, blepharophimosis, telecanthus and lower lid ectropion

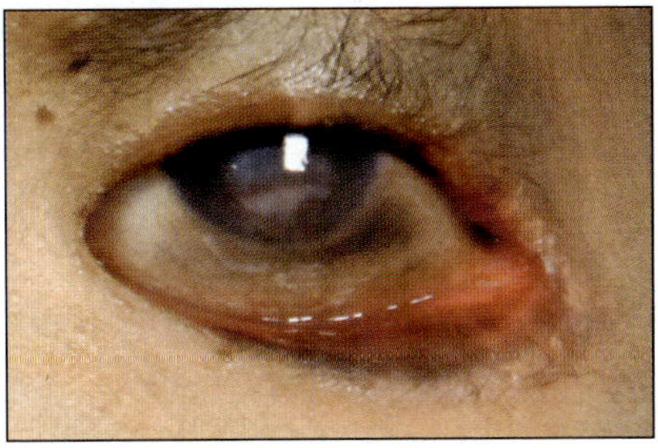

Figure 12B: The lower lid shows severe ectropion, vertical shortening of the anterior lamella, keratinization and pigmentation of the conjunctiva. The cornea shows exposure keratopathy

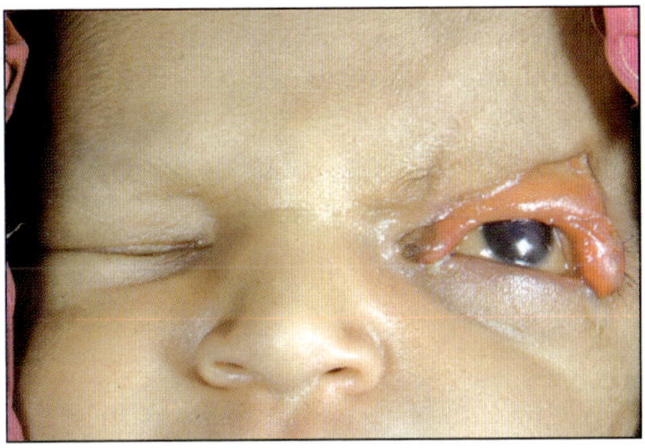

Figure 13: Left eye upper lid congenital ectropion, with complete eversion of eyelid

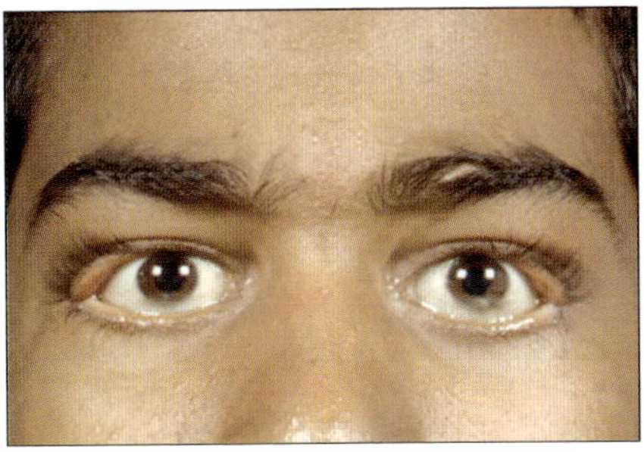

Figure 14A: Clinical photograph of patient with bilateral upper and lower lid lateral ectropion, with excess horizontal length

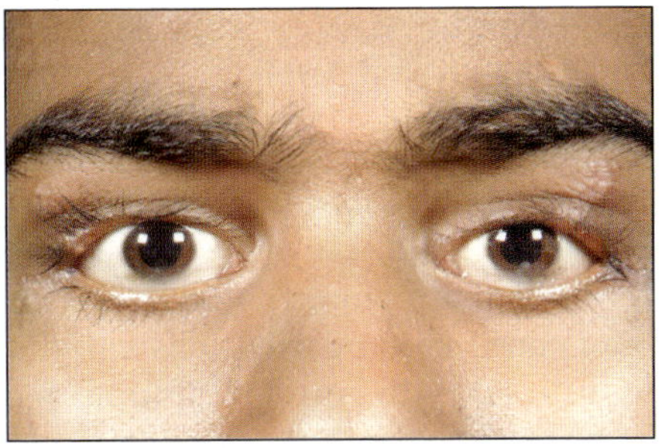

Figure 14B: Photograph of the same patient after surgical correction of the euryblepharon. The corneas are scarred due to exposure

Treatment

The treatment is surgical, anterior medial canthal tendon release, with medial canthoplasty or punctoplasty.

Distichiasis

Introduction, Signs and Symptoms

Distichiasis is an extra row of eyelashes behind the normal ciliary margin at the sites of meibomian glands. It may involve the whole length of the lid or only a segment. The distichiatic lashes rubbing on the ocular surface can induce epiphora or even keratopathy. Congenital distichiasis is associated with lower limb lymphedema; the gene responsible is FOXC 2.

Differential Diagnosis

Distichiasis is to be differentiated from other conditions with abnormal positions or abnormal directions of eyelashes, such as trichiasis, epiblepharon and entropion.

Investigation

Instillation of fluorescein in the eye will help to detect early keratopathy.

Treatment

If the patient is asymptomatic, observation alone suffices. A small number of lashes may be treated by electrolysis. In extensive distichiasis, the lid can be split along the grey line and cryo applied to the posterior lamella at the roots of the distichiatic eyelashes.

Epiblepharon

Introduction, Signs and Symptoms

Epiblepharon comprises a horizontal redundant lid fold of skin and orbicularis in the lower lid, causing vertical orientation of the eyelashes. There may be coexistent entropion. The eyelashes rubbing on the cornea cause epiphora, and may cause keratopathy. It is commoner in Mongolian features. It may be associated with inferior oblique weakness. Epiblepharon often resolves spontaneously by 3 years of age.

Differential Diagnosis

The condition is to be differentiated from congenital entropion and distichiasis.

Investigation

Instillation of fluorescein dye wil help to detect any keratopathy. Careful examination will rule out associated inferior oblique weakness.

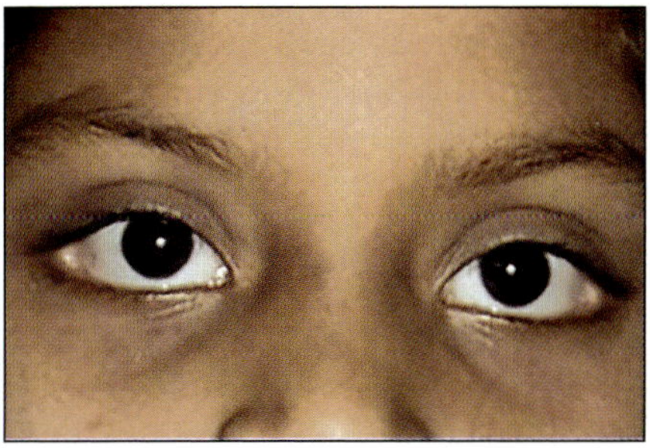

Figure 14C: Photograph of patient with mild degree of euryblepharon, with lateral ectropion of lower lid alone

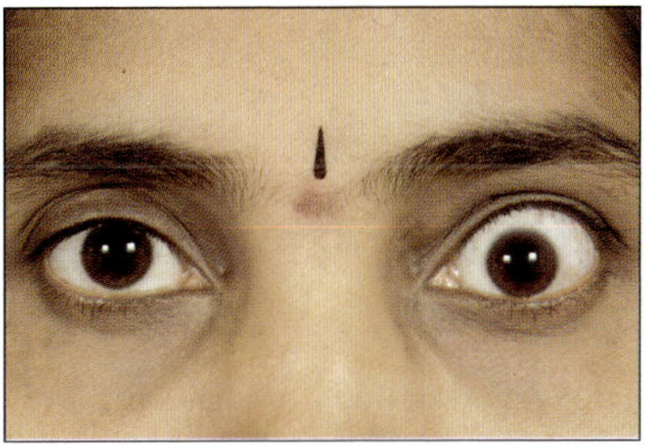

Figure 15A: Clinical photograph of patient with congenital retraction of left upper lid

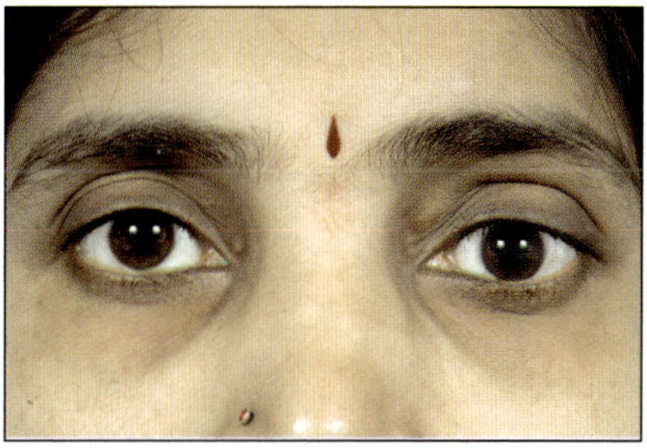

Figure 15B: Photograph of the same patient after surgical correction of the lid retraction

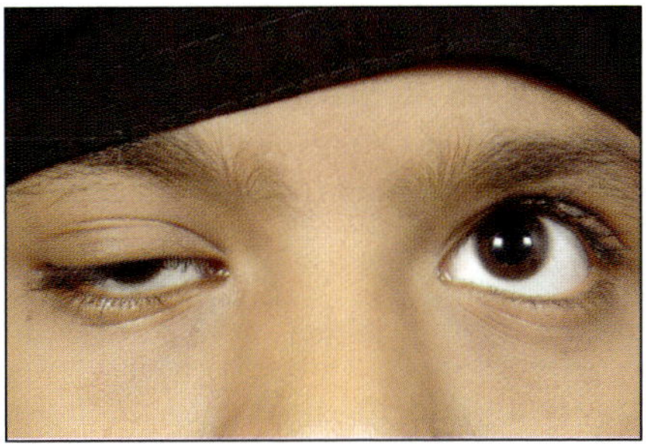

Figure 16A: Patient with right eye congenital ptosis

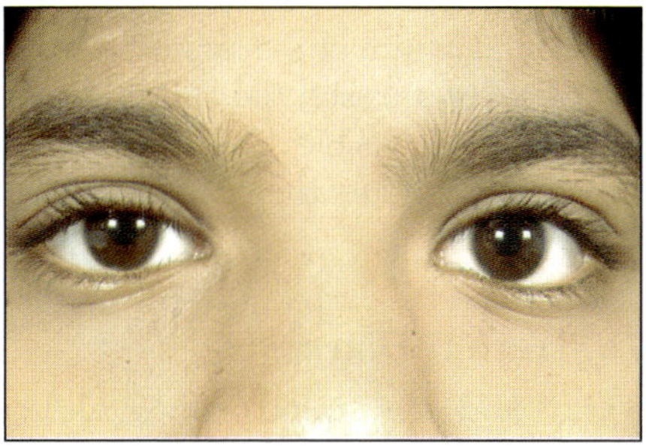

Figure 16B: Photograph of same patient after ptosis correction by frontalis suspension

Treatment

Epiblepharon may be treated with lubricants in the expectation of spontaneous resolution. If the cornea shows keratopathy, surgical intervention is required. The redundant skin and orbicularis oculi muscle is excised in the form of a spindle; usually 1-3 mm of excision would suffice. In severe cases everting sutures may be used in addition.

Congenital Entropion

Introduction

Congenital entropion affects the lower lid, and results from inadequate development of the lower lid retractors. This causes lower lid malpositions similar to that in senile entropion. The entropion is often accompanied by epiblepharon and epicanthus.

Signs and Symptoms

In congenital entropion the lower lid rolls inwards, and the eyelashes rub on the ocular surface. The patient may be symptomatic, with epiphora and keratopathy.

Differential Diagnosis

Congenital entropion must be distinguished from epiblepharon and distichiasis.

Management

Surgical correction is required if the patient develops keratopathy. The procedure of choice is reattachment of the lower lid retractors to the tarsus.

Tarsal Kink Syndrome

Introduction, Signs and Symptoms

Tarsal kink syndrome is a rare entity with horizontal fold along the entire horizontal length of the tarsus. Tarsal kink results in entropion of the upper lid; in the severest cases, the child presents within a few weeks of age, and the lid margin is not visible. The patient may have absent lid crease, blepharospasm, lid edema and keratopathy. The patient commonly presents with corneal ulcer in early infancy.

Differential Diagnosis

Tarsal kink syndrome with corneal infiltrate should be differentiated from patients presenting with other corneal ulcers.

Management

Surgical correction of the tarsal kink entails full-thickness blepharotomy the entire length of eyelid with marginal rotation. Due to the very early age of

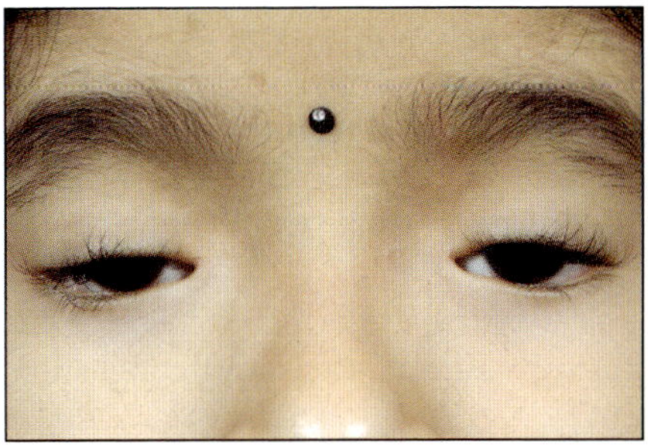

Figure 17A: Blepharophimosis Syndrome type 1, with ptosis, blepharophimosis, telecanthus and epicanthus inversus

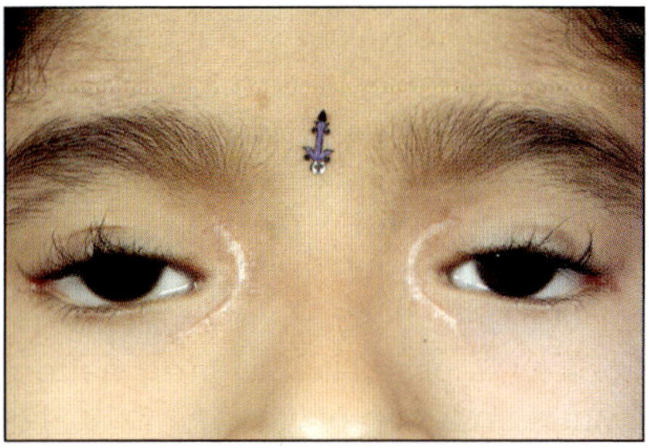

Figure 17B: Same patient after surgical correction of the epicanthus by C-U plasty

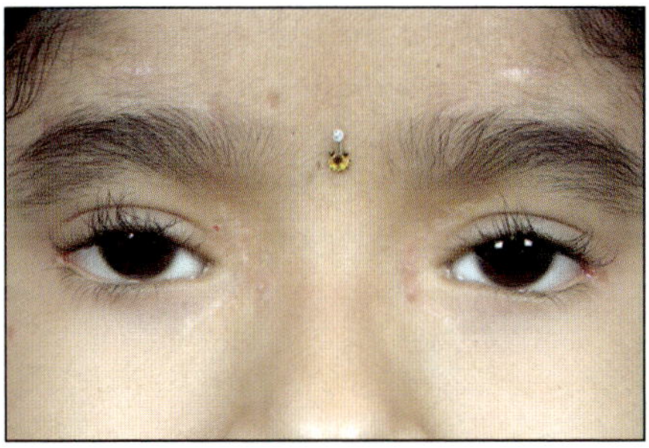

Figure 17C: Final surgical outcome of the same patient after ptosis correction

presentation and the associated corneal ulceration and scarring, amblyopia therapy is crucial after correction of the entropion.

Congenital Ectropion

Introduction, Signs and Symptoms

Congenital ectropion of the lower lid is rarely isolated; it is more likely to be a part of a syndrome such as Kohn-Romano syndrome. Congenital ectropion of the lower lid often has vertical shortage of skin. Severe ectropion will cause epiphora and exposure, and the tarsal conjunctiva may become keratinized.

Lamellar ichthyosis is a systemic condition which may result in cicatricial ectropion of upper and lower lid at birth.

Occasionally there is an isolated eversion of the upper lid, for which the etiology is postulated as birth trauma causing vascular stasis and congestion, leading to lid eversion.

Differential Diagnosis

The ectropion due to shortage of skin should be differentiated from euryblepharon, which also causes lateral ectropion of the lower lid.

Management

Congenital ectropion requires full-thickness skin grafting; the preferred donor site is the retroauricular area.

In lamellar ichthyosis, it may be difficult to identify any area of healthy skin as a potential donor site. Skin emollients should also be used liberally.

In the isolated upper lid eversion, one may escape surgery, and get by only with marginal traction suture to straighten the lid. If the ectropion persists, one may need to excise a part of the prolapsed conjunctiva to allow correction of the lid eversion.

Euryblepharon

Introduction, Signs and Symptoms

Euryblepharon presents with bilateral symmetrical enlargement of the horizontal palpebral apertures, with vertical shortage of eyelid skin, elongated lid margins, and downward and lateral displacement of outer canthi. The horizontal palpebral fissure length is increased to approximately 35 mm from the average of 28-30 mm. There is lateral ectropion, lagophthalmos and reduced blink rate with exposure keratopathy. The exposure and reduced blink rate may cause epiphora.

Differential Diagnosis

Euryblepharon should be distinguished from the congenital ectropion which has vertical shortage of skin, but not an elongated lid margin.

Other causes of epiphora in childhood should be differentiated from euryblepharon.

Management

Mild degrees may be managed conservatively, with lubricants. Moderate degrees will require tarsorrhaphy to protect the cornea. A lateral canthoplasty with shortening of the upper and lower lids laterally may be beneficial. The severest forms may require staged correction with augmentation of the posterior lamella and anterior skin graft.

Congenital Lid Retraction

Introduction, Signs and Symptoms

Congenital retraction of the upper lid may be unilateral or bilateral. A unilateral lid retraction may simulate contralateral ptosis. The condition is non-progressive. Other systemic features are usually normal.

Differential Diagnosis

Congenital lid retraction must be differentiated from other causes of lid retraction such as thyroid abnormalities, and Marcus-Gunn phenomenon. Children developing eyelid retraction must be investigated for intracranial space-occupying lesions, hydrocephalus and postencephalitic sequelae.

There has been a case report of accessory slip of levator palpebrae superioris causing lid retraction.

Investigation

Thyroid function tests may rule out endocrine-related lid retraction.

Management

Lid retraction may be treated by lid lengthening procedures.

Congenital Ptosis

Introduction, Signs and Symptoms

Congenital ptosis is the commonest of the congenital lid anomalies. The upper lid is at a lower level than normal, and the condition may be unilateral or bilateral. The affected eye may have limited elevation. A quick assessment of the severity of congenital ptosis is possible by looking at the red reflex of the pupil through distant direct ophthalmoscopy, and recording how much of the pupil is obscured by the lid. Other indicators of the severity of the ptosis are over-action of the frontalis muscles and chin elevation on inspection of the face. A greater palpebral fissure height in down gaze is seen in the unilateral ptosis, since the defective levator palpebrae muscle is also deficient in ability to relax.

A faint upper lid crease indicates weak levator action. Marcus-Gunn phenomenon, i.e. synkinetic elevation of the ptotic lid with jaw movement should be looked for. Amblyopia may develop due to visual deprivation, refractive error or associated strabismus.

Differential Diagnosis

Careful examination will rule out other causes of ptosis in the young.

Myasthenia gravis may rarely occur in a child. Variable ptosis, involvement of extraocular muscles and fatigability indicate myasthenic ptosis. The diagnosis may be confirmed by edrophonium test.

Chronic progressive external ophthalmoplegia may have an onset in the first decade of life, and show associated limitation of ocular movements.

Congenital ocular fibrosis presents with ptosis along with strabismus. The ocular movements are severely restricted.

Ptosis may be associated with weakness of the third cranial nerve.

Investigation

The child with ptosis requires careful cycloplegic refraction.

Ice test and edrophomnium test help to rule out ocular myasthenia.

Management

Severe ptosis with high-risk of amblyopia should be corrected early in life. Milder disease is corrected as the child reaches the school-going age. Severe ptosis with poor levator action is treated by a tarsofrontal sling; the material of the sling may be biogenic such as autogenous or preserved fascia lata or bovine pericardium, or synthetic such as mersilene, silicone, PTFE or polypropylene. Any associated strabismus requires correction before correction of the ptosis.

Ptosis with associated Marcus-Gunn phenomenon needs special consideration. Disinsertion of the levator aponeurosis from the tarsal attachment bilaterally with bilateral tarsofrontal sling has been advocated. An alternative is to disinsert the levator of the affected side alone, with bilateral sling surgery.

After correction of the ptosis, refractive error should be reassessed and correction provided. Amblyopia therapy should be instituted if required.

Blepharophimosis Syndrome

Introduction, Signs and Symptoms

Blepharophimosis syndrome presents as a combination of several features.

Blepharophimosis is characterized by a short horizontal palpebral fissure, 18-22 mm as opposed to the average of 28-30 mm. *Blepharoptosis* is severe, with poor levator function, absent lid crease and characteristic head posture with chin elevation and over-action of the frontalis. *Epicanthus inversus* shows a semilunar fold of skin at the medial canthus, extending from the lower lid to the upper lid. *Telecanthus* is an increased distance between the orbits. The inter-medial canthal distance is greater than half the inter-pupillary distance. The tetrad of Blepharophimosis, blepharoptosis, epicanthus inversus and telecanthus together comprise the Kohn-Romano syndrome. Blepharophimosis syndrome may, in addition, have inferiorly slanted palpebral apertures and lateral ectropion.

The Blepharophimosis, Ptosis, Epicanthus-Inversus Syndrome (BPES syndrome) has been identified to be autosomal dominant. There are two types of this syndrome: BPES Type I is associated with infertility, while BPES Type II is not. The gene involved in BPES Type I is FOXL2.

The Callahan classification of blepharophimosis is based on the particular combination of clinical features at presentation:

Blepharophimosis type I: Blepharoptosis, blepharophimosis, epicanthus inversus, telecanthus.

Blepharophimosis type II: Blepharophimosis and blepharoptosis, without epicanthus and normally spaced orbits.

Blepharophimosis type III: Blepharophimosis and blepharoptosis, with shortage of skin and palpebral apertures slanted inferiorly, with wide spaced orbits.

Differential Diagnosis

Blepharophimosis syndrome is to be differentiated from isolated congenital ptosis.

Management

Blepharophimosis syndrome requires staged repair. The epicanthus is corrected first, by Mustarde's double Z-plasty or by modified Y-V plasty. Any lateral ectropion causing lagophthalmos and exposure is corrected by lateral canthoplasty, and skin grafting if necessary. The ptosis is corrected by a tarso-frontal sling surgery.

Other Syndromes

There are several syndromes which are associated with lid anomalies. A few of the important ones are listed, with the responsible gene and clinical features mentioned in brief.

- Prader-Willi syndrome
  - Gene responsible—SNRP small nuclear ribonucleoprotein polypeptide)
  - Clinical features—almond shaped palpebral fissures, obesity, hypogonadism, mental retardation.
- Noonan syndrome
  - Gene responsible PTPN11 (protein tyrosinase phosphatase nonreceptor type)
  - Clinical features—hypertelorism, down slanting palpebral fissures, webbing neck, pulmonary stenosis, pectus excavatum.

- Rubinstein-Taybi syndrome
  - Gene responsible—CRE binding protein
  - Clinical features—heavy arched eyebrows, down slanting palpebral fissures, broad thumbs and toes, mental retardation.
- Fraser syndrome
  - Gene responsible—FRAS1(ECM protein)
  - Clinical features—cryptophthalmos, renal agenesis, syndactyly, laryngeal stenosis.
- Apert syndrome
  - Gene responsible—FGFR2
  - Clinical features—severe craniostenosis, syndactyly, hypertelorism, proptosis, strabismus.
- Crouzon syndrome and related syndromes (Pfeiffer and Jackson-Weis syndrome)
  - Gene responsible—FGFR2-FGFR
  - Clinical features—craniostenosis, limb anomalies (absent in JWS, PS), hypertelorism, proptosis, orbital asymmetry.
- Saethre-Chotzen syndrome
  - Gene responsible—TWIST
  - Clinical features—craniostenosis, limb and ear anomalies, ptosis.
- Waardenburg syndrome
  - Gene responsible—PAX3 (WS1), MITF (WS2)
  - Clinical features—iris heterochromia, deafness, white forelock, dystopia canthorum (WS1).
- Treacher Collins syndrome
  - Gene responsible—TCOF1
  - Clinical features—first branchial arch syndrome, down slanting palpebral fissures, eyelid colobomas.
- Coffin-Lowry syndrome
  - Gene responsible—RPS6KA3
  - Clinical features—X-linked mental retardation syndrome, hypertelorism, down slanting palpebral fissures.
- Stickler
  - Gene responsible—COL2A1, COL11A1, COL11A2
  - Clinical features—midfacial hypoplasia, cleft palate, hearing loss, spondyloepiphyseal dysplasia, proptosis.

Chapter 20

Congenital Nasolacrimal Duct Obstruction

Essam El Toukhy, Ibrahim Mosad (Egypt)

Pathophysiology

A very common condition in which the extreme end of the nasolacrimal duct underneath the inferior turbinate fails to complete its canalization in the newborn period. Canalization of the nasolacrimal duct usually completed by eight month of gestation.

Frequency

Rate: 2-4% of newborn
Race: No racial incidence.
Sex: No sexual difference.

Causes

Usually, these anomalies are sporadic, but genetics, prematurity, and maternal drug use can be possible influencing factors.

Ocular abnormalities are present in 20% of patients, and systemic abnormalities are present in almost 25% of patients with serious congenital nasolacrimal duct anomalies

Presentation

Amniotocele

This condition occurs in neonates as a distention in the lacrimal sac. Amniotic fluid enters the sac, is retained by a nonpatent nasolacrimal duct, and is trapped in the sac by the valve at the common canaliculus, the valve of Rosenmüller. Probing the nasolacrimal duct as an office procedure usually is curative.

Dacryocystitis (Acute Mucocele or Pyocele)

This condition exhibits acute distention and inflammation in the lacrimal sac region and may occur in the neonatal period. Probing is necessary in newborns with acute dacryocystitis to establish drainage as soon as possible. This procedure is performed with topical or local anesthesia only.

Tearing

Newborns who have congenital nasolacrimal duct obstruction may not develop acute dacryocystitis with a mucocele or pyocele of the sac in the early neonatal period but may simply have tearing with a chronic mucopurulent discharge, which usually manifests at 2 weeks. Topical antibiotics should be administered, and the parents must be instructed in the proper technique of lacrimal sac compression and massage. More than 90% of these cases clear and become asymptomatic with conservative management. Under normal circumstances,

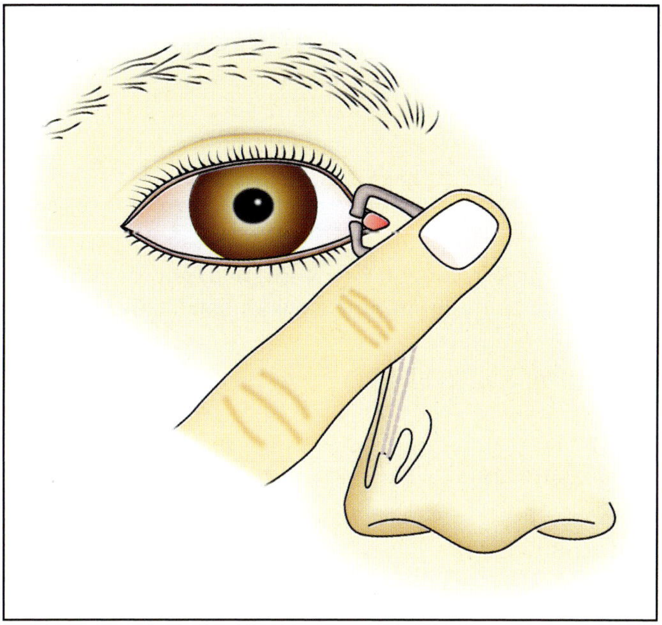

Figure 1: Massage technique for congenital nasolacrimal duct obstruction

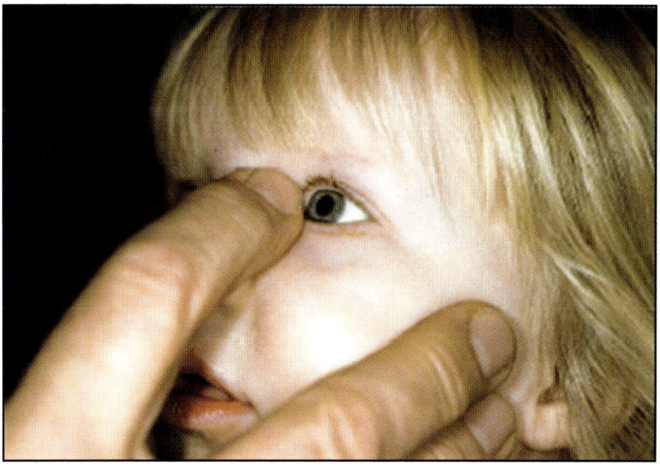

Figure 2: Massage technique for congenital nasolacrimal duct obstruction

these children with mild-to-moderate symptoms of epiphora and lid crusting can be monitored for the first nine months life without serious sequela. It is rarely necessary to make probing mandatory at an early age before 6 month.

Investigations

Diagnosis

- *Fluorescein dye disappearance test:* Grade as good, fair, or poor clearance
- *Jones dye tests:* Not as useful in practice with small children
- *Imaging Studies:*
  - Intubation dacryocystography
  - Scintillography

Differential Diagnosis

- Sinus mucocele
- Repeated conjunctivitis

Treatment

Medical Care

Congenital nasolacrimal duct obstructions resolves spontaneously in 90% of cases during the first year of life. Massage with digital pressure used as an aid to speeding up this natural resolution. Other than massage, topical antibiotics are useful for mucopurulent discharge, but the only treatment of efficacy for those patients who do not resolve spontaneously is surgery as follow.

Surgical Care

Probing

Probing cures 95% of congenital nasolacrimal obstructions. Prognosis for probing decreases with the increasing number of probings and the age of the patient. Rarely, it is successful after the third time or after 3 years.

Nasolacrimal Intubation

Success rates of 80-95% have been reported, inpatients have only been probed twice or less and are younger than 2 years. Prognosis is poor for those patients with previous dacryocystitis and for those patients in which an obstruction is encountered during the procedure. Increasing duration of intubation was not associated with increasing chance of success but with a significantly higher risk of failure if longer than 18 months. The retention of silicone tubes for longer than 12 months was associated with a significantly lower success rate (67%).

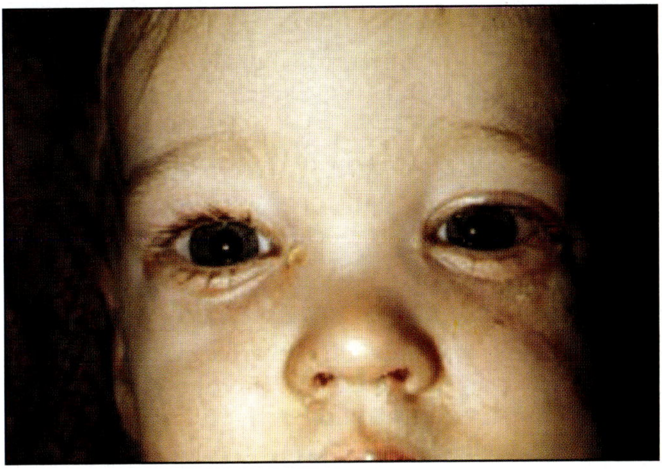

Figure 3: Congenital lacrimal obstruction presenting with persistent watering and mucopurulent discharge observed from the first month of life

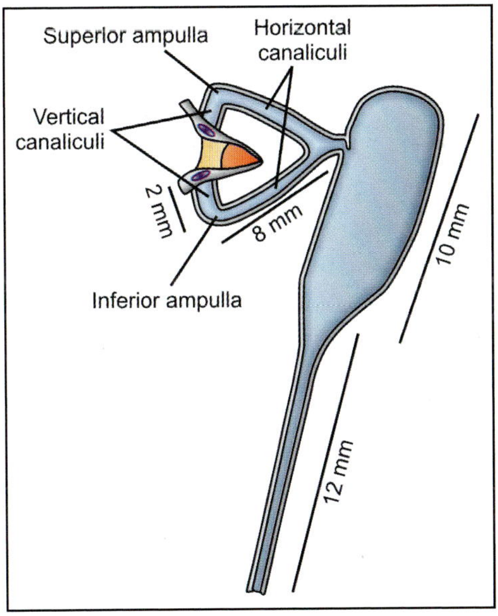

Figure 4: Important dimensions of the lacrimal drainage system

Balloon Catheter Dilatation

Balloon catheter dilatation of nasolacrimal system with or without silicone tubing: This procedure has slightly better results than intubation alone.

Dacryocystorhinostomy with or without Intubation

This treatment indicated when a patent canalicular system is present with failed previous treatnent.

Conjunctival Dacryocystorhinostomy

If the upper system is scarred or atretic then it can be bypassed using a prosthesis, such as a Lester-Jones' tube. This procedure probably should be avoided until the child is older than 10 years because the prosthesis requirs care from the patient and often has minor complications and revisions.

Complications and Prognosis

Bleeding

Serious bleeding is rare, occurring in only 1-2% of surgeries or postoperatively.

Surgical Failures

In these complicated conditions, a 10% rate of failure occurs.

Wound infections: These occur in 5-10% of patients, usually as wound abscesses on the fourth postoperative day.

Silicone or Polyethylene Tubing Complications

These complications occur in about 15% of cases and include the following: corneal abrasion, pyogenic granuloma, low-grade infection, chronic nasal irritation and congestion, epistaxis, sinusitis, and pharyngitis.

Bypass Tube Complications

These frequently occur in at least 40% of patients postoperatively and include tube loss or migration and tube obstruction.

Anesthesia Complications

In children, these complications are more frequent due to drugs, blood loss, malignant hyperthermia, and pseudocholinesterase deficiency.

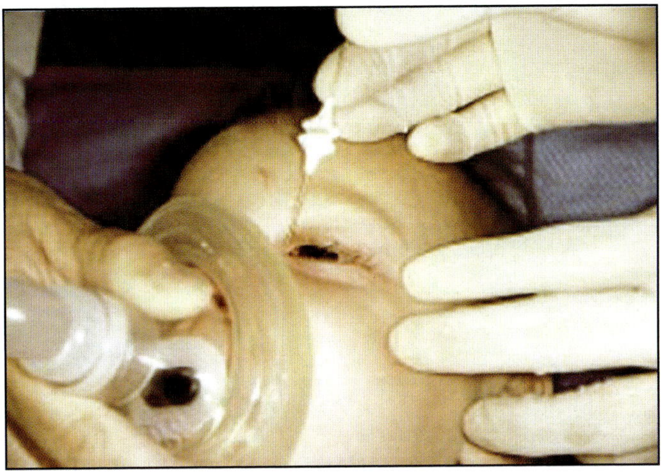

Figure 5: Probing of nasolacrimal duct under general anesthesia by mask

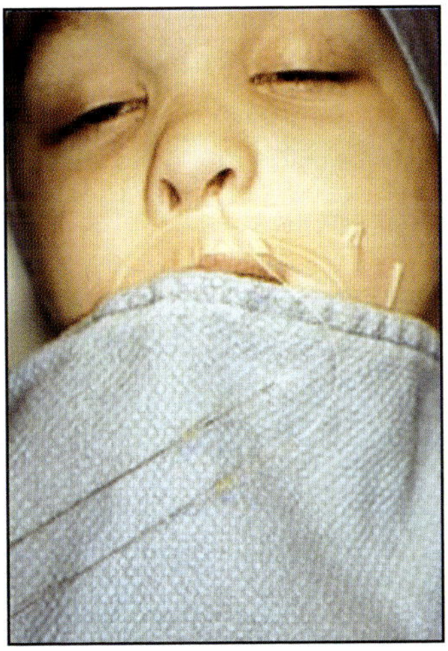

Figure 6: Both ends of the silicone tubing have been passed through canaliculus, sac, and duct, and have been retrieved from the nose

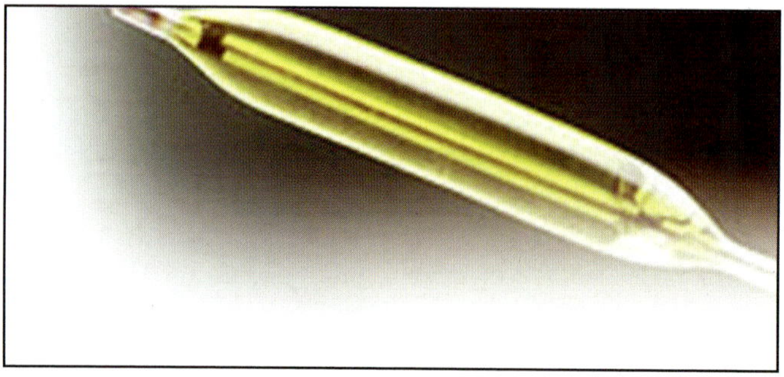

Figure 7: Catheter for patients older than 30 months of age (3 mm balloon diameter, 15 mm balloon length)

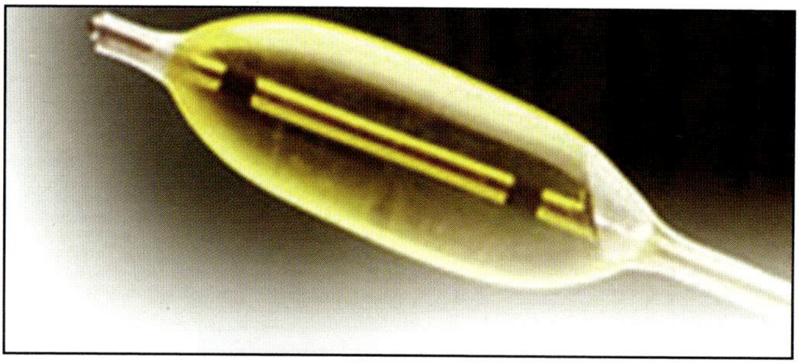

Figure 8: Balloon catheter for adults (5 mm diameter, 8 mm balloon length)

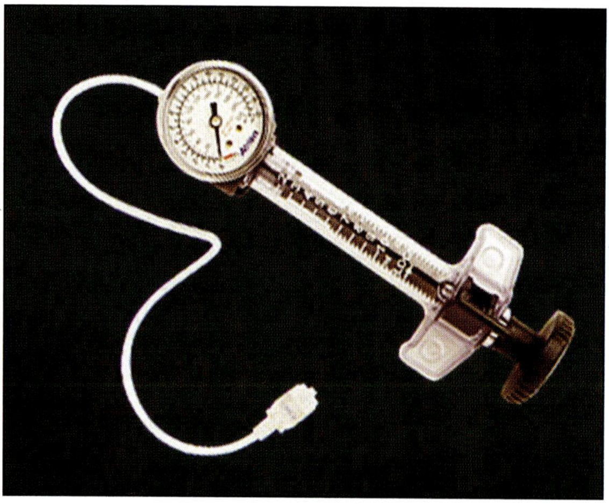

Figure 9: Balloon catheter inflation device

Chapter 21

Pediatric Epiphora

AK Grover, Shaloo Bageja
Malvika Bansal (India)

Introduction

Congenital nasolacrimal duct obstruction is the most common cause of epiphora in children, occuring in approximately 2-6% of infants. Ophthalmologists should however be aware of the other causes of epiphora in this age group. Thus, information of the developmental anatomy, abnormalities of the nasolacrimal system and other congenital disorders is essential for appropriate diagnosis and management of the conditions encountered.

Embryology of the Lacrimal System

Lacrimal system comprises the secretory and the excretory system.

Secretory System

It is ectodermal in nature. It begins as epithelial buds from basal cells of bulbar conjunctiva in the superotemporal fornix. These buds form cord of cells, which is later enclosed by the mesenchyme. At 60 mm stage lumen begins to form, though development continues 3-4 yr postnatally.

Accessory glands of Krause and Wolfring develop as non-keratinized buds of epithelium from conjunctiva.

Excretory System

The excretory system begins in the first trimester when two facial prominence derived from first branchial arch fuse. Fusion of lateral nasal prominence with maxillary process entraps two layer of surface ectoderm. The surface ectoderm forms solid epithelial lacrimal cord in rudimentary naso-optic fissure. The cord grows during fetal life and is later surrounded by mesenchyme. The canalization of cord begins at about 4th-5th month of fetal life. It extends both caudally and cephalad. The cephalic end forms canaliculi and sac while the caudal end grows towards the nasal cavity. The puncta open when eyelids separate. The last portion to canalize is the lower end of the duct at the inferior meatus. The valve of Hasner may rupture any time between 6th month of gestation to soon after birth or may be delayed to several months after birth.

Interruption in canalization at any stage of development may result in congenital nasolacrimal obstruction.

Developmental Abnormalities

Punctal and canalicular abnormalities include punctal agenesis, stenosis and membranous occlusion of punctum.

Lacrimal sac fistula or diverticula of sac may occur.

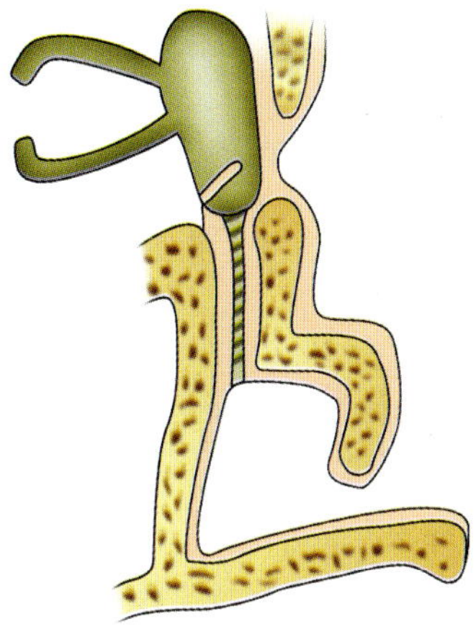

Figure 1: Nasolacrimal duct obstruction at or near the inferior meatus, due to non-perforation of the nasal mucosa

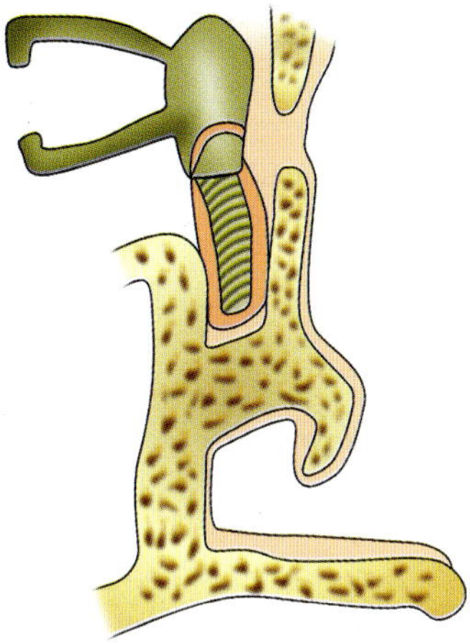

Figure 2: Almost complete absence of the nasolacrimal duct

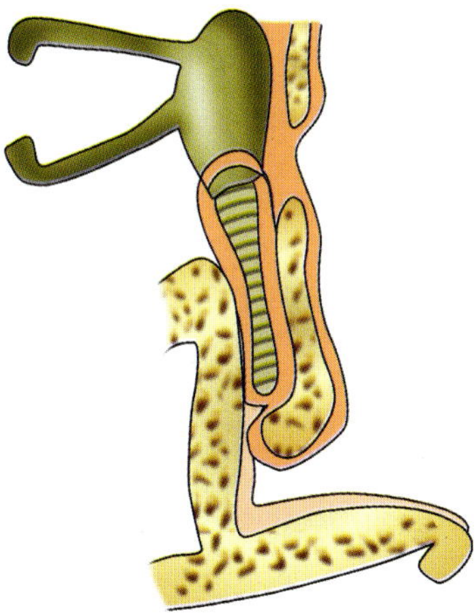

Figure 3: Obstruction at the lower end of the duct due to impaction of inferior turbinate

Nasolacrimal duct obstruction is the most common congenital abnormality, seen in 50% of infants at birth. The level of obstruction may vary in congenital nasolacrimal duct obstruction.

1. The most common obstruction occurring at the lower end of the duct where it fails to perforate the mucosa of the inferior meatus.
2. Absence of duct due to failure to the osseous nasolacrimal canal to form, commonly seen with cleft palate anomalies.
3. Blockage of duct due to impaction of anterior end of inferior turbinate.

Anatomy of Excretory System

The drainage system comprises of puncta, upper and lower canalicului, common canaliculus, lacrimal sac and nasolacrimal duct.

The excretory system begins with puncta which is about 0.3 mm in diameter. It is situated medially in line with meibomian glands orifice. The lower punctum is located lateral in position than the upper punctum. Both puncta are ringed by avascular fibrous tissue. The punctum leads into canaliculus which comprises of 2 mm verical and 8 mm horizontal limb. The two canaliculi may converge into common canaliculus in majority of cases. The two canaliculi or common canaliculus enter the lacrimal sac 3-5 mm from its apex. A fold of mucosa, i.e valve of Rosenmuller, at the junction of the canaliculi and sac prevents tear reflux from the sac back into the canaliculi.

The lacrimal sac lies within the lacrimal sac fossa, formed by the lacrimal bone and ascending frontal process of maxilla. The lacrimal fossa is enclosed by anterior and posterior crus of the medial canthal tendon. The lacrimal sac is about 15 mm in height.

The lacrimal sac drains into nasolacrimal duct. The intraosseous part of nasolacrimal duct is approximately 12 mm. The duct traverses downward, laterally and posteriorly. This is important to remember when surgeon is probing the lacrimal system, otherwise may create a false passage. The distal portion extends into the middle meatus forming the meatal portion of the duct, which is about 5 mm in length. The duct opens into the nose through the ostium under the inferior turbinate, which is covered by a mucosal fold called the valve of Hasner. The position of ostium may vary.

Important Points to Remember in Infants

1. Distance from punctum to the floor of the nose is approximately 20 mm .
2. Distance of the ostium from the tip of the inferior turbinate is about 15 mm and 25-30 mm from the external nares.

Physiology

Some amount of tear elimination occurs by evaporation along with physical factors like gravity and capillary action. However, the blink mechanism play

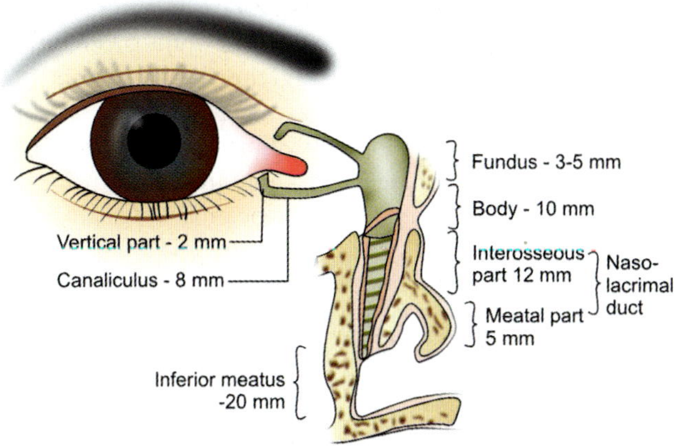

Figure 4: Anatomy of lacrimal excretory system

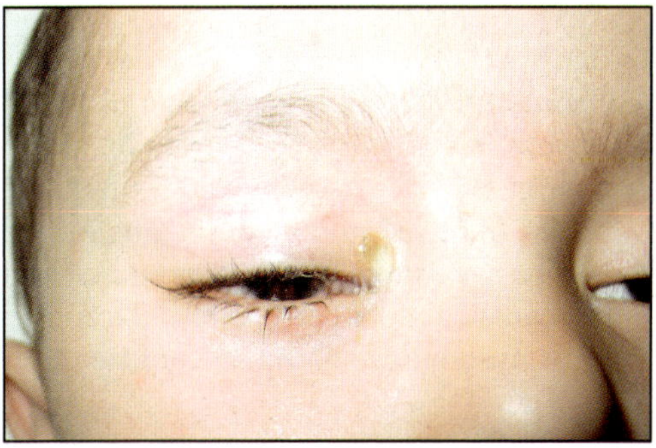

Figure 5: A 13-month-old child who presented with persistent watering and discharge

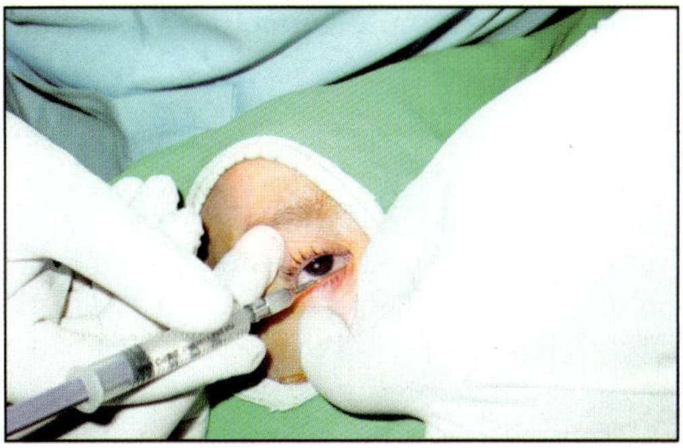

Figure 6: Syringing is performed prior to probing of the nasolacrimal duct to evacuate the lacrimal sac

an important role in the tear flow. Jones' description of lacrimal pump mechanism was well accepted in the past. It reported that blink mechanism propels the tears into nasolacrimal duct by altering the intrasac pressure. However, Rosengren-Doane has described a better explanation based on cinematographic studies. On blinking, the apposition of eyelids and contraction of orbicularis creates a positive pressure in the tear sac, thus drawing fluid into the nose. On opening of eyelids, the puncta separate and negative pressure draws tears into the canaliculi and the sac.

The valve of Rosenmuller at common canaliculus and the valve of Hasner at the lower end of naso-lacrimal duct ensure unidirectional flow of tears. Paralysis of orbicularis result in epiphora due to lacrimal pump failure.

Evaluation

In evaluating a patient of pediatric epiphora, it is important to obtain a detailed history and to carry out a careful examination of the patient.

History

A thorough history from child's parents is essential as the child is not co-operative for proper examination. Parent's usually present with complaint of persistent watering with or without mucopurulent discharge. Age of onset of symptoms is important as the tear production begins a couple of weeks after life. Thus, the child may be asymptomatic for a month or so. History of trauma is necessary to rule out canalicular or bony injury. Symptoms of photophobia, watering, corneal haze or nystagmus should be enquired to rule out congenital glaucoma.

Examination

Eyelid Margin

Eyelid margins are inspected for punctal position, its apposition to globe and its patency. It is important to exclude any lid abnormalities and any cause for reflex secretion like epiblepharon, conjunctivitis, trichiasis, blepharitis or meibomitis.

Medial Canthal Area

An ophthalmologist should look for any swelling over the medial canthal area like mucocele or congenital dacryocele. Pressure over the medial canthus may cause regurgitation of discharge from the punctum if blockage is distal to the sac. It is important to distinguish swellings above the medial canthal tendon which indicate conditions like anterior ethmoidal mucocele or encephalocele and one needs to perform a CT scan to identify the condition.

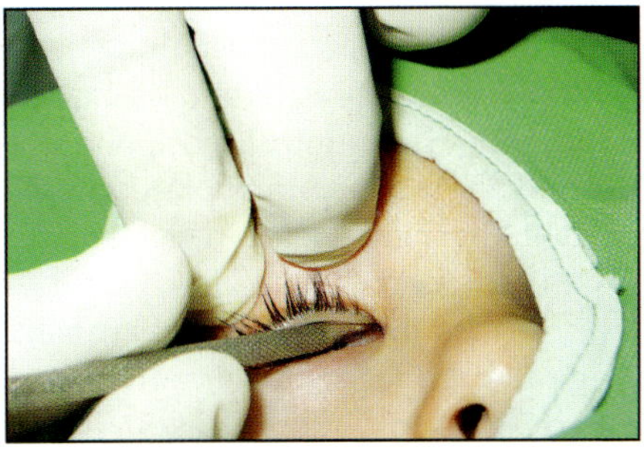

Figure 7A: A Nettleship dilator is used to gently dilate the punctum

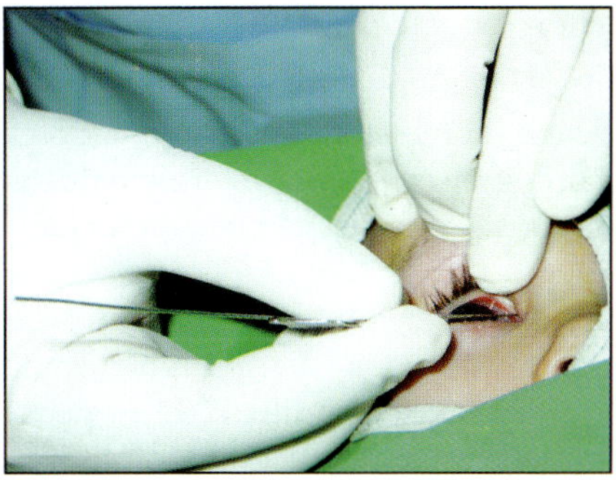

Figure 7B: Bowman probe size 00 is introduced into upper punctum perpendicular to eyelid margin

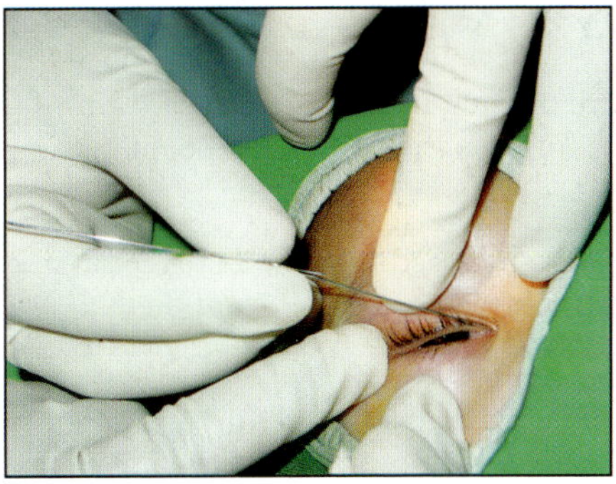

Figure 7C: Bowman probe is advanced horizontally while maintaining lateral traction of eyelid

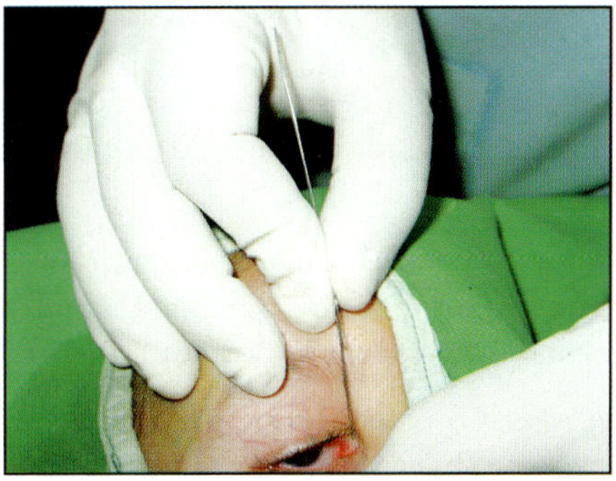

Figure 7D: Probe lies over the supraorbital notch at superior orbital rim and is advanced into the nasolacrimal duct

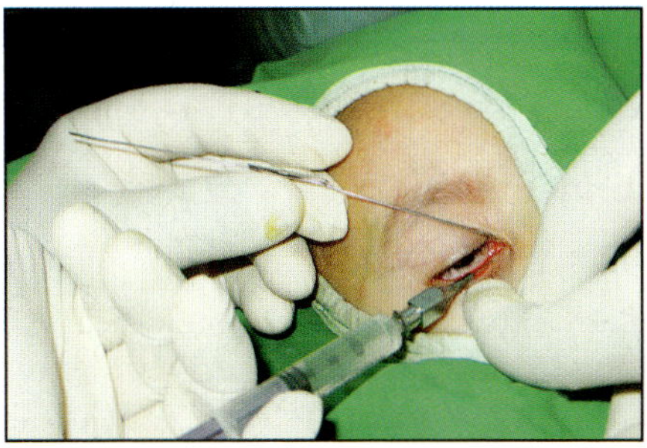

Figure 7E: Syringing of nasolacrimal system is done to check the patency

Investigations

In cases of congenital lacrimal system obstruction, the diagnosis is usually clear cut on history and examination as child present with watering, discharge, matting of eyelashes, inferior palpebral congestion. In doubtful cases, the dye disappearence test can be conducted. A drop of 2% fluorescein is placed in the inferior fornix. Tear film is observed with cobalt blue light. Delay in clearence of the dye after 5 minutes indicates outflow obstruction. This test is useful in children as diagnostic syringing cannot be performed in outpatient department.

Imaging has limited role in pediatric age though lacrimal scintigraphy or intraoperative dacryocystography can be performed in doubtful cases.

Management

Punctal and Canalicular Abnormalities

Punctal Agenesis

Agenesis of punctum results due to failure of conjunctival dehisence overlying a canaliculus during eyelid separation. Thus, leaving a persistent membrane across the punctum.

If papilla is visible, then the membrane can be punctured with a dilator. Syringing and probing following membrane rupture can restore the patency, if the remaining system is normal structurally.

If papilla is not seen, one may cut at the expected area of punctum and attempt probing. In case the passage is patent, intubation should of the lacrimal system is indicated. Canalicular agenesis is usually associated with punctal agenesis.

Single patent punctum, child may be asymptomatic especially in case of upper punctum involvement. If patient is symptomatic, surgeon should evaluate normal punctum and its passage.

Both punctum absent, requires conjunctivodacryocystorhinostomy when patient is old enough to take care of the tube.

Lacrimal Sac Abnormalities

Dacryocystocele

A dilated sac without any signs of inflammation indicate congenital dacryocele or amniotocele. It is due to entrapment of mucus or amniotic fluid within the lacrimal sac due to nasolacrimal duct obstruction. It presents within first few weeks of life. An infant presents with tense swelling at the medial canthus inferior to the medial canthal tendon. Gentle massage over the sac along with topical antibiotics may relieve the obstruction. Syringing and probing is required if infant is symptomatic even after massage. Probing is done as early as 6 wk of age.

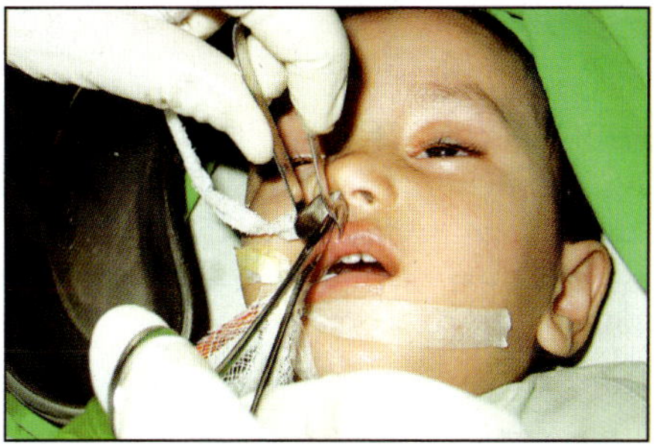

Figure 8A: Nasal cavity is packed before proceeding for inferior turbinate infracture

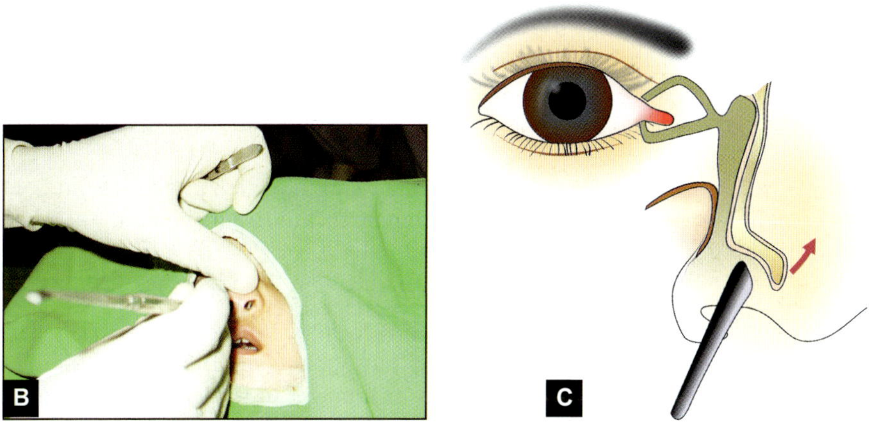

Figures 8 B and C: Inferior turbinate infracture with use of blunt spatula

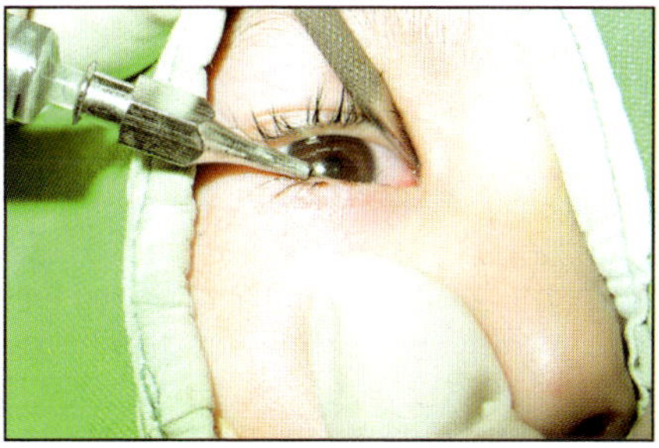

Figure 8D: Syringing through inferior canaliculus to check patency

Congenital Nasolacrimal Obstruction (CNLDO)

CNLDO is commonly due to membranous block of the opening into the inferior meatus at the valve of Hasner. Of the 50% of newborn infants who have obstruction at the inferior end of nasolacrimal duct, only 2-6% clinically presents with epiphora at 3-4 wks of age. Spontaneous resolution occurs in approximately 90% of all patients in first year of life. Conservative management is therefore recommended in all cases.

Conservative Management

Parents are educated regarding maintenance of lid hygiene and lacrimal sac massage (Criggler massage).

Criggler massage: Surgeon should demonstrate the proper technique of massage to the mother. It should be emphasized to use the little finger for this maneuver. One should first palpate the medial canthal tendon and move the finger downwards, feeling the anterior lacrimal crest. Massage is done with firm strokes over the lacrimal sac at least twice a day. Approximately, 90% of the infants respond to massage in first year of life and 60% respond in their second year of life.

Topical antibiotics are advised at least thrice a day to reduce mucoid discharge. Infants who do not respond to conservative management are taken up for probing.

Acute dacryocystitis: Some cases of CNLDO may present with an acute episode of inflammation of lacrimal sac. It is often associated with cellulites and needs to be managed vigorously with systemic intravenous antibiotics. One should not attempt to drain the pus in acute stage as it may lead to lacrimal – cutaneous fistula. Early syringing and probing is indicated once the acute stage subsides.

If lacrimal sac abscess is developed, surgical drainage is required.

Syringing and Probing

Timing of Probing

Timing of probing is controversial, most of the surgeons now prefer to wait till one year of age, while some surgeons advocate early probing.

Anesthesia

It is performed under general anesthesia with protected airway. Laryngeal mask may be used instead of endotracheal intubation depending on the choice of the anesthesiologist.

Technique

Before starting the procedure it, the lacrimal sac needs to be evacuated either by performing massage over the sac area or syringing with saline.

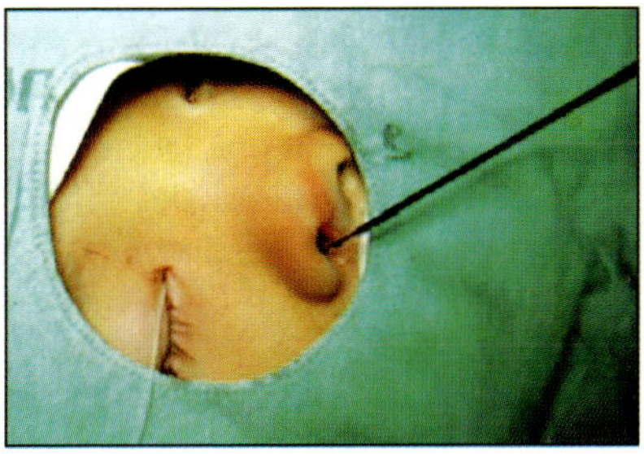

Figure 9A: Silicone tube is passed through the canaliculus into the nasolacrimal duct

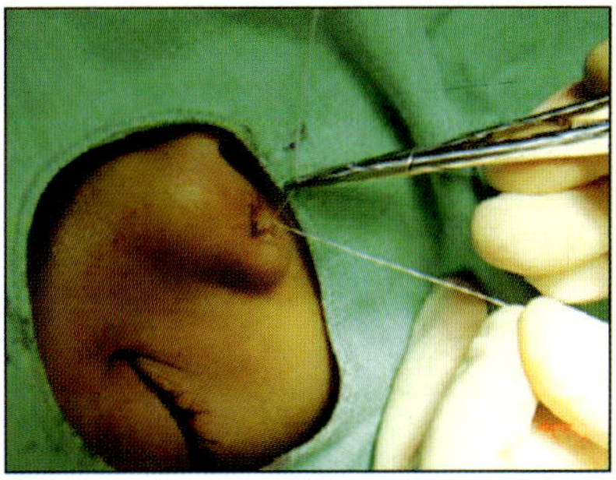

Figure 9B: Silicone tubing are tied together in the nose

Upper punctum is generally preferred for probing to prevent any damage to the lower punctum during the manipulation. Punctum is dilated with Nettleship dilator and then Bowman probe (size 0 or 00) is introduced into the punctum perpendicular to the eyelid margin. It first traverses the vertical 2 mm of the canaliculus and then the horizontal part while maintaining a lateral traction of eyelid is maintained. The lateral traction of skin stretches the canaliculus and avoids any chance of damage to the canalicular mucosa and decreases the probability of creation of a false passage. If one feels the resistance while passing the probe medially, it may be due to kink of the canaliculus. Surgeon should withdraw the probe slightly and then proceed medially maintaining the lateral traction. As the tip reaches the medial wall of lacrimal sac and lacrimal bone, surgeon will feel a hard stop.

The probe is then slightly withdrawn and rotated superiorly against the brow and should come to rest over the supraorbital notch at the superior orbital rim. The probe is then passed downwards, posteriorly and slight laterally down the nasolacrimal duct. The probe should slide down smoothly. In case of any feel of resistance, withdraw the probe slightly and proceed forward. If the surgeon feels the firm stop at a distance of about 12 mm (distance from punctum to nasolacrimal duct) and cannot manipulate further, it indicates a bony obstruction and absence of nasolacrimal duct. Dacryocystorhinostomy is indicated in such a situation. If probe pass down the nasolacrimal duct to about 20 mm, it indicates that it has reached the inferior meatus. Some resistance is felt due to membranous obstruction. Firm pressure passes the probe into the nasal cavity with a slight " pop up" sensation. Successful probing is verified by syringing. Some surgeons confirm the patency by passing a spatula under the inferior turbinate to have a metal on metal feel.

Availability of nasal endoscopes, may also assist in verifying the correct passage of probe. It aids rupturing of the membrane under direct visualization and thus avoids creation of false passage. Position of inferior turbinate can be visualized and infracture of the turbinate can be done if inferior turbinate is impacted at the ostium.

Postoperatively, steroid – antibiotic drops four times a day for 2 weeks along with nasal decongestant drops are prescribed.

Failure

Probing may fail due to formation of small opening through the membrane, leading to closure postoperatively or due to impaction of inferior turbinate.

Repeat probing is attempted at least 6 weeks after the initial one.

Inferior Turbinate Infracture

It is performed under general anesthesia. The nasal cavity is packed before proceeding for turbinate infracture.

Lens spatula is passed under the inferior turbinate, the anterior end of turbinate is rotated medially and superiorly towards the septum. Then the spatula is passed backwards and then the middle and the posterior part of turbinate are fractured. Patency is checked by syringing. Nasal cavity is packed for 24 hours as there may be a risk of slight bleed.

Postoperatively, steroid-antibiotic drops and nasal decongestants are prescribed.

Silicone Intubation

Indication

Silicone intubation is indicated in cases of recurrent failed probing with or without inferior turbinate infracture or in older children.

Various types of intubation sets like Crawford, Ritleng and others are available for the purpose.

It is performed under general anesthesia. Before intubation nasal packing is done to constrict the mucosa of the inferior turbinate. These silicone tubings have metal bodkins attached at each end. Punctum is dilated. If metal tube cannot be easily passed through the punctum, one or three snip procedure may be performed. The metal tubings are passed through each canaliculus into the nasolacrimal duct. They can be pulled into the nasal cavity with the help of an artery forceps. The silicone tubings are tied together in the nose near inferior meatus after removing the metal bodkins.

The procedure can be combined with inferior turbinate infracture. Stents are left in position for atleast six months.

Balloon Dacryoplasty

This is a new technique of management, where collapsed catheter is introduced into the nasolacrimal duct by a procedure similar to probing. The balloon is inflated with saline to 8 atm for 90 seconds, deflated, and then reinflated for 60 seconds with the catheter at the sac—Nasolacrimal duct junction and at the lower nasolacrimal duct. The balloon should not be inflated in the lacrimal sac as it may rupture the system. The procedure is not so popular due to dependence on the requirement of a catheter and its high cost.

Dacryocystorhinostomy (DCR)

Indication

DCR is indicated in cases of repeated failed probing with inferior turbinate infracture or silicone intubation or in cases where on the initial probing a bony obstruction is diagnosed. It is also indicated in traumatic cases leading to canalicular scarring or injury to intraosseous part of nasolacrimal duct and in craniofacial abnormalities, associated with nasolacrimal abnormalities.

Timing

Surgery is usually not performed before 3 years of age except in cases of persistent episodes of acyte dacryocystitis.

Anesthesia

The procedure is performed under general anesthesia. Mild hypotensive anesthesia may be preferred to minimize blood loss intraoperatively.

DCR in children is may be difficult owing to smaller size of the structures. The technique requires some modifications due to some anatomical differences from the adult lacrimal system. The anterior lacrimal crest and the lacrimal fossa are pooly developed and it is sometimes difficult to locate the site for osteotomy. Medial canthal tendon insertion provides an important landmark to identify the superior part of anterior lacrimal crest.

Due to thin bones, osteotomy is easily performed. One should prefer to have a larger osteotomy as there may be postoperative bony regrowth which may be a cause of failure.

Failures have been observed in the pediatric age group due to less well-defined anatomy, postoperative bony growth and greater scarring.

Mitomycin C have also been tried intraoperatively by applying a soaked piece of cotton to the osteotomy site to reduce fibrosis and scarring postoperatively.

Endonasal DCR

Endonasal DCR, though technically difficult in young children offers a number of advantages over the external approach. It avoids the need for a skin incision and consequent scarring, enables creation of a large ostium even when the lacrimal sac is small and scarred. It has additional advantage of limited intraoperative bleeding.

Summary

Abnormalities of lacrimal system are encountered frequently in the pediatric age group. Epiphora is a common condition in infancy and early childhood. Congenital nasolacrimal duct obstruction resolves spontaneously in 90-95% cases in first year of life. Inital management includes massage of lacrimal sac and application of topical antibiotics. Syringing and Probing alone or in combination with inferior turbinate infracture is performed in cases who does not respond to conservative therapy after one year of age. Silastic intubation is performed for repeated failed probing and finally DCR is indicated in cases of failed probing after 3 years of age.

Chapter 22

Congenital Anomalies of the Anterior Segment

Hala Elhilaly, Rania El Essawy
Hoda MH Mostafa (Egypt)

Anophthalmos/Microphthalmos

Anophthalmos and Microphthalmos are major congenital structural ocular malformations that occur as a result of insults to the developing eye during the first 8 weeks of gestation. It could be isolated or associated with other congenital anomalies.

Prevalence

The ***prevalence*** of both anophthalmos and microphthalmos is estimated to lie between 1 and 3.5 per 10,000 with no predilection to sex or race, however, an increased incidence has been noticed in low socioeconomic societies, and consanguinity is a known predisposing factor.

Anophthalmos is the congenital absence of the globe. True anophthalmos may be difficult to differentiate both clinically and radiologically from extreme microphthalmos (clinical anophthalmos) where a very small globe can only be detected by serial histological sections of the orbital contents.

Mann classified Anophthalmos into three distinct types:

Primary anophthalmos: Caused by failure of development of the optic vesicle from the forebrain before 2 mm stage of embryonic life. It is usually bilateral and sporadic.

Secondary anophthalmos: An extremely rare and lethal anomaly due to complete suppression or grossly anomalous development of the entire anterior neural tube: the forebrain and its derivatives, the optic vesicles.

Consecutive or degenerative anophthalmos: Occurs when the optic vesicle forms but subsequently degenerates due to insults during the second stage of development: 4-8 weeks of embryonic life.

Anophthalmos is most commonly bilateral, sometimes occurring on one side and microphthalmos on the opposite side. The orbit and eyelids are formed but small (micro-orbitism and micro-blepharism), the eyelids are shortened in all directions, often with a dystrophic levator muscle, the fornices are shallow, the extraocular muscles are present but may be maldeveloped.

Infants with true bilateral anophthalmia show an absence of the optic nerves and optic chiasma with maldeveloped optic foramina. Lack of properly established connections from the developing eyes to the optic pathways results in hypoplasia or absence of the related white matter tracts and lateral geniculate ganglia. Dysgenesis or absence of the corpus callosum may also be seen suggesting an anomalous formation of the lamina terminalis which is a precursor of the forebrain and the corpus callosum.

Microphthalmos is a condition in which the affected eye is smaller than 15 mm in greatest diameter at birth (normally16-19 mm), less than 19 mm at 1 year or 22 mm in adulthood.

Microphthalmos occurs between 7 and 14 mm stages of embryonic development when the primary optic vesicle already has invaginated but the fetal cleft (embryonic neuroectodermal fissure) has not closed. It is due to

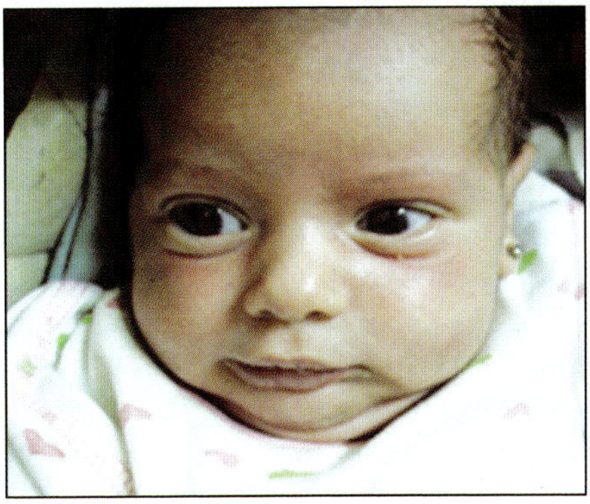

Figure 1: Left microphthalmos

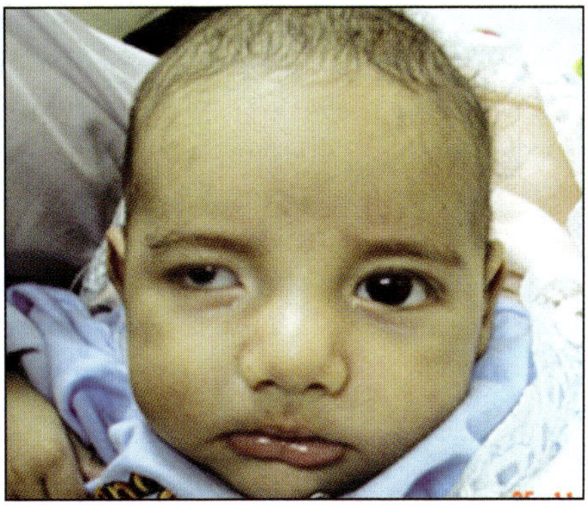

Figure 2: Right microphthalmos

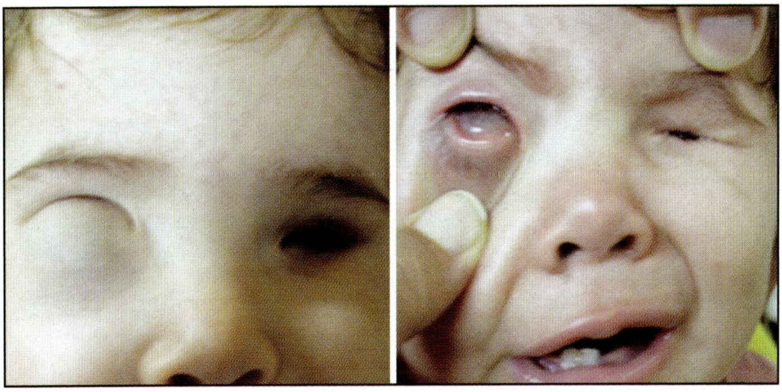

Figure 3: Right microphthalmos with cyst and left clinical anophthalmos

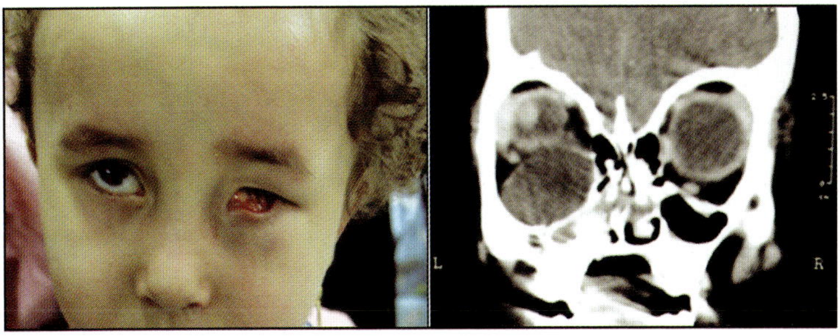

Figure 4: Left microphthalmia with a cyst and its CT scan appearance

intrauterine involution of the optic vesicle and interference with the normal fusion of that fissure. Three types of microphthalmia are recognized:

Simple microphthalmos (nanophthalmos) is a very rare form. The eye is small, but normal, with no other gross abnormalities; however, the relative lens/eye volume is high making it susceptible to acute and chronic angle closure glaucoma. Also there is hypermetropia, thick sclera and a tendency towards postoperative or even spontaneous uveal effusion and secondary choroidal or retinal detachment.

Microphthalmos associated with other ocular anomalies or more generalized systemic malformations as in congenital Rubella and Trisomy 13. The eye is reduced in size with a microcornea often an iris, ciliary body, choroidal or optic nerve coloboma, and may be corneal opacities, posterior synechiae, cataract or retinal detachment.

Microphthalmos with a cyst (colobomatous microphthalmos) where the sclera is thin and ectatic appearing as a cyst of variable size that may grow to become bigger than and obscuring the microphthalmic globe itself. The microphthalmic eye is usually displaced upwards behind the upper lid by a cyst located inferiorly and presenting as a bulge in the lower eyelid. Rarely the cyst is located posteriorly causing proptosis.

Duke Elder described three categories of cysts associated with microphthalmos: a relatively normal eye with a small cyst not apparent clinically; an obvious cyst associated with a grossly deformed eye; a large cyst which has pushed the globe backwards so that it is no longer visible clinically. The condition is usually unilateral but frequently the other eye shows the evidence of a coloboma.

Histologically there is an eversion of the retina through the unclosed fissure to form a lining of rudimentary neuroectodermal tissue covered with a fibrous outer coat of variable thickness which may be continuous with the sclera but the choroid is absent. The cavity of the cyst is usually in direct continuity with the vitreous cavity and is filled with a clear fluid.

Differential Diagnosis

Differential diagnosis is from *congenital cystic eyeball* where there is failure of invagination of the primary optic vesicle occurring between 2 and 7 mm stage of embryonic development. The orbit shows a cystic structure of a bluish color due to contained fluid and uveal pigment. In some instances, invagination occurs but is incomplete leading to a condition known as *congenital nonattachment of the retina.*

Etiology

Anophthalmos/Microphthalmos may be due to genetic or nongenetic factors that cause the disease to occur in isolation or as a part of a syndrome. All patterns of inheritance are observed: autosomal dominant, autosomal recessive, X-linked dominant and recessive or sporadic. Chromosomal aberrations commonly in the form of trisomy (Trisomy 13, 18 and 22) and deletions may account for 16% of all cases of anophthalmia and microphthalmia. *Nongenetic*

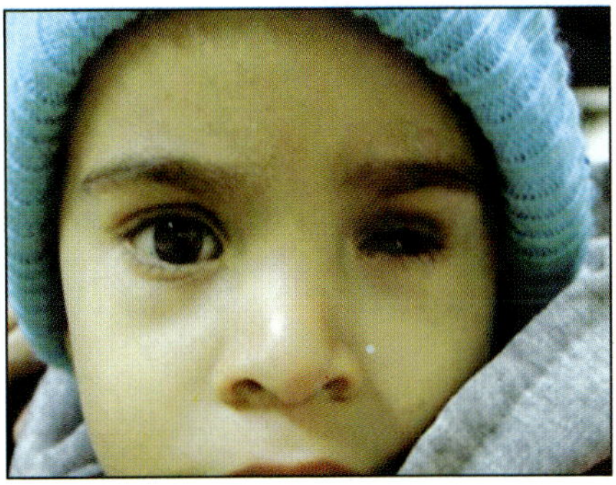

Figure 5: Left anophthalmia with an artificial eye and a right iris coloboma

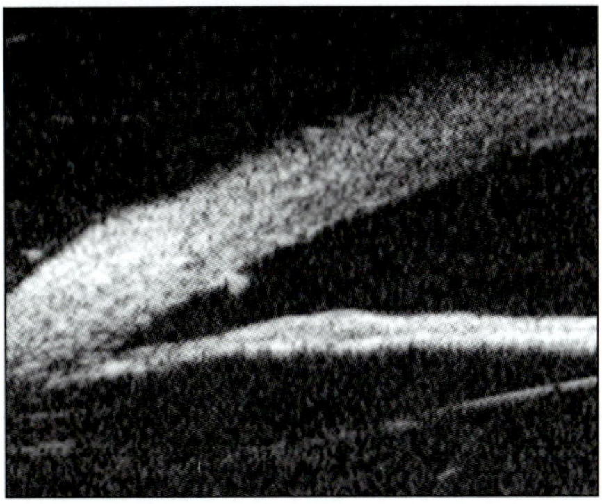

Figure 6: Posterior embryotoxon may not be not easily detected clinically, but with the high resolution of UBM, its detection may be easier (*UBM image courtesy of ZEl Sanabary, MD, Cairo University)*

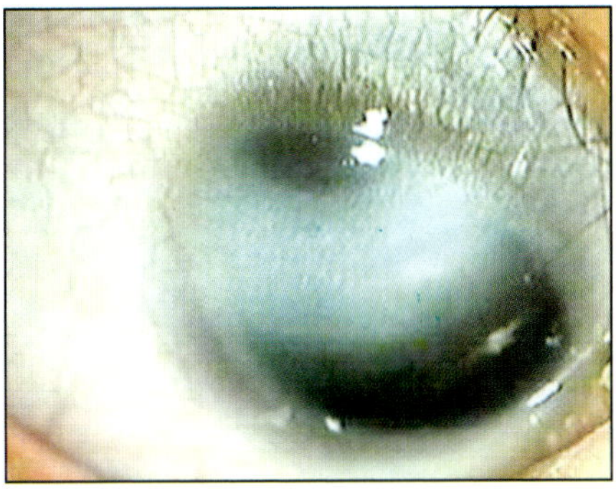

Figure 7: Color image of a patient with Peter's anomaly

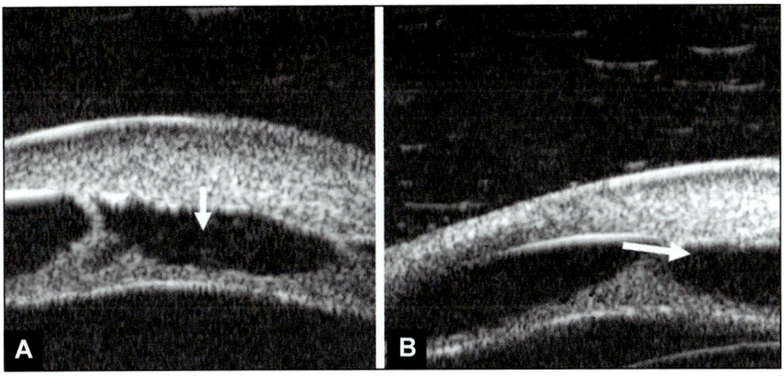

Figures 8A and B: Typical Peter's anomaly with defective central Descemet's membrane (down arrow) and iridocorneal synechiae at the edges of the defect (right arrow) (*UBM image courtesy of Z El Sanabary, MD, Cairo University)*

factors include maternal exposure to infections as Rubella, Toxoplasma and Cytomegalovirus, influenza and fever. A number of potential environmental teratogens have been proposed including: alcohol, drugs such as thalidomide, retinoids, warfarin, and carbamazepin, vitamin A deficiency, hyperthermia and exposure to X-rays or agricultural pesticides; the evidence in their support however, is only preliminary and the condition may result from a variety of different exposures alone or in combination. It is also probable that a background of genetic susceptibility is required.

Ocular and Systemic Associations

The condition may be associated with microcornea, sclerocornea, Peter's anomaly, cataract, persistent fetal vasculature (posterior hyperplastic primary vitreous), iris coloboma. aniridia, choroidal, retinal or optic nerve colobomata. *Systemic Associations* differ according to the syndrome (see Table 1), there may be syndactyly or polydactyly; ear anomalies; nasal anomalies such as a thin-pinched nose; orodental anomalies such as thin lips, high-arched palate, macrostomia, micrognathia, bifid tongue or delayed eruption of teeth; hypoplastic or ambiguous external genitalia. Also cardiac anomalies, oesophageal atresia and skin defects in the form of hypo or hyperpigmentation. Both cranial and intracranial anomalies may be seen as: microcephaly, hydrocephaly, hemifacial atrophy, facial clefting, hypogenesis of corpus callosum and cerebellar hypoplasia.

CT scan and MRI are of value in:

1. Demonstration of anophthalmia or microphthalmia by showing an absent or a small globe,
2. Assessment of associated craniofacial anomalies
3. Detection of associated intracranial anomalies.

Management

The management is a challenge especially in cases of anophthalmia and severe microphthalmia. Treatment could be long and complicated with multiple orbital, conjunctival and eyelid reconstruction surgeries required throughout the child's life, and even then results may be disappointing because a perfectly normal-looking orbit will not be achieved. Psychological support for both the parents and the child is necessary.

Examination and management of other ocular anomalies wherever possible such as associated cataract, exclusion of other system malformations by the pediatrician and genetic counseling when required are all appropriate measures.

The *timing* of surgery differs according to the severity of the condition: early interference is only required in cases of large orbital cysts protruding through the palpebral fissure and in anophthalmia where the results are much better if treatment is initiated in the first year. Recent studies have confirmed that enucleation in childhood compromises orbital growth, cases with small or

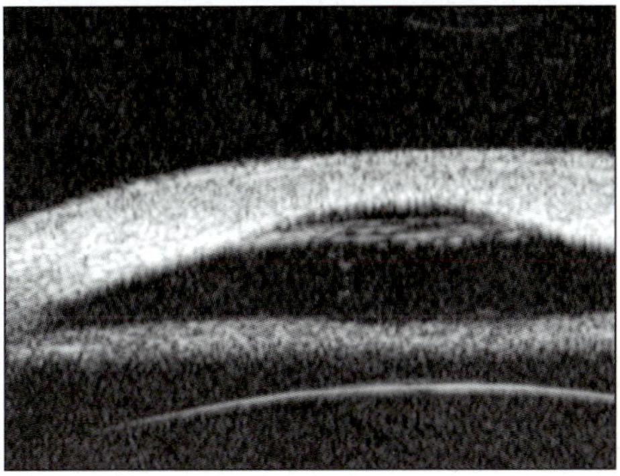

Figure 9: Variant of Peter's anomaly with poorly developed DM (*UBM image courtesy of Z El Sanabary, MD, Cairo University)*

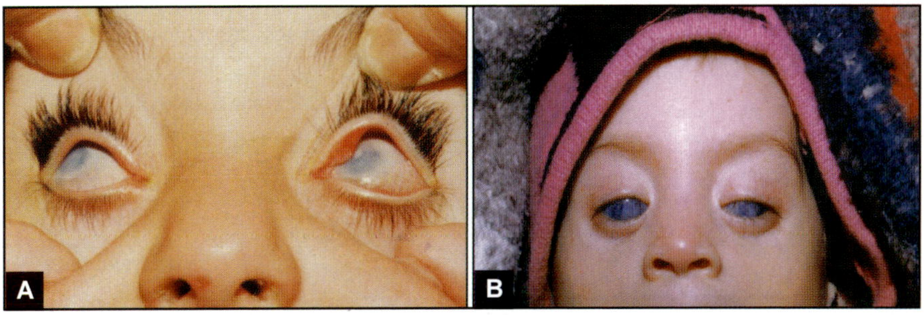

Figures 10A and B: Showing bilateral corneal opacification consistent with sclerocornea

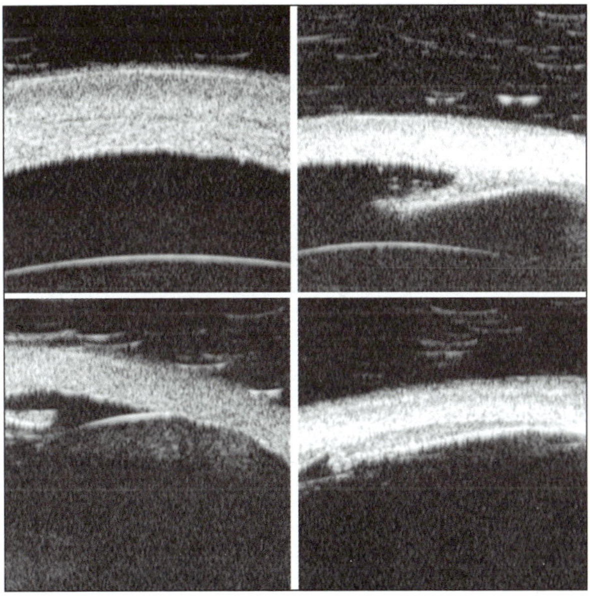

Figure 11: Sclerocornea with different lenticulo-corneal relationships (*UBM image courtesy of Z El Sanabary, MD, Cairo University)*

Table 1

Syndrome	*Ocular associations*	*Systemic associations*
Trisomy 13 (Patau's syndrome)	Iris or ciliary body colobomata, cataract, persistent fetal vasculature, corneal dysgenesis, retinal dysplasia	Mental retardation, low set ears, cleft palate, cleft lip, polydactyly, cryptorchidism
Trisomy 18 (Edward's syndrome)	Narrow palpebral aperture, ptosis, epicanthus, hypo or hypertelorism, proptosis, nystagmus, rarely corneal opacities, colobomata, cataract	Mental retardation, low set ears, micrognathia, prominent occipit, narrow pelvis and may be hip subluxation, flexed overlapping fingers, cardiac and renal anomalies
Lenz microphthalmia's syndrome		Mental retardation, malformed ears, skeletal anomalies, urogenital anomalies.
Fryns' anophthalmia plus syndrome		Nasal deformity, choanal atresia, bifid uvula, facial cleft
Anophthalmia-esophageal-genital syndrome		Esophageal atresia, cryptorchidism
Fetal Rubella's syndrome	Corneal opacity, cataract, glaucoma, chorioretinitis,	Deafness, cardiac anomalies
Fetal alcohol syndrome	Short palpebral fissures, ptosis	Microcephaly, cardiac anomalies
CHARGE'S syndrome	Colobomata most commonly retinal	Cardiac anomalies, choanal atresia, ear anomalies, deafness, genital anomalies
Aicardi's syndrome	Chorioretinal lacunae	Infantile spasms, agenesis of corpus callosum
Focal dermal hypoplasia (Golz's syndrome)		Skin anomalies, skeletal anomalies, dental anomalies
Microphthalmia and linear skin defect syndrome (MLS)	sclerocornea, chorioretinal abnormalities	Skin anomalies, agenesis of corpus callosum, hydrocephalus, infantile seizures, mental retardation, cardiac anomalies
Goldenhar's syndrome	Epibulbar dermoids, accessory auricular appendages,	Vertebral anomalies
Hallermann-Streiff's syndrome	Microcornea, cataract	Mandibular hypoplasia, parrot-beak nose, bird-like facies.

medium-sized cysts with an associated ocular remnant help stimulate orbital expansion better than any artificial orbital implant, so, although parents are often keen to have the microphthalmic eye or the cyst removed to improve cosmoses, elective enucleation is better postponed to school age.

Management of Anophthalmos

Orbital surgery

Orbital expansion can be achieved by:

1. Progressively increasing the size of a *Solid Conformer,*
2. An *Inflatable Silicone Expander* reconstituted with saline through a tube placed at the lateral orbital rim.
3. *Osmotic Tissue Expander* which is a recently introduced self-inflating Hydrogel or HEMMA expander. Once expansion of the orbit and fornices permits, fitting of an ocular prosthesis improves the appearance. More volume enhancement can be achieved by orbital implants when feasible.

In cases of late referral with severe micro-orbitism or insufficient orbital volume, a *three dimensional orbital bone expansion* surgery for the bony orbit with or without bone grafts to augment the deficient contours is needed.

Eyelid surgery

Fitting of the prosthesis is often limited by the palpebral fissure and eyelid shortening. The palpebral fissure may be widened by a lateral and/or a medial canthotomy or canthoplasty. Additional lengthening of eyelids can be accomplished by a combination of skin, mucosal or cartilage grafts, but this is best postponed until maximum expansion has been achieved by conformer therapy as early treatment may lead to cicatricial tissue formation.

Management of Microphthalmos

Patients with poor orbital volume can achieve very good cosmetic results if treated with conformers as early as possible, microphthalmic eyes with some residual vision can be treated with clear conformers that do not obscure the visual axis, cosmetic scleral shells with optical correction have also been recently introduced. Cysts may be aspirated but this is frequently followed by fluid re-accumulation, in this case surgical excision and orbital implantation is indicated. Silicone, acrylic, hydroxyappatite and other implants may be used but the Dermis fat graft has the advantage of being autogenous and with the ability to enlarge as the child grows.

Anterior Segment Dysgenesis

Anterior segment dysgenesis (ASD) constitutes a spectrum of developmental disorders involving the cornea, angle, iris and lens. It most likely represents an abnormal embryonic development of the cranial neural ectoderm. Many theories on the pathogenesis of ASD have been proposed. A developmental arrest, late in gestation, of certain anterior segment structures derived from neural crest cells is the most likely mechanism. First, abnormal retention of the primordial endothelial layer on the surface of the iris and anterior chamber angle, with subsequent contraction, is believed to account for the iris changes and the tissue strands in the anterior chamber angle. Furthermore, deposition of basement membrane by these cells is felt to result in a prominent Schwalbe's line. Secondly, a developmental arrest in the posterior recession of the iris root during the third trimester, results in a high insertion into the posterior aspect of the trabecular meshwork. Lastly, incomplete development of the trabecular meshwork and Schlemm's canal represents further evidence of developmental arrest occurring during the third trimester.

Posterior Embryotoxon

Posterior embryotoxon is a prominent, anteriorly displaced Schwalbe's line. It can be found in up to 15% of normal eyes without any clinical significance or may represent a form fruste of anterior segment dysgenesis.

On slit-lamp examination, it appears as a whitish, irregular arcuate ridge located 0.5 to 2 mm central to the limbus. The majority of posterior embryotoxon is seen temporally and limited to a few clock hours, but in some patients, it can be seen for 360 degrees.

Alagille's syndrome or arteriohepatic dysplasia is an autosomal dominant condition involving jaundice caused by a developmental scarcity of intrahepatic bile ducts. It has characteristic cardiovascular, skeletal, facial and ocular features. A prominent Schwalbe's line occurs in 90% of cases of Alagille's syndrome and is identified as an important marker. Early recognition of the syndrome is helpful in establishing the proper diagnosis to avoid unnecessary abdominal surgery and institute vitamin therapy.

Axenfeld-Rieger's Syndrome

The presence of posterior embryotoxon in association with numerous iris processes is known as Axenfeld's anomaly. If there is iris hypoplasia in addition to Axenfeld's anomaly, then the condition is referred to as Rieger's anomaly. If systemic features are present it is referred to as Rieger's syndrome. Many eponyms exist for Axenfeld-Rieger syndrome (ARS) including anterior cleavage syndrome and anterior segment mesodermal dysgenesis disorders.

The historical classification of ARS based on phenotypes has been challenged with the advent of the Human Genome Project and more of the molecular biology mechanisms underlying development are being unravelled. It has now become apparent that ARS shares genotypic and phenotypic overlap with other anterior segment dysgenesis such as iridogoniodysgenesis anomaly, iridogoniodysgenesis syndrome, iris hypoplasia and familial glaucoma iridogoniodysplasia. It has been proposed that all these overlapping groups of conditions should be classified under the umbrella term of ARS to eliminate the confusing sub-classification and to facilitate communication between clinicians.

Axenfeld-Rieger's syndrome is inherited in an autosomal dominant pattern. Three chromosomal loci (4q 25, 6p 25, 13q 14) have recently been demonstrated to link to ARS and related phenotypes. The PITX2 gene, on chromosome 4q 25, and the FOXC1 gene, on chromosome 6p 25, have been implicated. These are genes coding for paired-like homeodomain and forkhead/winged-helix transcription-factor families. Mutation in DNA binding domain of these genes can cause a wide variety of phenotypes that share features with ARS. Mutation resulting in increased PITX2 activity has been found to correlate with more severe ARS ocular phenotype. A plyomorphism in the GJA1 gene has been recently identified in association with ARS and raises the possibility of its participation as a modifier gene.

In ARS, gonioscopic examination reveals that the anterior chamber angle is open and the trabecular meshwork is visible, but the scleral spur is obscured by the more anterior insertion of the peripheral iris into the posterior portion of the trabecular meshwork.

In Rieger's anomaly, iris pathology can range from mild stromal thinning (iris hypoplasia) to marked atrophy with hole formation, corectopia and ectropion uvea. When corectopia is present, the pupil is displaced towards a prominent peripheral iridocorneal adhesion; the atrophy and hole formation occurs in the quadrant away from the direction of the pupil.

Abnormalities of the anterior chamber angle do not appear to progress after birth except for occasional thickening of iris strands. Abnormalities of the central iris are usually stable, but have been observed to progress during the first years of life. These changes consist of distortion or displacement of the pupil and occasional thinning and hole formation of the iris. Other associated ocular anomalies include sclerocornea, persistent pupillary membrane, microphthalmos and typical iris coloboma.

Glaucoma develops in 50 to 60% of patients with ARS. It may manifest itself during infancy but more commonly appears in childhood or young adulthood. Glaucoma is felt to occur more often in patients with centric iridic changes and in those with more-pronounced anterior peripheral iris insertion into the trabecular meshwork.

Rieger's syndrome is associated with many systemic anomalies, in particular, those involving developmental defects of the teeth and facial bones. Dental defects may include a reduction in crown size (microdontia), a decreased but evenly spaced number of teeth (hypodontia), and a focal absence of teeth (oligodontia or anodontia). Facial anomalies may include maxillary hypoplasia with flattening of the midface and a receding upper lip and prominent lower lip. Hypertelorism, telecanthus, and broad flat nose have also been described.

Other nonocular associations of ARS include congenital lip abnormalities, hydrocephalus, empty sella syndrome, middle ear deafness, kidney abnormalities, hypospadias, umbilical skin folds and heart defects. There is considerable variation in nonocular features, even among family members with ARS.

All associated ocular and systemic anomalies appear to arise from the maldevelopment of the neural crest cells. Patients with ARS should be examined for the presence of anomalies in the tissues of neural crest origin.

Management of glaucoma in patients with Axenfeld-Rieger's syndrome is difficult. Medications, particularly aqueous tumor suppressants may be effective, although many patients will require surgery. Goniotomy is reported to be effective in some younger patients , but this procedure can be complicated by extensive iris processes and should probably be avoided inpatients with large areas of contact between the iris and cornea. Trabeculotomy, too has a high-risk for substantial bleeding, endothelial cell damage, and inflammation in eyes with thick iridocorneal adhesions. Some authors believe that filtering surgery with anti-metabolites is the best surgical procedure for these patients. Eyes that fail trabeculectomy may require an aqueous shunt, or ultimately diode cyclophotocoagulation.

Peter's Anomaly

Peter's anomaly is a congenital, mostly bilateral condition in which a central corneal opacity is present with corresponding defects in the posterior corneal stroma, Descemet's membrane and endothelium. The condition is usually sporadic, although autosomal recessive and autosomal dominant transmission both have been reported. Approximately, 50% of patients will have associated glaucoma. Some cases can have the peripheral anterior chamber angle abnormalities of Axenfeld-Rieger syndrome since they are both defects of neural crest cell origin which may lead to diagnostic confusion.

Peter's anomaly is often classified into three groups: (1) posterior corneal defect with leucoma alone; (2) posterior corneal defect with leucoma and adherent iris strands; (3) posterior corneal defect with leucoma, adherent iris strands, and keratolenticular contact or cataract.

The corneal opacity in Peter's anomaly is usually central, oval and well-defined, but it may sectorial and have diffuse margins. The affected cornea is rarely vascularized and the peripheral cornea is usually clear although scleralization of the limbus may occur in Peter's anomaly type II, the lens either lies in juxtaposition to the corneal surface or is in normal position with an intact surface but cataract is present. In contrast to the first two forms of Peter's anomaly, the last variant may occur in eyes with microphthalmia, persistent hyperplastic primary vitreous (PHPV) and retinal dysplasia.

Peter's plus syndrome is a multiple malformation syndrome characterized by a combination of Peter's anomaly of the eye and other extraocular defects, including short-limb dwarfism, a thin upper lip, hypoplastic columella, and a round face. Hypothyroidism, multiple midline defects such as cleft lip and palate, cardiac anomalies, an atretic cranial meningocele as well as malformations of the ear have also been reported.

Histopathology in Peter's anomaly shows an abnormal, immature or absent Descemet's membrane and attenuated, endothelial cells in the area of the corneal opacity, in addition to thinning or even complete absence of Bowman's membrane. It has been suggested that there is failure of the normal differentiation of the mesoderm into normal endothelium and trabecular meshwork.

Differential diagnosis of Peters anomaly includes causes of corneal opacities that may be seen in children. These include sclerocornea, where the entire cornea is opacified, aniridia, trauma assocciated with forceps delivery during birth, congenital glaucoma, mucopolysaccharidoses, congenital hereditary endothelial dystrophy (CHED) and a perforated corneal ulcer.

Ultrasound biomicroscopy (UBM) has proved to be useful in confirming the diagnosis of Peter's anomaly. It also acts as a preoperative guide in cases undergoing penetrating keratoplasty by detecting keratolenticular and iridocorneal adhesions.

Management of Peter's anomaly primarily relies on controlling glaucoma, when present and preventing amblyopia. Detection of glaucoma is complicated by the corneal opacity, which affects the accuracy of tonometry and obscures the clinician's view of the anterior chamber angle and optic nerve head. Although some cases may respond to medical management, many cases ultimately may require filtering surgery. Multiple procedures and adjunctive medical therapy are often required to achieve and maintain adequate IOP control. Visual results are poor due to uncontrolled glaucoma, amblyopia, and other anterior and posterior segment anomalies that may accompany Peter's anomaly. Patients undergoing keratoplasty after adequate pressure control are reported to have long-term graft clarity in 36% of cases.

Sclerocornea

Sclerocornea is one of the common causes of corneal clouding or opacification in the newborn. It presents at birth by nonprogressive, noninflammatory opacification of the peripheral and to a lesser degree the central cornea with vascularisation. Despite its characteristic presentation it should be differentiated from other pathologies such as congenital glaucoma, trauma, infectious diseases, dystrophies, metabolic causes and other forms of ocular dysgenesis.

The sclera and choroid develop from mesenchymal tissue of neural crest origin. Sclerocornea results from mesenchymal dysgenesis leading to anomalous development of this portion of the anterior segment. It has been suggested that the wave of mesenchymal tissue that normally forms the corneal stroma fails to form the clear cornea and forms tissue resembling sclera instead. This wave of tissue remains as homogenous sheets throughout the 7th-10th week of gestation until the limbal anlage develops. Failure of the limbal anlage to develop or its central displacement may be responsible for various forms of sclerocornea.

Most cases are sporadic however, inheritance patterns have been demonstrated. Autosomal dominant patterns as well as autosomal recessive traits have been reported. Cases with an autosomal dominant pattern are invariably less severe.

Sclerocornea is usually bilateral and affects male and female newborns equally. Sclerocornea presents in a newborn with opacification of the peripheral cornea with vascularization. Although the axial portion of the cornea may also be involved to a varying degree, the peripheral opacification is usually denser. The limbus is indistinct and blends with the surrounding sclera. Some cases may present with involvement of only a small arc at the periphery. Where relatively clear cornea is present it is invariably flatter than normal. Accurate visualization of the anterior segment is often hindered by the opaque cornea. It should be noted that in cases of total sclerocornea the relative clarity of the central cornea as compared to the periphery can be important in differentiating sclerocornea from Peter's anomaly.

Histologically there is thickened collagen fibers in the superficial stroma of the cornea as compared to the posterior stroma. This is a pattern similar to that seen in the sclera. Recent evidence however, suggests that sulphation patterns of interfibrillar keratan sulphate proteoglycan within the tissue matrix may resemble cornea rather than sclera as previously postulated.

Ultrasound Biomicroscopy (UBM) has proven to be a vital tool in assessing the nature and extent of structural defects as well as confirming the presence of associated anterior segment anomalies in cases of sclerocornea thus aiding in the surgical decision making process.

Differential diagnosis of sclerocornea is that of causes of a cloudy cornea in a newborn, this includes infantile glaucoma, forceps injury, congenital hereditary endothelial dystrophy, congenital rubella, and congenital syphilis. Other conditions presenting with corneal opacities such as Peter's anomaly, congenital hereditary stromal dystrophy, mucopolysaccharidosis, mucolipidosis and cystinosis may also be confused with sclerocornea.

Laterality, intraocular pressure and associated findings will usually aid in determining the pathology underlying the corneal opacification. However, although many of these entities may seem quite different, the various degrees of affection in sclerocornea may sometimes make an accurate diagnosis difficult. UBM is a useful tool in such cases.

Ocular associations may commonly be encountered in cases of sclerocornea. microphthalmia, iris anomalies, anterior chamber irregularities have been documented in cases of sclerocornea. UBM has dramatically improved the clinician's ability to diagnose associated ocular anomalies which may not be readily diagnosed by routine anterior segment examination.

Systemic associations may be encountered in cases of sclerocornea such as skeletal anomalies, various cerebellar, cranial and cardiac anomalies.

Sclerocornea may also present as part of the a documented syndrome such as the MIDAS (microphthalmia-dermal aplasia-sclerocornea) syndrome. This syndrome is synonymous with the microphthalmia with linear skin defects (MLS) syndrome. This syndrome includes linear areas of erythematous skin dysplasia involving the chin, neck, and head, occurring in association with microphthalmia, corneal opacities, and orbital cysts. Additional findings may include agenesis of corpus callosum, sclerocornea, chorioretinal abnormalities, hydrocephalus, seizures, mental retardation, and nail dystrophy. Some features of the phenotype of this syndrome overlap those of Aicardi and Goltz' syndromes.

As with the majority of congenital corneal opacities the ultimate aim in the absence of extensive associated ocular anomalies is to clear the visual axis by performing a penetrating keratoplasty. Associated conditions such as anterior segment anomalies and glaucoma must also be addressed. The timing of this intervention is a debatable issue however in most cases a single or sometimes multiple keratoplasties are indicated to prevent deprivation amblyopia.

Chapter 23

Developmental Lens Abnormalities

Arturo Perez Arteaga (Mexico)

Introduction

Developmental cataract is a type of small cataract in youth, resulting from heredity, malnutrition, toxicity, or inflammation, seldom affecting vision. Types are as follows:

1. Punctate.
   a. Blue dot.
   b. Sutural.
   c. Central Pulvurental.
2. Zonular.
3. Fusiform.
4. Nuclear.
5. Coronary.
6. Anterior Capsular (Polar).
7. Posterior Capsular (Polar).

Investigations

Etiology can include maternal (and infantile) malnutrition, maternal viral infection (e.g. Rubella), placental hemorrhage causing deficient fetal oxygenation, hypocalcaemia, chromosomal abnormality (e.g. Down's syndrome) and metabolic disorders (e.g. galactosemia). In some cases the cause can remain unknown.

Clinical Signs and Symptoms

Symptoms: The informant, usually parents talk about a history of white spot at the pupillary area. The child is usually brought with history of diminution of vision referring that is unable to follow or recognize objects and parents. Some other symptoms can be unsteady and deviated eyes. Associated symptoms of systemic disease, if present, are usually recognized.

Signs: Decreased visual acuity, many times difficult to establish in very young children, lenticular opacity (leukocoria), nystagmus, deviation of eye, usually convergent strabismus. There may be other ocular and systemic abnormalities in cases of rubella nuclear cataract or other systemic conditions.

Diagnosis

1. *Detailed clinical history:* Because many times developmental cataracts can be part of a systemic disorder, clinical history is of vital importance.
2. *Detailed clinical examination:* It should include visual status, intraocular pressure, fundus examination (when possible), B-scan ultrasonography to exclude posterior segment abnormality like a retinoblastoma or other causes of leukocoria, A-scan to determine axial length of the eye, retinoscopy and cover test.
3. *Laboratory investigations:* Blood test including blood glucose, calcium and phosphorus, RBC transferase and galactokinase levels, TORCH test

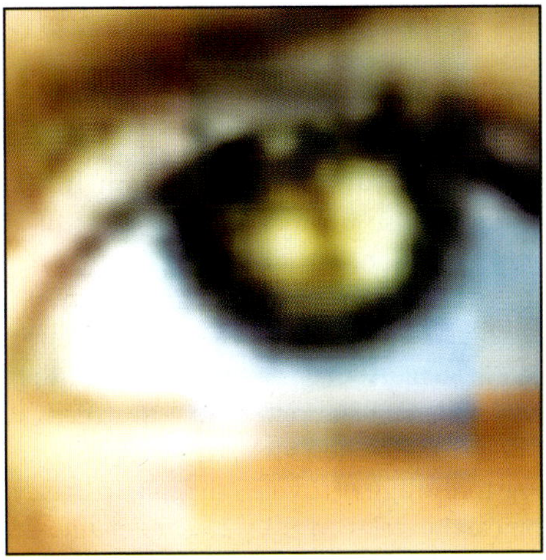

Figure 1: Developmental cataract

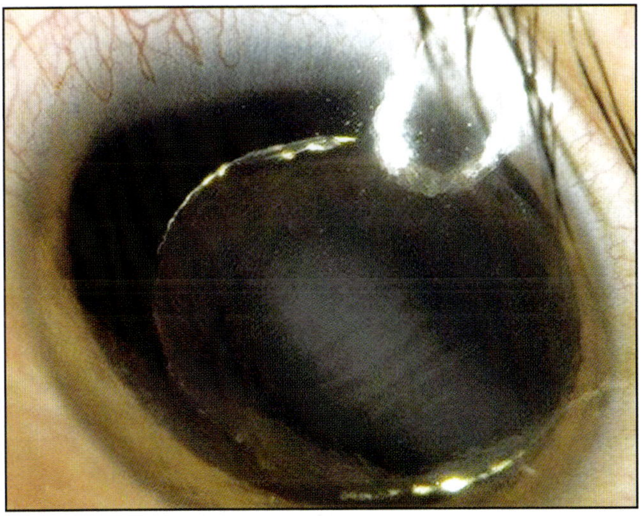

Figure 2: Homocystinuria

and hepatitis B virus. Urine analysis includes reducing substance for galactosaemia and for amino acids (to exclude Lowe syndrome in suspected cases).

Treatment

It can include different options according the case, described as follows:

a. *No treatment at all:* No treatment is an option if vision is not affected significantly. Sometimes use of mydriatics if opacity is central and vision improves with pupil dilation.
b. *Surgery:* Timing of surgery is of particular importance. In case of a bilateral dense cataract the time is 6 weeks. In case of bilateral partial, if vision is not significantly affected, surgery may be delayed up to the age of 2 years or up to puberty. Uniocular dense cataract, oblige to urgent surgery within days. In partial uniocular cataract, when vision is not significantly affected, surgery may be delayed up to the age of 2 years or up to puberty. In cases in Rubella cataract, operation can be delayed till 1-2 years of age. But early surgery may be indicated if cataract is total, or if eye deviation and/or nystagmus are present.
c. *Surgical technique:* Operative procedures available are aspiration and irrigation (ECCE), lensectomy (Pars plana or anterior route), aspiration and irrigation (ECCE) with primary posterior capsulotomy with partial anterior vitrectomy; it all depending the particular case.
d. *Rehabilitation:* Posterior chamber IOL, contact lens, aphakic spectacles, occlusion therapy for treatment and prevention of amblyopia. Long life-term follow-up is mandatory.

Prognosis

It depends upon the particular case, the associated damage and the systemic disease.

Marfan's Syndrome

Introduction

Marfan's syndrome is inherited as a dominant trait. It is carried by a gene called FBN1, which encodes a connective protein called fibrillin-1. Parents have a 50/50 chance of passing on the gene to their children. People with Marfan's are typically tall, with long limbs and long thin fingers. The most serious complication is defects of the heart valves and aorta artery but it also affects the lungs, eyes, dural sac and hard palate. In addition to being a connective protein that forms the structural support for tissues outside the cell, fibrillin-1 binds to another protein. Researchers now believe that the inflammatory effects of transforming growth factor beta (TGF-β), at the lungs, heart valves, and aorta, weaken the tissues and cause the features of Marfan's syndrome.

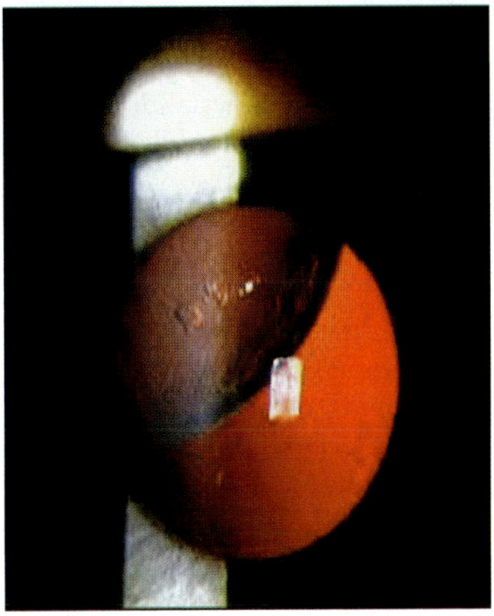

Figure 3: Marfan's syndrome

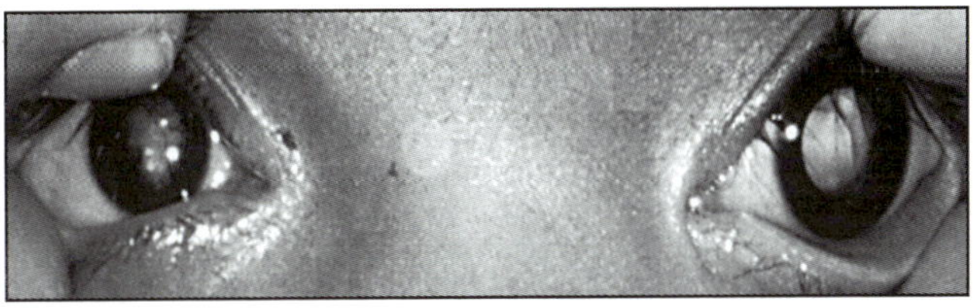

Figure 4: Persistent fetal vasculature

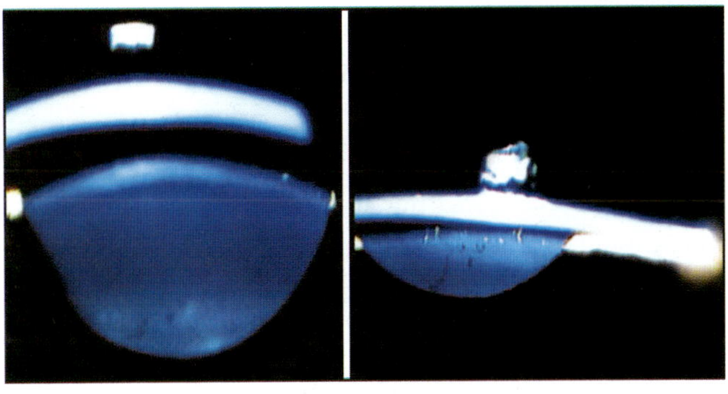

Figure 5: Weill-Marchesani syndrome

Clinical Signs and Symptoms

Although there are no unique signs or symptoms of Marfan's syndrome, the characteristics of long limbs, dislocated crystalline lenses, and aortic root dilation is sufficient to make the diagnosis with confidence. There are more than thirty other clinical features that are variably associated with the syndrome most of them involving the locations of connective tissue like skeleton, skin, and joints. There is a great deal of clinical variability even within families that carry the identical mutation.

Marfan's syndrome affects the eyes and vision in many characteristic ways. Myopia (particularly high myopia) and astigmatism are common, but hyperopia can be present in some patients. Subluxation (dislocation) of the crystalline lens in one or both eyes can occur in 80% of the patients. In Marfan's the dislocation is typically superotemporal whereas in the similar condition called homocystinuria the dislocation is inferonasal. Retinal detachment and early onset glaucoma can decrease the visual prognosis in these patients.

Investigations

Marfan's syndrome is caused by mutations in the *FBN1* gene on chromosome 15, which encodes a glycoprotein called fibrillin-1, a very important component of the extracellular matrix. The fibrillin-1 protein is essential for the proper formation of the extracellular matrix including the biogenesis and maintenance of the elastic fibers. The extracellular matrix is critical for both the structural integrity of connective tissue and recently has been involved as a reservoir for growth factors. Elastin fibers are found throughout the body but are particularly abundant in the aorta artery, ligaments and in particular at the zonular ligament; so, as a consequence these areas are among the more affected.

Diagnosis

The following conditions may result from Marfan's syndrome but may also occur in people without any known underlying disorder. A diagnosis of Marfan's syndrome is based on family history and a combination of major and minor indicators of the disorder, rare in the general population, that occur in one individual. For example, four skeletal signs with one or more signs in another body system such as ocular and cardiovascular in one individual. Aortic aneurysm, arachnodactyly, bicuspid aortic valve, dural ectasia, crystalline lens subluxation, flat feet, gigantism, glaucoma, hernia, mitral valve prolapse, myopia, obstructive lung disease, pneumothorax, retinal detachment, scoliosis and stretch marks.

The differential diagnosis must take in count the following disorders that have similar signs and symptoms of Marfan's syndrome: Congenital contractural arachnodactyly, Ehlers-Danlos syndrome, homocystinuria, Loeys-Dietz syndrome, MASS phenotype, Sticler's syndrome and multiple endocrine neoplasias.

Figure 6: Developmental cataract

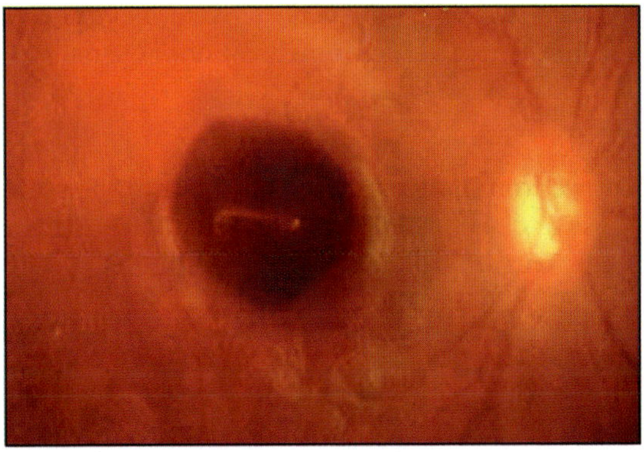

Figure 7: Homocystinuria

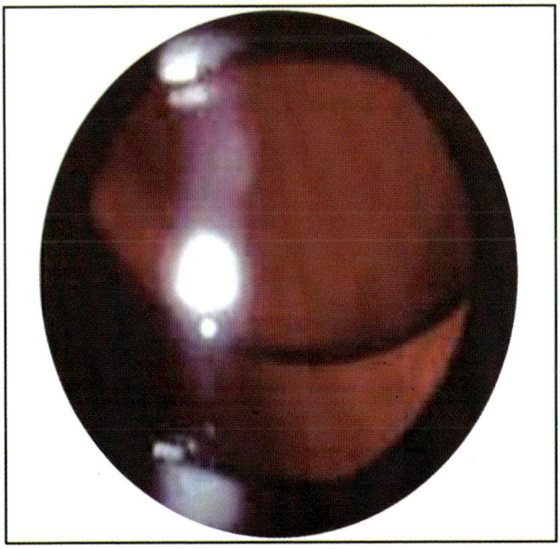

Figure 8: Marfan's syndrome

Treatment

There is no cure for Marfan's syndrome, but life expectancy has increased significantly over the last few decades, and clinical trials are underway for promising new treatments. The syndrome is treated by addressing each issue as it becomes clinically significant, and, in particular, considering preventive medication, even for young children, to slow progression of aortic dilation.

In ophthalmology the surgical treatment of ectopia lentis must be consider. If vision is unaffected no surgery is indicated, only refractive correction is used. When an important subluxation is present, surgery can be useful. Many approaches can be done according the surgeon: Intracapsular extraction with anterior chamber IOL, or a posterior chamber IOL fixated to sulcus or to iris; phacoemulsification with endocapsular rings and sometimes sutures, to preserve the capsular bag and "in the bag" IOL implantation; pars plana vitrectomy with lensectomy. In every case, a particular care of the retina is mandatory. Retinal detachment is treated as usual; nevertheless the prognosis is not good. Glaucoma is treated with medication as usual.

Prognosis

It may have variations from patient to patient according the severity of the case, the time of diagnosis and the onset of the particular treatment. A long-life term of follow-up must be carried by many physicians.

Homocystinuria

Introduction

Homocystinuria is an inherited autosomal recessive defect in methionine metabolism that is caused by a deficiency in the enzyme cystathionine synthase that leads to a multisystem disorder of the connective tissue, muscles, central nervous system, and cardiovascular system. These groups of hereditary metabolic disorders are characterized by an accumulation of homocysteine in the serum and an increased excretion of homocysteine in the urine.

Clinical Signs and Symptoms

Even that an infant with homocystinuria is usually healthy when newborn, three important systems involved, representing the landmark of the disease (neurological, vascular and ophthalmic). The neurologic features include thromboembolic complications of the central nervous system and psychomotor delay occurring during the first year of life. A developmental delay is noted when patients are aged 2-3 years. Psychiatric symptoms are present in approximately one-half of patients with homocystinuria. Pyramidal symptoms are occasionally observed in areas like as the legs. In the skeletal and muscular apparatus the characteristic long and thin extremities with arachnodactyly may not appear until late in childhood or until adolescence. Sometimes osteoporosis is already present for some time before. Vascular occlusive disease

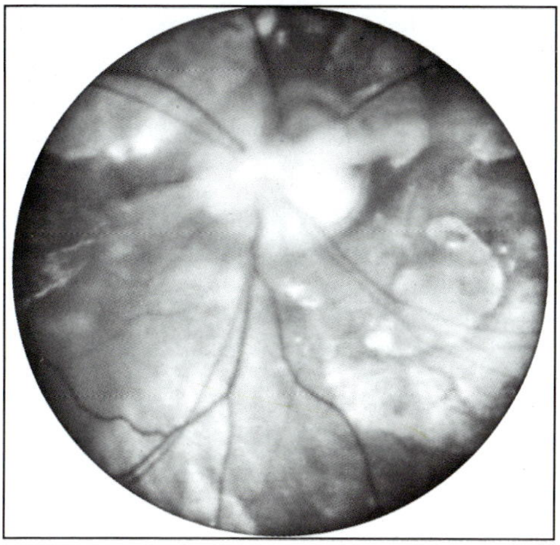

Figure 9: Persistent fetal vasculature

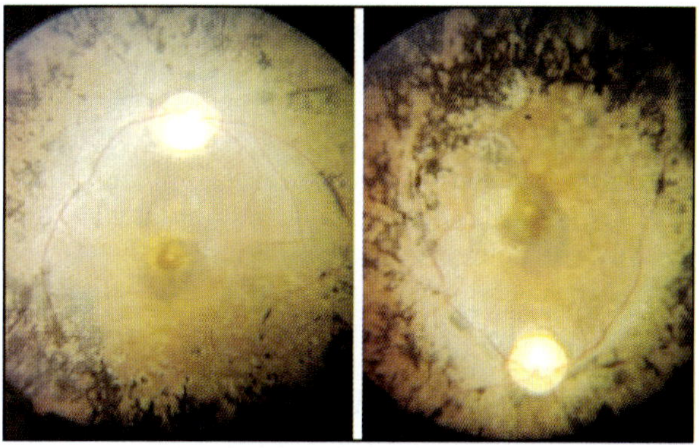

Figure 10: Weill-Marchesani syndrome

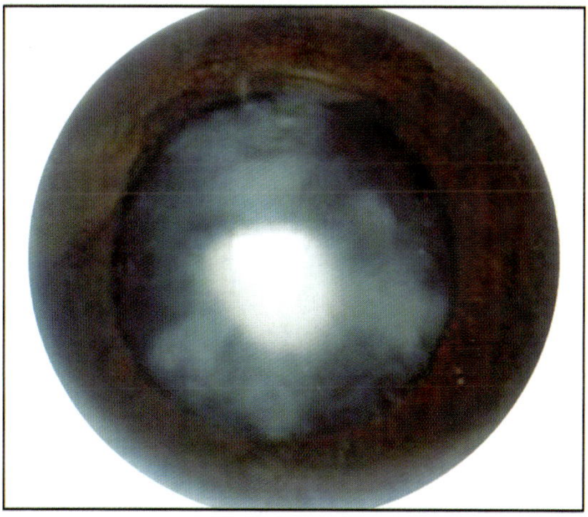

Figure 11: Developmental cataract

is an important and serious feature. Thromboembolic events, such as cerebrovascular occlusions or pulmonary emboli, usually do not occur until adulthood but are reported sometimes in childhood and infancy.

The ophthalmologic features include severe myopia and the characteristic sign of ectopia lentis that may precede lens dislocation. Once established, ectopia lentis progresses, even when good biochemical control of the disease is performed. The ophthalmologic findings are similar to those in patients with Marfan's syndrome. Ectopia lentis is an almost universal feature in patients older than 10 years (the dislocation of the ocular lenses usually occurs in patients aged 4-10 years) and it can even be present in newborns. Other findings can include myopia, iridopathy (atrophy), cataracts, secondary glaucoma, and retinal degeneration. Atrophy of the optic nerve, strabismus, nystagmus, or diminished convergence is less frequent findings.

Investigations

On the basis of the type of homocystinuria, the following 3 nosologic units are distinguished as follows: Homocystinuria can be caused by the deficiency of cystathionine synthase; can be caused by insufficient vitamin B_{12} synthesis resulting from a defect in the remethylation of homocysteine to methionine; can be caused by a deficiency in methylenetetrahydrofolate reductase. The methionine level is within the reference range. In all cases the basis of the disease is a defect of the gene coding for L-serine dehydratase cystathionine synthase, which converts homocysteine and serine into cystathionine. Deficient activity of this enzyme has been demonstrated in liver extracts, in brain tissue, and in cultured skin fibroblasts and lymphocytes. The deficiency leads to an accumulation of homocysteine and methionine and to its conversion into homocysteine, which is excreted in the urine. The accumulation of homocysteine leads to damage of the collagen and elastic fibers. The binding of homocysteine to lysine residues results in the formation of thiazine bonds.

Differential Diagnosis

The diagnosis is based on the clinical picture and the results of laboratory analysis. The cyanide nitroprusside reaction in the urine is used as the Brand reaction. The reference range methionine level is less than 1 mg/dL (30 μM). Homocysteine levels of up to 0.2 μmol/mL and methionine levels of up to 2 μmol/mL characterize cystathionine synthetase deficiency.

Marfan's syndrome is the primary differential diagnosis. Clinical features of homocystinuria, such as ectopia lentis, dolichocephalia, and chest and spinal deformities, are similar to the features found in patients with Marfan's syndrome, although the cerebral symptoms, the changes in the hair, and the disorders of mental development are absent in patients with Marfan's syndrome. Generalized osteoporosis, arterial and venous thrombosis, and mental retardation, which are features of homocystinuria, do not occur in patients with Marfan's syndrome. In addition, and as a final feature, homocysteine is not detectable in the urine of patients with Marfan's syndrome.

Treatment

Neonates in whom homocystinuria is diagnosed have had a benign course when they are fed on methionine-restricted cysteine-supplemented diets. Homocysteine Reduction Formula, a special nutritional supplement created by Brimhall, can also lower homocysteine levels. Cysteine can be supplemented to a maximum of 500 mg per day. The administration of pyridoxine in high doses (300-600 mg/d) has demonstrated to be effective in some patients. Other possible treatments include the use of folic acid.

Surgical treatment should be considered, especially in patients with pupillary-block glaucoma or in those with recurrent lens dislocation into the anterior chamber. Other ophthalmologic or orthopedic disorders should be corrected.

Prognosis

The diagnosis should be established as early as possible. The prognosis is favorable if patients use adequate diet alimentation; even so, nearly 25% of patients die before age 30 years.

Weill-Marchesani Syndrome

Introduction

In 1932, Georges Weill reported eight patients with dislocation of the lens and other dysmorphic features. Several of these persons had arachnodactyly and were regarded as having the Marfan's syndrome, but two were of stunted stature with short, stiff digits.

Some years after, in 1939, Marchesani documented a boy aged eight years and three siblings in another family, all of whom had ectopia lentis. He recognized that although ectopia lentis was a feature of the Marfan's syndrome, the patients whom he had studied had short fingers rather than arachnodactyly. He emphasized this point by including comparative photographs in his article, in which he termed the disorder "brachydactyly and congenital spherophakia". The condition was first named for Marchesani, but when Weill's earlier report was recognized, the conjoined eponym came into general use.

Investigations

The precise mode of inheritance of Weill-Marchesani syndrome is still uncertain. Most of the reports support an autostomal recessive pattern of inheritance. The heterozygous patients may have short stature or brachydactyly and may suffer from refractive errors (mostly myopia) but not ectopia lentis. The consanguinity among parents suggests autosomal recessive inheritance. However, a high degree of inbreeding in some family pedigrees makes it difficult to decide the type of inheritance.

Clinical Signs and Symptoms

Typically, these patients have small shallow orbits, mild maxillary hypoplasia, narrow palate, small spherical crystalline lenses, and myopia with or without glaucoma, frequent ectopia lentis, occasional blindness, malformed and misaligned teeth, and cardiac defect. Late ossification of the epiphyses is a constant feature. The typical clinical findings are enough to establish the diagnosis.

Diagnosis

Diagnosis is made when several characteristic clinical signs are observed. There is no single test to confirm the presence of Weill-Marchesani syndrome. Exploring family history or examining other family members may prove helpful in confirming this diagnosis. Even so, a variety of manifestations of Weill-Marchesani syndrome can present a diagnostic problem. A diagnosis should be based only on the combination of specific ocular and skeletal abnormalities. The physician should take in count that isolated ocular or skeletal features can occur as isolated familial anomaly or as a part of some other diseases.

The main differential diagnosis is with Marfan's syndrome, because both present similar features but also sharp contrast. A typical Marfan patient is tall, lean, with high arm span, arachnodactyly and hyper-extensible joints, while Weill-Marchesani individuals are short in stature, with brachymelia, brachydactyly, stubby spade-like hands and feet, and limitation of mobility of joints.

Treatment

Physical therapy and orthopedic treatments are generally prescribed for problems stemming from mobility from this connective tissue disorder. However, this disorder has no cure, and generally, treatments are given to improve quality of life.

Despite the systemic features ophthalmic surgery has been documented to help those with ocular diseases, such as some forms of glaucoma; however, long-term medical management of glaucoma associated with this disease has not proven to be successful. To maintain vision, an early diagnosis is necessary. Peripheral iridectomy, lens extraction and recently laser iridotomy are used in the treatment.

Prognosis

It may have variations from patient to patient according the severity of the case, the time of diagnosis and the onset of the particular treatment. A long-life term of follow-up must be carried by many physicians.

Persistent Fetal Vasculature

Introduction

Persistent fetal vasculature syndrome (PFVS) is a new term that has replaced the older name of persistent hyperplasic primary vitreous. This new name is better than older because it recognizes that two parts of the fetal vasculature can persist leaving the eye with an opaque lens and vascular stalk of tissue. One of the changes that the name does not imply is that the retina may also be altered (retinal dysplasia) either in larger or microscopic amounts.

Clinical Signs and Symptoms

Usually, PFVS is found in one eye that is somewhat smaller than the better eye (dominant) and has a white pupil reflex (leukocoria) and elongated ciliary processes. This set of findings does not assure whether retinal dysplasia is present or not. In some eyes the stalk of persistent fetal vessels may not opacify the visual axis of the lens (some part of the light rays may pass through the lens allowing vision). This stalk can pull on the retina and disturb it as well as pull on the lens causing it to be poorly shaped (posterior lenticonus). This child that usually does not have the white pupil, is often diagnosed at a later age, decreasing this way the visual prognosis.

Investigations

Ultrasound studies, visual evoked potential response or electroretinography testing are helpful in evaluation but finally the clinical evaluation should be performed. At this time there are no other known systemic problems associated. At this time no genetic mutations have been associated with the typical unilateral PFVS. About 10% of infants affected by PFVS have both eyes involved. These children more frequently have retinal dysplasia. Bilateral PFVS is also not associated with systemic changes.

Differential Diagnosis

The disease that can be indistinguishable from bilateral PFVS with extensive retinal dysplasia is called Norrie's disease. In this process the child may be affected with hearing loss or other central nervous system problems. Genetic testing is available for Norrie's disease. As with many diseases known to be under genetic control, there may be several mutations. Norrie's disease testing will confirm the diagnosis in 80% of the cases, leaving 20% of children where a mutation cannot be found, but clinical examination confirms the diagnosis of Norrie's disease.

Treatment

Treatment for PFVS is surgical, usually with removal of the lens and persistent vascular stalk tissue. It can accomplish several things. It may reduce the risk of glaucoma and usually clears the opaque tissue out of the eye allowing light to reach the retina. It also can relieve pulling or distortion of the retina because of tractions. When the media are clear the physician can form an opinion as to the amount or absence of retinal dysplasia. The flourescein angiography and OCT testing in infants under anesthesia can be much more accurate about microscopic retinal dysplasia; it can be done during the same surgical procedure.

Prognosis

If the eye has no retinal dysplasia the visual prognosis improves; even so there still is a great challenge to overcome occlusive amblyopia. This can often be helped by contact lenses and occlusive therapy.

Chapter 24

Disorders of Eyelid

Essam El Toukhy, Mohamed El Badri
Ali Saeed Odadi Assiri (Egypt)

Entropion

Introduction

Entropion or turning of the lid margin is one of the most common lid malpositions encountered in clinical practice.

The most common type of entropion is involutional entropion.

Clinical Picture of Entropion

- Irritation, tearing and scaring
- Ulceration of conjunctiva or cornea
- It can eventually lead to visual loss from corneal opacities.

Classification of Entropion

- Involutional entropion
- Congenital entropion
- Spastic entropion
- Cicatricial entropion.

Congenital Entropion

- Is a rare entity that is present at birth
- The entire lower lid and lashes turn inward
- There is absence of the lower lid crease.

Pathophysiology

It is due to disinsertion of the lower lid retractors or secondary overaction of marginal orbicularis muscle.

Treatment

Reattaching or plicating of the lower lid retractors.

Differential Diagnosis

- Epiblepharon in which a fold of skin pushes the lashes against the globe and tends to correct itself with growth of facial bones

Spastic Entropion

Causes

- Recent ocular surgery
- Inflammatory eye condition.

Pathophysiology

Acute lid swelling and orbicularis spasm.

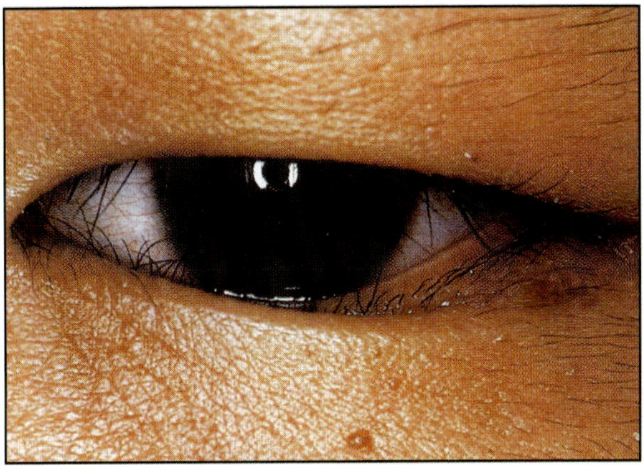

Figure 1: Epiblepharon

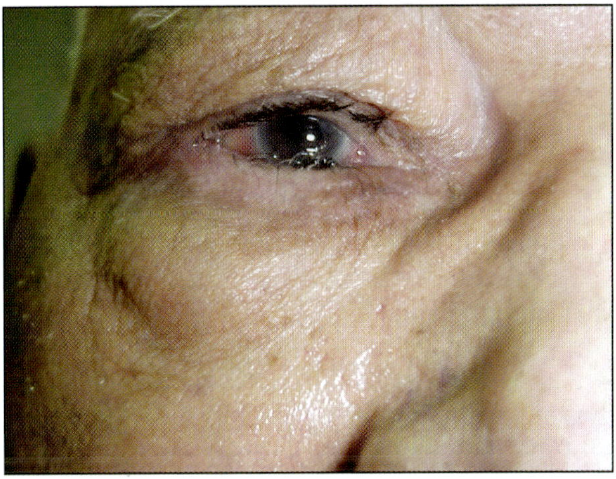

Figure 2: Involutional entropion

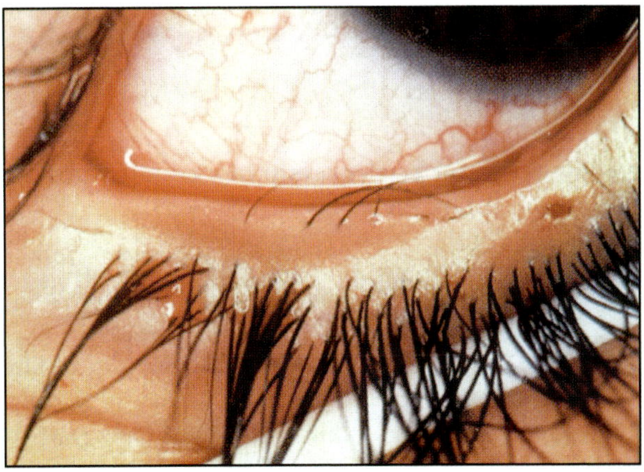

Figure 3: Distichiasis

In which preseptal orbicularis muscle over-rides pretarsal orbicularis and lid margin turns inward.

Treatment

- Treatment of inflammatory eye by antibiotic and steroids
- Taping of lid
- local anesthesia infiltration
- Botulinum injection in orbicularis muscle will break the cycle of ocular irritation and orbicularis spasm and lid malposition will resolve.

Prognosis

Botulinum toxin treatment has proven successful in temporarily elimination of the spasm.

Cicatricial Entropion

Pathophysiology

Caused by contracture in the conjunctiva and the tarsus or both leading to shortening of posterior lamella of lid.

Causes

Secondary to
- Acids and alkali
- Burns
- Trachoma
- Steven Johnson's syndrome
- Mechanical trauma
- Cicatricial pemphigoid
- Viral

Clinical Picture

- Blepharoconjunctivitis
- Meibomitis
- Rounding of posterior lid border and posterior migration and keratinized epithelium and secondary trichiasis.
- Keratoconjunctivitis sicca.

Treatment of Cicatrizing Entropion

- Trichiasis is treated by electrolysis, cryosurgery, argon laser therapy or excision of lash follicles.
- Cicatricial entropion is treated by mucous membrane graft.

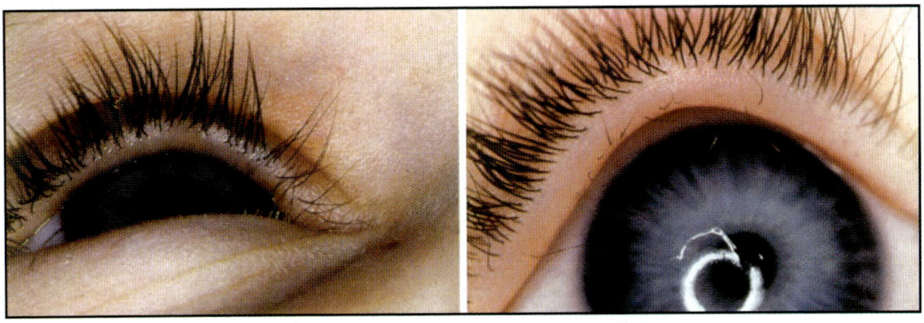

Figure 4: Trichiasis without entropion

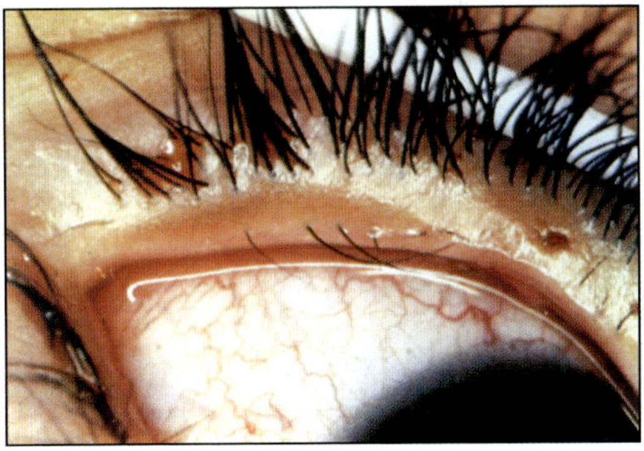

Figure 5: Trichiasis

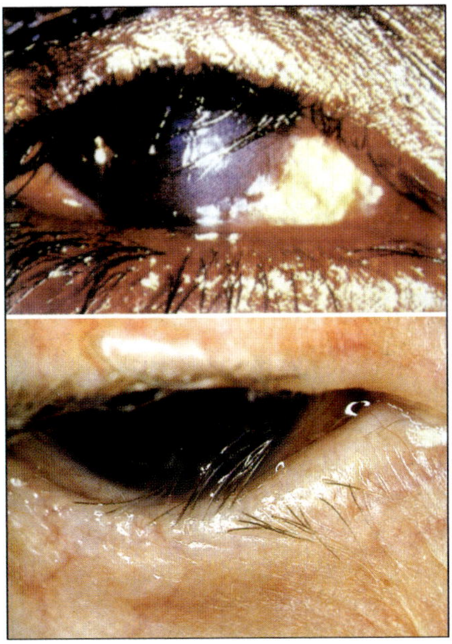

Figure 6: Upper and lower lid entropion

Involutional Entropion

Is the most common variety encountered.
It affects only the lower lids and is associated with aging.

Pathophysiology

It is due to

- Laxity of the tarsal ligaments
- Weakness of retractors.
- Over-riding and preseptal on pretarsal orbicularis.

Medical Treatment

- Patients with blephritis and meibomitis should by treated.
- Patients with dry eyes should by treated by artificial tears.

Surgical Treatment

1. Three suture technique.
2. Direct anatomic surgical approach.
3. Weis procedure.
4. Weis procedure with lateral tarsal strip.

Three Suture Technique

- It is best suited for poor risk patients at the bedside or in the office.
- The lid should not be too lax.
  A. Suture technique, sagittal view of 5-0 vicryl sutures passed through the retractor complex.
  B. The suture is brought out just anterior to the inferior tarsal border through orbicularis muscle to emerge 3 to – 4 mm below the lower lid cilia. This brings the retractors back to their normal anatomic position.

Direct Anatomic: Surgical Approach

This approach seeks to correct the three main causative factors

- Over-riding of orbicularis
- Weakness of retractors
- Horizontal lid laxity.

Direct anatomic approach:

A. A subciliary incision exposing the tarsal plate, dehisced edge of the lower eyelid retractors, preaponeurotic, fat, orbital fat, and orbicularis muscle.
B. A lateral tarsal strip is fashioned and sutured to periosteum of the inner aspect of the frontal process of the zygoma.
C. The edge of the lower eyelid retractor is advanced and sutured to the inferior tarsal border or to the cut edge of the pretarsal orbicularis with 6-0 silk.

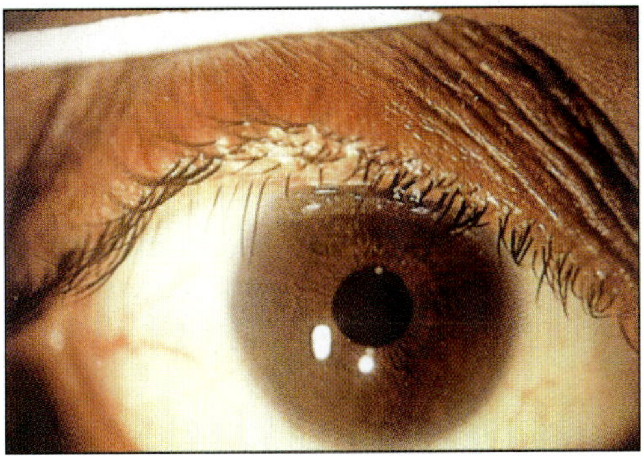

Figure 7: Upper lid entropion

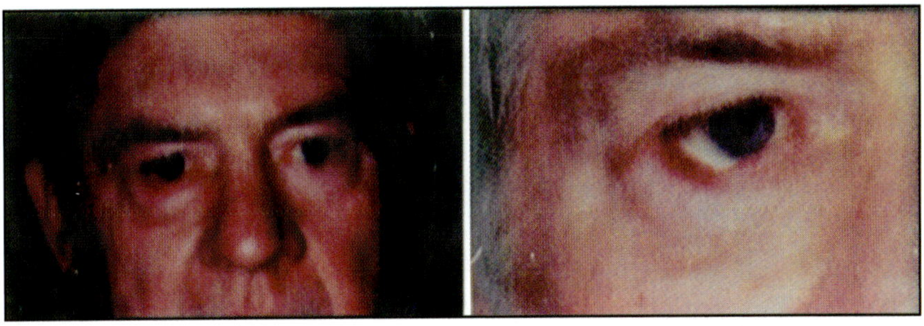

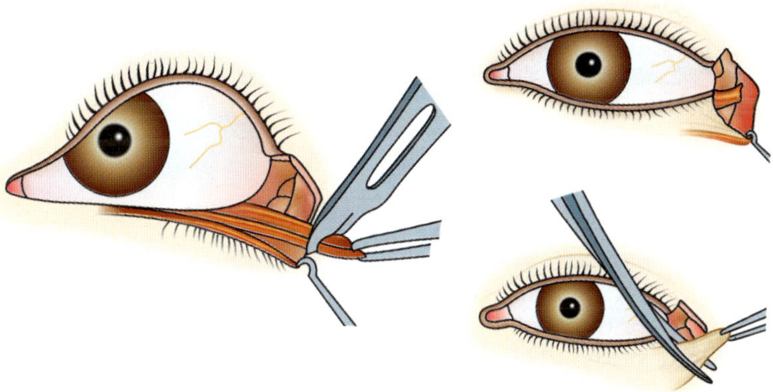

Figure 8: Lateral tarsal strip procedure

Weis Procedure

A. Three double—armed 5-0 vicryl
Sutures are placed along the lower eyelid, through conjunctiva and retractors, anterior to the tarsal plate, exiting through the orbicularis and skin at the level of the lashes.
B. The tarsal edge of the horizontally shortened lid is sutured to periosteum. The **5-0** vicryl sutures have already been preplaced through conjunctiva and retractors, exiting anterior to the trasal plate through orbicularis and skin.

Weis procedure with lateral tarsal strip :
Used in weakens of retractors combined with congenital lid laxity.

Lateral Tarsal strip procedure
- Horizontal canthotomy.
- Inferior cantholysis.
- Excision of a part of skin and orbicularis
- Excision of a part of lid margin—according to lid laxity.
- Peeling of conjunctiva to prevent postoperative inclusion cyst.
- Suturing of tarsal strip by double armed vicryl 5-0 to the periosteum of frontal process of the zygoma.
- Closure of skin by interrupted sutures.

Ectropion

Introduction

It is one of the most common malpositions of the eyelid, defined as rolling-out "eversion" of the lid margin away from the eye-ball. The lower lid is commonly involved.

Pathophysiology

According to the mechanism of the defect "pathological factor" the ectropion was classified to different types.
1. When the anterior lamella is shortened either postoperatively, trauma (burns or injuries), or ulceration, the resultant cicatricial ectropion will take place.
2. Supporting of the lower eyelid in its normal position depending on the orbicularis oculi muscle tone and loss of this support will lead to paralytic ectropion as in case of facial nerve palsy.
3. Senile or involutional which is caused by a horizontal lid laxity as a result of lengthening of medial and lateral canthal tendons with ageing changes, it is the most common type of ectropion and has a continuous pathological process that is aggravated by conjunctivitis and epiphora.
4. When the eyelids are well-supported by a big eyeball relative to its orbital cavity in presence of blepharospasm well cause a spastic ectropion and on the other hand when eyelids are less supported by a less prominent inferior

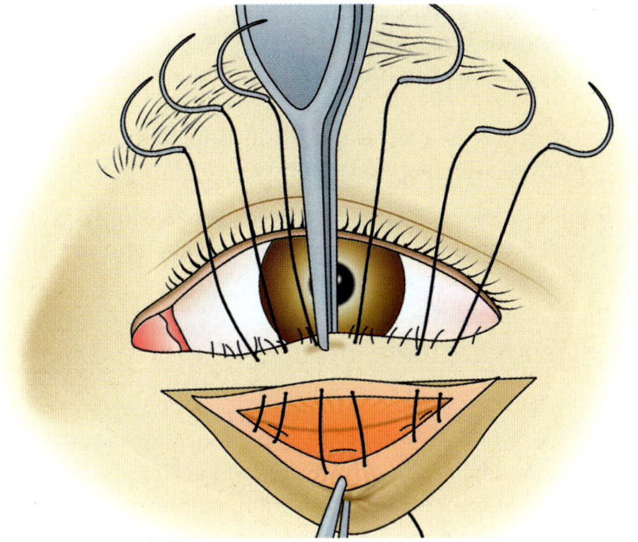

Figure 9: Weis procedure 1

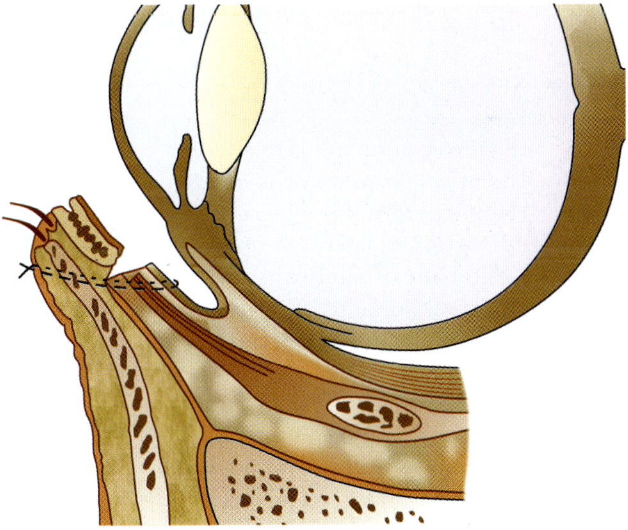

Figure 10: Weis procedure 2

orbital rim will lead to a midfacial hypoplasia with resultant ectropion as in case of exophthalmos and children.

5. Mechanical ectropion is caused by eversion of the lower lid by a tumor or a mass.
6. Congenital ectropion is a rare condition due to shortage of skin as in congenital ichthyosis or blepharophimosis.

N.B: The condition of ectropion "during sleep" due to floppy eyelid syndrome should be suspected by exclusion in which the skeleton of lids "tarsus is lengthened and become more lax".

Clinical Signs and Symptoms

History

Patients with ectropion will complain of tearing, burning sensation and redness of the involved eye, however the age of the patient is an important clue in which the congenital ectropion is an infancy condition, epiphora is a less complaint of the elderly, but more common with young patients due to adequate tears production. Involutional ectropion is the most common type with patients while paralytic ectropion is more apparent in elderly rather than youngs with 7th CN Palsy.

Examination

It should be directed towards recognition of the ectropion and its severity .

1. *Severity of ectropion:*
   - *Mild* : The lower punctum is everted.
   - *Moderate* : The tarsal conjunctiva is exposed.
   - *Severe* : The lower fornix is exposed.
2. *Extent of ectropion:* Medial or lateral or involving the entire lower eyelid.
3. Presence of any traumatic or surgical scar tissue.
4. Presence of a horizontal lid laxity. Which is demonstrated by:
   a. *Eyelid snap test:* Pull the eyelid inferiorly.
      - If the eyelid springs to its normal position without a blink it means no lid laxity.
      - If it remains away from the eye for a time; it means a lax lid. Then the degree of lid laxity will be determined by the number of blink required to bring the lid on contact to the eye.

   b. *Eyelid distraction test:* By pulling the eyelid away from the eye, the lower lid should not move more than 6 mm from the eye.
5. Signs of lower facial nerve palsy as brow ptosis, lid retraction with incomplete blink, lagophthalmos and absence of nasolabial fold.
6. Weakness of the preseptal orbicularis oculi is tested by closure of the eyelids.
7. Examination of corneal sensation is a must.

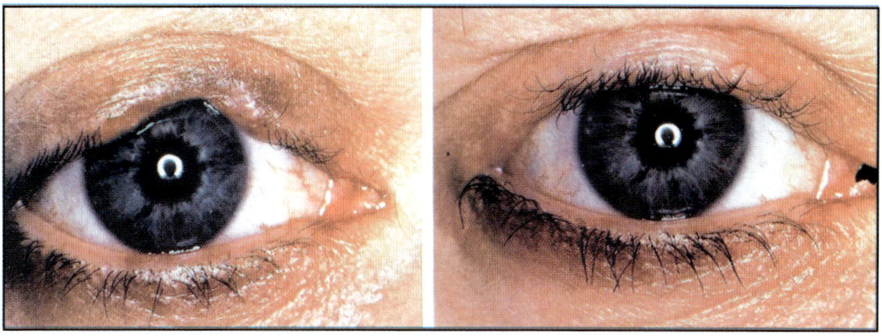

Figure 11: Lid notching after extensive electrolysis

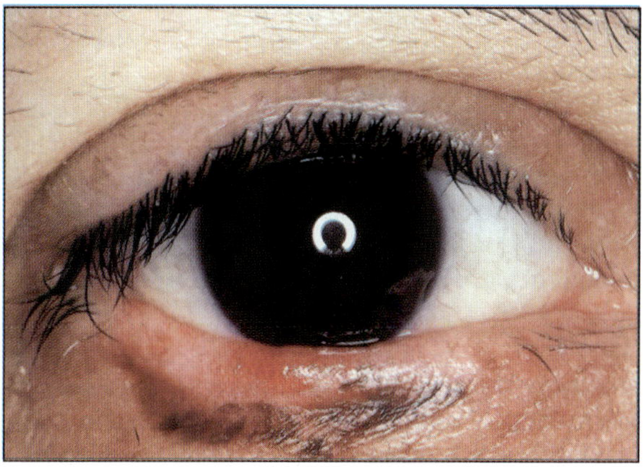

Figure 12: Madarosis and pigmentation after cryo

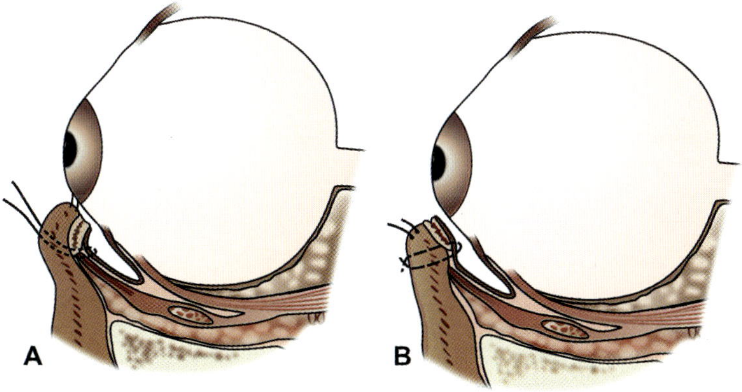

Figures 13A and B: Suture techniques sagittal view

Treatment of Ectropion

The management of ectropion depends on the cause, extent and presence or absence of a horizontal lid laxity.

1. *Involutional ectropion:*
   A. *With no horizontal lid laxity:*
   Medial conjunctivoplasty (medial spindle operation)
   " Excision of a diamond of tarsoconjunctiva"
   - With mild horizontal laxity:-lazy-T procedure (medial conjuncto-voplasty and full thickness lid excision)
   - With severe horizontal laxity; medial canthal tendon plication.

   B. *Entire lid ectropion*
   - If no excess skin; horizontal lid shortening .
   - If with excess skin; horizontal lid shortening plus blepharoplasty.
   - Lateral tarsal strip procedure.
2. Treatment of cicatricial ectropion
   a. If mild: Z-plasty
   b. If severe; skin grafts or flaps
3. Treatment of paralytic ectropion.
   A. *Temporary method:*
   - Conservative (artificial tears and ointment).
   - Surgical (Tarrsorhaphy)

   B. *Permanent methods:*
   - With ectropion
     1. Medical canthoplasty.
     2. Lateral canthoplasty.
     3. Medial canthoplasty with lateral tarsal strip.
     4. Encirclement (with prosthetic silicon sling).
   - *Without ectropion*
     1. Upper lid weight (gold).
     2. Graded levator recession.
     3. Brow lift to correct brow ptosis .
4. Treatment of mechanical ectropion: Removal of the cause.
5. *Treatment of congenital ectropion:* Skin graft ± horizontal lid shortening as appropriate.
6. *Treatment of spastic ectropion:*
   A. Treatment of blepharospasm (Botulinum toxin injection).
   B. Snellen's sutures : In which three double-armed sutures are passed from the lower fonix through the periostium of the inferior orbital margin to emerge on the skin of cheek and tied over small pieces of rubber of removed after 2 weeks.

Prognosis

Is usually good with preservation of corneal wetting and clarity. Surgery results in long-term cure in functional obstruction.

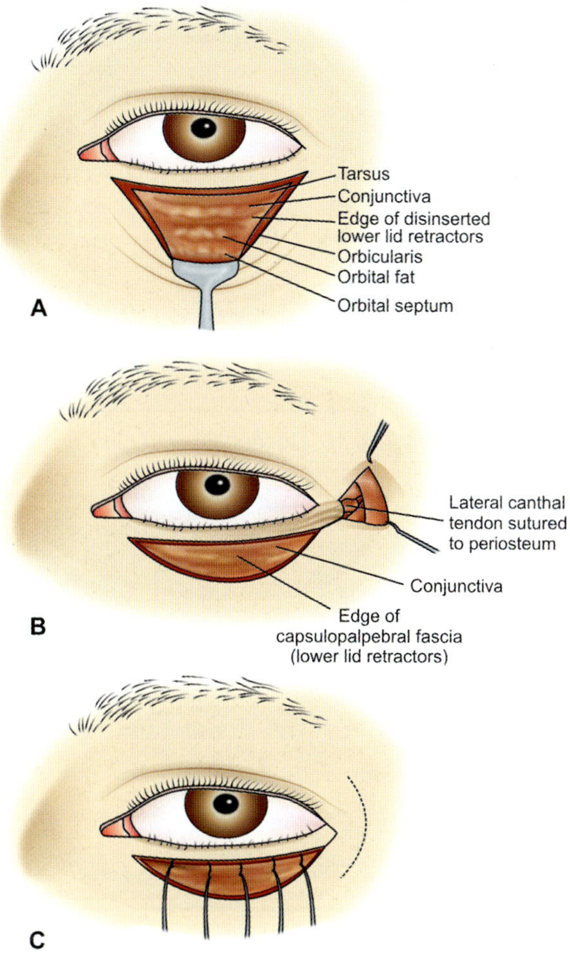

Figures 14A to C: Causative factors for surgical approach

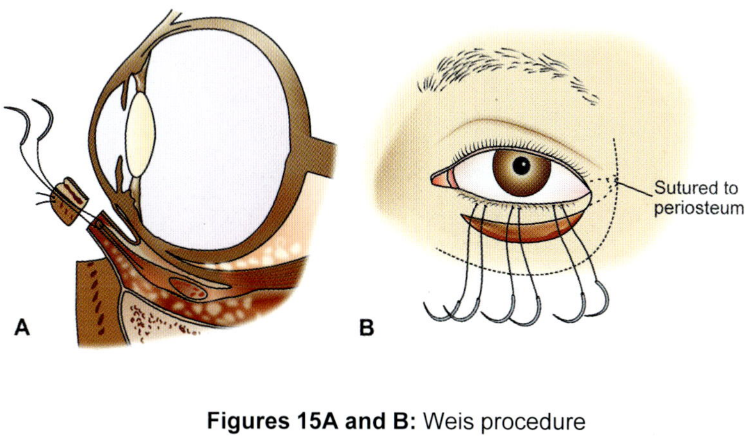

Figures 15A and B: Weis procedure

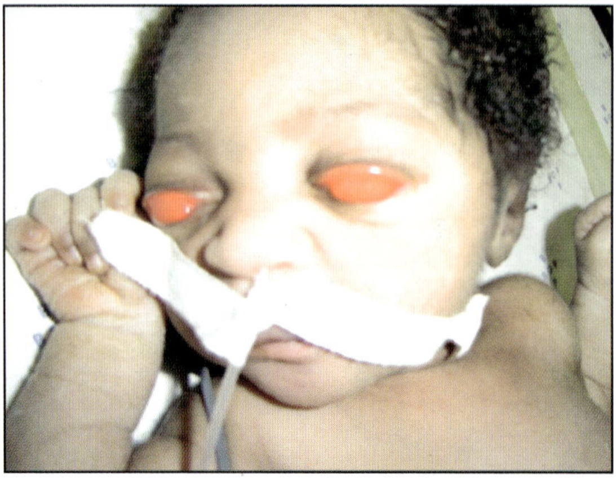

Figure 16: Congenital ectropion

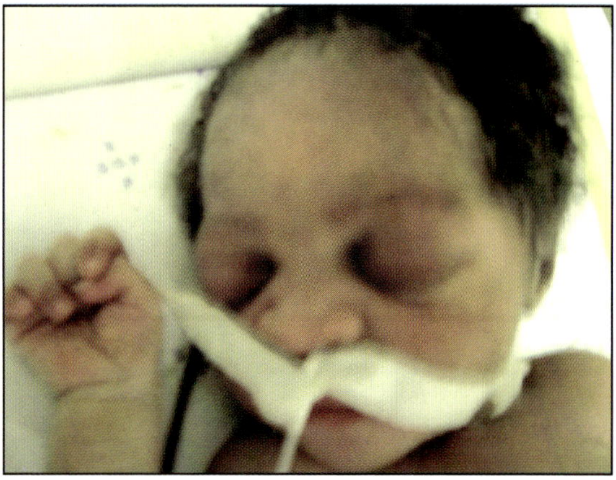

Figure 17: Congenital ectropion; immediate postoperative

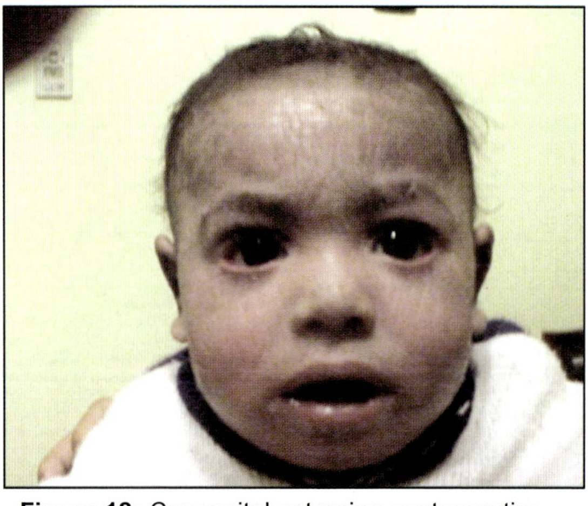

Figure 18: Congenital ectropion postoperative

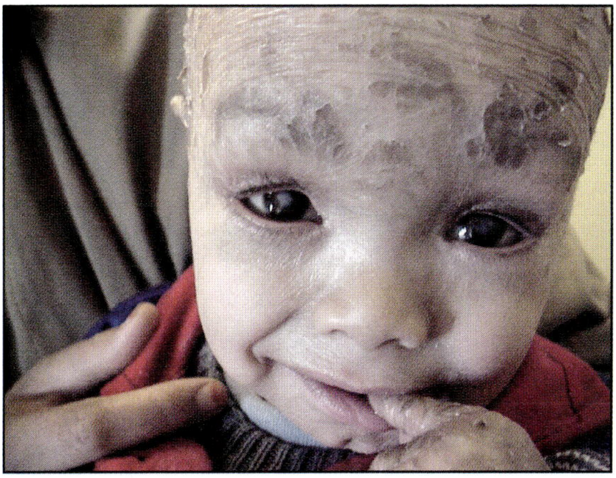

Figure 19: Congenital ectropion postoperative 1

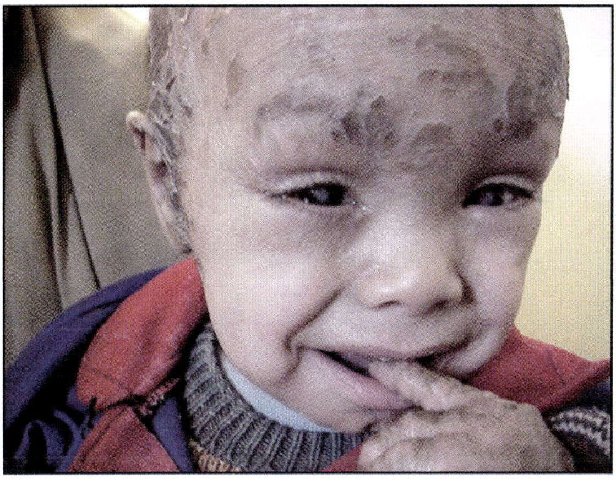

Figure 20: Congenital ectropion postoperative 2

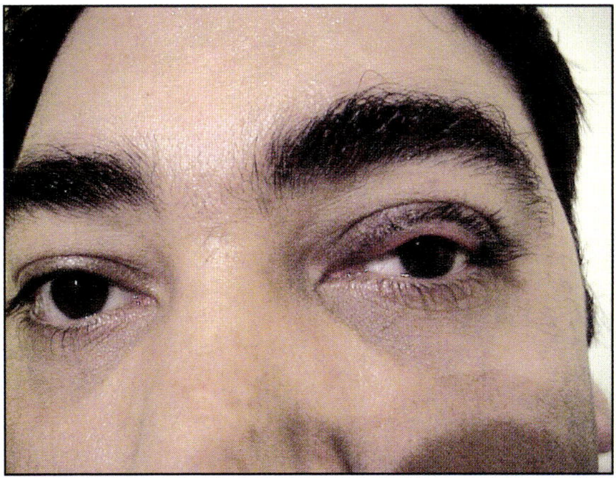

Figure 21: Floppy eyelid syndrome

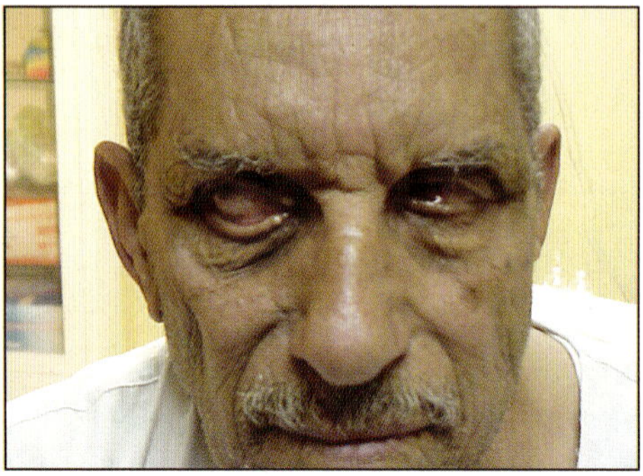

Figure 22: Ectropion preoperative

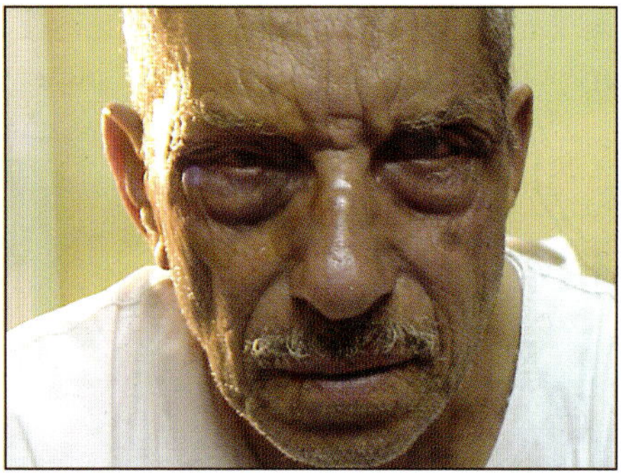

Figure 23: Ectropion postoperative

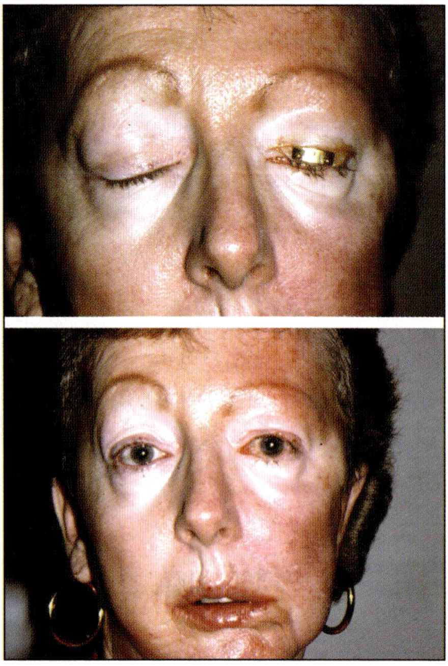

Figure 24: Gold weight implant preoperative

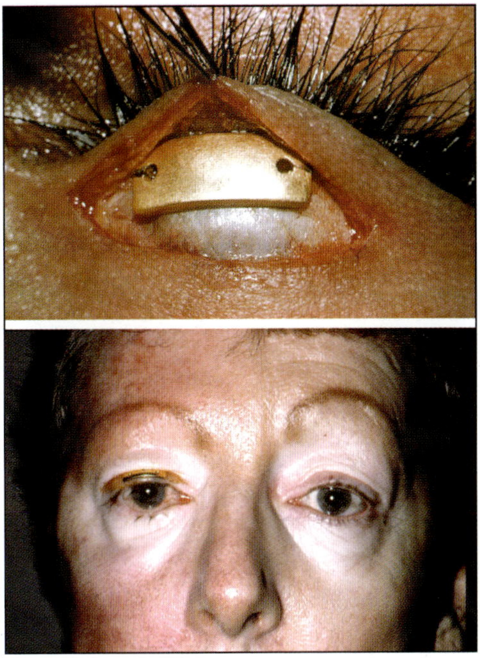

Figure 25: Gold weight implant trial and implantation

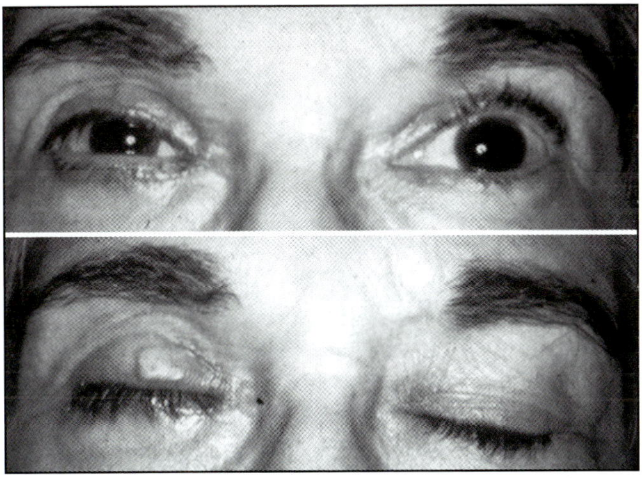

Figure 26: Gold weight implant postoperative

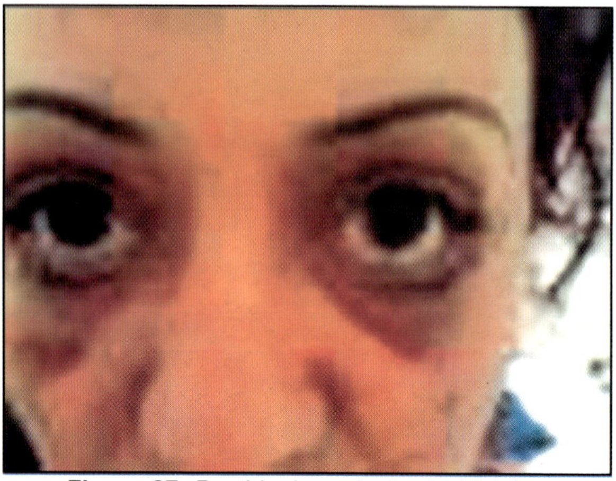

Figure 27: Postblepharoplasty cicatricial ectropion preoperative

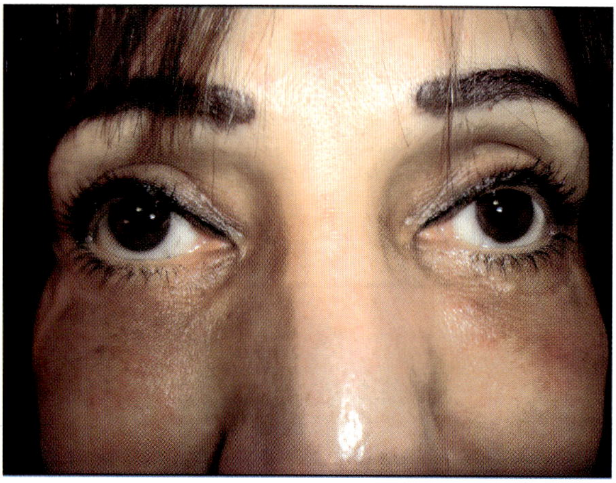

Figure 28: Postblepharoplasty cicatricial ectropion postoperative

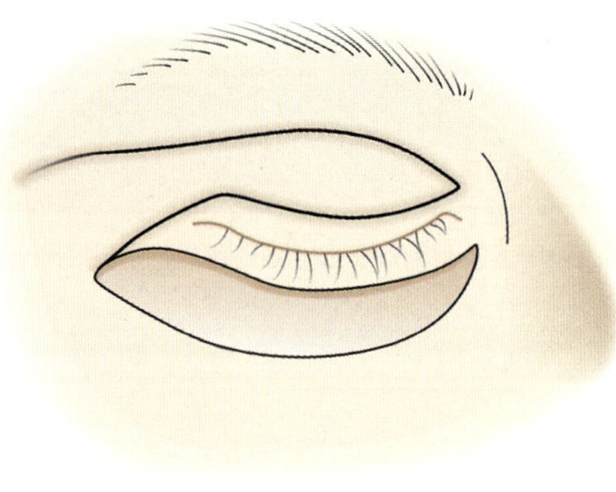

Figure 29: Transposition flap 1

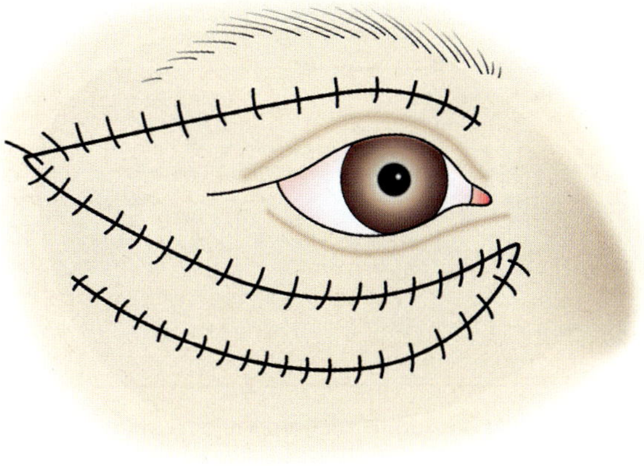

Figure 30: Transposition flap 2

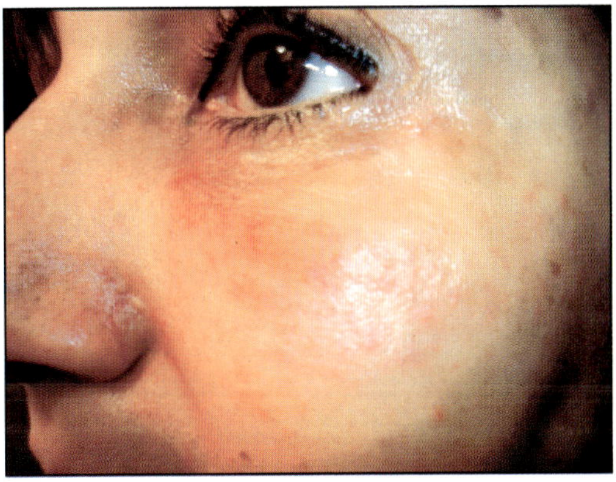

Figure 31: Transposition flap, magnified

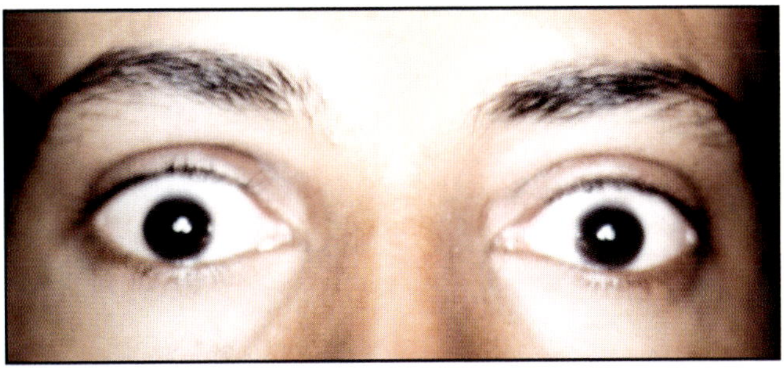

Figure 32: Lid retraction preoperative

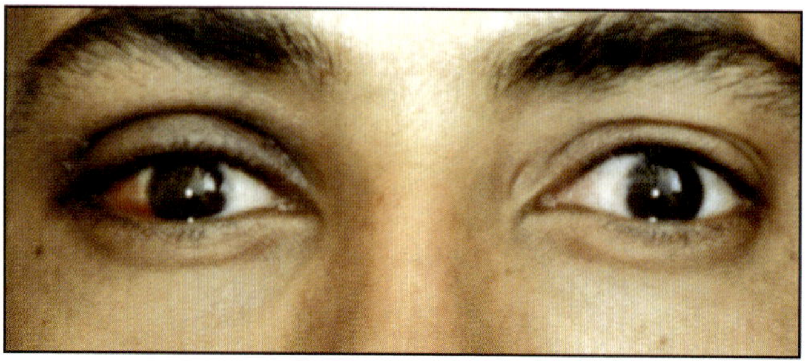

Figure 33: Lid retraction postoperative

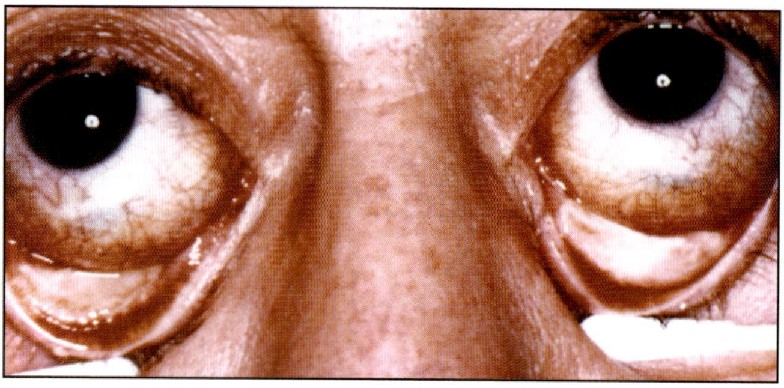

Figure 34: Hard palate graft

Chapter 25

Diseases of the Lids

Ashok Garg (India)

Stye (Hordeolum Externum)

Introduction

- Stye is an acute purulent infection (abcess) of Lash follicles and its associated gland of Zeiss or Moll.
- It is mainly Staphylococcal infection.
- Stye is generally seen in patients with Staphylococcal Blepharitis.

Clinical Signs and Symptoms

- Stye presents as a painful inflamed swelling in lid margin pointing anteriorly through the skin.
- Symptoms are out of proportion to the disease process.
- Redness and heat are present. After this a pus point develops at the root of the cilium and gets evacuated spontaneously.
- One lesion present can infect the surrounding follicles leading to a crop of lesions (Multiple minute abcesses).

Investigations

- Subjective ocular examination is sufficient to make the diagnosis and no specific investigations are indicated.

Differential Diagnosis

- International hordeolum
- Cyst of Zeiss and Moll

Treatment

- Most Styes either resolve spontaneously or evacuates anteriorly close to the eyelash roots.
- Resolution may be supported by removing the eyelash associated with the infected follicle followed by hot compresses helps in localization of the lesion and relief of symptoms.
- Application of local antibiotic ointment to the lid margin prevent the spread of the disease to the surrounding area.
- Systemic antibiotics and anti-inflammatory drugs are also advocated for reduction of infection and inflammation and relief of pain which in advanced stage is quite severe.
- Pus can also be evacuated once the lesion is localized and points on the surface under the cover of systemic broad spectrum antibiotics.
- Surgical incision is required only in case of large abcess under local anesthesia.
- Recurrence is prevented by the treatment of Chronic Blepharitis.

Prognosis

- Good

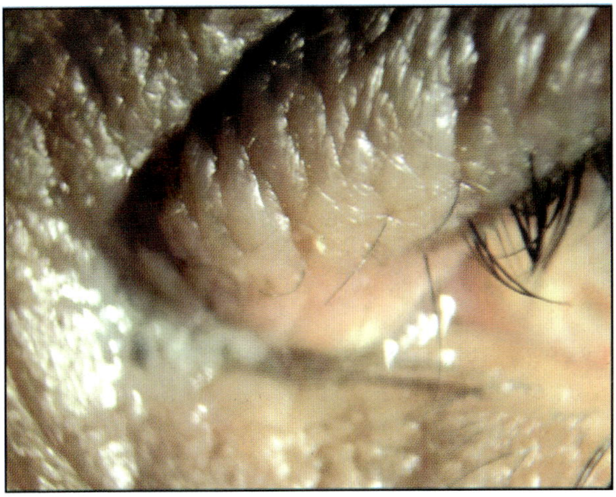

Figure 1: Hordeolum externum (Stye)

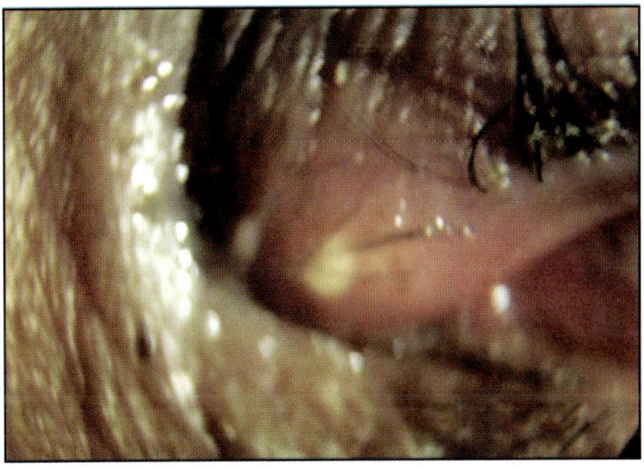

Figure 2: Hordeolum externum (Stye)

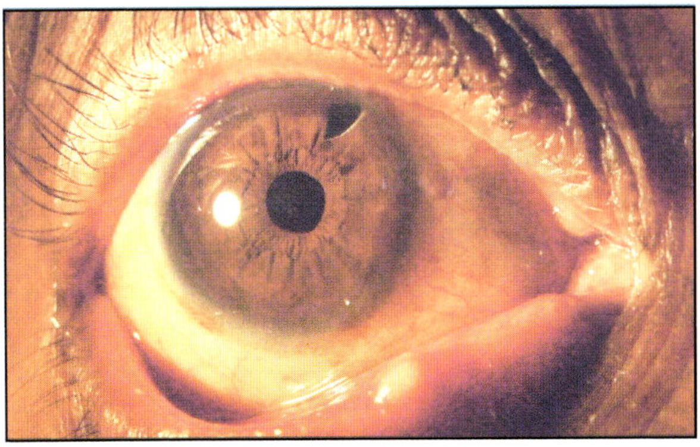

Figure 3: Marginal Chalazion lower lid

Chalazion (Meibomian Cyst)

Introduction

- Chalazion is a chronic inflammatory lipogranuloma of the tarsal glands.
- It is caused by infection of retained sebaceous material inside the meibomian gland due to obstruction of duct.
- Chalazion are common in patients with meibomian gland dysinfection.
- Chalazion is truly not a cyst as it's walls consist of granulomatous tissue and are not lined by epithelium.

Clinical Signs and Symptoms

Clinically it starts slowly and without symptoms. In the beginning it is small and hard free from overlying skin.

- It is more common in upper lid and seen frequently in adults.
- Chalazion present as a painless, slowly enlarging roundish, firm lesion in the tarsal plate.
- Mostly the lesions remain stationary after growing to a certain size but sometimes spontaneous regression or secondary infection can take place.
- Sometimes Chalazion of upper lid presses on the cornea causing blurred vision from induced astigmatism.
- Pathologically, there is a unique inflammation of the meibomian glands producing granulation tissue. It affects the area around the acini and leads to fibrosis. There is infiltration of lymphocytes, plasma cells and epithelioid cells. In the center of the mass there is deposition of lipid producing a picture of lipogranuloma.
- There is a chronic low grade infection producing accumulation of sebaceous material in the acini which results in development of granulation tissue due to toxic irritation.

Investigations

- Subjective ocular examination is adequate to clinch diagnosis.
- Eversion of the eyelid may show the presence of an external conjunctival granuloma in the region of the cyst.

Differential Diagnosis

- Stye
- Cyst of Zeiss and Moll.

Treatment

- If Chalazion is small and asymptomatic, it can be left alone.
- Medical management includes hot compresses and expressing out the material by massaging the lid.
- Intralesional injection of 1 mg triamcinolone is successful in mild to moderate cases.

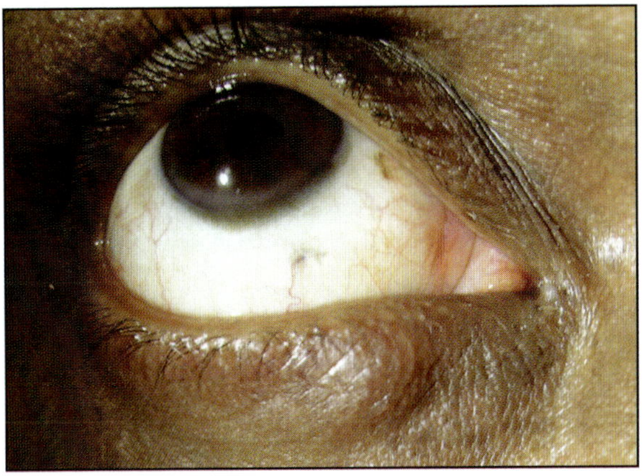

Figure 4: Chalazion lower lid

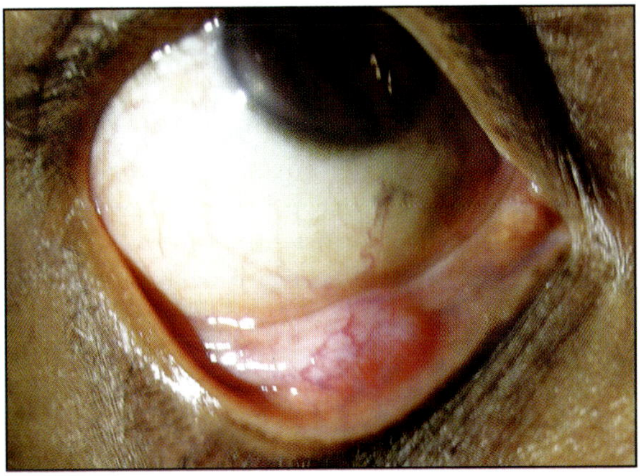

Figure 5: Chalazion lower lid

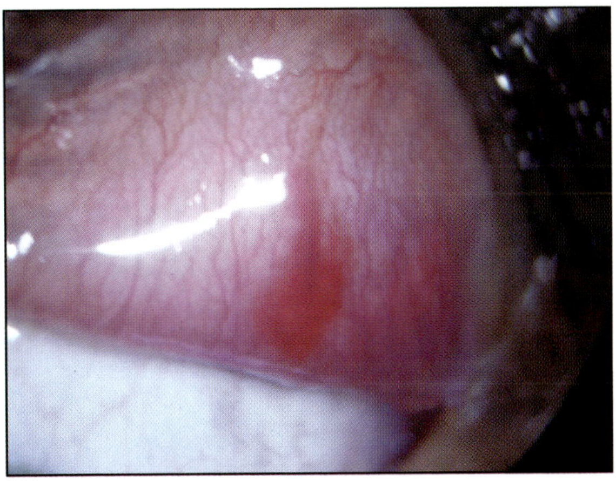

Figure 6: Incision and curettage for Chalazion upper lid (1st day post op.)

- In majority of cases incision and curettage under local anesthesia is required.
- The lid is then everted with a special Chlazion clamp.
- An incision is then made through the conjunctiva into the cyst, the contents are curetted and any associated external granulomatous tissue is excised with scissor. Evacuation of the granulation tissue is done with scoop.
- After proper evacuation, an antibiotic ointment is instilled and the eye is padded for about 6 hours. Systemic broad spectrum antibiotic and anti inflammatory drugs are given.

Prognosis

- Generally prognosis is good.
- Recurrently occurring Chalazia should be closely watched and tissue must be examined for any malignancy.

Blepharitis

Introduction

- Blepharitis is chronic inflammatory condition of the eye lid margin which leads to secondary changes in the conjunctiva and cornea.
- It is quite common but most of the time patient ignore it and goes undiagnosed.
- Etiology is varied one, but the most common causes are staphylococcal infection, seborrhea and meibomian gland dysfunction.

Clinical Signs and Symptoms

- Itching in the eye specially at the lid margin is most common complaint of the patient.
- Red eye with watering and burning sensation may also be present.
- This condition is more common in young females and is generally associated with Dandruff of the scalp.
- Lid margin is thickened, edematous and may have dilated vessels. Gray or yellowish white scales are often observed along the lid margin, scraping of it may lead to tiny ulcers of fine points of bleeding.
- In chronic conditions cilia fall of (Madrosis) with fibrosis at the site. New misdirected cilia may grow (trichiasis).
- Infection can lead to recurrent stye and angular blepharitis – conjunctivitis.
- In some cases secondary changes are seen in the conjunctiva and cornea due to hypersensitivity to staphylococcal exotoxins. They may develop into chronic papillary conjunctivitis, punctate epithelial erosions in the lower part of the cornea. Marginal corneal ulcers or Phlycten.
- In some cases cystic nodules are seen at the openings of meibomian gland ducts and a foamy discharge is floating over the tear meniscus.
- Tear film is disturbed causing dryness of the conjunctiva and cornea (Sicca).

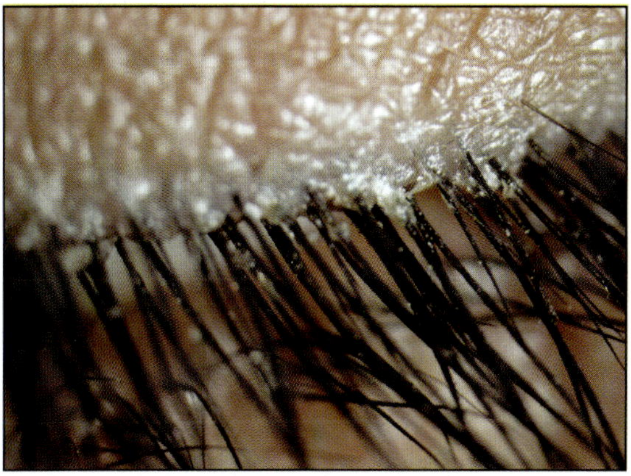

Figure 7: Seborrheic blepharitis

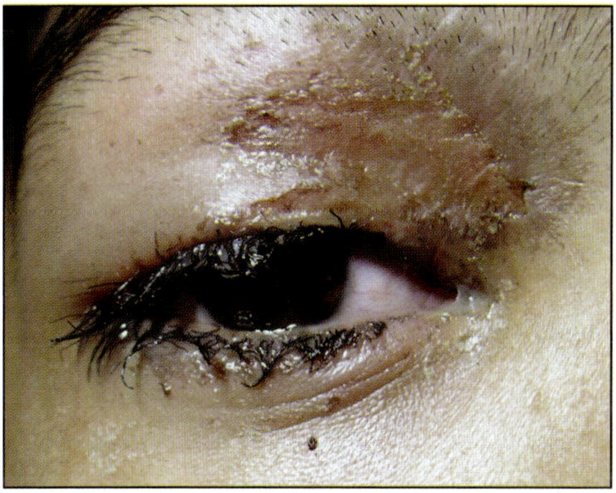

Figure 8: Blepharitis (After thermal burns)

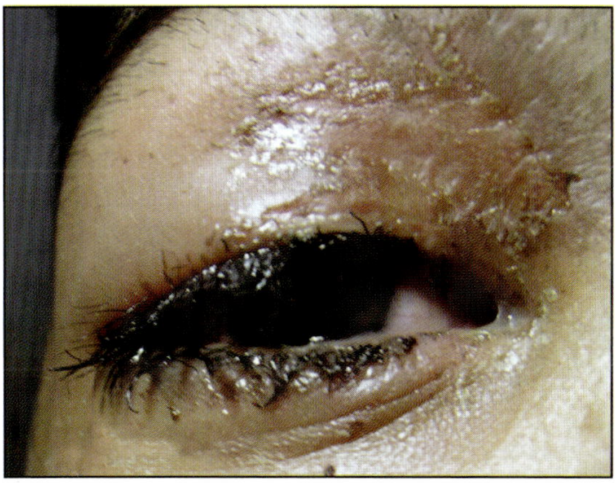

Figure 9: Blepharitis (After thermal burns)

- This peculiar condition is known as triple 'S' syndrome, a combination of Staphylococcal infection, Seborrhea and Sicca.

Investigations

- Subjective ocular examination is adequate to make the diagnosis.
- In cases of Seborreheic Blepharitis careful slit-lamp examination reveals minute oil globules at the orifices of the meibomian glands.

Treatment

Conservative long-term treatment is indicated as total eradication may not be possible.

Hot compresses are prescribed in melting solidified white deposits.

Hygeine of the Lid margin with antiseptic soap with warm water atleast twice a day is important mechanical expression of excessive secretion from meibomian glands is advised.

- Local and systemic antibiotics are indicated to control the infection. Scales are softened by wetting with boric acid and then mechanically removed by gentle scraping.
- Once the primary infection is under control, local steroids can be prescribed to treat secondary effects in the conjunctiva and cornea.
- Treatment with antibiotics and astringents should be continued for at least 2-3 weeks after visible cure.
- Simultaneous treatment of seborrheic dermatitis and dandruff with medicated Shampoo is necessary.
- Improvement of General health with vitamins and antioxidants is essential to prevent relapses.
- In parasitic infection, mechanical removes of the organisms is most sufficient.

Prognosis

Generally prognosis is good however, sustained medical treatment and compliance is required from the patient.

Dermatitis

Introduction

- Skin of the eyelid is a very common site for inflammation even with very mild irritants as it is thinnest and most extensible in the body.

Clinical Signs and Symptoms

- Acute dermatitis is characterized by erythema, vesiculation and crusting with burning sensation and itching.

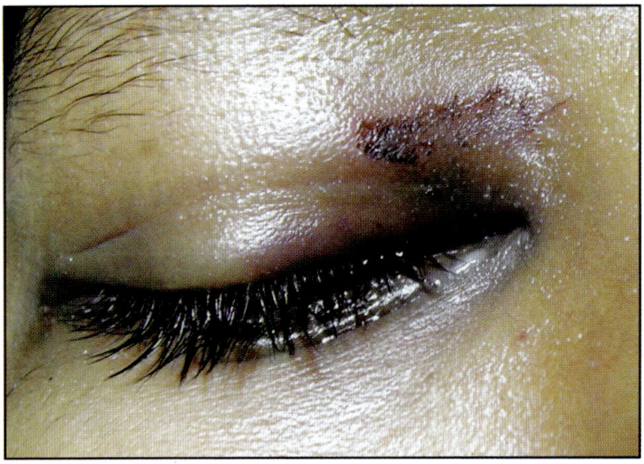

Figure 10: Blepharitis (After injury)

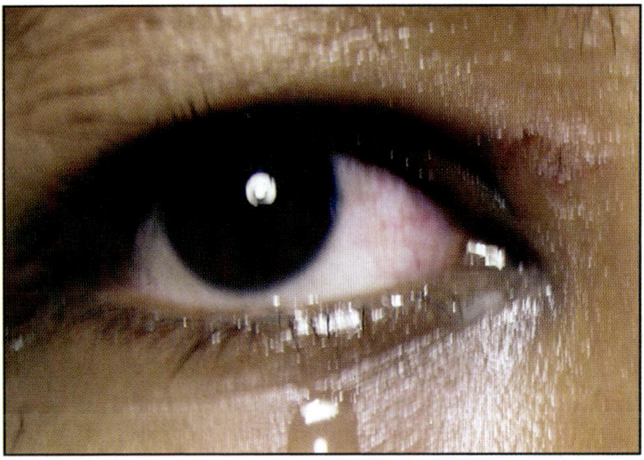

Figure 11: Blepharitis

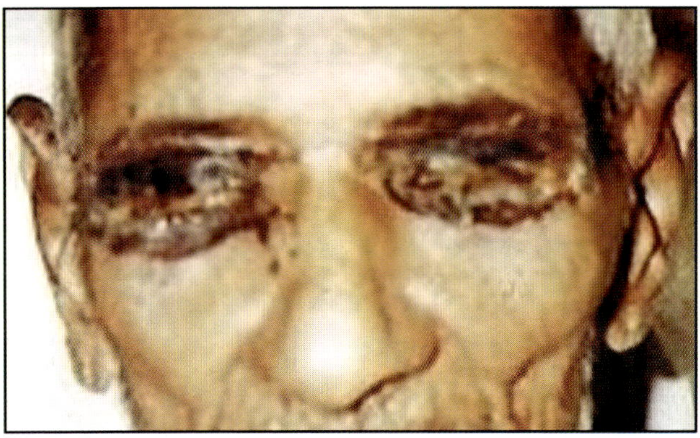

Figure 12: Drug induced dermatitis—Front profile

- Chronic dermatitis is shown by thickening of the skin and itching with minimal erythema. Local drugs (Drops and ointments) and cosmetics are the common irritants.
- In atopic dermatitis patient is sensitive to allergants to much greater degree than normal. They may have a past history of hay fever or asthma. Chronic, Keratoconjunctivitis, Keratoconus and Lenticular opacities may be associated with atopy.
- Contact dermatitis involving the eyelids are common. It is caused by transmission of irritating substances to the lids by fingers. Failure to rinse the hands adequately following transfer of irritating chemicals in soaps or detergants is the most common cause.

Investigations

- Subjective ocular examination is required to make the diagnosis.

Treatment

- Conservations management involves patch testing in order to identify the irritant and then its removal from the patients surrounding.
- Acute dermatitis is best treated with cold compresses and nonfluorinated short-term corticosteroids like hydrocortisone are helpful. Long-term use of corticosteroids is contraindicated as it may aggravate the dermatitis.

Prognosis

Good.

Warts (Verruca Vulgaris)

Introduction

- Warts are small elevated lesions with a papillomatous surface.
- It is a virus infection caused by wart virus belonging to PAPOVA group.
- Sometimes it erupts as a crop of lesions which appear simultaneously.

Clinical Signs and Symptoms

It appears as elevated lesion in the form of cyst either from upper and lower eyelid protruding anteriorly without any symptoms generally.

Investigation

Subjective ocular examination is generally recommended.

Treatment

Generally cryoapplication is recommended for the regression of wart.

Surgical excision is also indicated but it often leads to recurrence.

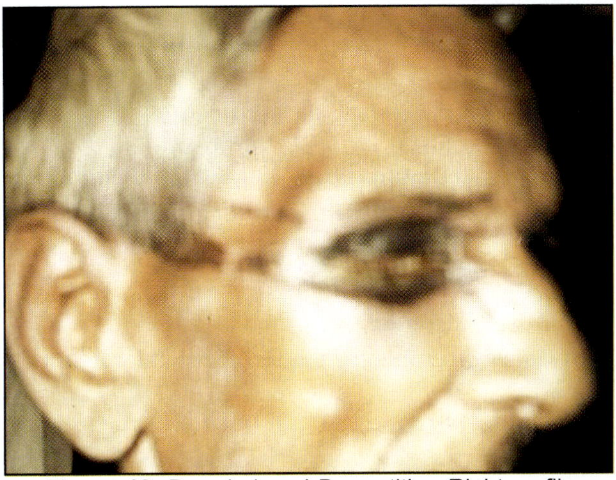

Figure 13: Drug induced Dermatitis—Right profile

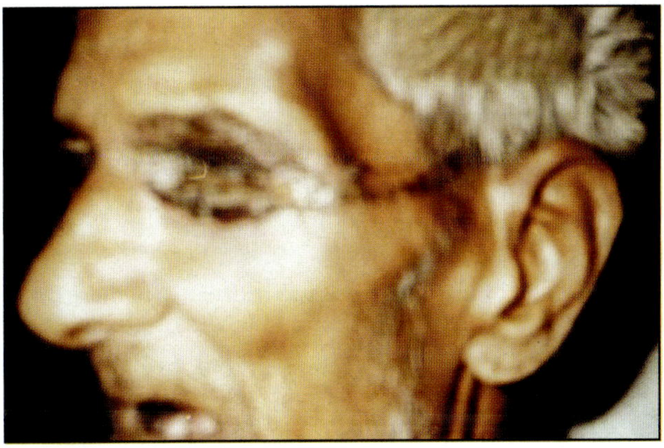

Figure 14: Drug induced Dermatitis—Left profile

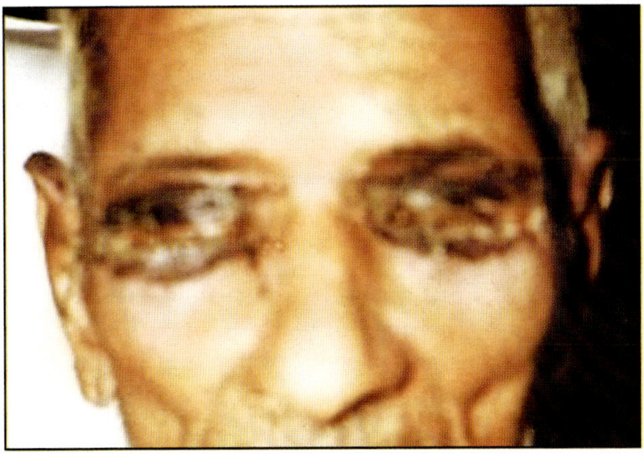

Figure 15: Drug induced Dermatitis—Zoomed in

Molluscum Contagiosum

Introduction

- It is a caused by a viral infection and mostly affects children.
- The typical lesions multiple, skin colored dome shaped nodule measuring from 1-3 mm sometimes umblicated are seen.
- It is due to infection caused by viruses belonging to a group of poxviruses.

Clinical Signs and Symptoms

- Lesions when present close to the lid margin can produce follicular conjunctivitis due to liberation of the virus into the conjunctival sac.

Investigation

- Subjective ocular examination.
- Microscopically intracytoplasmic inclusion bodies can be seen which can displace and compress the nucleus to one side.

Treatment

Skin lesion treatment is recommended by expression or cauterization.

Prognosis

- Generally it is good.
- Immunocompromised patients including those of AIDS are prone to develop this virus infection.

Trichiasis

Introduction

- Trichiasis is an inward misdirection of the lashes. In this condition few cilia are misdirected backward and they rub against the cornea.
- Trichiasis is caused by trachoma, ulcerative blepharitis, ocular burns, membranous conjunctivitis, injury or operation on the lid margin. It can also be seen in congenital distichiasis.

Clinical Signs and Symptoms

- Patient complain of Foreign body sensation, irritation, lacrimation, photophobia and pain. The misdirected lashes may rub against the cornea or cause corneal erosions and vascularization and in severe long standing cases corneal pannus may develop.

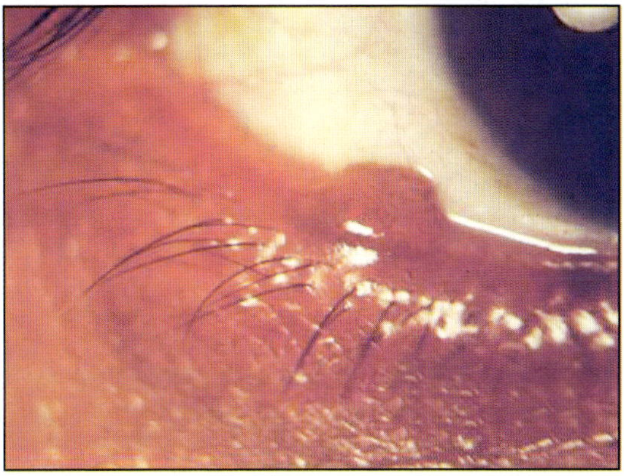

Figure 16: Verruca vulgaris lower lid

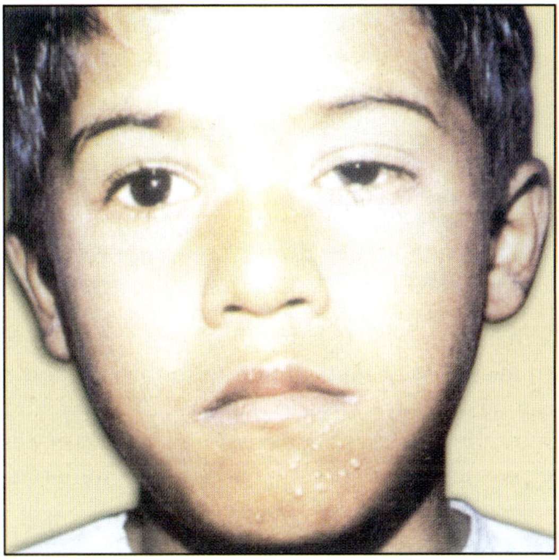

Figure 17: Molluscum contagiosum involving lids and face

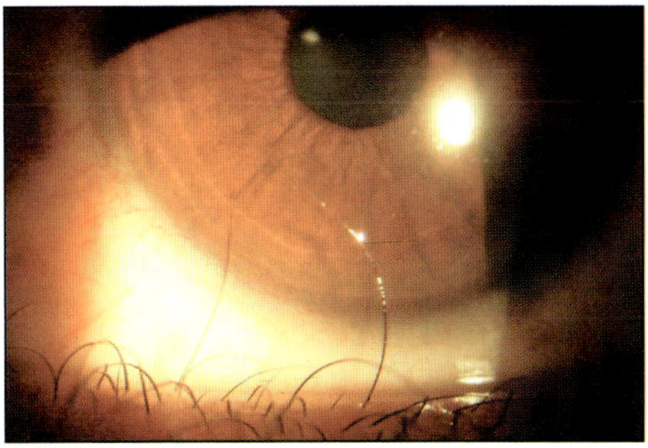

Figure 18: Trichiasis lower eye lid

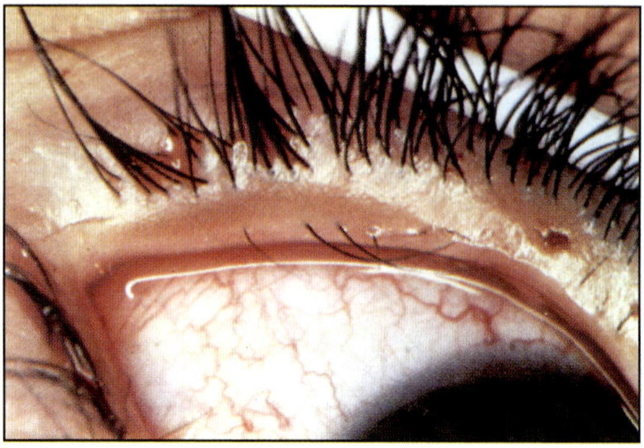

Figure 19: Trichiasis upper eye lid

Investigation

- Subjective ocular examination and slit-lamp examination clinch the diagnosis.

Differential Diagnosis

- Pseudotrichiasis secondary to entropion.

Treatment

- Epilation (Mechanical removal of cilia with forceps) is effective but recurrence with in 4-8 weeks is common with this method.
- Hair follicles can be destroyed by electrolysis. This procedure is not simple and frequent multiple treatments are required to obtain desired results. In this procedure passage of an electric current (3-5 milliamperes) is passed through a fine needle inserted into the root of the eyelash. Then eyelash is removed with the help of forcep. It is a painful procedure.
- Hair follicles can also be destroyed by passage of a current of 30 milliampere for 10 seconds through a diathermy needle.
- Cryotherapy is Safe and effective method for destroying the misdirected lashes. The cryoprobe with –20°C temperature is applied on to the root of the eyelash, a freeze-thaw-freeze technique is used. It destroys the hair follicles but leaves a depigmented area after healing.
- Trichiasis can also be corrected with argon laser but it is less effective than cryotherapy.
- Surgical correction may be required in patient with severe trichiasis.

Prognosis

- Generally prognosis is good if proper and adequate treatment is given.

Chapter 26

Congenital Tumors

AK Grover, Shaloo Bageja (India)

Pigmented Lesions

Naevi

These are benign congenital tumors. They may vary in size and may be sessile or pedunculated. The commonest location is along the lid border. Risk of malignancy is low. However in large tumors, there will be 4-6% risk of malignant transformation. Sudden increase in size and increase in pigmentation suggests concern regarding malignant transformation and requires excision.

Management

Shave off flush with the lid margin if it involves the lid margin or .

If naevus does not involve the lid margin excision with direct repair with margin repair can be done.

Naevus of Ota (Oculodermal Melanocytosis)

It is characterized by patchy bluish or brownish pigmentation of periocular skin and sclera. The lesion is composed of dermal melanocytes and has malignant potential. Increased intraocular pigmentation contributes to risk of glaucoma. It is occasionally associated with Sturge-Weber syndrome.

Management

Ruby laser has been tried to lighten the cutaneous component.

Angiomatous Tumors

Portwine Stain (Naevus Flammeus)

This condition is characterized by telangiectasia of the deeper skin capillaries. It involves the part of the face which is innervated by the trigeminal nerve. It is often associated with Sturge-Weber syndrome. Congenital glaucoma and choroidal hemangioma have strong association.

Strawberry (Capillary) Hemangioma

These are benign tumors present at birth. 90% of these clinically manifest by age of 1 month.

Symptoms and Signs

The child may present with ptosis, refractive error, amblyopia and proptosis.

Prognosis

These tumor grow for 3-6 months after birth and slowly regresses by second year of life. Spontaneous resolution occurs in 40% by 4years of age and 80% by 8 years.

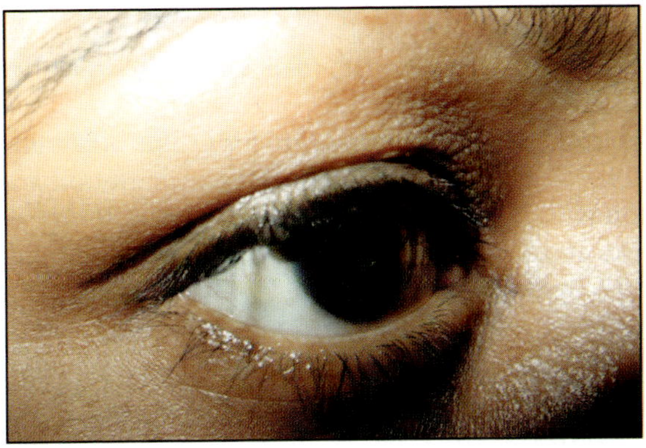

Figure 1: Showing naevus in upper eyelid

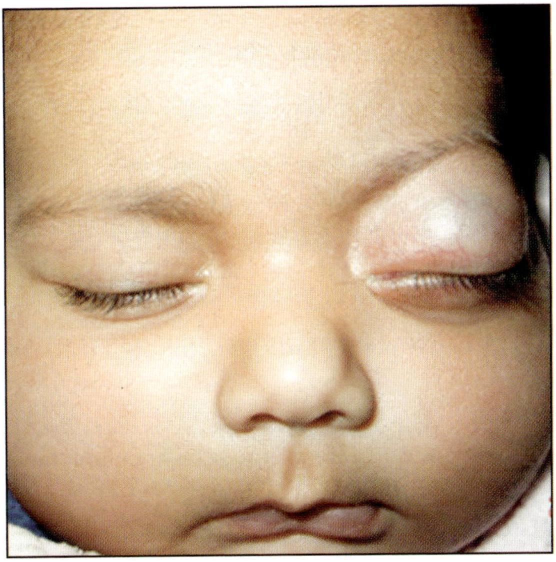

Figure 2: An infant with capillary hemangioma

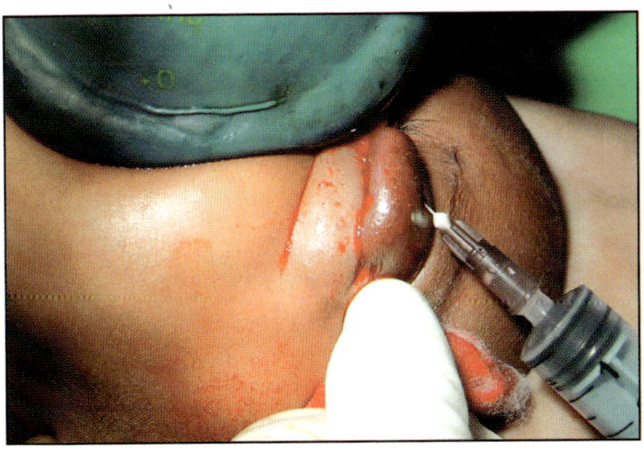

Figure 3: Injecting corticosteroid in the hemangioma

Management

Surgery is indicated in cases of total ptosis obscuring the visual axis and induced astigmatism and for better cosmesis.

Intralesional injection of 1-2 ml of corticosteroid. Betamethasone 6mg/ml and Triamcinolone 40 mg/cc combined in 1:1 concentration and is injected all around the lesion with 26G needle deep into the lesion. Rapid shrinkage occurs in first two weeks and then continues slowly for several months. Injection may be repeated after 6 weeks in case of residual mass. Depigmentation of overlying skin, eyelid necrosis and rarely central retinal artery occlusion are few complications seen with steroid injection.

Dermoid and Epidermoid Cyst

Abnormal sequestration of surface ectoderm beneath the skin during embryonic development results in the cyst formation. Lids are usually secondarily involved due to extension of the tumor from the orbits.

Signs

They are clinically evident by first year of life. Most common location is superonasal. On palpation, these are firm in consistency, non tender and are attached to underlying periosteum.

Investigation

Imaging is necessary to know the extension.

Management

Surgical excision is required in case of progressive enlargement of mass.

Plexiform Neurofibroma

Involvement of the lid with plexiform neuroma in cases of neurofibromatosis. Café au lait spots are characteristic of neurofibromatosis.

Management

Surgery is indicated in cases of significant mechanical ptosis and to improve cosmesis. Surgical debulking of the mass along with ptosis correction and lateral shortening may be performed.

Prognosis

These tumors cannot be fully excised and recurrence is common.

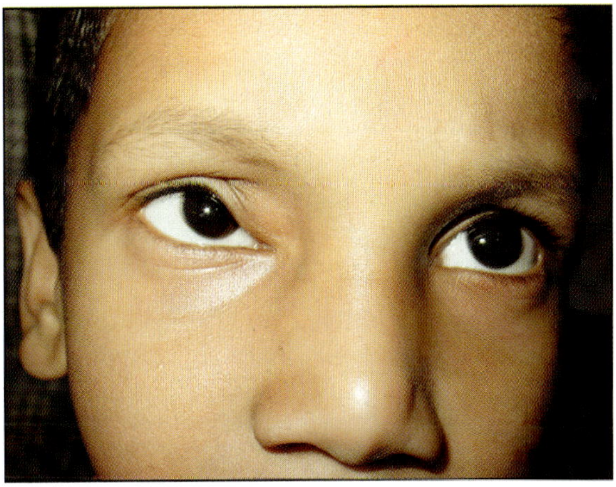

Figure 4: Showing swelling superonasally of dermoid

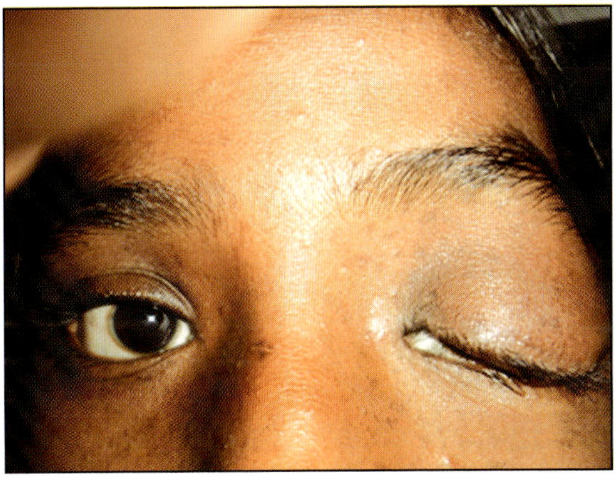

Figure 5: Showing plexiform neurofibroma of let upper lid

To conclude, pediatric abnormalities poses challenges for an Ophthalmologist. Patient's co-operation is a limitation for adequate assessment in pediatric age group. Cosmetic consideration is also critical for child's psychological development. It is important to carefully assess and plan the technique of intervention for gratifying results.

Chapter 27

Congenital Ptosis: Evaluation and Management

AK Grover, Shaloo Bageja (India)

Introduction

Congenital Ptosis is a common entity managed by the oculoplastic surgeons. It results from a developmental dystrophy of the levator muscle of unknown etiology. Management of the condition requires a thorough understanding of the surgical anatomy and a meticulous surgical technique based on a proper evaluation.

Surgical Anatomy of the Upper Eyelid and Eyebrow

The thorough understanding of the surgical anatomy of eyelid is necessary to give good functional and cosmetic results.

The layer of upper eyelid from anterior to posterior are skin, subcutaneous tissue, orbicularis muscle, submuscular tissue, orbital septum and preaponeurotic pad of fat, levator aponeurosis, Müller muscle, tarsal plate and conjunctiva.

Skin of the upper lid is thinnest in the body. The skin is attached loosely over the eyelid, but firmly over the brow, lid margins and canthi.

Orbicularis muscle is responsible for blinking and lid closure. It originates from medial palpebral ligament and the fibers spread in elliptical fashion. It is divided into orbital and palpebral portion. The palpebral portion runs from medial canthal ligament to lateral palpebral raphe.

Submuscular layer is corrected with the submuscular layer of the brow and thus the infection can spread through this plane. Most of the blood vessels and nerve lie in this area.

Orbital septum and tarsal plate—form a continuous layer of fibrous tissues and is mainly responsible for the stability of the eyelid.

Levator muscle – is the main retractor of the upper eyelid. It originates above the optic foramina under the lesser wing of sphenoid. It moves forward under the orbital roof and above the superior rectus muscle. Near the equator of the globe it is transformed into fibrous aponeurosis, which travels forwards and inferiorly and gets inserted into the upper 2/3rd of the anterior tarsus. The other attachments of the levator aponeurosis are to skin of the upper lid after penetrating the orbicularis muscle forming the lid crease. Its medial and lateral extensions are known as 'horns'. The lateral horn attaches to the orbital tubercle. by the canthal ligament. It is important to remember that the lateral horn separate the lacrimal gland into palpebral and orbital part. The medial horn forms the medial canthal ligament.

Müller muscle—is a thin sheet of non-striated muscle which arises near the junction of the levator and its aponeurosis from its under surface and attaches to the superior forward border of tarsus. The superior transverse ligament (Whitnall's ligament) arises from the under surface of the levator. It assists in suspension of the levator muscle.

Conjunctiva—is inner most layer of the lid. The palpebral conjunctiva is transparent, highly vascular and is strongly attached to tarsus of upper lid. It is continuous with the bulbar conjunctiva via superior fornix.

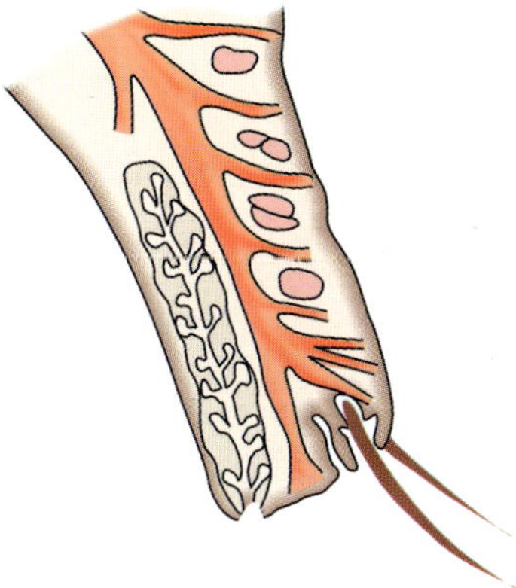

Figure 1: Showing surgical anatomy of the eyelid

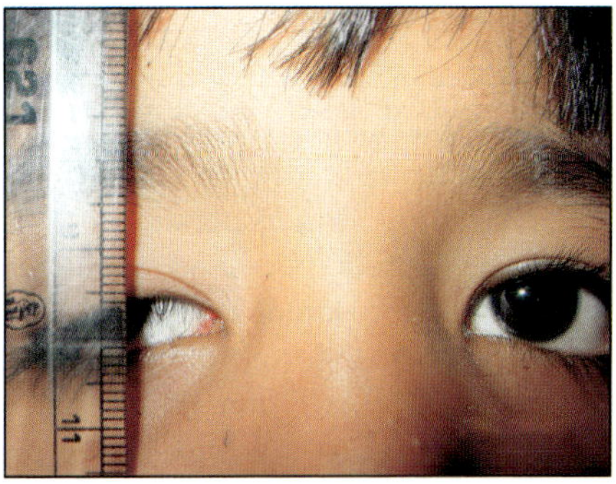

Figure 2: Measurement of Margin reflex distance 1 (MRD1)

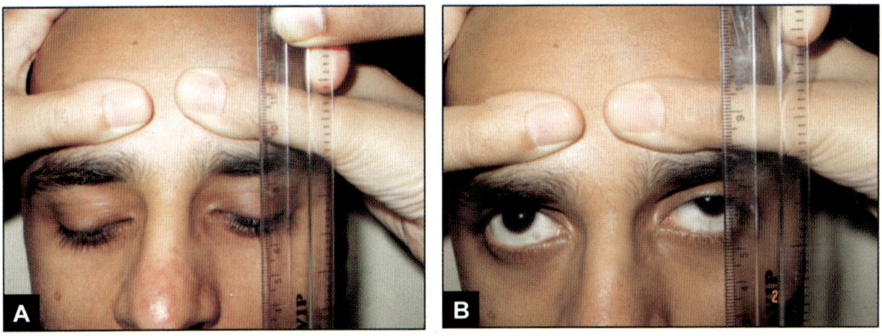

Figures 3A and B: Measurement of levator action by Berke's method

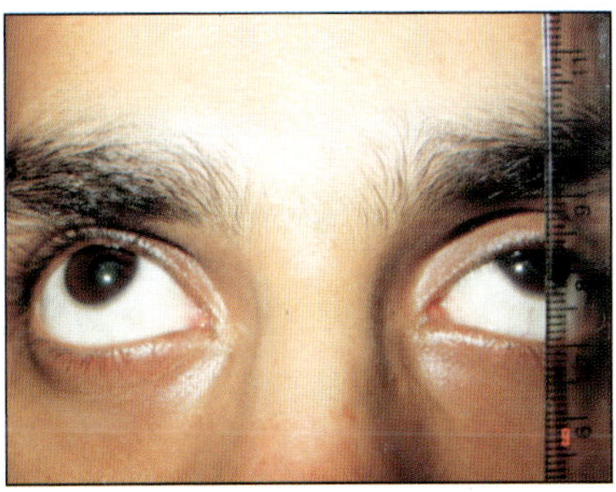

Figure 4: Measurement of Margin limbal distance (MLD)

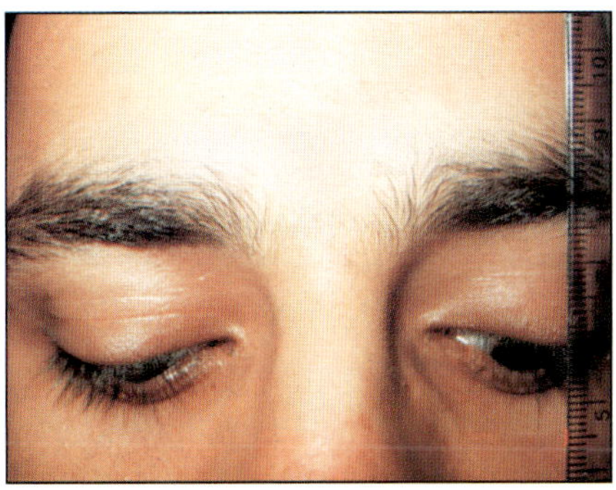

Figure 5: Measurement of Margin crease distance (MCD)

Frontalis muscle—originates from epicranial aponeurosis anterior to the coronal suture and inserts into skin and subcutaneous tissue of the eyebrow. It helps in elevation of upper lid by drawing the scalp, raises the eyebrow and form the crease on forehead.

Classification of Congenital Ptosis

Congenital ptosis may be classified as:

- Congenital simple ptosis
- Complicated
  - With oculomotor abnormalities
  - With blepharophimosis syndrome synkinetic ptosis
    - Marcus Gunn Jaw Winking
    - Misdirected third nerve ptosis.

Clinical Evaluation

Preoperative history and examination are vital because these decide the choice of surgery.

History

It is important to determine whether the condition is congenital or acquired. Relevant history should be elicited in all patients regarding the time of onset, any variation of the ptosis during the day, associations with any jaw movements or abnormal ocular movements and head posture. Photographic records of childhood often reveal important information.

A family history of similar conditions should be determined. Any history of previous surgery or trauma or use of steroid should be recorded. History of any reactions to previous anesthesia both by the patient and his relatives need to be asked. Any bleeding tendencies should also be recorded.

Ocular Examination

Visual Acuity

Best corrected visual acuity should be checked to record the presence of amblyopia in the ptotic eye.

Palpebral Aperture

The measurement of the palpebral aperture is necessary as the difference between the two eyes gives the measurement of the ptosis in unilateral cases or the difference from the normal in the bilateral cases. Should be seen in up gaze, down gaze and primary gaze.

Normal—9-10 mm in primary gaze.

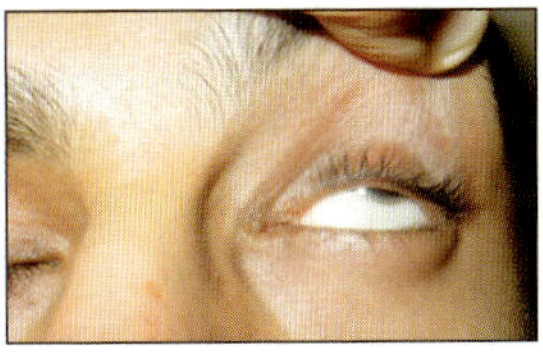

Figure 6: Assessing the Bell's phenomena

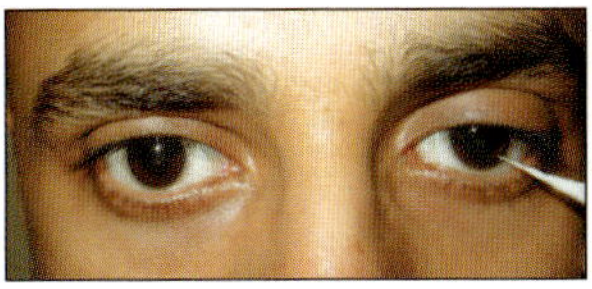

Figure 7: Assessing the corneal sensation

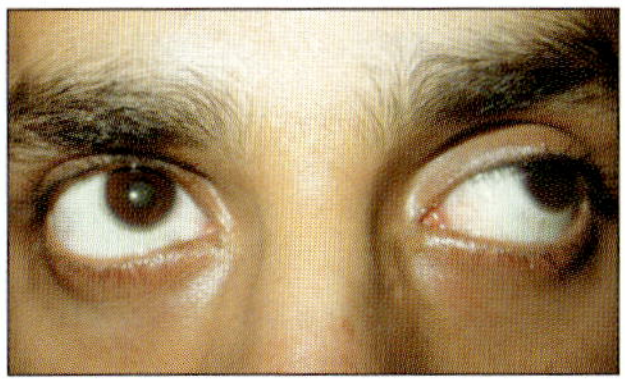

Figure 8: Assessing ocular motility especially the elevators

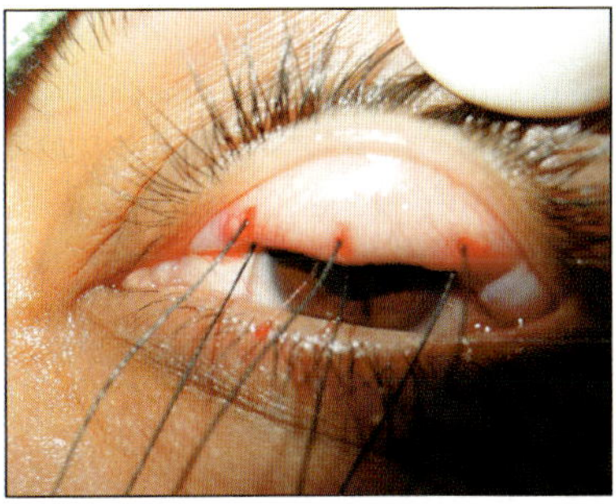

A. Lid everted and sutures passed through the superior margin of the tarsal plate

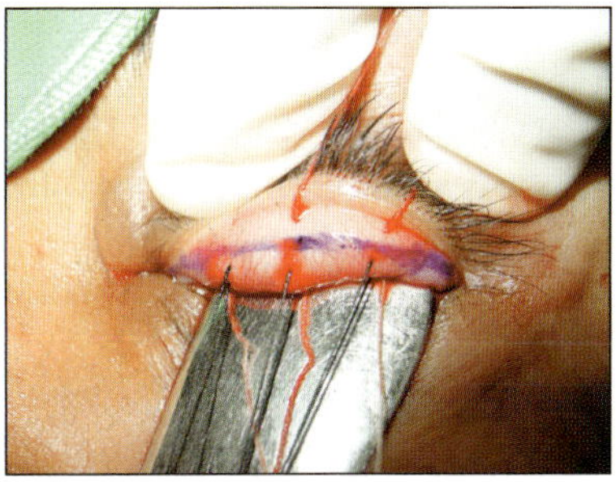

B. Marking along the proposed line of excision. Corresponding sutures passed close to everted lid margin

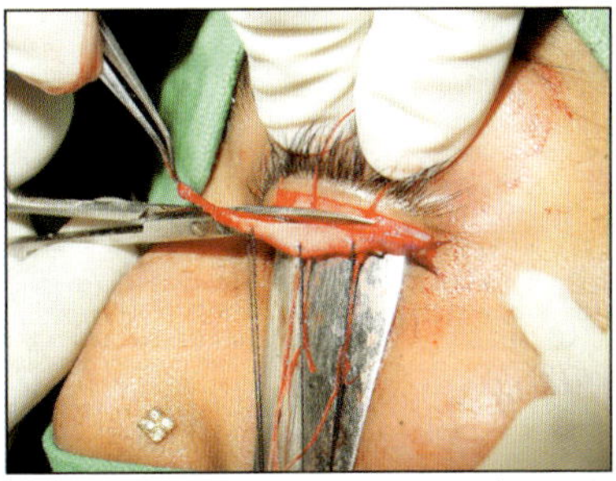

C. A scissor is used to cut along the groove created by the knife

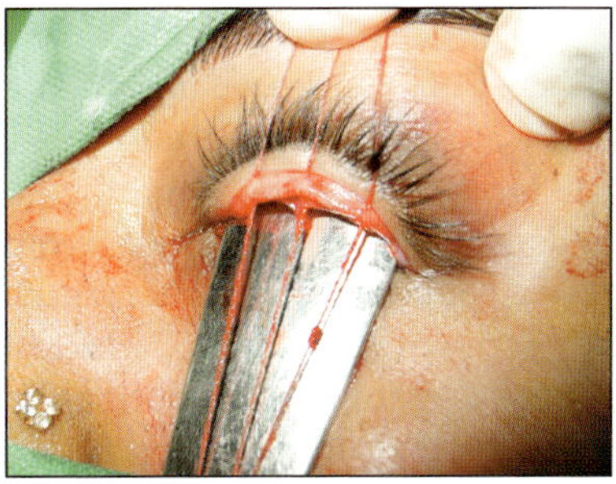

D. Excision is completed. Conjunctival and tarsal edges are raised with the aid of the traction sutures, to assist in suturing

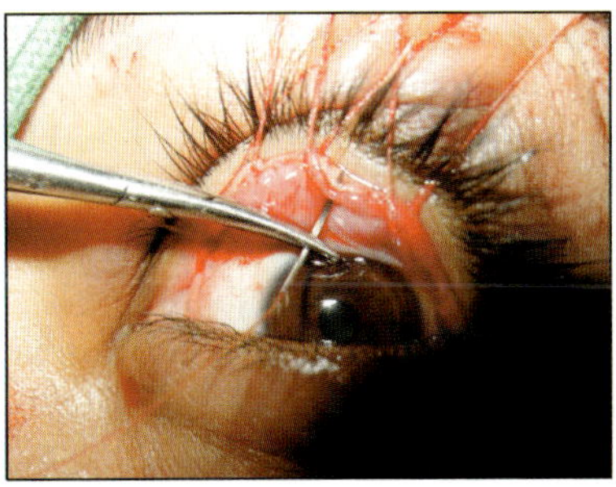

E. Continuous sutures with 5'0 plain catgut, with knots buried within the wound

Figures 9A to E: Modified Fasanella Servat surgery

However, judging the amount of ptosis by difference in the size of palpebral aperture has limitations due to possible alterations in the position of lower eyelid.

Margin Reflex Distance

Hold the light source directly in front of the patient looking straight ahead. The distance between the center of the lid margin of the upper lid and the light reflex on the cornea would give the MRD 1. If the margin is above the light reflex the MRD 1 is a +ve value. If the lid margin is below the corneal reflex in cases of very severe ptosis the MRD 1 would be a –ve value. The latter would be calculated by keeping the scale at the middle of upper lid margin and elevating the lid till the corneal light reflex is visible. The distance between the reflex and the marked original upper lid margin in –ve sign would be the MRD 1.

Margin reflex distance 1 (MRD 1): Normal 4-5 mm

The mean measurement in Indian eyes is 4.1 ± 0.5.

Amount of ptosis

The difference in MRD 1 of the two sides in unilateral cases
or
the difference from normal in bilateral cases
gives the amount of ptosis.

Amount of ptosis may be classified as:

Mild ptosis	2 mm or less
Moderate ptosis	3 mm
Severe ptosis	4 mm or more

It must be remembered that ptotic lid in unilateral congenital ptosis is usually higher in down gaze due to failure of levator to relax. While in acquired ptosis it is invariably lower than normal lid in down gaze.

Levator Function

Berke's Method (Lid Excursion)

Measures the excursion of the upper lid from extreme down gaze to extreme up gaze with action of frontalis muscle blocked. The patient is positioned against a wall while the surgeon's hands press the forehead above the eyebrows ensuring that there is no downward or upward push. The patient is then asked to look at extreme downgaze and then in extreme upgaze and the readings are recorded in millimeters. The measurements need to be accurate. The levator action of the two eyes is compared. In our study in a North Indian population levator action in normal eyelids was 13.8+0.1 mm. Crowell Beard reported normal eyelid excursion to be between 12-17 mm.

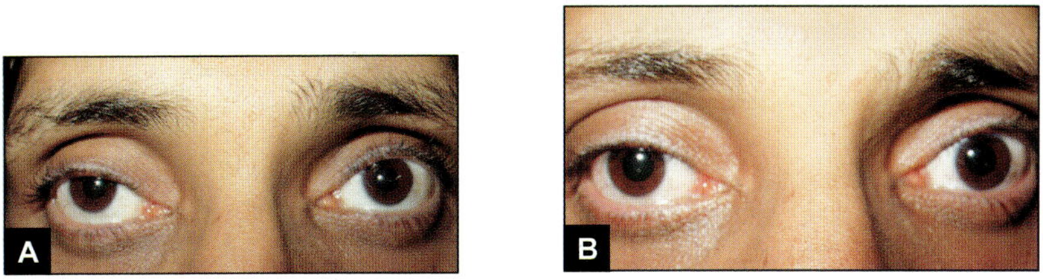

Figures 10A and B: Preoperative and postoperative photograph following modified Fasanella Servat surgery

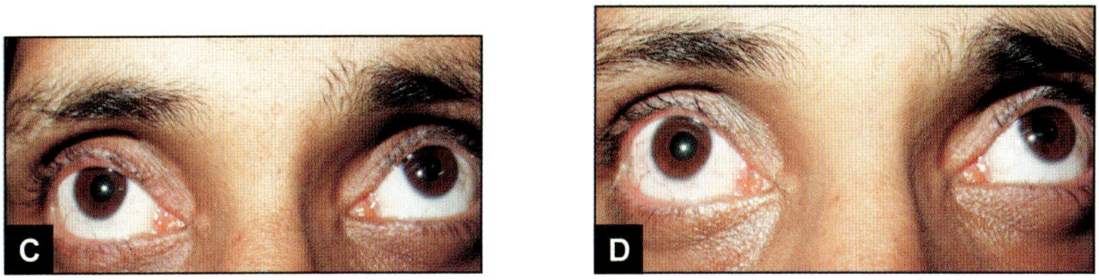

Figures 10C and D: Preoperative and postoperative photograph in upgaze

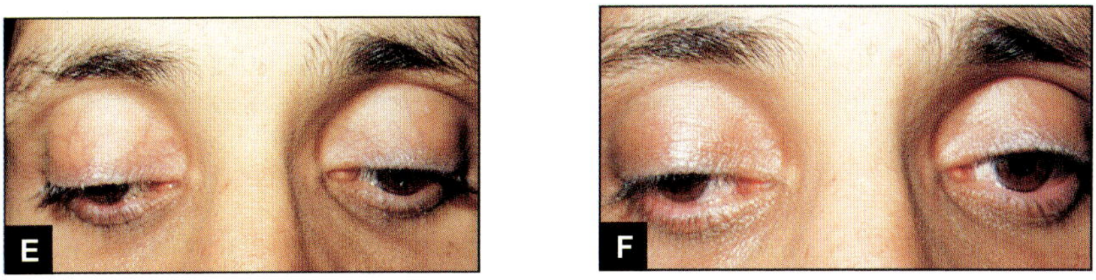

Figures 10E and F: Preoperative and postoperative photograph in downgaze

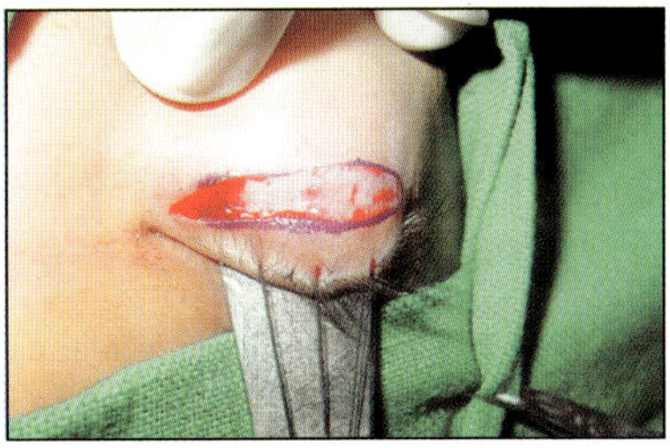

A. Matched lid crease is marked. Skin and orbicularis are incised

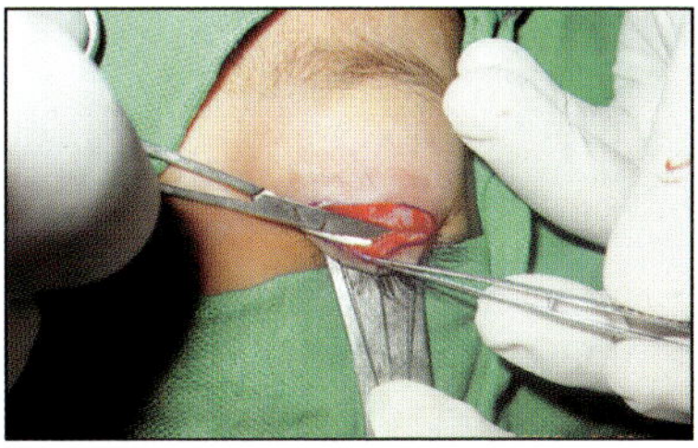

B. Skin and orbicularis dissected from tarsal plate

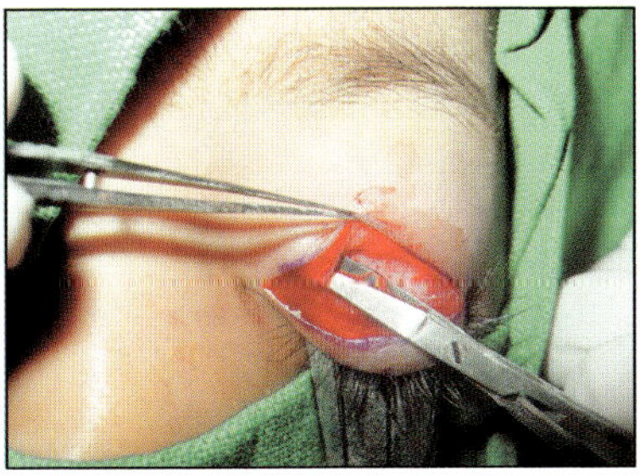

C. Dissection done superiorly from the orbital septum

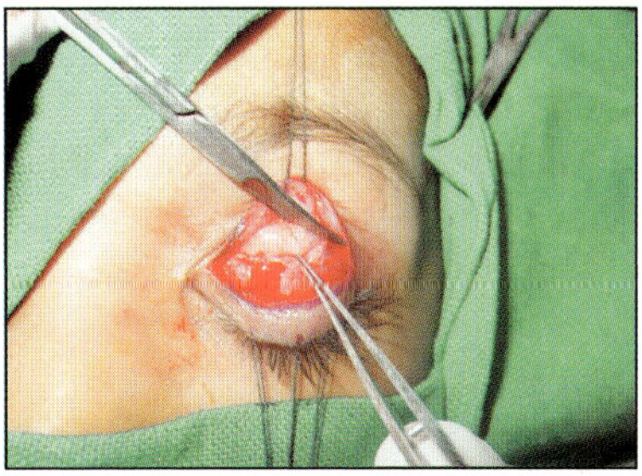

D. Orbital septum cut exposing the preaponeurotic fat

The levator function is classified as:

8 mm or more	Good
5-7 mm	Fair
4 mm	Poor

Putterman's method

This is carried out by the measurement of distance between the middle of upper lid margin to the 6'o clock limbus in extreme up gaze. This is also known as the Margin limbal distance (MLD).

Normal is about 9.0 mm

The difference in MLD of two sides in unilateral cases
or
the difference with normal in bilateral cases multiplied by three would give the amount of levator resection required.

Assessment in Children

Measurement of levator function in small children is a difficult task as no formal evaluation is allowed by the child. The presence of lid fold and increase or decrease on its size on movement of the eyelid gives us a clue to the levator action. Presence of anomalous head posture like the child throwing his head back suggests a poor levator action.

Iliff Test

This is another indicator of levator action. It is applicable in first year of life. The upper eyelid of the child is everted as the child looks down. If the levator action is good lid reverts on its own.

Margin Crease Distance (MCD)

Measurement of the margin crease distance (MCD) is the next important step in examination. The height of the crease on the normal side should be measured and compared to the ptotic eyelid in the downgaze. In case of a very faint lid crease it can be made prominent by using a cotton tipped applicator below the lid margin. In patients, when more than one lid creases are present, the most prominent one should be considered.

MCD in Normal eyes is 5-7 mm.

The distance of the lid crease from the margin is measured as it helps in planning the surgical incision. Also presence of a distant lid fold in a case of moderate to severe ptosis with good levator action indicates a levator aponeurotic dehiscence.

Bell's Phenomenon

It is the upward rotation of eyeball on closure of the eye. This is referred to as Bell's positive.

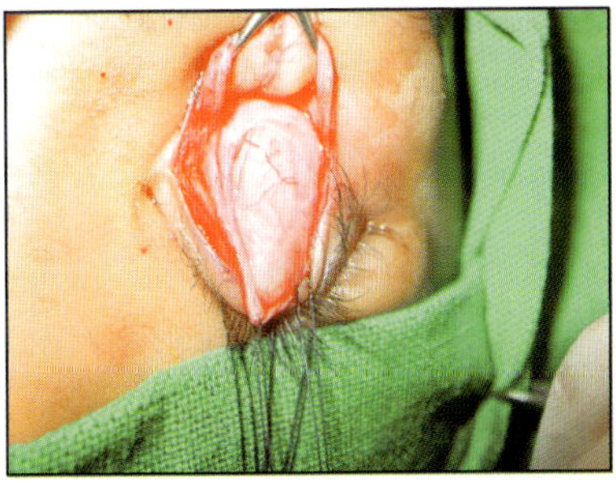

E. Levator is free from the adjoining structures

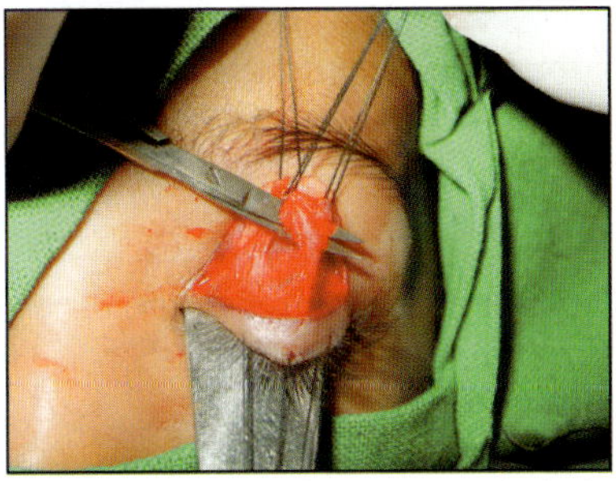

F. Levator fibers of aponeurosis being cut from its insertion in the inferior half of the anterior surface of tarsus

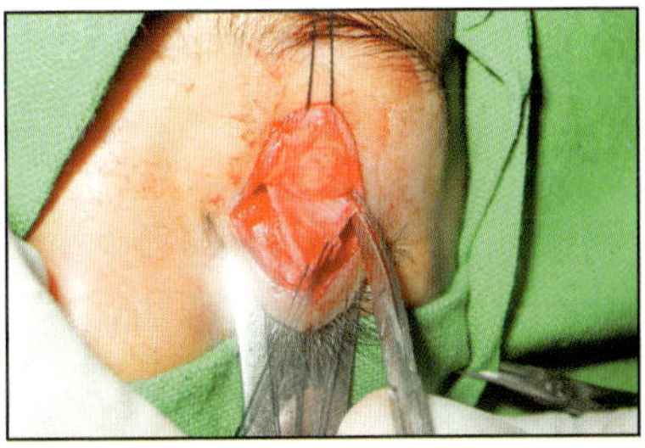

G. Lateral horn being cut

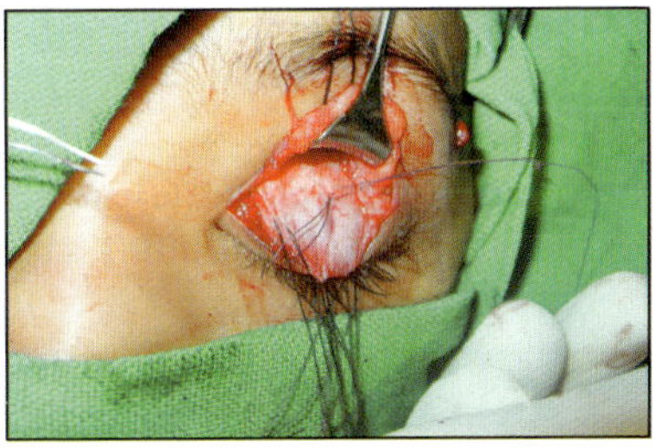

H. Double armed 5'0 vicryl sutures passed through the tarsus

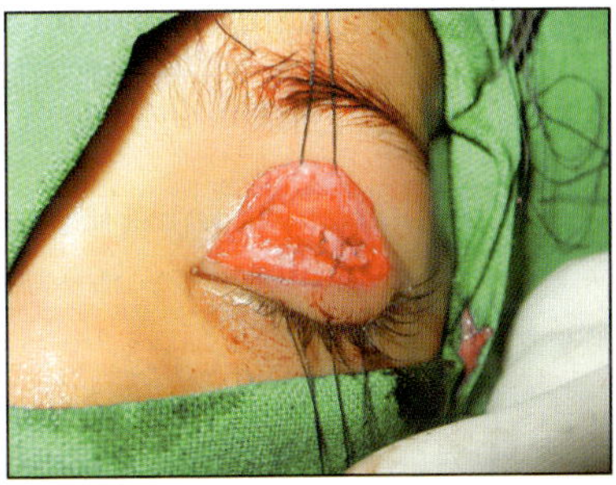

I. Three double armed suture passed through the levator and tightened

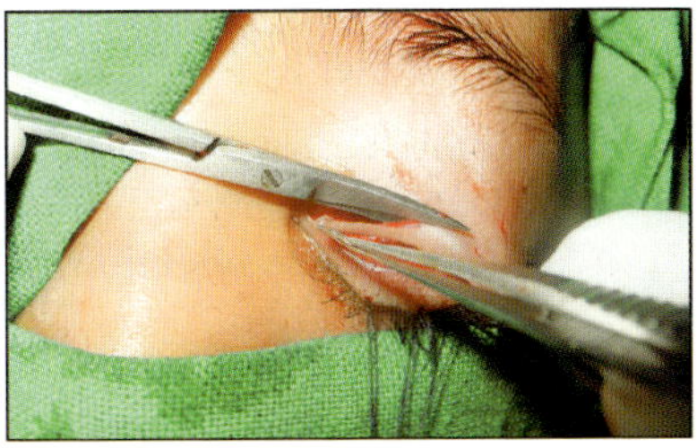

J. Strip of excess skin removed

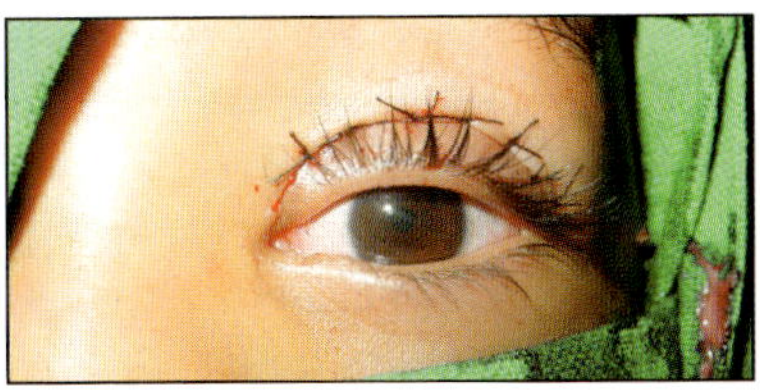

K. Skin sutures applied

Figures 11A to K: Levator resection: Skin approach

Confirmation of presence of Bell's phenomenon is important before undertaking any surgical procedure to avoid risk of postoperative exposure keratopathy.

Corneal Sensation

The presence or absence of corneal functions should be noted using a cotton wisp.

Ocular Motility

The extraocular muscle functions especially the elevator muscles should be recorded. Any association of eye movements with change in degree of ptosis should be looked for.

Tensilon Test

This test is done in doubtful cases where an acquired ptosis due to *Myasthenia gravis* is suspected. In adults 1 mg of neostigmine is injected I/M. The ptosis improves in 5 to 15 minutes if *Myasthenia gravis* is the cause. Edrophonium is more faster and effective than neostigmine. It is loaded in a tuberculin syringe and 2 mg injected slowly in 15-30 seconds. The needle is left *in situ* and rest 8 mm is injected slowly if no untoward incident is observed within 1 minute. The effect occurs in 1 to 5 minutes if myasthenia is the cause. If cholinergic reaction occurs 0.5 mg of atropine sulphate is given intravenously.

Phenylephrine Test

Phenylephrine 10% drops are used to assess mild cases of ptosis as in Horner's syndrome. Positive phenylephrine test suggests that patient would respond well to Müller's muscle resection.

Associations

The presence of jaw winking oculomotor anomalies and blepharophimosis syndrome should be noted. The presence of any other associated ocular anomaly should also be recorded.

The presence of jaw winking is assessed by moving the jaw from side to side (chewing movements), opening and closing the mouth. Before considering for the surgery the possible causes for pseudoptosis should be excluded viz. hypothalmos, enophthalmos, epicanthus, overhanging skin, etc.

It is advisable to wait till 3-4 years of age when the tissues are mature enough to withstand the surgical trauma and as better assessment and postoperative care is possible due to patient's co-operation. There should be no delay in surgical management in cases of severe ptosis where pupil is obstructed and the possibility of the development of amblyopia is high. In these cases a temporary procedure may be opted early on followed by definitive surgery later.

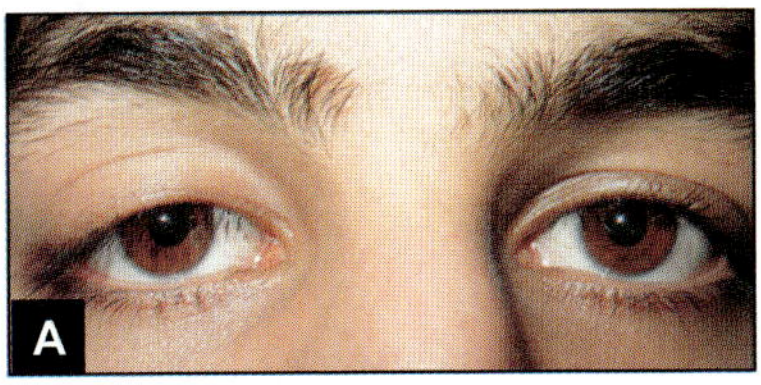

Figure 12A: Preoperative simple ptosis

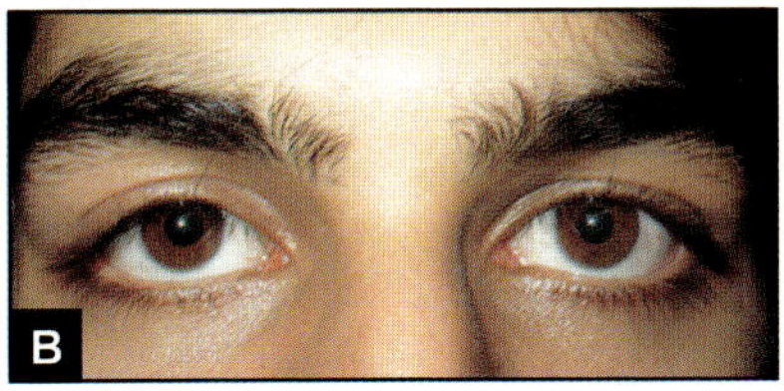

Figure 12B: Postoperative following levator resection. Note the symmetrical lid crease and contour

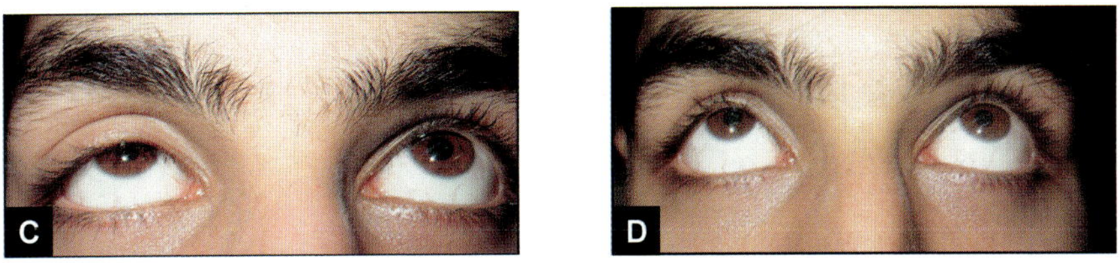

Figures 12C and D: Preoperative and postoperative: Upward gaze

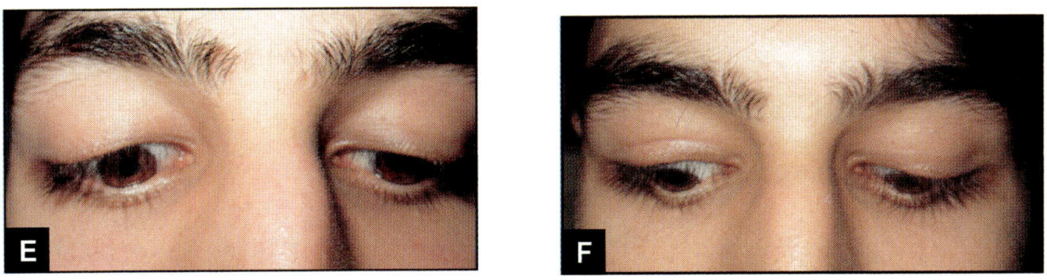

Figures 12E and F: Preoperative and postoperative: Downward gaze

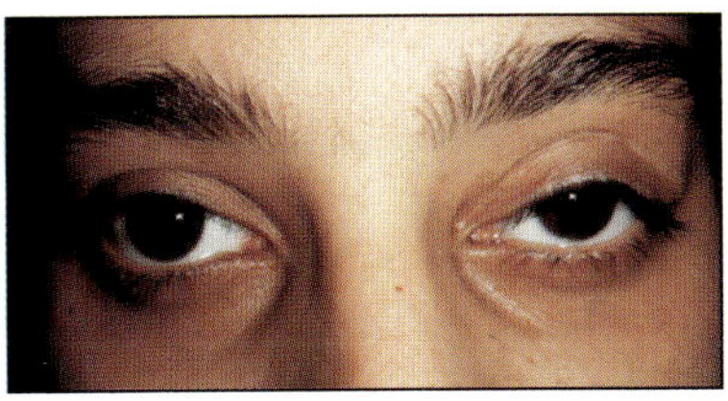

Figure 13: Showing residual ptosis following levator resection

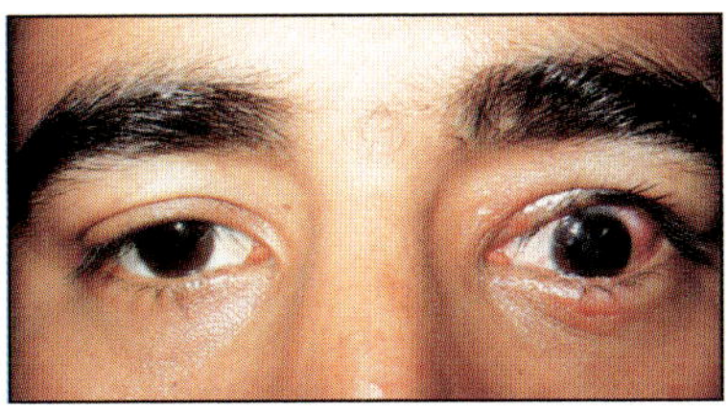

Figure 14: Showing overcorrection following surgery

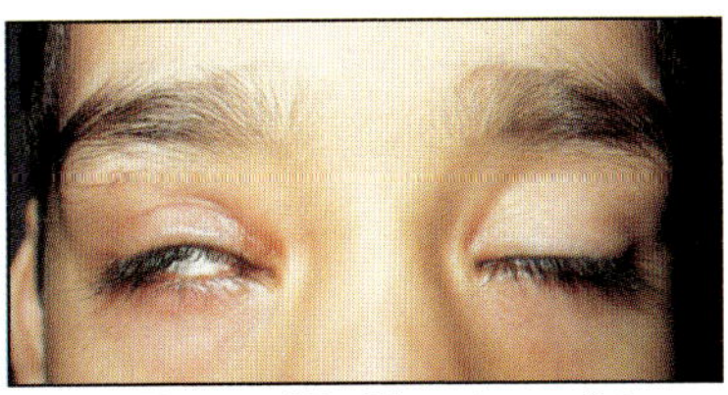

Figure 15: Showing mild lagophthalmos

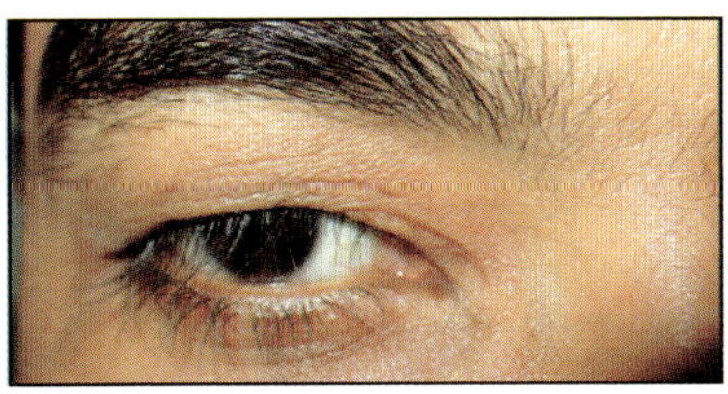

Figure 16: Showing excess skin with entropion

Surgical Approaches

Surgical approach depends on:

1. Ptosis is unilateral or bilateral
2. Severity of ptosis
3. Levator action
4. Presence of abnormal ocular movements, jaw winking phenomena or blepharophimosis syndrome.

The choice of surgical procedure for congenital ptosis depends primarily on:

1. Amount of ptosis as determined on the basis of MRD
2. Levator action.

Commonly Performed Surgeries

- Fasanella Servat Operation
- Levator resection
- Brow suspension ptosis repair.

Indications for the Choice of Different Surgical Procedures

Ptosis	*Levator action*	*Surgery*
Mild	> 10 mm	Fasanella Servat or small levator resection
	< 10 mm	Levator resection
Moderate	Good	Levator resection
	Fair	Levator resection
	Poor (rare)	Whitnall's sling or Brow suspension
Severe	Fair	Levator resection or Brow suspension ptosis repair
	Poor	Brow suspension ptosis repair

Bilateral Ptosis

In cases of bilateral ptosis, bilateral surgery is preferred to ensure a similar surgical intervention in the two eyes. However in cases where gross asymmetry exists between the two eyes the eye with a greater ptosis may be operated first and the other eye is operated after 6-8 weeks when the final correction of the operated eye can be assessed.

Surgical Techniques

Modified Fasanella Servat Surgery

It is the excision of tarsoconjunctiva, Müller's and levator. We use a simple modified technique that avoids the use of hemostat or any special clamp.

Xylocaine with adrenaline is used for local anesthesia in adults but general anesthesia is necessary for children.

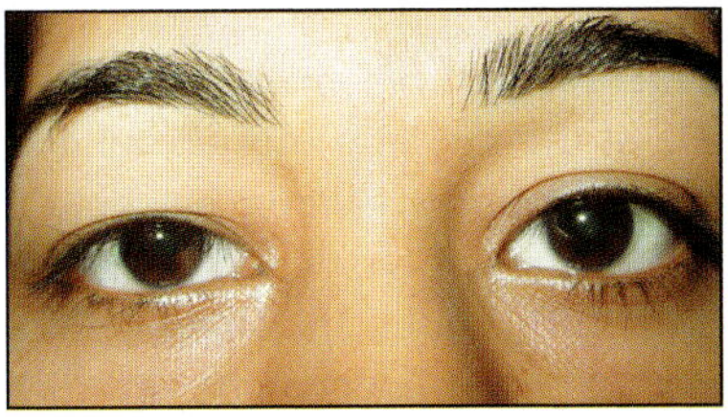

Figure 17A: Showing excess skin with poor lid fold

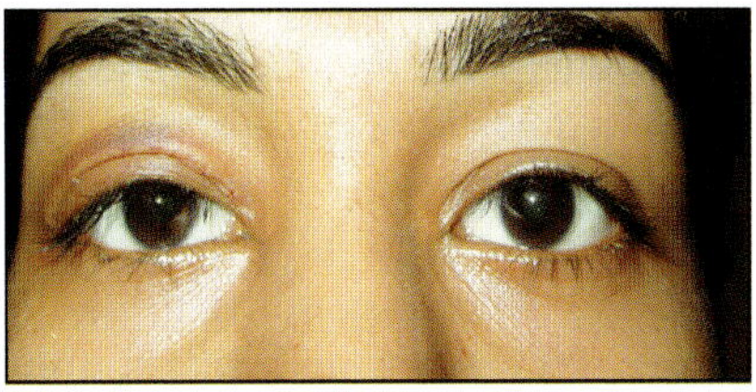

Figure 17B: Postoperative skin removal with lid fold creation

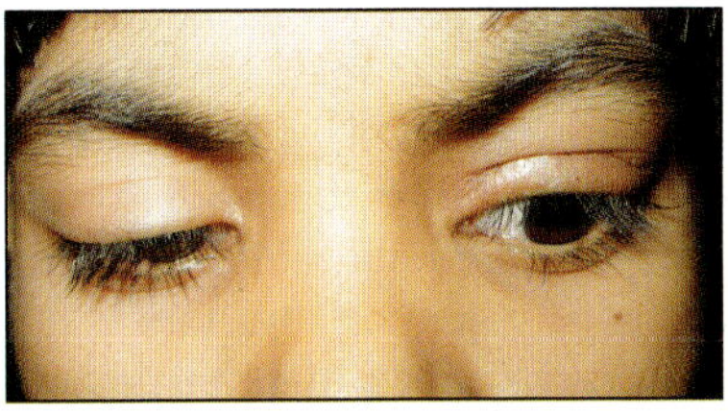

Figure 18: Showing lid lag which is an inevitable association of levator surgery

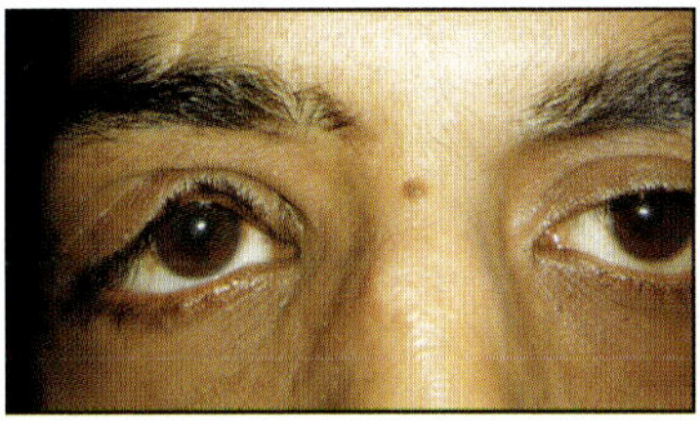

Figure 19: Showing lid notching

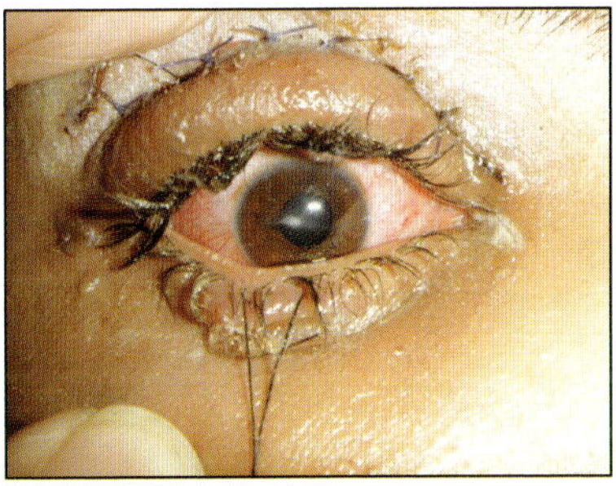

Figure 20A: Showing exposure keratitis following levator surgery

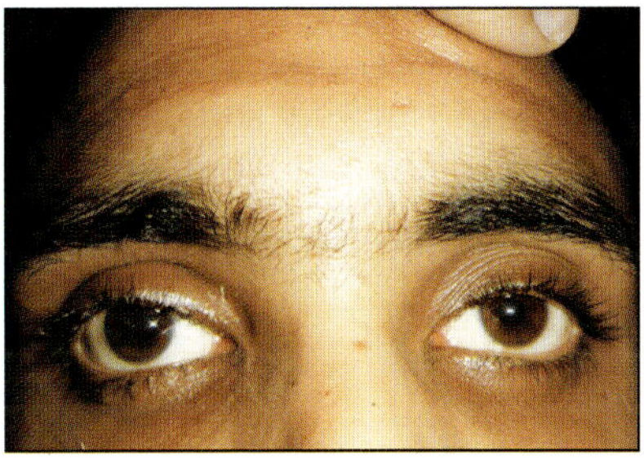

Figure 20B: Exposure keratitis responded to tear substitutes and lid taping

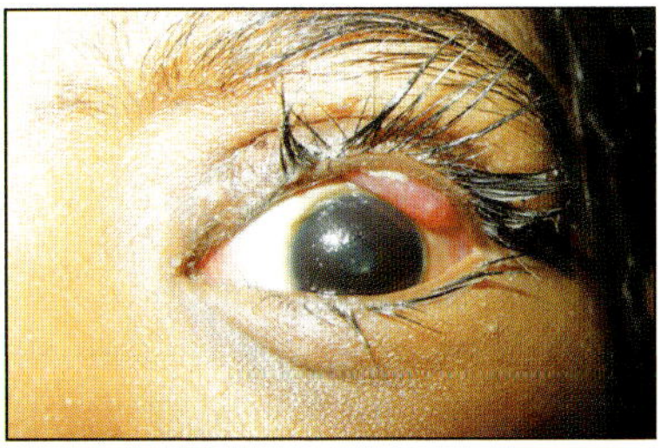

Figure 21: Showing fornix prolapse

Surgical Steps

Eyelid is everted and tarsal plate is exposed. Three sutures are passed close to the folded superior margin of the tarsal plate at the junction of middle, lateral and medial one third of the lid. Three corresponding sutures are placed close to the everted lid margin starting from conjunctival aspect near the superior fornix in positions corresponding to the first 3 sutures. Proposed incision is marked on the tarsal plate such that a uniform piece of tarsus, decreasing gradually towards the periphery is excised. This is necessary to avoid the central peaking. A groove is made on the marked line of incision and the incision is completed with the scissors. The first set of sutures help in lifting the tarsal plate for excision. The second set aids suturing by lifting and supporting conjunctival and tarsal edges during suturing. The tarsal plate not more than 3 mm in width is excised.

5-0 plain catgut is used for continuous suturing and the knot is buried within the wound. Postoperatively the patients are kept on antibiotics and anti-inflammatory agents and cornea is observed for any sign of abrasion.

The preoperative and postoperative photographs of a patient taken up for Fasanella servat surgery in the primary, up and down gaze are shown in Figures 10A to F.

Complications of Fasanella Servat Surgery

1. Under or overcorrection—If the lid is too low then reoperate. If the lid is too high, in early postoperative traction might help otherwise reoperate.
2. Dry eye—Surgery should be avoided in patients with dry eye symptoms as the procedure removes some of the accessory lacrimal glands. The patient should be treated with lubricating drops and ointment.
3. Keratopathy— Results due to the suture or scar beneath the lid and abrades the cornea.

Levator Resection

This is the most commonly practiced surgery for ptosis correction. It may be performed by skin or conjunctival route but the former is preferred by most surgeons because it allows a good titration/assessment on the table and creates a good lid fold.

2% xylocaine with adrenaline is locally infiltrated. The injection is also used in cases being operated in general anesthesia to achieve hemostasis.

Surgical Steps

The proposed lid crease is marked to match the normal eye considering the margin crease distance of the normal eye as well as the amount of skin show measured in the primary position. In bilateral cases highest forming crease is used which is usually at the superior border of the tarsus or standard measurements can be used.

Three 4-0 silk sutures are passed near the lid margin to provide traction. A lid spatula is placed under the lid and incision through the skin and orbicularis

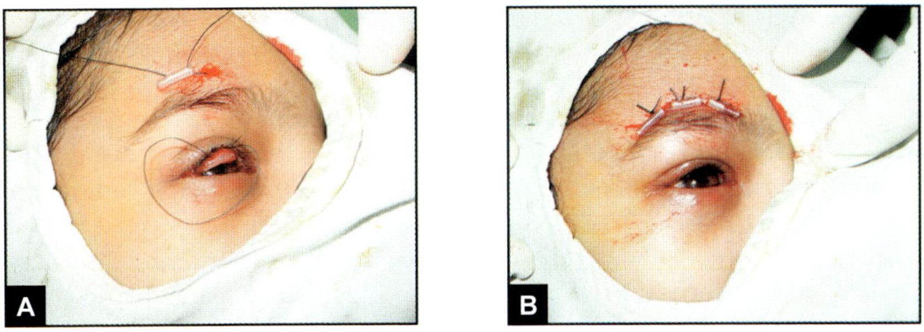

Figures 22A and B: Double armed 4'0 silk suture is passed through prolapsed fornix

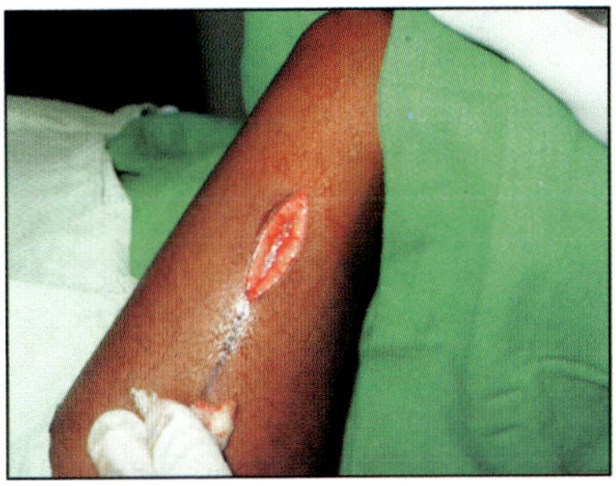

A. Incision marked. 2 inch above the lateral condyle

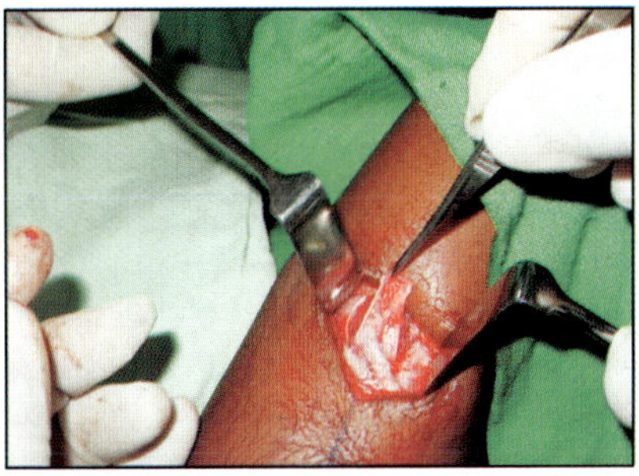

B. Fascia lata is exposed

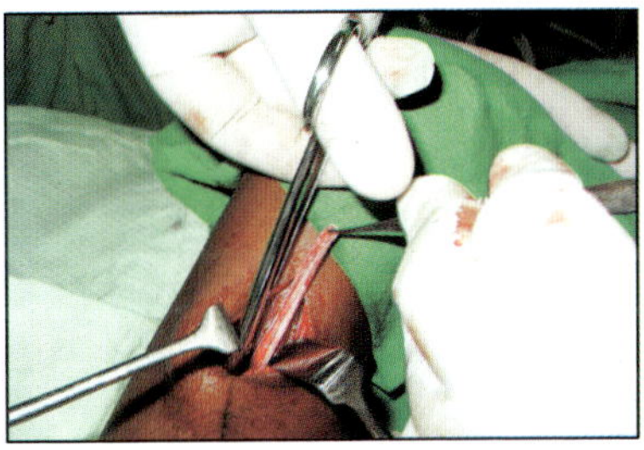

C. 12 mm fascia lata strip being removed

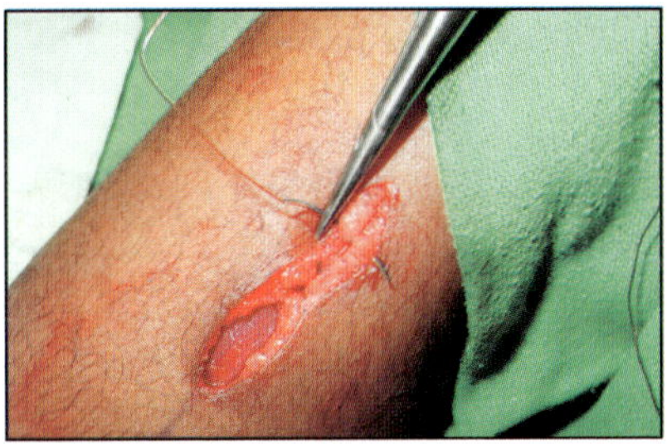

D. Subcutaneous tissue closed with 4'0 catgut

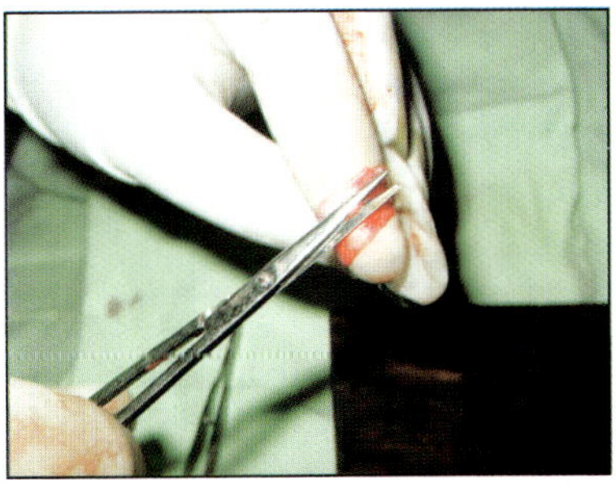

E. Trimming of the strip, fat removed

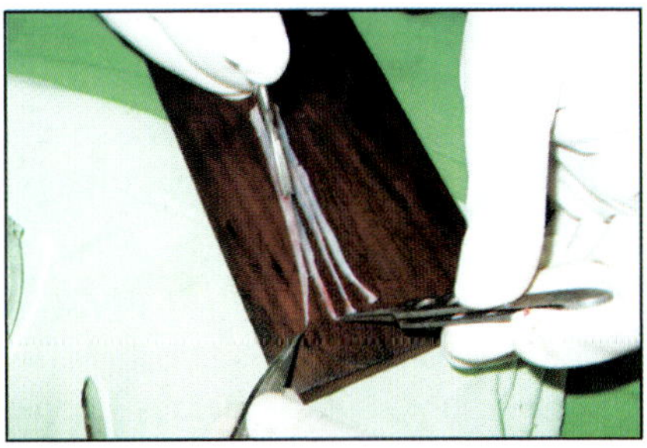

F. Strip placed on a wooden board and divided into 4 strips of 3 mm width each

Figures 23A to F: Harvesting fascia lata

made along the crease marking. The inferior skin and orbicularis are dissected away from the tarsal plate. The upper edge is separated from the orbital septum. The orbital septum is cut completely across exposing the preaponeurotic fat. Fat is retracted posteriorly exposing the whole tendinous aponeurosis. Three partial thickness traction 4-0 silk suture are passed through the distal end of the aponeurosis. The fibers of the aponeurosis are cut from their insertion in the inferior half of the anterior surface of the tarsus. The levator is freed from the adjoining structures. The lateral and the medial horn are cut. The direction of the cut should be vertical to avoid damage to the lacrimal gland laterally or the pulley of superior oblique muscle medially. Care should be taken that Whitnalls ligament is not damaged which is visualized as a whitish fascial condensation running across the junction of the muscular and aponeurotic part of the levator about 15 mm from the insertion. A double armed 5-0 vicryl is passed through the center of the tarsal plate by a partial thickness bite. It is then passed through levator aponeurosis and intraoperative assessment is made. Two more double armed vicryl 5-0 sutures are passed through the tarsus about 2 mm from the upper border in the center and at the junction of central third with the medial and lateral thirds. These sutures are then placed in the levator and intraoperative assessment made. The lid level and contours are evaluated. The eyelid is left at the position determined preoperatively based on the levator action.

Excess levator is excised. If required a strip of skin is removed from above the lid crease. A piece of orbicularis may be excised inferior to the lid crease to debulk the lid. Four to five lid fold forming sutures are placed. The sutures pass through skin edges taking a bite through the cut edge of levator. An inverse frost 6-0 silk suture is passed through the lower lid margin over a bolster.

We use a modification of Berke's criteria based on our postoperative observations.

The position of the lid aimed at during the table assessment should be as follows:

Levator action	*Recommended placement of lid*
2-4 mm	1 mm above the limbus (when levator resection is chosen to be undertaken)
5-7mm	1 mm below the limbus
8 mm or more	2 mm below the limbus

Patients are prescribed oral antibiotics and anti-inflammatory agents. Preoperative and postoperative photographs are demonstrated on Page 341.

Complications of Levator Surgery

Undercorrection: Multiple factors may be responsible for undercorrection. It may either be due to inadequate resection of levator or due to a thin friable or fibrotic levator muscle associated with poor levator action where even a large levator resection may prove inadequate. In these cases even where a good correction is achieved in early postoperative period, there may be a late development of

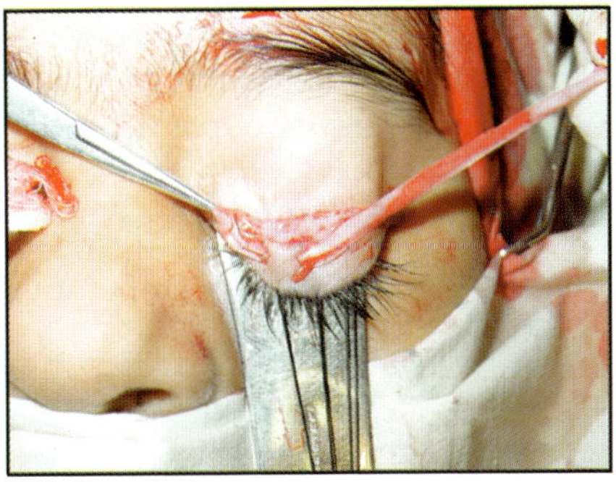

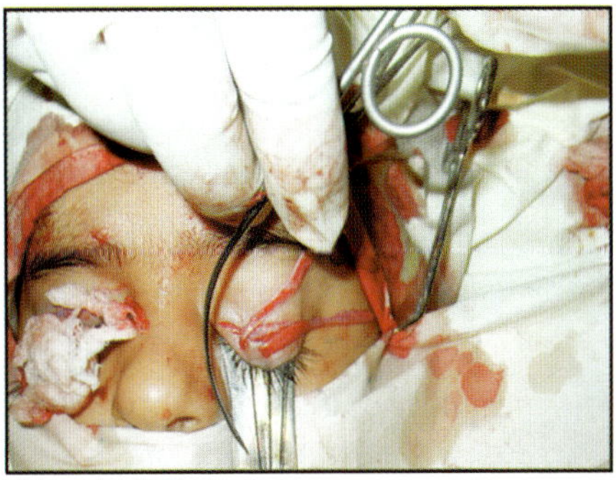

A and B. Fascia lata needle is passed through submuscular plane on medial side and strip pulled

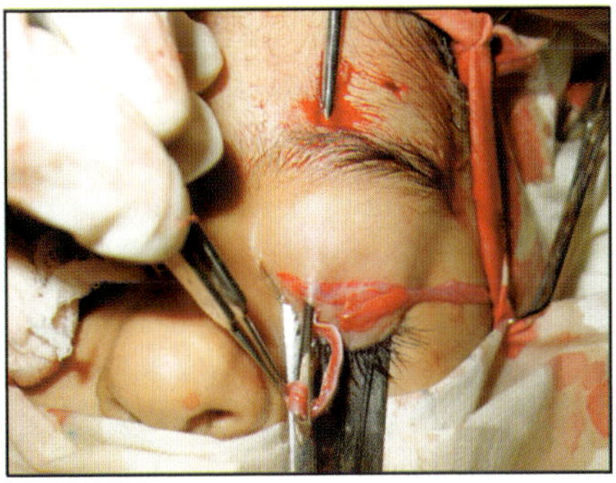

C. Needle passed from brow incision to medial lid incision

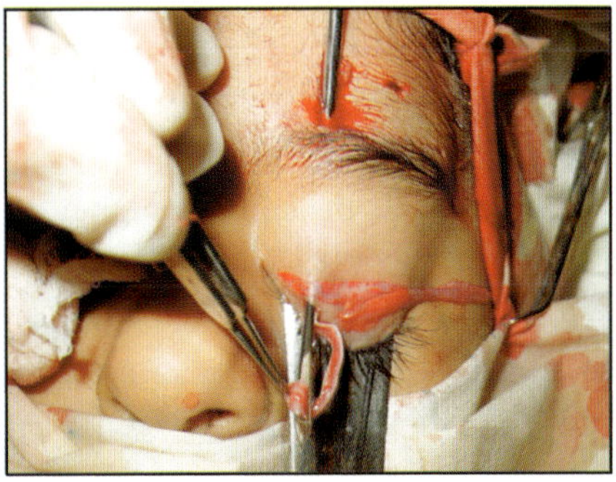

D. Fascial strips pulled from both medial and lateral brow incisions

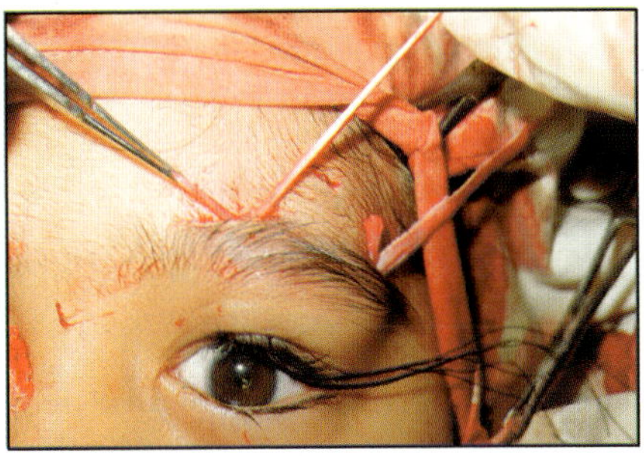

E. Knot tightened and secured to get proper lid position

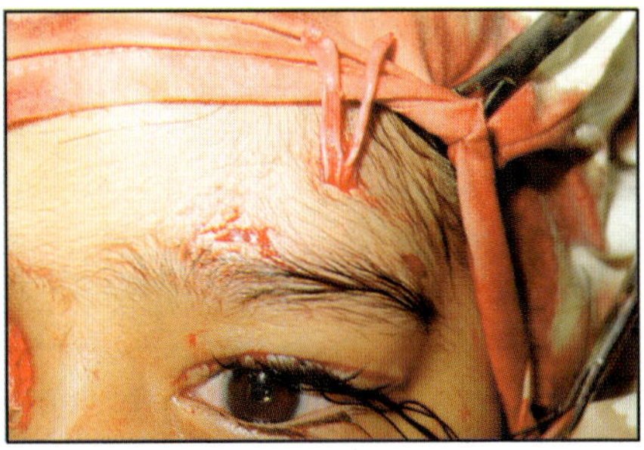

F. One end of fascial strip passed through central brow incision and tightened

Figures 24A to F: Fascia lata sling surgery by modified Crawford double triangle technique

drooping in a few months time. **The surgeon should wait for a couple of months before considering for re-surgery.**

Overcorrection: Overcorrection may be due to too large a resection of the levator or due to advancement of the levator too far down on the tarsus.

Massage and traction on the lashes can be tried in the early postoperative phase. But in late phase tarsotomy, levator recession or recession with a spacer such as scleral graft is required depending on the amount of overcorrection.

Lagophthalmos: Lagophthalmos is usually severer in the early postoperative period and diminishes with the passage of time.

Entropion: Entropion occurs due to surgical shortening of the tarso-conjunctival layer as compared to anterior skin muscle lamina.

Ectropion: Massage can be tried in early phase otherwise surgical correction is carried out by advancement of skin and muscle flap.

Lid fold: Lid fold may be placed asymmetrically due to appropriate position of the skin incision. The correction may require recreations of the lid crease.

Lid lag: This is an inevitable association of levator resection as the levator resection raises the lid to a higher position, but does not alter the tone of the muscle.

Notching of the lid margin: Notching of the lid margin may occur due to irregular resection of the tarsus or due to improper placement of sutures for levator resection.

Exposure keratitis: Keratopathy can occur after any type of ptosis surgery as it is accompanied by lagophthalmos. The milder forms usually respond to tear substitute drugs and taping of eyelids.

Conjunctival prolapse: This is usually due to separation of fibers of levator attaches to the superior fornix in large resections of levator. Reposition of prolapsed conjunctiva is done in early phase. If this fails, it can be corrected by passing the suture from prolapsed conjunctiva through the lid or by excision of excess conjunctiva.

Brow Suspension Repair

This surgery is the procedure of choice in simple congenital ptosis with a poor levator action. A number of materials like nonabsorbable sutures, muscle strips, banked or fresh fascia lata strips, extended Poly tetra fluoro ethylene (ePTFE) have been used for suspension. We prefer Poly tetra fluoro ethylene (ePTFE) sutures for temporary thread sling procedure and fresh autogenous fascia lata for permanent brow suspension.

Temporary Sling

Thread sling is carried out in very young children with severe ptosis where prevention of amblyopia and uncovering the pupil is the main aim. We use

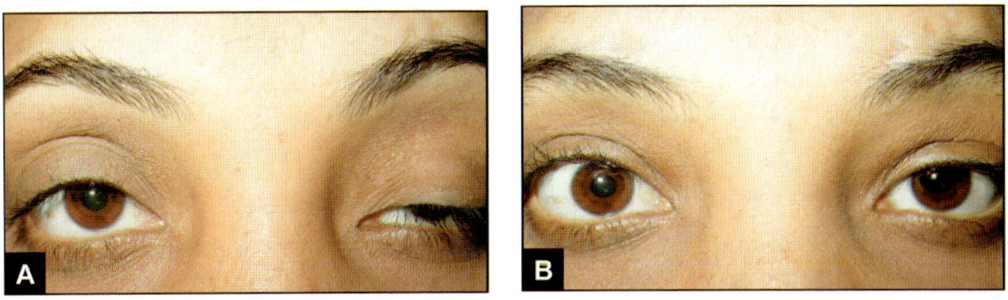

Figures 25A and B: Preoperative and postoperative: Primary gaze following fascia lata sling surgery

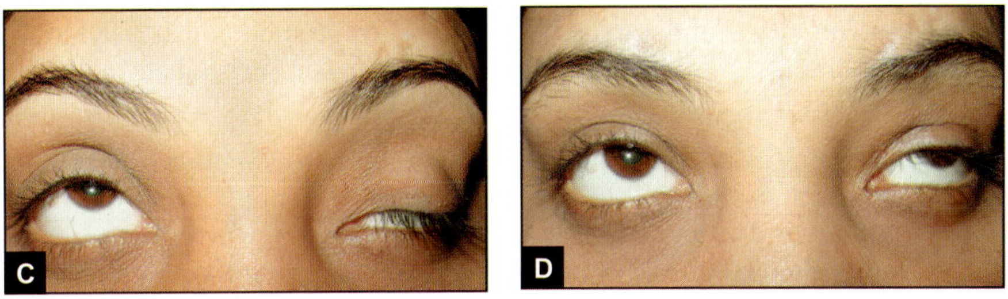

Figures 25C and D: Preoperative and postoperative: Upward gaze

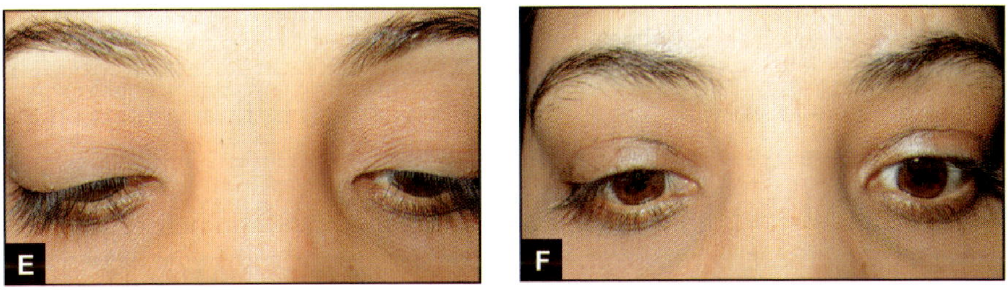

Figures 25E and F: Preoperative and postoperative: Downward gaze

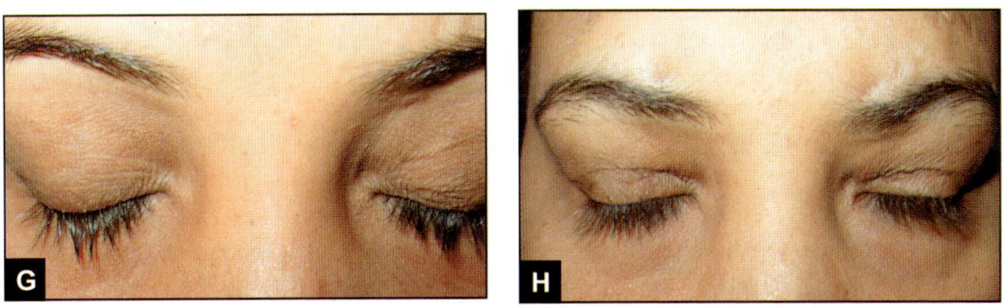

Figures 25G and H: Preoperative and postoperative: On lid showing minimal lagophthalmos

CV 0 ePTFE (Goretex) sutures by modified Crawford technique for brow suspension. The suture sling procedures have a relatively higher recurrence rate of 20–30% or may show formation of suture granuloma. Definitive surgery may be performed at a later date when a fascia lata sling is carried out.

Fascia Lata Sling

It is considered in children above four years of age having severe congenital simple ptosis with poor levator action. We prefer fresh autogenous fascia for suspension. Even in cases of unilateral severe ptosis a bilateral procedure is preferred because a unilateral surgery causes marked asymmetry in down gaze. Results of bilateral surgery are more acceptable.

All cases are done under general anesthesia. Infiltration with 2% xylocaine and adrenaline is done in the region of the proposed incision in the thigh, eyelid and the eyebrow region.

Harvesting of fascia lata: A line joining the lateral condyle of femur to the anterior superior iliac spine is marked. A lower thigh incision about 2 inches above the lateral condyle on the marked line is site of incision. However due to lower thigh scar we often use the upper thigh for past 2 years which is about one inch in size. The skin incision is deepened through the fat till the glistening fascia is visible. The fascia is then cleared of the overlying tissue for a length of four inches upwards from the incision. A 12 mm incision is then given at the lower end of the exposed fascia lata. Dissection is carried out beneath the fascia lata separating it from the underlying vastus lateralis muscle along the whole length of the previous dissection. Two linear incisions are given 12 mm apart on the fascia along the length of dissection using a long scissors. The superior end of the fascia is made free by making horizontal cut using a long bladed scissors while the assistants retract the skin and the subcutaneous tissue. The subcutaneous tissue is closed using 4-0 chromic catgut and the skin is closed using 4-0 silk sutures. We now have an autologous fascia lata four inches long and 12 mm wide. It is kept in a bowl containing Ringer lactate and 1 cc of gentamicin.

The fat is trimmed from the fascia lata strip.

The fascia lata strip is kept on a wooden board, stretched and fixed. It is divided into four pieces each of about 3 mm width by a scalpel blade.

Fascia lata sling suspension: Three traction sutures are passed along the lid border. Four incisions are made 2-4 mm above the margin.The placement of these determines the position of lid fold. The two central incisions are on either side of the center of the lid while the other two are at the junction of middle and lateral thirds and middle and medial thirds of the lid. A lid crease incision is also given.

The eyebrow incisions are marked next. They are made at a line perpendicular to the intersection of two lateral eyelid incisions and the two medial incisions while the eyelid is placed in the desired normal position. A

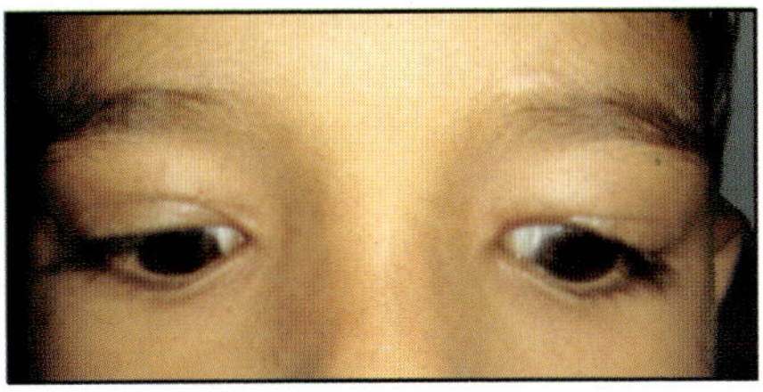

Figure 26: Showing lagophthalmos, inevitable complication of fascia lata sling

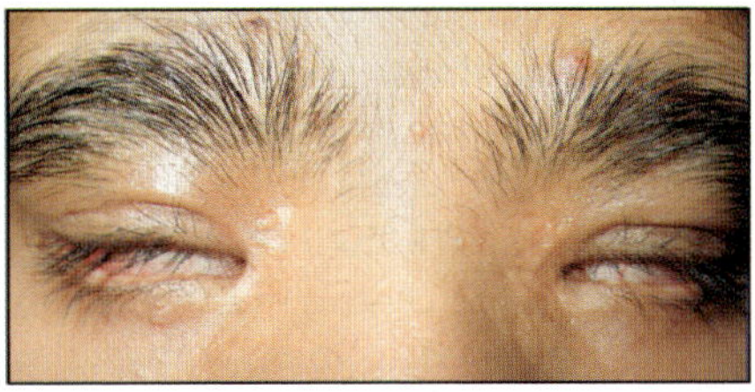

Figure 27: Showing lid lag following sling surgery

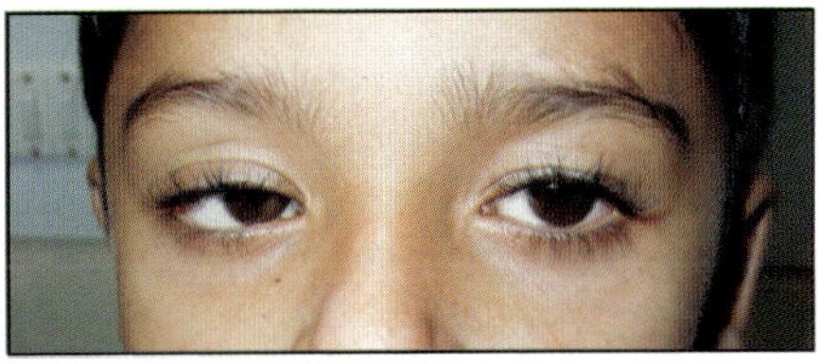

Figure 28: Showing undercorrection

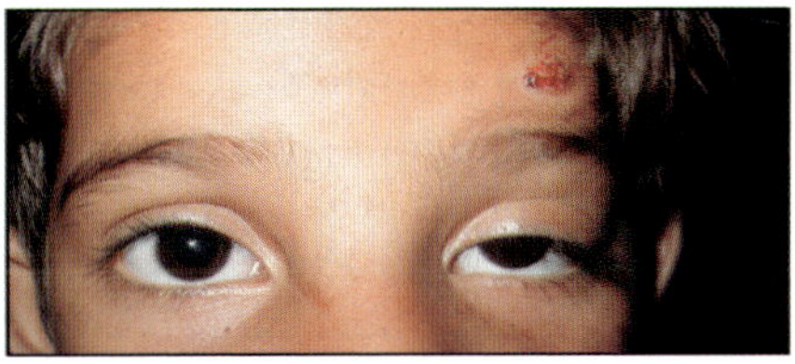

Figure 29: Showing suture granuloma with synthetic material

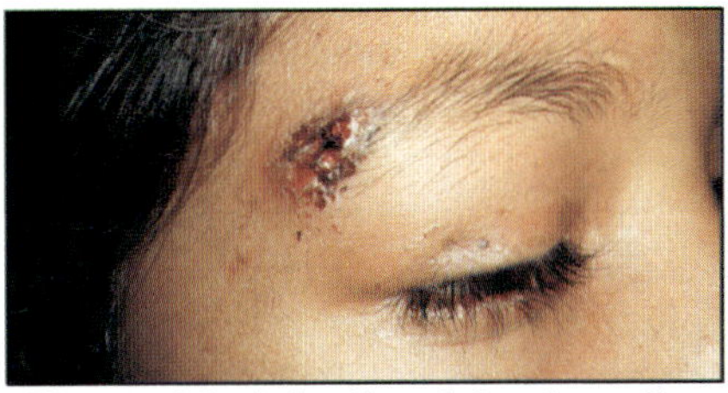

Figure 30: Infection following sling surgery, more common with synthetic material

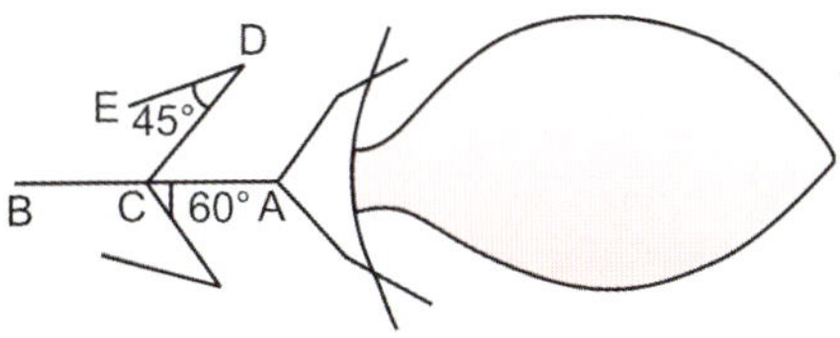

Figure 31: Z-plasty

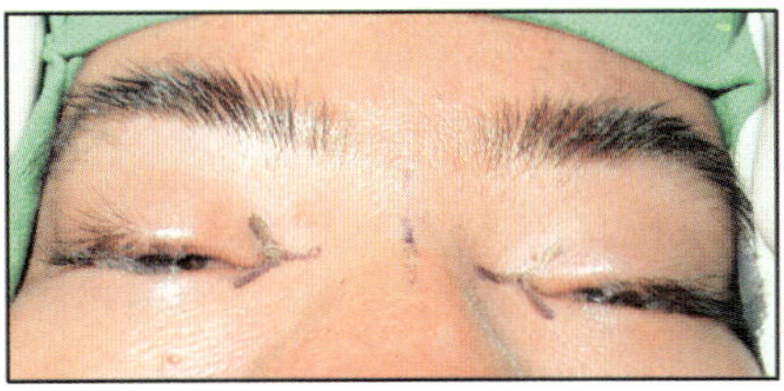

Figure 32A: Markings of Y-V plasty

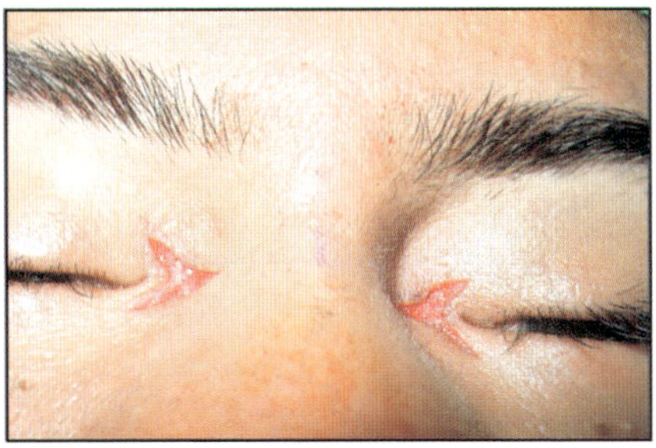

Figure 32B: Incision given and flap undermined

third incision is made in the middle of the first two but 4-6 mm higher than the first two incisions.

The eyelid incisions are made down to the tarsus and the brow incisions are made upto the frontalis. Blunt dissection is carried out to make pockets for the fascial knots. The two ends of a strip are then passed from the outer eyelid incisions to the central eyelid incision using a Wright's fascia lata needle. The needle is passed in the submuscular plane from the lateral brow incision to emerge from the lateral incision in the lid. The fascia is threaded through the eye of the needle and is pulled through. The Wright's needle is again passed from the lateral incision to the second eyelid incision threaded with fascia and drawn up. The procedure is repeated on the medial side. The fascial strips are pulled up and a single tie is made so as to place the eyelid margins as high as possible without lifting the eyelid from the globe. After a single tie the position and contour of the eyelid is assessed. Required adjustments are made. Presence of good lid crease is ensured at this stage. The knots are then secured using 5-0 vicryl. A second tie is made and secured.

One end of fascial strip from each brow incision is pulled-through the central brow incision. Knots are tied and secured. All the knots are buried in the pockets prepared for them. The excess of skin created by shortening of the posterior lamina is judged and excised by removing a spindle of skin from above the eyelid crease. Eyelid incisions require no closure. The brow incisions are closed with 5-0 silk and the eyelid crease incision by 6-0 silk.

Patients are prescribed oral antibiotics and anti-inflammatory agents. An appropriate selection and meticulous execution of surgical technique hold the key to obtain excellent functional and cosmetic results in patients with ptosis.

The preoperative and postoperative photographs of patient with severe ptosis corrected by bilateral fascia lata sling are shown in Figure.

Complications of Frontalis Sling

Though the sling surgery is much simpler than levator surgery, but it is accompanied by some complications.

Unavoidable Complications

1. Lid lag: Lid lag is more prominent in uniocular cases, thus the bilateral sling is preferred to maintain the synchronicity between the two eyelids. The patient can be taught to bend his head down instead of turning the eyes down.
2. Lagophthalmos: Normally the patient has little difficulty with lid closure as the eyeball rolls upward sufficiently to protect the cornea though the sclera may remain exposed.

   The frequent use of lubricants and ointment at night time is prescribed for longer duration.

Avoidable Complications

1. *Undercorrection:* Usually due to failure to raise the lid sufficiently high or due to placement of lid at a lower position due to improper judgement under GA.

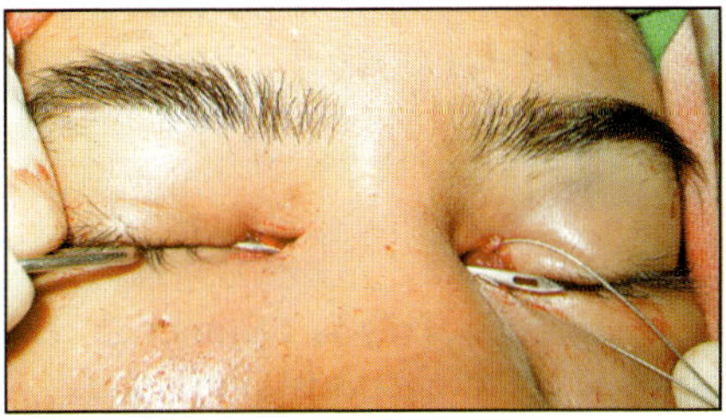

Figure 33: Transnasal wiring

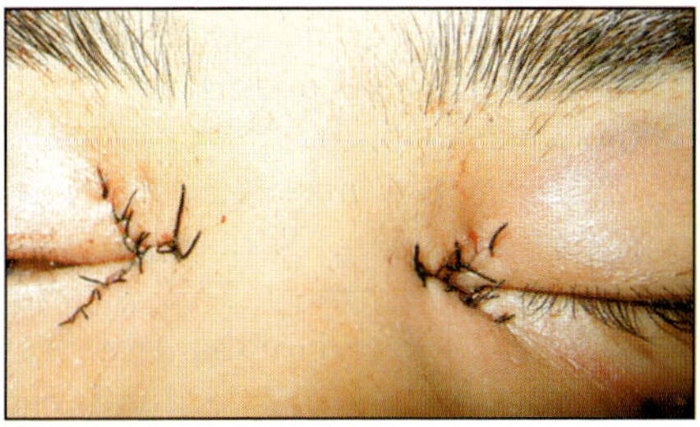

Figure 34: Skin sutured

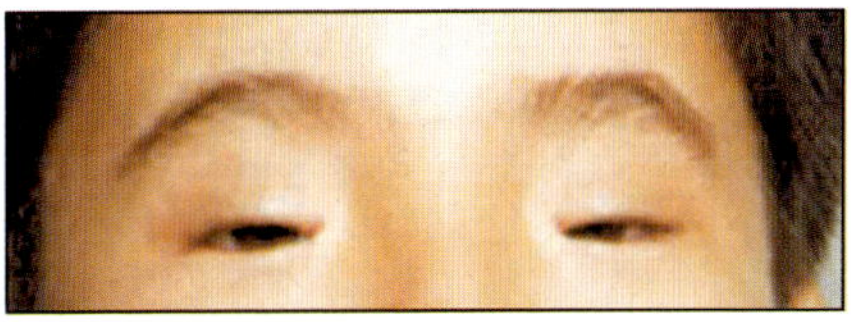

Figure 35A: A patient with blepharophimosis syndrome

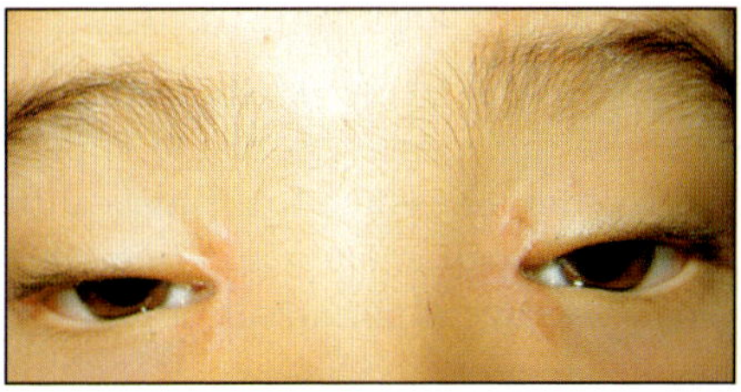

Figure 35B: Postoperative photograph following Y-V plasty and transnasal wiring

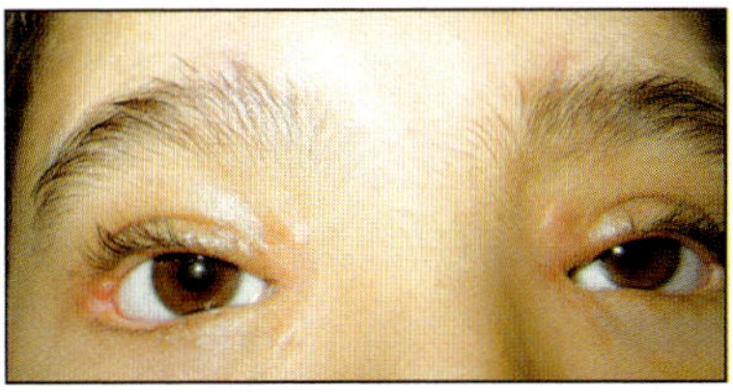

Figure 35C: Postoperative photograph following fascia lata sling surgery

2. Overcorrection: Overcorrection is not a common complication. It results due to excessive tightening of the sling. The management is difficult and requires the loosening of subcuticular tissue sufficiently to allow drooping down of lid.
3. *Notching or Tenting:* Usually occurs due to high position of one of the fascial strips. This can be corrected intraoperatively by loosening of the strip so that lid curve is maintained.
4. *Recurrence:* It is possible due to release of suture ends or rupture.
5. *Ectropion:* Ectropion may occur due to too much tightening of the strip.
6. *Exposure keratitis:* Requires use of lubricants and patching at night.
7. *Granuloma formation:* This is commoner with synthetic material.
8. *Infection:* Infection either early or later may occur. This is commoner with synthetic material. Infection is rare with use of autogenous fascia lata.

Management of Complicated Ptosis

Ptosis with Oculomotor Abnormalities

It is necessary to correct the ocular motility problem before correction of ptosis because the restriction of the superior rectus and accompanying hypotropia makes the assessment of ptosis difficult. Secondly, the hypotropic eye with poor Bell's penomenon is extremely vulnerable to exposure keratopathy due to postoperative lagophthalmos.

Congenital Ptosis with Superior Rectus Weakness

- Superior weakness is a common association as both muscles develop from the same myotome. The hypotropia is corrected by an inferior rectus recession at times combined with superior rectus resection as the first procedure. Ptosis correction is then carried out using the procedure indicated by evaluation.

Ptosis Associated with Double Elevator Palsy

- Knapps procedure may be done for ptosis associated with double elevator palsy. The lateral and medial rectus tendons are transposed to the sides of superior rectus insertion. This does not cause significant limitation of adduction or abduction. Ptosis is corrected 3 months later.

Blepharophimosis Syndrome

The blepharophimosis syndrome comprises of ptosis, epicanthus inversus, telecanthus, horizontal shortening of palpebral aperture, flattened supraorbital ridges, arching of the eyebrow and lateral ectropion of the lower eyelid.

- Mustarde's double "Z" plasty or Y-V plasty with transnasal wiring is done as a primary procedure. This gives a good surgical result both in terms of correction of telecanthus as well as deep placement of the medial canthus. The results are long lasting.

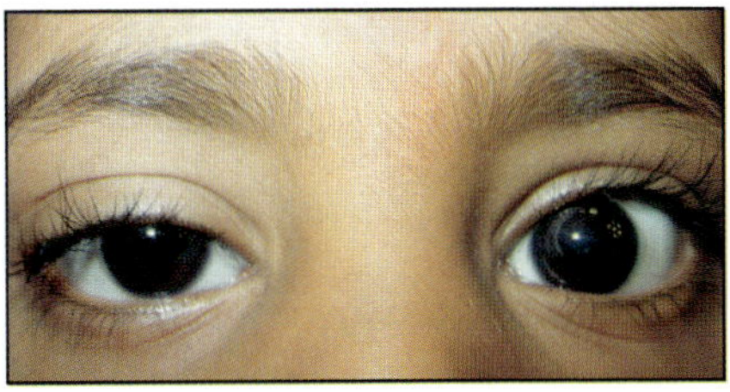

Figure 36A: A patient with moderate ptosis with Marcus Gunn phenomenon

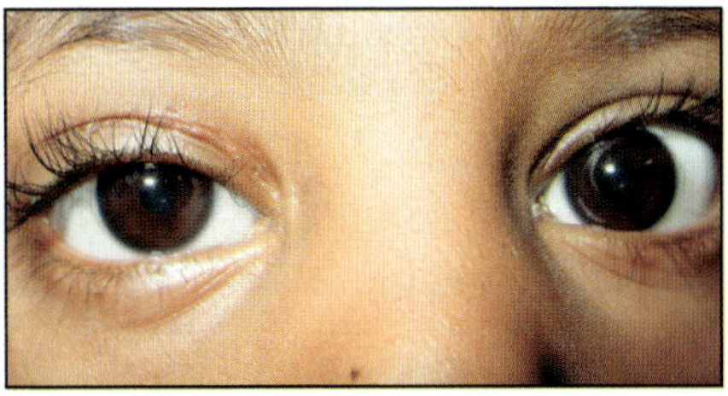

Figure 36B: Postoperative photograph following bilateral levator excision with fascia lata sling surgery

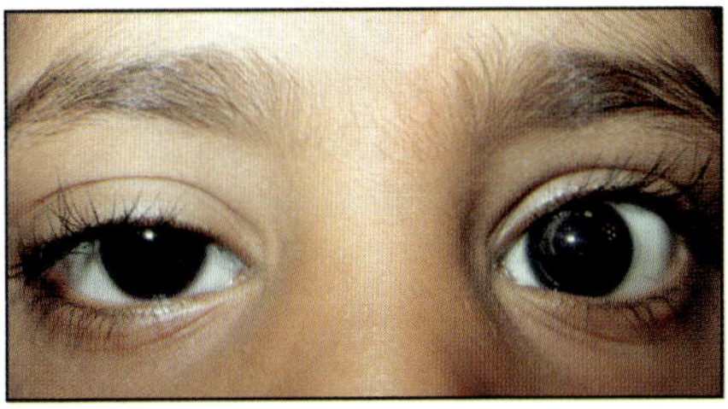

Figure 36C: Marcus Gunn phenomenon elicited on opening of mouth

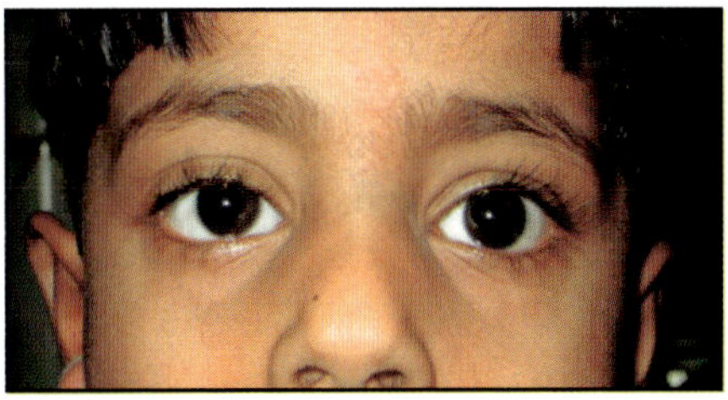

Figure 36D: Postoperative photograph. Marcus Gunn phenomena is eliminated

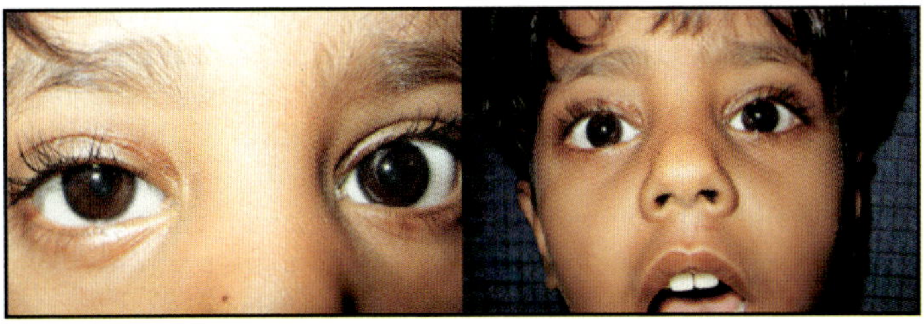

Figure 36E: Pre- and postoperative photographs

- Brow suspension is carried out 6 months after the first procedure for correction of ptosis.

Double Z Plasty or Y to V Plasty with Transnasal Wiring

Lateral canthotomy and canthoplasty may be carried out before the skin incision is made.

The markings for double Z plasty are made as shown in Figure. The first mark is made just medial to the medial canthus (A). The proposed canthal site (B) is marked such that intermedial canthal distance is half that of interpupillary distance. The two marks are joined. All the other lines drawn are 2 mm smaller than the line AB. Two lines are drawn from A parallel to upper and lower lid margins. From the center point of AB(C), a line is drawn medially at 60° both above and below (CD). Another line is drawn outwards at an angle of 45° from the point of D (DE).

The markings for Y-V plasty are shown in Figure. The incision are made through the skin down to the orbicularis. The flaps are undermind. The site of proposed canthus is cleared of all tissue upto the periosteum and the medial palpebral ligament is exposed. The periosteum is incised medial to the insertion of MPL and is reflected along with the lacrimal sac.

A large bony opening 12-15 mm high and 10-12 mm wide is made as for dacryocystorhinostomy but located more posterior and superior. The edges of the bony opening are smoothened. A similar procedure is performed on the opposite side.

Medial palpebral ligament (MPL) of one side is wired with 24 G stainless steel wire close to its attachment to the tarsus and the two ends of the wire are passed to the opposite side through the bony opening with the aid of an aneurysm needle or a Wright's fascia lata needle. The wire is threaded into the opposite MPL by a similar double bite. The two ends are tightened and a single twist given to the wires . The position of the medial canthus is assessed from the front, above and the sides. Once the desired position is obtained the wire is twisted several times and cut. The ends of the wire are pushed into the bony opening. After achieving the hemostasis the incision is closed in several layers. The skin flaps may need to be trimmed before they are tranposed and sutured with 6-0 silk.

Lateral Canthoplasty

Thee lateral canthus is crushed by a straight hemostat for a few seconds. A lateral canthotomy is performed. The bulbar conjunctiva at the lateral canthus is undermined. The apex of the conjunctiva is sutured to the proposed new position of the canthus which is short of the end of the skin incision . The skin edges distal to the new lateral canthus are apposed with 6-0 silk sutures. The similar procedure is repeated on other side.

The bandage is removed after 24 hours and sutures are removed between 5-7 days.

Stage II

The second stage is performed after 6 months. A bilateral fascia lata sling is performed.

Marcus Gunn Ptosis

Ptosis associated with lid retraction on opening the jaw or its movement to the opposite side is classical marcus gunn phenomenon. An inverse Marcus Gun phenomenon is also known.

Management depends on the cosmetic significance of the jaw winking. Where jaw winking is not significant the choice of procedure depends on the amount of ptosis and the levator action, as in any case of congenital simple ptosis. A larger levator resection is necessary and undercorrection is common. In case with significant jaw winking bilateral levator excision with a fascia lata sling surgery is the procedure of choice.

Misdirected Third Nerve Ptosis

- In cases of misdirected third nerve ptosis where treatment is indicated levator excision with bilateral fascia lata sling is the procedure of choice.
- Ptosis associated with third nerve palsy is difficult to manage because of poor Bell's phenomenon. A crutch glass may be prescribed or a conservative sling surgery may be performed.

Chapter 28

Disorders of the Conjunctiva

Marek E Prost (Poland)

Pathologic Responses of the Conjunctiva

Some features of conjunctival disorders seen in slit-lamp or during examination with side illumination may be specific for various types of conjunctival diorders. They include:

Conjunctival Hyperemia

It is produced by dilation of blood vessels and is classified as superficial (dilation of conjunctival vessels seen as a reddish flush of the conjunctiva) and deep (dilation of ciliary of episcleral vessels seen as a bluish subconjunctival flush). Superficial hyperemia disappears after instillation of phenylephrine drops or touching with glass rod. The extent and location of conjunctival hyperemia depends on underlying pathology. Diffuse, superficial hyperemia of both the bulbar and tarsal conjunctivae is typical of conjunctivitis. It is usually the most pronounced in viral conjunctivitis. Circumcorneal conjunctival hyperemia of deep vessels that extend 1 to 3 mm out from the limbus, without significant hyperemia of the bulbar superficial conjunctival vessels is seen in iritis and acute glaucoma. Diffuse or circumscribed areas of both superficial and deep hyperemia involving 20 to 100% of the bulbar conjunctiva without hyperemia of the tarsal conjunctiva is typical of episcleritis and scleritis.

Conjunctival Vessels Tortuosity

General tortuosity of all, small conjunctival vessels without any inflammatory signs is typical feature of Fabry disease, ataxia telangiectasia (Louis Bar syndrome), mucolipidosis I and blood hyperviscosity disorders. Dilated large vessels are seen in Sturge-Weber syndrome and especially in carotid-cavernous sinus fistula and dural shunts (corkscrew, aterialized venous vessels). Segmental dilatation and tortuosity of vessels can be seen as a secondary signs of various conjunctival disorders including melanocytic lesions, choristomas, epithelial cysts, pterygium and pinguecula.

Telangiectasis

These vascular lesions are segmental alterations of the conjunctival vessels structure with aneurysmal dilatation. They are typical signs of Goldenberg syndrome (galactosialidosis), Rendu-Osler-Weber syndrome and ataxia telangiectasia (Louis Barr syndrome). Very rarely they can be found in lymphangiectasia. Conjunctival telangiectasis have been also described in morphea coup de saber syndrome (congenital linear groove in scalp or forehead skin spreading to the lids and eye).

Conjunctival Hemorrhages

Can be found in conjunctivitis (the most frequently in viral – picornaviral and herpetic infections), after trauma, rise of central venous pressure (after the birth, after the activity involving Valsalva type maneuvers, after a seizures) and disorders with thrombocytopenia.

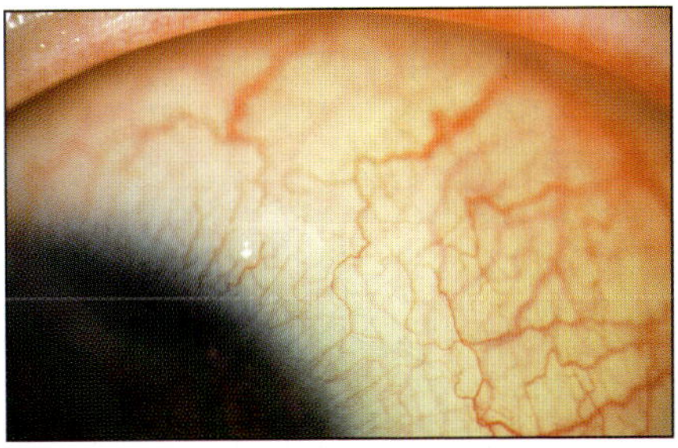

Figure 1: Superficial conjunctival hyperemia in bacterial conjunctivitis

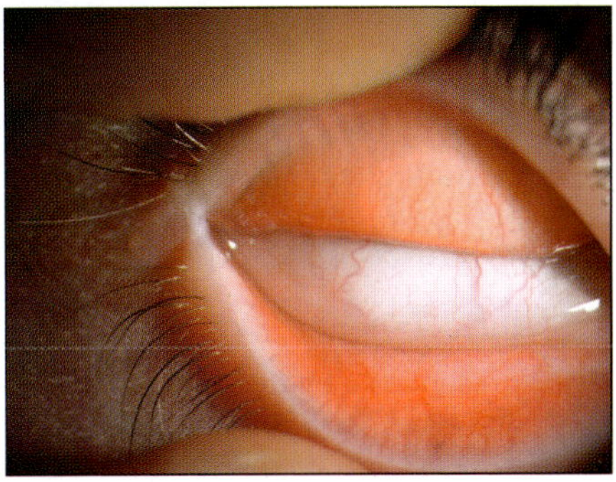

Figure 2: Significant conjunctival hyperemia in epidemic keratoconjunctivitis

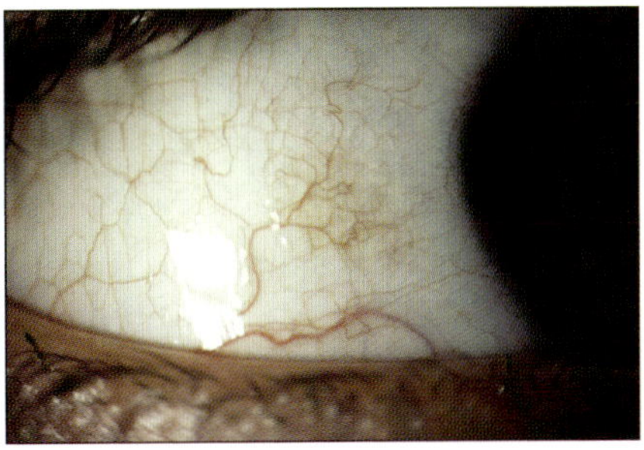

Figure 3: Vascular tortuosity in ataxia telangiectasia

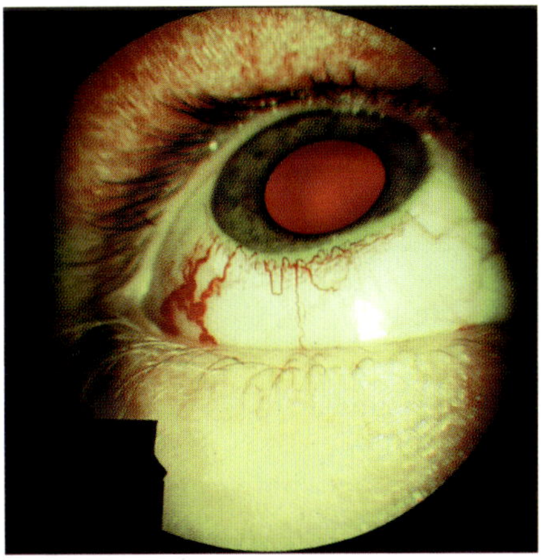

Figure 4: Dilated large conjunctival vessels in Sturge-Weber syndrome

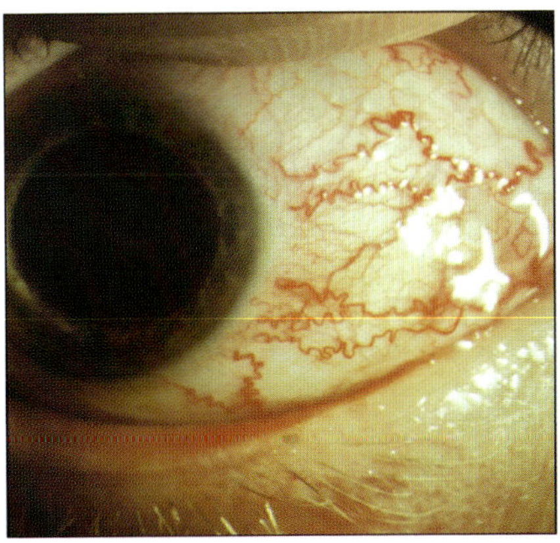

Figure 5: Corkscrew, aterialized venous vessels in carotid-cavernous sinus fistula

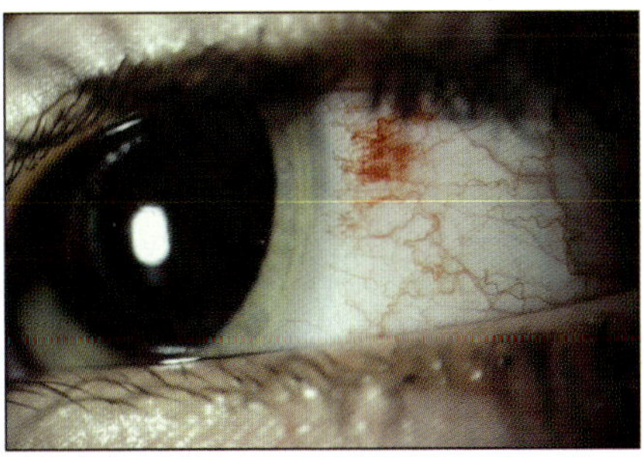

Figure 6: Conjunctival telangiectasia in ataxia telangiectasia

Edema

It is caused by edematous thickening of conjunctiva. Gross edema with ballooning of the conjunctiva often leading to its prolapse between the eyelids is known as chemosis. It can be associated with allergy, trauma (including surgery), acute infections and orbital inflammations.

Papillae

They present as elevated, polygonal, hyperemic areas separated by pale channels with central vessel erupting into a spoke-like pattern. The connective tissue septa that anchor the epithelium to the deeper collagenous tissue limits the size of papilla to less than 1 mm. Papillae are non specific sign occurring in any kind of inflammation (mainly in bacterial and allergic).

Giant Papillae

They are formed by the disruption of the connective tissue septa and coalescence of 2-4 papillae. Its size is greater than 1 mm. They are usually manifestation of ocular allergy not infections, typically found in vernal conjunctivitis, atopic keratoconjunctivitis, and giant papillary conjunctivitis (reaction to contact lenses, sutures, prostheses).

Follicles

There are numerous, smooth, yellowish elevation of the conjunctiva, 2-4 mm of diameter, similar to small grain of rice, with no vessels inside them. Follicles represent hyperplasia of subconjunctival lymphoid tissue. They are common presentation of viral (acute inflammation lasting less than 3 weeks), chlamydial conjunctivitis (chronic inflammation with exacerbation lasting more than 3 weeks) and can be found in benign lymphoid hyperplasia (folliculosis), Parinaud's oculoglandular syndrome and in toxic reactions (medications, molluscum contagiosum).

Membranes or Pseudomembranes

True membranes develop when conjunctival epithelium becomes necrotic and firm adhesions are formed between necrotic cells and the overlying coagulum. Membrane removal leaves raw, bleeding surface. Pseudomembranes are formed by inflammatory cells and exudates that are loosely adherent to the underlying epithelium and can be peeled away without bleeding and damage to ocular surface. Membranes and pseudomembranes are usually manifestations of beta hemolytic streptoccocal conjunctivitis, herpetic keratoconjunctivitis, chlamydial conjunctivitis in newborns, ligneous conjunctivitis, candida infections and can be found in diphtheria, Stevens-Johnson syndrome and after chemical burns.

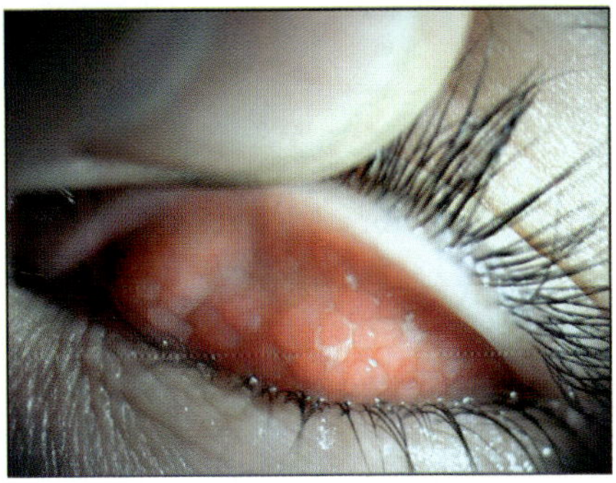

Figure 7: Conjunctival papillae in bacterial conjunctivitis

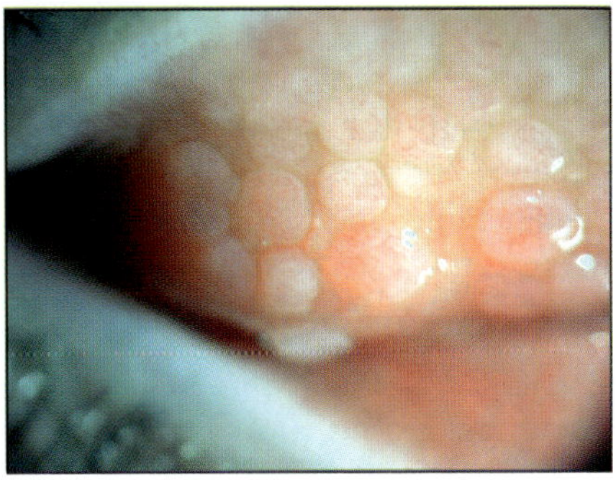

Figure 8: Giant papillae in giant papillary conjunctivitis

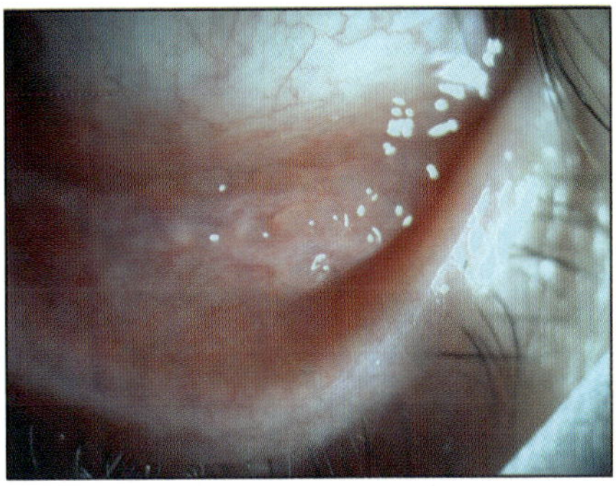

Figure 9: Follicles in inclusion conjunctivitis in adolescent

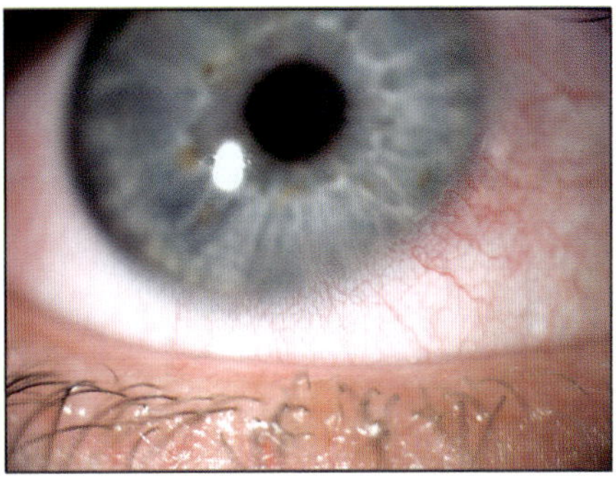

Figure 10: Micro-pannus in staphylococcal blepharoconjunctivitis

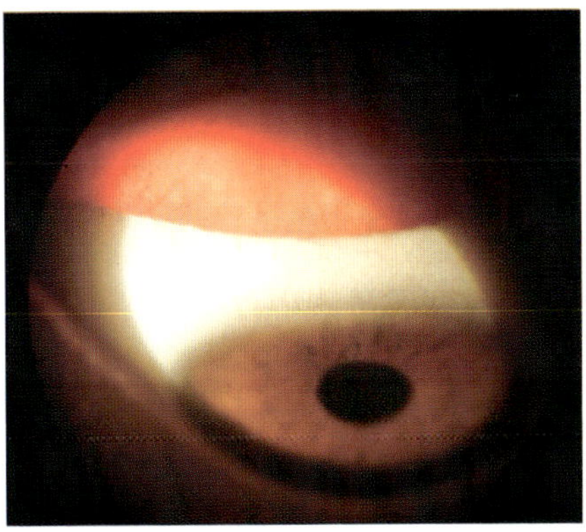

Figure 11: Gross-pannus in trachomatous keratoconjunctivitis *(Courtesy: Dr Mohamed Higazy, Cairo, Egypt)*

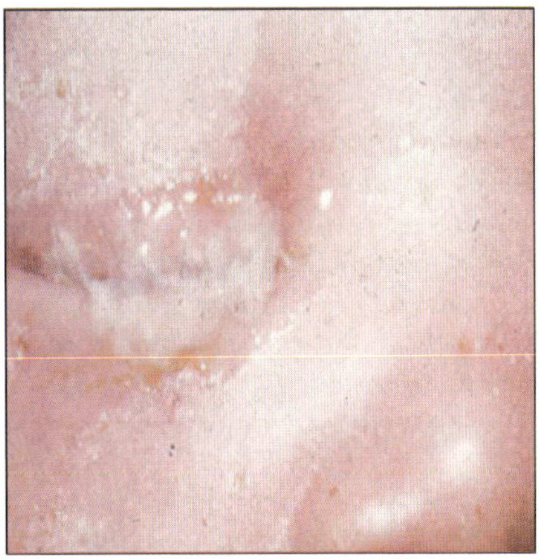

Figure 12: Neonatal gonococcal hyperacute conjunctivitis

Micro-pannus

It is subepithelial proliferation of fibrovascular tissue from limbus into the cornea that extends 1-2 mm beyond the normal vascular arcade. It can be found in chlamydial, conjunctivitis, staphylococcal blepharoconjunctivitis, vernal conjunctivitis and after contact lens wear.

Gross-pannus

Extends more than 2 mm beyond the normal vascular arcade. Superior pannus is typical manifestation of trachoma but can be occasionally seen in staphylococcal blepharitis, herpetic keratoconjunctivitis, atopic keratoconjunctivitis and in rosacea.

Conjunctival Scarring

It can occur in a variety of inflammations (infectious, immunological, allergic, posttraumatic). Raw and denuded surfaces of conjunctiva can adhere and scar leading to symblepharon and shortening of the conjunctival fornices. The most pronounced scarring occurs in trachoma, chemical burns and in erythema multiforme, Stevens-Johnson and toxic epidermal necrolysis.

Infections

Neonatal Conjunctivitis (Ophthalmia Neonatorum)

Neonatal conjunctivitis requires special diagnosis and therapy because of frequent corneal and systemic involvement. Therefore treatment should be performed in cooperation with pediatrician because of possibility of life-threatening systemic manifestations of infections. Most of neonatal conjunctivitis develops as a result of vaginal delivery by infected mother and is indicative of inadequate prenatal care. The conjunctivitis can be prevented by prophylaxis of the neonates at birth (Crede's procedure). It includes the use of topical 1% silver nitrate solution or 1 % silver acetate in single-dose ampules (long-term standard prophylactic agent but no more available in many countries), 0,5% erythromycin or 1,0% tetracycline ointments or 2,5% povidone-iodine solution. Silver nitrate solution is effective against *Neisseria gonorrheae* but has limited spectrum of activity against other bacteria and is not active against Chlamydia and viruses. Erythromycin and tetracycline are effective against bacteria and Chlamydia and povidone-iodine spectrum including bacteria, Chlamydia and some viruses such as herpes or HIV.

The cause of conjunctivitis can be correlated with the onset of clinical signs. Slide stains and cultures of conjunctival smears or scrapings are indicated in all cases of suspected neonatal conjunctivitis.

It is necessary to exclude obstruction of nasolacrimal duct in all neonates with conjunctivitis.

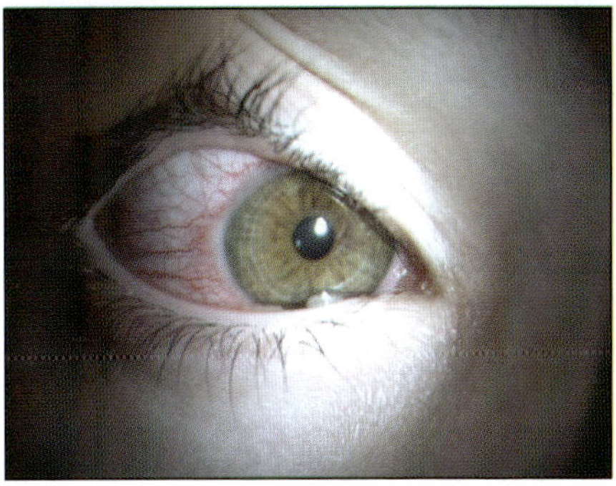

Figure 13: Acute bacterial conjunctivitis with purulent discharge and conjunctival hyperemia

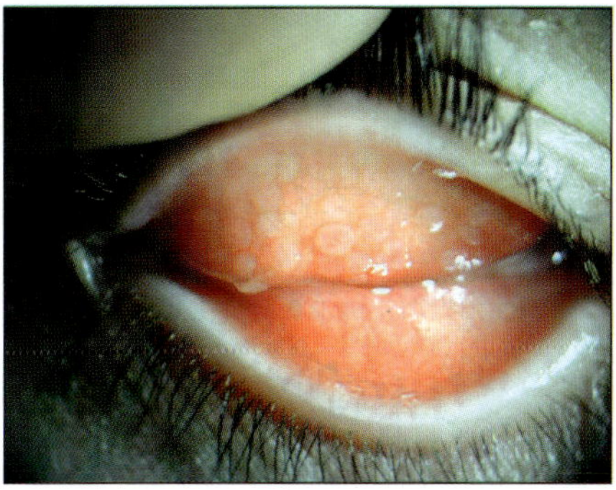

Figure 14: Conjunctival papillary reaction in chronic bacterial conjunctivitis

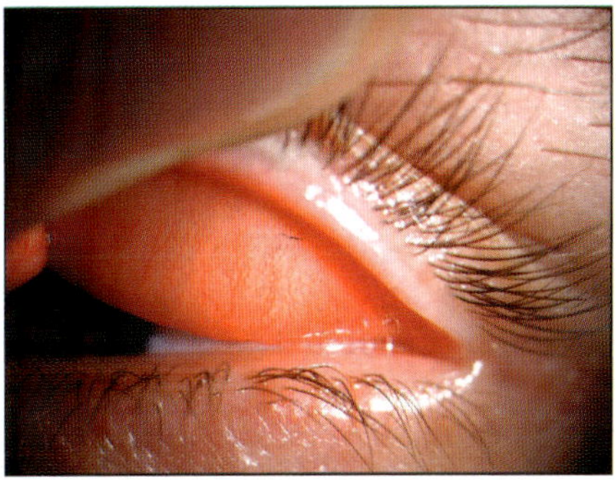

Figure 15: Conjunctival hyperemia and lid edema in viral conjunctivitis

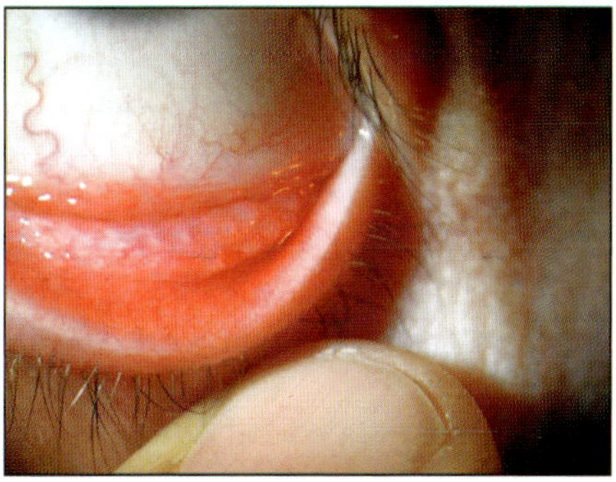

Figure 16: Typical follicular reaction in lower palpebral conjunctiva in viral conjunctivitis

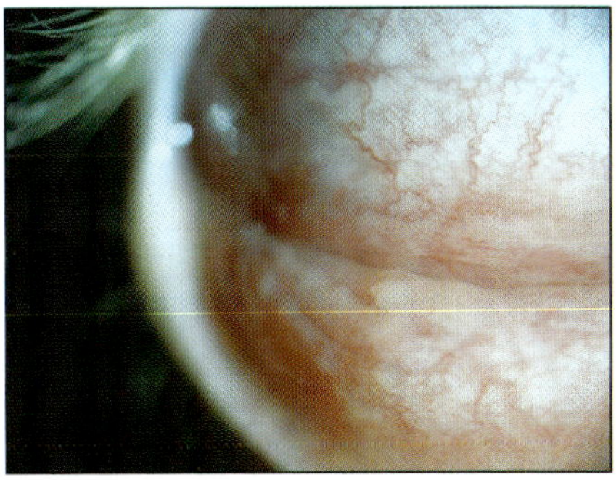

Figure 17: Conjunctival hyperemia and follicles in epidemic adenoviral keratoconjunctivitis

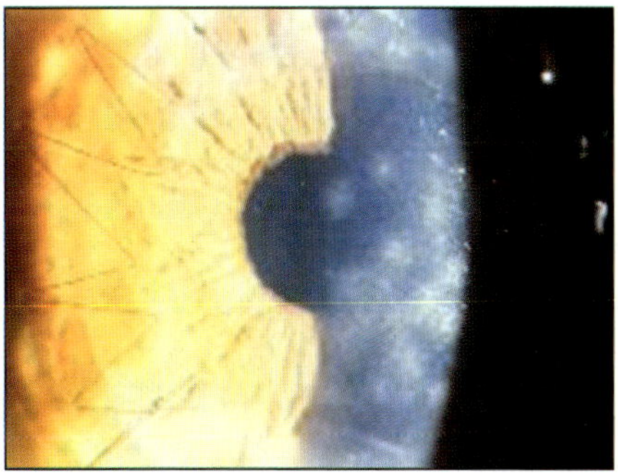

Figure 18: Small, round, grayish, subepithelial infiltrates in the cornea of patients with epidemic keratoconjunctivitis

Chemical Conjunctivitis

This type of conjunctivitis results from instillation of silver nitrate drops used for prophylaxis. It begins some hours after the delivery and is characterized by mild conjunctival hyperemia, watery discharge. It resolves spontaneously after 24-36 hours. Chemical conjunctivitis develops primarily in neonates in whom silver nitrate from large, multiuse eye-drop container was used. It occurs much less frequently since single-use ampules are in more common use.

Gonococcal Hyperacute Conjunctivitis

This type of conjunctivitis is caused by *Neisseria gonorrhoeae*, a gram-negative diplococcus. *N gonorrhoeae* can penetrate intact corneal epithelium and cause corneal ulceration and perforation. Its occurrence decrease significantly since introduction of prophylaxis and nowadays is rare in many countries but in some of them it is still one of major causes of neonatal blindness.

The infection develops 2-4 days after the birth and presents as hyper-acute conjunctivitis with bilateral severe profound lid edema, copious purulent, yellow-green discharge and marked chemosis. Conjunctival membranes may form. If infection is not treated immediately or treated inadequately diplococus can penetrate epithelium and severe corneal ulceration with perforation can occur.

Ocular infection could be part of systemic infection with septicemia, meningitis and arthritis.

Neonates with gonococcal conjunctivitis can be coinfected with Chlamydia trachomatis.

Because gonococcal conjunctivitis is vision threatening disease prompt diagnosis with slide stains and cultures of conjunctival smears is mandatory in all cases.

Treatment should be started immediately with systemic (basic therapy) ceftriaxone 25-50 mg/kg/day (not to exceed 125 mg) IM or IV for 7 days. In case of cephalosporin allergy intravenous penicillin G can be used but this antibiotic is nowadays less frequently used because of reported penicillin resistance of *Neisseria gonorrhoeae*. Topical therapy is additional to systemic treatment and consists of fluoroquinolones drops or erythromycin ointment administered every hour and saline lavage of copious purulent discharge.

Patient should be seen daily.

Treatment should be performed with cooperation with pediatrician and/or venerologist. It is mandatory to examine and treat mother and her sexual partner.

Other Bacterial Conjunctivitis

Streptococcus pneumoniae, Staphylococcus aureus, Staphylococcus epidermidis, Proteus species, Klebsiella pneumoniae, Pseudomonas species, Serratia marcescens are the most common pathogens of neonatal bacterial conjunctivitis. Infection may occur at any time during neonatal period and has typical picture of bacterial conjunctivitis with purulent discharge, lid edema and conjunctival hyperemia.

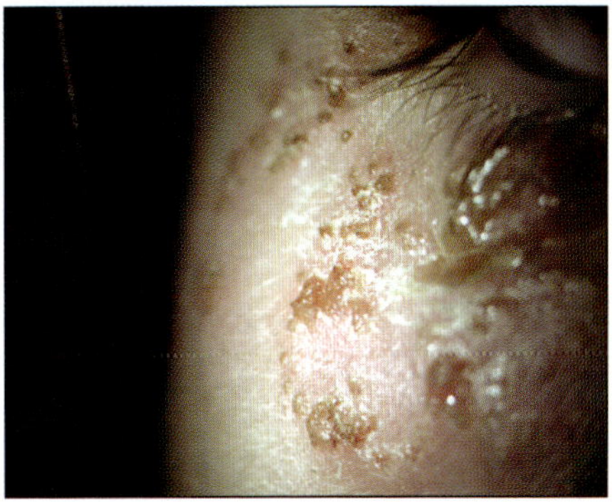

Figure 19: Vesicular eyelid rash in child with herpetic conjunctivitis

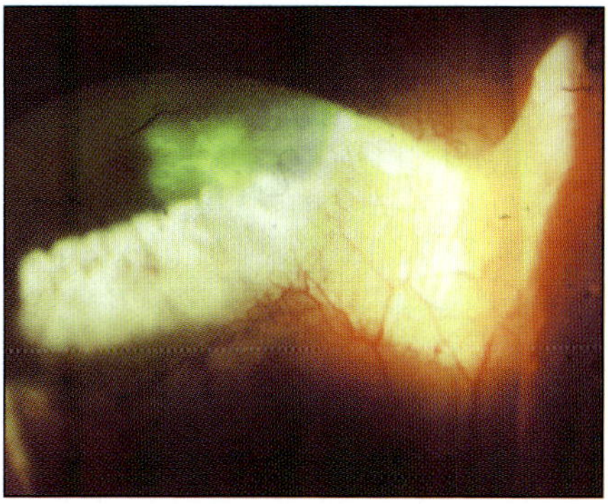

Figure 20: Typical picture of linear branching figures of epithelial corneal lesions (dendritic keratis) in epidemic keratoconjunctivitis

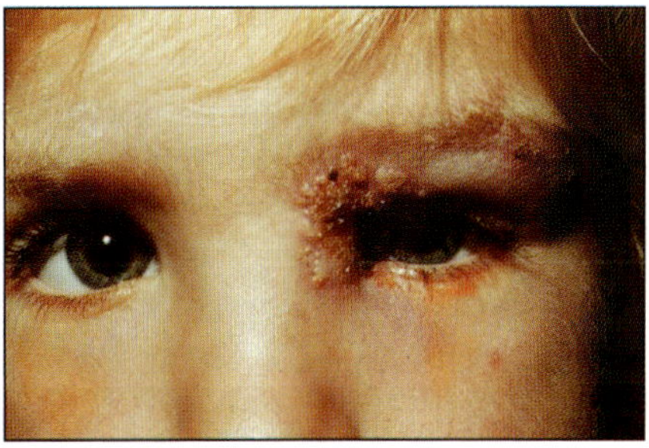

Figure 21: Eyelid vesicular skin eruptions in a child with varicella-zoster conjunctivitis

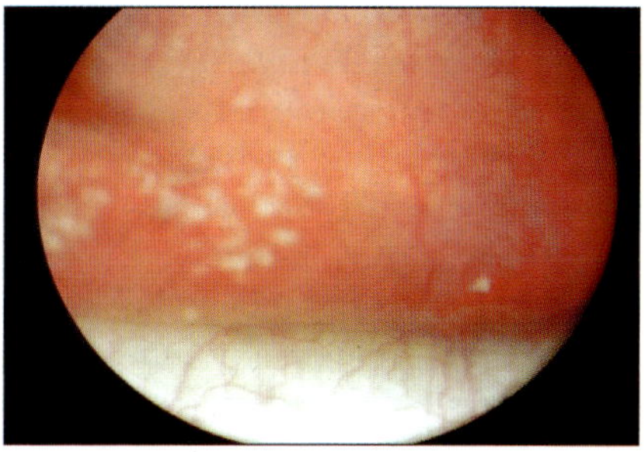

Figure 22: Follicles in the superior tarsal conjunctiva in active trachomatous inflammation – follicular (TF) *(Courtesy: Dr Mohamed Higazy, Cairo, Egypt)*

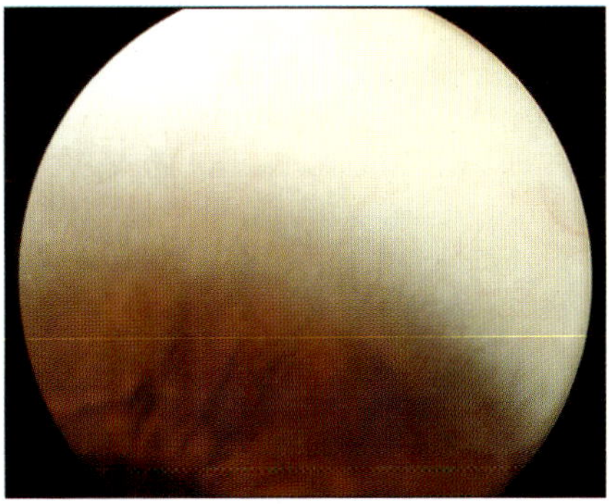

Figure 23: Vascularized superior corneal pannus in active trachoma. *(Courtesy: Dr Mohamed Higazy, Cairo, Egypt)*

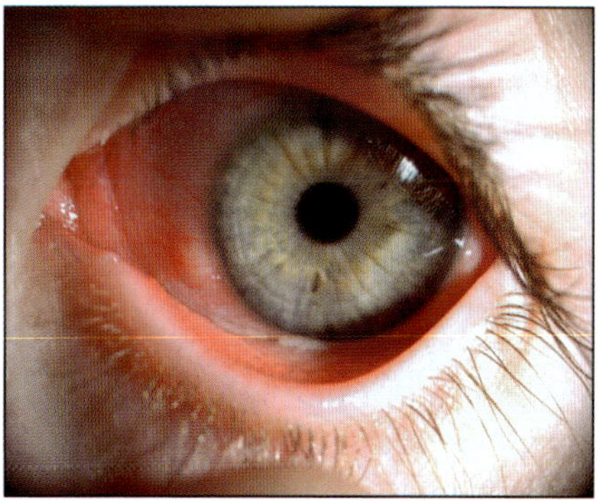

Figure 24: Chlamydial inclusion conjunctivitis in adolescent. Note mucopurulent discharge and follicular reaction.

Corneal involvement is extremely rare (Pseudomonas). In neonatal conjunctivitis it is advisory to perform slide stains, cultures and antibiotic sensitivity.

Usually treatment starts with topical aminoglycosides or fluoroquinolones although sulfacetamide, erythromycine and tetracycline are still in use. If it is not effective after 5-7 days switch to newer topical fluoroquinolones.

It is obligatory to exclude obstruction of nasolacrimal duct in all neonates with purulent discharge.

Chlamydial Conjunctivitis

This infection is one of the most frequent causes of neonatal conjunctivitis and has been estimated to occur in 2% to 6% of all newborns. The high incidence of infection may also be related to the ineffectiveness of silver nitrate in preventing chlamydial infection. It is usually caused by Chlamydia. trachomatis subtypes D-K.

Neonatal chlamydial conjunctivitis is characterized by the onset of a mild to moderate unilateral or bilateral mucopurulent conjunctivitis 5 to 10 days after the birth. Typical signs are eyelid edema, chemosis, mucopurulent discharge and conjunctival membranes or pseudomembranes. Follicular reaction (typical of pediatric or adult conjunctivitis) is not observed because subconjunctival lymphoid tissue does not mature before 3 months of age. Sometimes cornea is involved, including punctate opacities and micropannus formation. Systemic chlamydial infection (pneumonia nasopharyngeal infection and otitis) can develop in more than 50% of neonates.

The recommended treatment is oral (basic therapy) erythromycin 50 mg/kg/day in four divided doses for 2 weeks and topical erythromycin or tetracycline ointments for two weeks.

Untreated cases may persist 3-12 months. Important aspect of treatment is concurrent therapy of the mother and her sexual partner.

Viral Conjunctivitis

Neonatal viral conjunctivitis is usually caused by herpes simplex virus type 1 (transmitted during vaginal delivery by infected mother) or less frequently by type 2 (transmitted by a kiss from an adult). Infection may be local or disseminated. Ocular signs develops 5-12 days after the birth and include lid edema, conjunctival hyperemia, serous discharge and occasionally vesicular lid eruptions. Follicular reaction (seen in pediatric or adult conjunctivitis) is not observed because subconjunctival lymphoid tissue does not mature before 3 months of age. Conjunctivitis is often associated with corneal involvement. Typical manifestation is dendritic or geographic keratitis. More serious complications include cataract, chorioretinitis, optic neuritis. Disseminated herpetic infection (encephalitis and skin sores) should be ruled out because of high mortality rate in neonates.

Acyclovir 3% ointment 4 times a day is topical treatment of choice. Recently introduced ganciclovir 0,15% ocular gel is comparably effective to acyclovir in treatment of ocular herpetic infections but there are limited information about

Table 1: Differential diagnosis in infections of the conjunctiva in neonates

Causes	Time of Onset	Clinical Features	Comments and Treatment
Chemical	1-2 day	Mild hyperemia and serous discharge	Treatment not necessary
Neisseria Gonorrhoeae	2-4 days	Hyperacute conjunctivitis, severe purulent, yellow-green discharge, lid edema, chemosis, rapidly progressive, corneal ulcer, risk of corneal perforation in hours. Can cause blindness.	Check for sepsis, meningitis, arthritis. **Urgent case**, treatment with systemic (basic therapy) ceftriaxione 25-50 mg/kg/day (not to exceed 125 mg) IM or IV for 7 days. Topical saline lavage, fluoroquinolones or erythromycin every hour. Treat mother and her sexual partner
VIral (HSV 2)	5-12 days	Lid vesicles, copious serous discharge, lid edema, possibility of corneal changes	Check for cataract, uveitis and disseminated infection (encephalitis, skin sores). Topical acyclovir. Systemic acyclovir treatment may be necessary in intra-ocular or disseminated infections
Chlamydia	5-10 days	Mucopurulent discharge, marked hyperemia, sometimes micropannus, pseudomembranes and rarely corneal opacity No follicular reaction	Check for pneumonia, nasopharyngitis and otitis. Treatment with oral (basic therapy) erythromycin 50 mg/kg/day in four divided doses for 2 weeks and topical erythromycin or tetracycline ointments for two weeks. Treat mother and her sexual partner
Other Bacterial S. Pneumoniae Staphyl aureus **Proteus, Klebsiella, Pseudomonas, Serratia marces**	1-30 days	Purulent discharge, no corneal changes	Start treatment with topical aminoglycosides or fluoroquinolones. If not effective switch to newer topical fluoroquinolones Exclude obstruction of nasolacrimal duct
Nasolacrimal duct obstruction	ca. 21 days	Bacterial conjunctivitis	Lacrimal sac massage if not effective perform probing. Topical aminoglycosides for prophylaxis of keratitis

its use in neonates. Systemic acyclovir treatment should be considered in neonates with intraocular or disseminated infections.

Pediatric Conjunctivitis

Bacterial Conjunctivitis

In children bacterial conjunctivitis is usually caused by *Haemophilus influenzae* and less frequently by Streptococcus and Staphylococcus species. The sources of the infection are usually a skin or respiratory tract pathogens. Usually one eye is involved but infection of second eye may develop in some days.

Bacterial conjunctivitis can present as hyperacute, acute, subacute or chronic.

Hyperacute conjunctivitis is very rare but sight threatening form of bacterial conjunctivitis caused by Neisseria species (N. gonorrheae or meningitides) and less often Pseudomonas aeruginosa infections. The disease is usually bilateral and is characterized by sudden, rapid onset, fulminating conjunctivitis with marked eyelid swelling, severe hyperemia, chemosis and profuse, thick, yellow-green purulent discharge. Typically, the purulent discharge is copious and quickly recurs when wiped or washed away. There is high risk of a corneal infiltration and corneal necrosis and perforation in hours which can lead to blindness. The gonococcal conjunctivitis develops usually in newborns and less often in pediatric patients. In children septicemia with arthritis and pelvic inflammatory disease is rarely occuring. *Neisseria gonorrhoeae* infections are transmitted sexually and therefore it is mandatory to examine and treat not only the patient but also his/her parents. *Pseudomonas aeruginosa* infection spreads by direct contact with infected individual.

Acute bacterial conjunctivitis is the most frequently caused by *Haemophilus influenzae* or *Streptococcus pneumoniae*. It usually begins suddenly in one eye with hyperaemia and moderate to copious purulent or purulent discharge, but infection of second eye may develop in some days. Patients initially complain of unilateral then bilateral tearing and vague irritation. Associated mild to moderate eyelid edema and erythema may give the appearance of pseudoptosis. Purulent discharge may accumulate on the eyelashes, resulting in eyelids sticking together in the morning on awakening. Some bacteria are able to cause conjunctival membranes or pseudomembranes (beta hemolytic Streptococcus, Bordetella pertussis—diphtheria). Very rarely acute conjunctivitis can progress to keratitis and infection of orbital tissue (preseptal cellulites). Rare systemic associated findings are sinusitis, rhinitis and otitis media.

Subacute or chronic conjunctivitis: In this stage the most frequent cause are Streptococcus, Staphylococcus and Moraxella species. The duration of infections is on average 5-7 days and is usually mild and self-limiting. The patients present with moderate purulent discharge, mild conjunctival hyperemia and crustings on the eyelids and/or eyelashes (dried purulent discharge). Sometimes conjunctival papillary reaction may be seen in chronic bacterial conjunctivitis. Corneal involvement is very rare in subacute and chronic bacterial conjunctivitis

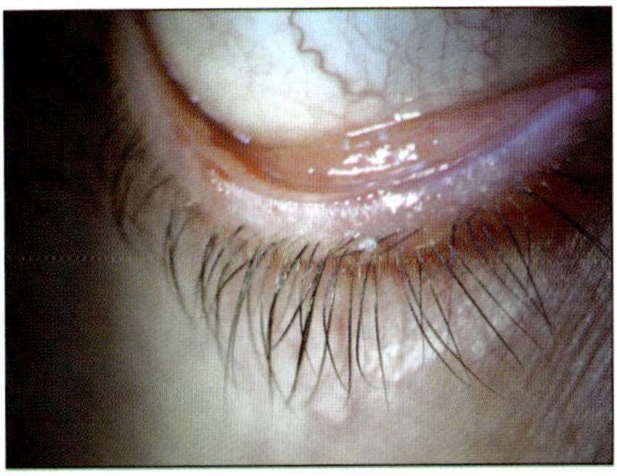

Figure 25: Crustings, edema and small ulcerations of the lid margin in a girl with staphylococcal blepharoconjunctivitis

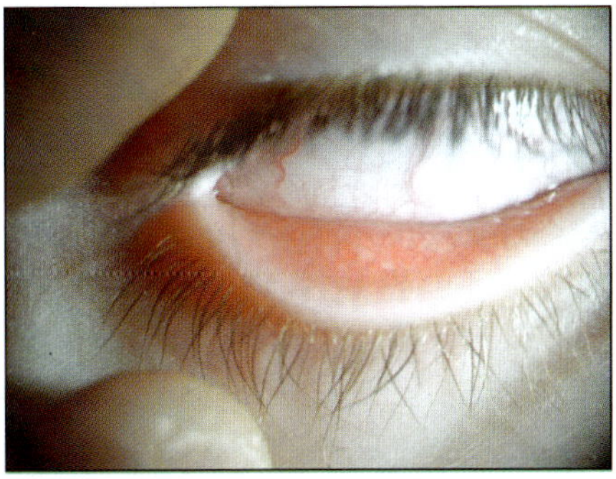

Figure 26: Follicular toxic reaction in patient with prolonged neomycin therapy

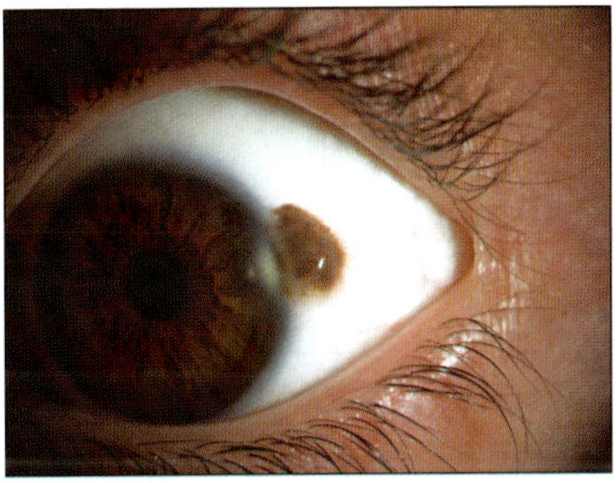

Figure 27: Congenital melanotic melanocytic limbal nevus

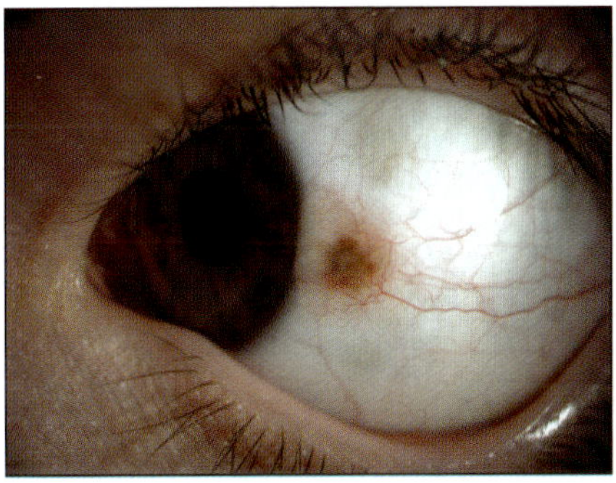

Figure 28: Partly pigmented congenital limbal nevus

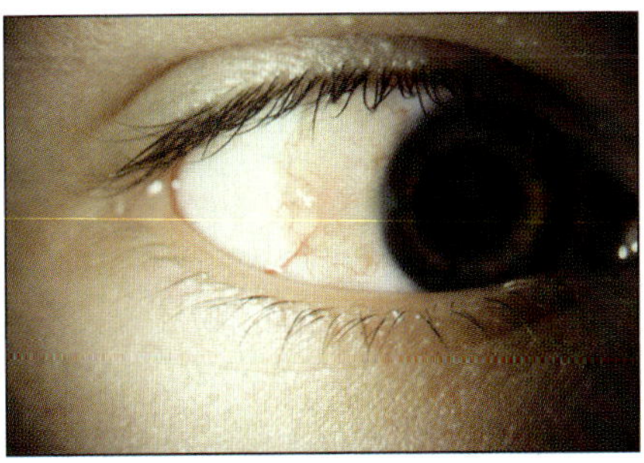

Figure 29: Slightly pigmented acquired limbal nevus

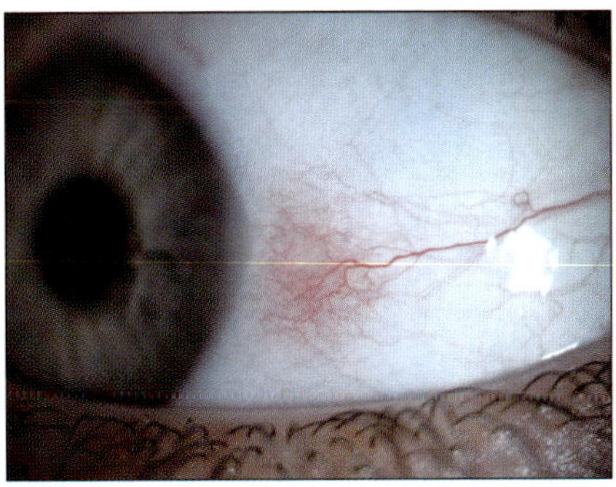

Figure 30: Amelanotic acquired limbal nevus

in children but marginal conjunctivitis may occur in staphylococcal conjunctivitis as an result of an immune-mediated reaction to staphylococcal toxins. Pre-auricular lymph nods are not enlarged.

In children it may very rarely progress to keratitis and infection of orbital tissue (preseptal cellulites).

The most typical sign of bacterial conjunctivitis is purulent discharge and eyelids sealing in the morning upon awakening.

In neonate and infants it is necessary to exclude nasolacrimal duct obstruction as a cause of bacterial conjunctivitis.

Diagnosis of bacterial conjunctivitis: In hyper-acute conjunctivitis it is mandatory to perform promptly slide stains, cultures and antibiotic sensitivity. In acute, subacute or chronic conjunctivitis diagnosis is made on the basis of medical history and eye examination. Usually slide stains, cultures or cytology are not necessary to prove the diagnosis. Diagnostic tests are indicated in difficult clinical cases, recurrent conjunctivitis and in patients not responding to medication. One have to remember that in patients with bacterial conjunctivitis treated previously with antibiotics the results of slide stains and cultures are very often negative.

Usually Gram stain is used for direct identification of causative bacteria. The conjunctival smears and scrapings can be cultured on various media, the most popular is blood agar. (see below)

In infants it is necessary to exclude nasolacrimal duct obstruction as a cause of bacterial conjunctivitis.

Treatment of bacterial conjunctivitis: Patient with **hyper-acute bacterial** conjunctivitis patient should be admitted to the hospital and slide stains, cultures and antibiotic sensitivity are performed. Treatment is started immediately with systemic antibiotics (basic therapy) – in children with weight less than 45 kg—ceftriaxone (125 mg IM) or spectinomycin 40 mg/kg (maximum dose 2 gm) single doses. In older children single doses of 1 gm of ceftriaxone IM, 500 mg orally of ciprofloxacin or spectinomycin 2 gm IM have been proved to be effective. Topical last-generation fluoroquinolones every 1 hour can also be administered. Afterwards therapy is adjusted according to sensitivity of the cultured organism. Lavage of purulent discharge from the infected eyes should be considered.

In acute, subacute and chronic conjunctivitis treatment is started with broad spectrum topical antibiotics. Antibiotic therapy usually speeds the resolution and lessens the severity of the disease. Since ordinary bacterial conjunctivitis very often is self-limited less expensive option like aminoglycosides may be selected but fluoroquinolones are used more and more frequently nowadays. If this therapy is not effective after 7 days switch to topical fluoroquinolones. If conjunctivitis does not improve during next 7- 10 days perform cytology and consider other diagnosis:

- Other types of conjunctivitis: chlamydial or viral with secondary bacterial infection,
- Nasolacrimal duct obstruction
- Chronic blepharoconjunctivitis

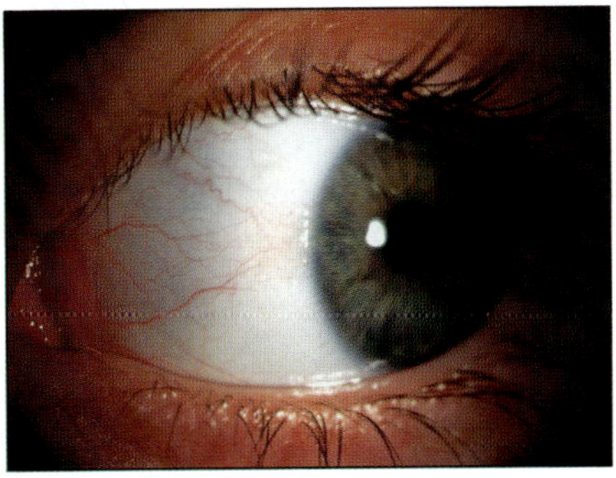

Figure 31: Amelanotic acquired limbal, nevus with cystic degeneration

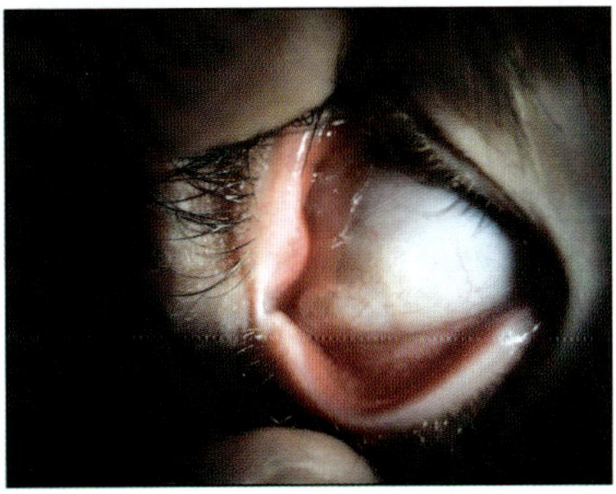

Figure 32: Subconjunctival lymphangiectasis in patients with neurofibromatosis

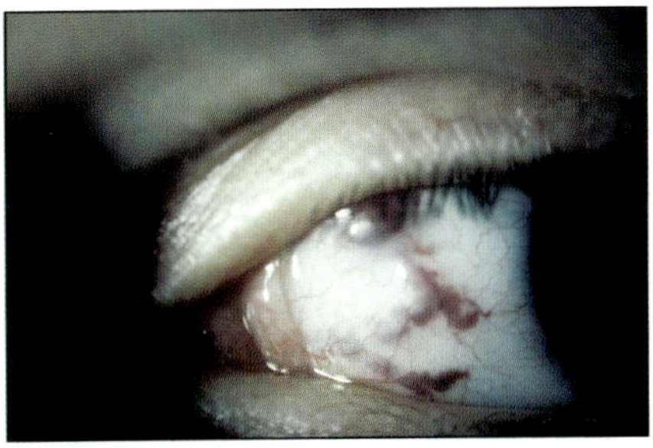

Figure 33: Subconjunctival lymphangiectasis with lymph vessels filled with blood

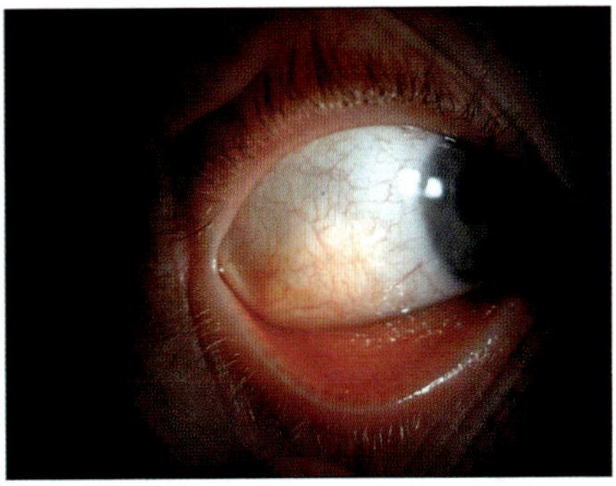

Figure 34: Dermolipoma penetrating into the orbit

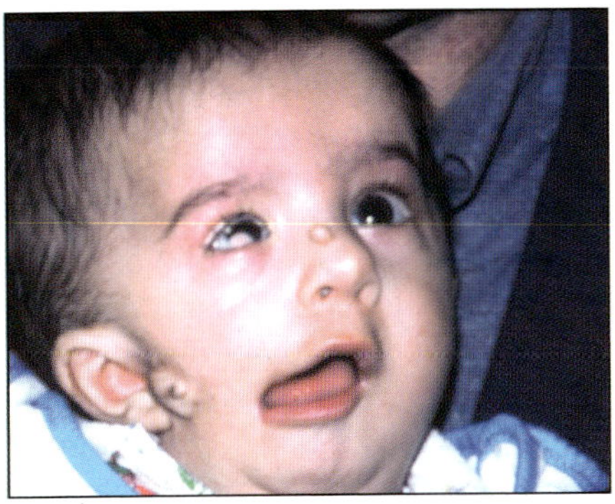

Figure 35: Dermolipoma in a child with Goldenhar syndrome

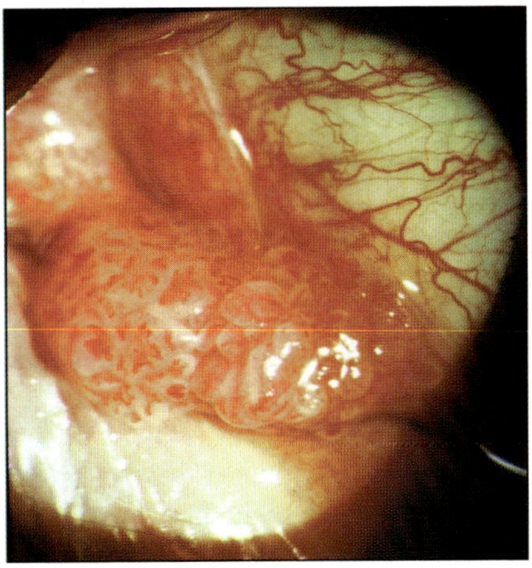

Figure 36: Inner canthus conjunctival papilloma

Because antibiotic resistance is becoming growing problem it is advisable to select bactericidal and not bacteriostatic antibiotics to diminish probability of development of antibiotic-resistant bacterial isolates. It is also recommended to maintain adequate dosing (e.g. aminoglycosides at least 3 times/day, fluoroquinolones 4 times/day) to decrease the possibility of exposure bacterial populations to repeated, sublethal doses of antibiotics which can stimulate development of mutations responsible for the increased resistance.

Viral Conjunctivitis

Usually caused by adenoviruses (epidemic keratoconjunctivitis and pharyngoconjunctival fever) or herpes simplex, less frequently by varicella-zoster virus, picornaviruses, pox and papilloma viruses or moluscum contagiosum infections. The infections are transmitted by hand to eye contact, contact with upper respiratory droplets, infected swimming pools or infected ocular instruments like tonometers. Viral conjunctivitis usually has acute onset and is unilateral at first with involvement of second eye after some days. Typical signs are conjunctival hyperemia, copious, clear, serous, watery discharge, lid edema and follicular conjunctival reaction. It follows longer course than bacterial conjunctivitis, usually 2-3 week. Conjunctival and subconjunctival hemorrhages may occur in viral conjunctivitis most frequently and commonly in acute hemorrhagic conjunctivitis (picornaviruses infection). To the smaller extent they may occur in epidemic and herpetic keratoconjunctivitis. Preauricular lymph nodes are usually involved. Sometimes history of recent fever, upper respiratory tract infections or pharyngitis helps to establish diagnosis.

Adenoviral infections are usually highly contagious and occur in epidemics. Patients usually give a history of recent exposure to an individual with red eye at home or work. The onset of infection is abrupt and second eye is involved in 1-2 days. The disease presents with usually significant conjunctival injection, copious, clear, watery, serous discharge, eyelid edema and follicular conjunctival reaction. Distinctive signs of adenoviral infection are: follicular conjunctivitis with abrupt onset, watery discharge, lid edema, subepithelial corneal infiltrates and preauricular lymph nodes enlargement. Patients with adenoviral conjunctivitis are contagious to others for 3 weeks after beginning of infection. Subtypes of adenoviral conjunctivitis include epidemic keratoconjunctivitis (EKC) caused by serotypes 3, 4 and 7 and pharyngoconjunctival fever (PCF) caused by serotypes 8, 9 and 37.

1. *Epidemic keratoconjunctivitis (EKC)* is characterized with sudden onset of signs and symptoms, significant irritation, soreness, red eye, photophobia, foreign body sensation, and excessive watery discharge. Marked eyelid swelling and erythema is often present. In severe cases conjunctival membranes, pseudomembranes and subconjunctival hemorrhages and chemosis may develop. Typical complication of EKC is development small, round, grayish subepithelial infiltrates in the cornea. They appear about 2 weeks after onset of the conjunctivitis and may persist for weeks to months, sometimes to years eventually resolving spontaneously without scarring.

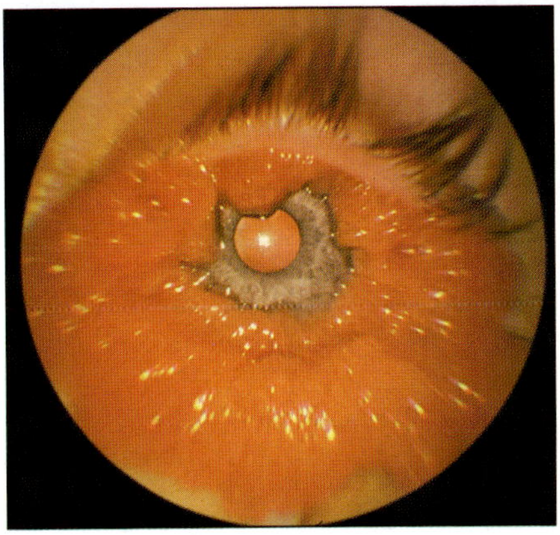

Figure 37: Exuberant papilloma involving whole bulbar conjunctiva

They may decrease visual acuity and cause glare. Preauricular lymph nodes are usually enlarged. Sometimes concurrent upper respiratory infection is observed.

2. Pharyngoconjunctival fever (PCF) is characterized by fever, pharyngitis, acute follicular conjunctivitis, regional lymphoid hyperplasia with tender, enlarged preauricular adenopathy. Usually clinical sign and symptoms are less severe than in EKC and there corneal involvement is rare.

Herpes simplex conjunctivitis in children is caused by HSV type 1, much less frequently with HSV type 2. Conjunctival signs are typical for viral conjunctivitis but sometimes vesicular eyelid rash may accompany herpetic conjunctivitis and is distinctive sign of this infection. Herpetic conjunctivitis is often associated with corneal involvement. Typical manifestation is dendritic keratis with typical picture of linear branching figures. Other forms of corneal involvement are less frequent (epithelial keratitis, neurotrophic keratopathy, interstitial keratitis, necrotizing stromal keratitis, disciform stromal keratitis, endothelitis). Other complications occur much less common and include uveitis or trabeculitis. Preauricular lymph nodes are usually involved. Fever, upper respiratory tract infections may precede or accompany herpes simplex conjunctivitis. Distinctive signs of herpetic infection are: vesicular eyelid rash and dendritic epithelial keratitis.

Varicella-zoster conjunctivitis is caused by VZV virus and is unilateral. It is characterized by typical vesicular skin eruptions involving the tissues innervated by the ophthalmic division of the trigeminal nerve (eye, ear, mouth, tongue, skin), fever, headache, significant ocular pain and sometimes extraocular signs and symptoms (hyperesthesia, pain in affected dermatome, vertigo, hearing loss, taste alteration, paralysis of the facial nerve). Conjunctivitis is associated with corneal involvement in 40-60 % of the cases, iridocyclitis in up to 40 % and elevated IOP in 40%. These complications usually cause decrease of visual acuity. Recurrence is a characteristic feature of herpes zoster ophthalmicus. Vesicular eyelid and face rash and significant pain that accompany varicella-zoster infection is distinctive sign of this infection.

Acute hemorrhagic conjunctivitis is caused by picornaviruses (usually enterovirus 70 and coxsackievirus A 24) and has been described in Egypt and other African countries, China, India, Japan and Cuba. As EKC it is rapidly progressive and highly contagious infection and tends to occur in epidemics. Its signs include ocular pain, swollen lids, conjunctival follicles, chemosis and typical subconjunctival hemorrhages, which can range from petechiae to coalescent, large areas of hemorrhages. Superficial epithelial changes can be seen sometimes in the cornea. The infection usually resolves after 7 days without sequel although hemorrhages may persist longer. In infants and children poliolike paralysis, aseptic meningitis and involvement of different organ systems ranging from myocardium to CNS, respiratory system and skin have been described.

Molluscum contagiosum is a cutaneous or conjunctival pox viral infection, that causes a raised waxy, umbilicated, filled with cheesy material lesions on the eyelids, near the lid margin and face. Immunocompromised state may predispose to multiple and/or large lesions. Virus and its toxins that is shed into the tear film from eyelid lesions may cause a toxic reaction of the conjunctiva and cornea, resulting in a chronic, follicular conjunctivitis and sometimes punctate corneal epithelial defects with subepithelial corneal opacities and mild superior keratitis. Conjunctivitis is usually unilateral less often bilateral. Infrequent complications include conjunctival scarring and occlusion of the lacrimal puncta. Usually there is no enlargement of lymph nodes. Typical umbilical eyelid lesions help to establish the diagnosis.

Verrucae, commonly known as warts, are produced by human papillomavirus. If skin lesions grow on the eyelid margin and among the lashes, the viral particles and desquamated epithelium cells may cause a secondary, mild toxic, follicular conjunctivitis. Human papillomavirus can also cause conjunctival papilloma (see further).

Diagnosis of viral conjunctivitis

Usually clinical diagnosis is used. Viral cultures and immunodiagnostic tests are not very helpful ad are infrequently used in clinical practice. They are only performed in diagnostic difficult cases. The results of viral cultures are delayed for several weeks.

Treatment of viral conjunctivitis

1. **In adenoviral infections** treatment is only supportive. Recently introduced ganciclovir 0,15% ocular gel has antiviral activity against some serotypes of adenoviruses causing adenoviral conjunctivitis. Topical antibiotics can be used to prevent bacterial superinfection.
2. **In herpetic and varicella-zoster infections** topical acyclovir (3% ointment) is treatment of choice in prevention of corneal involvement or in patients with simultaneous keratitis. Newly introduced drug ganciclovir (0,15% ocular gel) is comparably effective to acyclovir in treatment of ocular herpetic infections. Topical idoxuridine (IDU), vidarabine and trifluridine are nowadays less available. Oral acyclovir 200 to 400 mg five times per day until the conjunctivitis resolves is sometimes used in more severe cases.

3. **In molluscum contagiosum and papilloma** treatment is by surgical excision, incision, cauterization, cryotherapy or curettage. The conjunctivitis and keratitis typically resolve after removal of skin lesions. Spontaneous resolution is usually seen in 3 to 12 months in immunocompetent patients.

Topical corticosteroid should be used with caution in viral conjunctivitis. They can enhance resorption of corneal subepithelial infiltrates but can worsen underlying viral infection.

Chlamydial Conjunctivitis

The chlamydiae are obligate intracellular organisms, depending on the host cell to carry out metabolic biosynthesis, counted among the gram-negative bacteria. The species consists of three subgroups: *C. trachomatis*, *C. pneumoniae* and *C. psittaci*. Humans are the reservoir of *C. trachomatis* and *C. pneumoniae*; *C. psittaci* causes zoonosis. By serologic typing C. trachomatis can be divided into subtypes, whereby A, B, Ba and C induce trachoma, subtypes D-K cause inclusion body conjunctivitis (adult and neonatal) and urethritis, prostatitis, cervicitis and salpingitis, subtypes L 1-2-3 produce lymphogranuloma venerum.

Although *C. trachomatis* is the infectious agent of both trachoma and inclusion conjunctivitis (adult and neonatal), the clinical presentations and the epidemiologic characteristics of the two diseases are very different.

The incidence of trachoma is highest in unhealthy, dirty, crowded, poor hygienic conditions. Transmission generally occurs with contact of conjunctival exudates directly or via flies.

Subtypes D-K, as well as the L varieties are transmitted sexually and therefore cause veneral disease, in which ocular involvement represents secondary infection.

Chlamydial conjunctivitis consists from 3 clinical syndromes: trachoma, adult inclusion conjunctivitis (occurring also in adolescents) and neonatal chlamydial conjunctivitis (see above).

Trachoma

Trachoma and its complications still represent a serious world health problem and remains a major cause of preventable blindness in parts of Africa, the Middle East, India and Southeast Asia. Trachoma affects approximately one-seventh of the world's population. Active stage of this disease is frequently found in children with peak prevalence in 3-5 years of age. The occurrence falls rapidly in school period. The disease is transmitted through close personal contact (through hands, clothing), tends to occur in clusters. It may be also carried by flies that have come in contact with discharge from the eyes or nose of an infected person. Therefore it can affect entire families and communities. It is estimated that currently 6 million people are visually impaired as a result of trachoma and 150 million suffer from active infection. It can ruin the economic well-being of entire communities.

Trachoma manifests gradually as a repeated cycle of infections and its complications. In its early active phases the disease presents as a follicular conjunctivitis with predilection for the superior tarsal conjunctiva. Presence of 5 or more follicles in this area is indicative of active trachoma. Symptoms are photophobia, tearing, mucopurulent discharge. Conjunctival follicles at the limbus are characteristic of more advanced trachoma. Primary corneal involvement is frequent and includes superior corneal pannus formation and punctate keratitis. Corneal infiltrates (superior, diffuse, limbal) and marginal ulceration may occur. In the most advance phases there is pronounced inflammatory thickening of the upper tarsal conjunctiva obscuring the normal deep tarsal vessels. Cicatrization of limbal follicles leads to the development of sharply delineated depressions (Herbert pits)—characteristic signs of trachoma. Corneal pannus eventually regress but can cause diffuse haze of the superior cornea.

In cicatricial phase progressing conjunctival and subconjunctival scarring can result in palpebral fibrosis and deformities, entropion, ectropion and trichiasis. Typical sign is Arlts line—horizontal line forming as a result conjunctival scarring at the junction of the anterior one third and posterior two-thirds of upper tarsal conjunctiva. Conjunctival and eyelid deformities cause repeated damages of the cornea resulting in corneal ulceration, neovascularization and sometimes perforation. End result of these lesions is opacification of the cornea. Corneal changes are the major blinding complication of trachoma. The conjunctival scarring may also cause many other secondary complications, including severe dry eye syndrome and punctal stenosis.

Practical, simple grading scheme of clinical signs in trachoma was prepared by World Health Organization.

Ocular disease may be associated with infections of other extraocular mucous membranes, commonly nasopharynx.

Adult Inclusion Conjunctivitis

This type of conjunctivitis is sexually transmitted and can develop also in adolescents. Ocular infection commonly occurs by autoinoculation (sexual contact or by hand to eye contact) with infected genital and urinary secretion.

The disease usually is unilateral, but may be bilateral too. It is chronic, prolonged (lasting many months) recurrent conjunctivitis with exacerbations and remissions. Patients complain of ocular irritation, photophobia, redness. Typical signs include mucopurulent discharge, moderate conjunctival hyperemia and follicular conjunctival reaction particularly on the inferior fornix. Chlamydial conjunctivitis can be associated with corneal involvement (punctate epithelial keratitis, subepithelial infiltrations and small superior pannus) which can cause diminished visual acuity. Preauricular lymph nodes are usually enlarged and tender. Girls often have chronic vaginitis or cervicitis, boys symptomatic or asymptomatic urethritis. All patients with suspected or confirmed chlamydial conjunctivitis should be evaluated and co-managed with a gynecologist or urologist.

Table 2: World Health Organization trachoma simple grading scheme

	Grading	*Clinical manifestations*
ACTIVE	**TF** Trachomatous inflammation – follicular	The presence of 5 or more follicules at least 0,5 in diameter in the central part of the upper tarsal conjunctiva
	TI Trachomatous inflammation – intense	Pronounced inflammatory thickening of the upper tarsal conjunctiva obscuring more than half of the normal deep tarsal vessels
CICAT-RICIAL	**T S** Trachomatous scarring	Presence of visible scarring in the upper tarsal conjunctiva
	TT Trachomatous trichiasis	At least one eyelash rubs on the eyeball, or evidence of recent removal of in-turned eyelashes
	CO Corneal opacity	Easily visible corneal opacity over the pupil, so dense that at least part of the pupil margin is blurred when view through the opacity

Diagnosis of Trachoma

If diagnosis cannot been made on the clinical basis performance of cytology with Giemsa stain (basophilic intracytoplasmic inclusion bodies in epithelial cells—Halberstaedter–von Provazek bodies), direct immunofluorescent antibody tests (DFA, IFA), ELISA and PCR tests of ocular specimens may be helpful.

Treatment of Trachoma

Because of frequent concomitant systemic infections oral azithromycin (one time dose 1 gm p.o.) or clarithromycin, tetracycline, doxycyline or erythromycin for 3 weeks for the patient and his or her sexual partner is basic therapy for chlamydial conjunctivitis. Tetracycline should not be used in children younger than 7 years. Therapy of both patients and his/her sexual partner is necessary. In some countries only topical treatment is used as follows: topical sulphamethacin eyedrops 10% 30% 4 times/day, together with erythromycin 0.5% ointment or tetracycline ointment during night for 2 weeks although some authors claim that topical therapy is relatively ineffective in the treatment of eye disease. The effectiveness of topical treatment additional to systemic therapy is not proven.

Acanthameba Keratoconjunctivitis

Acanthameba keratoconjunctivitis is uncommon but sight-threatening condition that mainly affects contact lens wearers. It is caused by free-living protozoans (amebas), that may be found in soil, dust, fresh water, tap water, hot tubs and swimming pools. Contact lens wearers using poor sterilization and storage techniques of lenses (instead of commercially produced solutions) are at particular risk. Very rarely it can occurs after minor corneal abrasions infected with soil or ground waters. Typical classic clinical picture of Acanthameba keratoconjunctivitis include multifocal, patchy, corneal stroma infiltrates coalescing to form a central or paracentral non-suppurative ring in patient with severe ocular pain out of proportion to the clinical findings. Visual acuity is significantly decreased. Conjunctivitis is always secondary to keratitis.

Fungal Keratoconjunctivitis

Fungal keratoconjunctivitis can be caused by nonfilamentous fungi e.g. *Candida* species or filamentous fungi e.g. *Aspergillus* or *Fusarium* species. It should be suspected in cases of patients with bacterial or herpetic keratits unresponsive to standard treatment. It usually develops after trauma with vegetable matter (such as wood) and sometimes in immunocompromised patients. Clinical picture consists with gray, stromal, corneal infiltrate with indistinct, feathery borders. Visual acuity is significantly decreased. Sometimes satellite lesions surround the primary infiltrate. Purulent discharge in lower part of anterior chamber can also be found. Conjunctivitis in fungal infection is always secondary to keratitis.

Blepharoconjunctivitis

Blepharoconjunctivitis (inflammation of the eyelid margin and conjunctiva) is common ophthalmological disorder in children as well as one of the most difficult conditions to treat. It can be related to skin or lid diseases. Usually the anterior lid margin is affected but occasionally the inflammation of posterior lid margin is more pronounced (chronic meibomitis). The causes, clinical features and treatment are presented in Table 3. Complications of blepharoconjunctivitis are: recurrent chlazions, loss of eyelashes (madarosis) and thickening of lid margins (tylosis ciliaris).

Diagnosis of Conjunctival Infections

Slide stains of smears or scrapings: Direct identification of causative micro-organisms can be performed with slide stains smears and scrapings. Usually the material is obtained with conjunctival smears. Deep corneal scrapings are necessary for identifications of *Acanthamoeba* and fungi. The most frequently used stains are listed in Table 5.

Table 3: Pediatric infectious conjunctivitis: Main clinical diagnostic guidelines

Cause	Main causing factor	Duration	Main ocular manifestations	Systemic manifestations
Bacterial	Usually *Haemophilus* less frequently streptococci and staphylococci and enteric gram-negative organisms	5-7 days	Sticky purulent discharge, moderate conjunctival hyperemia, crustings on the eyelids and/or lashes, lids sealing in the morning upon awakening by purulent discharge. Some bacteria are able to cause conjunctival membranes or pseudomembranes (beta hemolytic *Streptococcus*, *Bordetella pertussis*).Very rarely acute conjunctivitis can progress to keratitis and infection of orbital tissue (preseptal cellulitis).	Very rarely sinusitis, rhinitis and otitis media. Preauricular lymph nods not enlarged
Hyper-acute bacterial	Often caused by *Neisseria* species (*N. gonorrhoeae*, meningitides) less often by other bacteria e.g. *Pseudomonas aeruginosa*		Develops usually in newborns and less often in pediatric patients. Bilateral, severe, fulminating conjunctivitis with profuse lid and conjunctiva edema, very copious, yellow-green, purulent discharge. There is high risk of a corneal infiltration and corneal perforation in hours. Can lead to blindness due to corneal opacification.	Septicemia with arthritis and pelvic inflammatory disease (rarely). Examine patient and his/her parents (veneral disease).
Viral	Usually adenoviruses, herpes simplex viruses less frequently varicella-zoster viruses, picornaviruses, molluscum contagiosum, or pox and papilloma viruses	2-3 weeks	Significant conjunctival hyperemia, copious, clear, watery, serous discharge, eyelid edema, follicular conjunctival reaction, sub- and conjunctival hemorrhages (picornaviruses). Typical vesicular eyelid rash in herpes simplex and vesicular skin eruptions in zoster, umbilical eyelids lesions in molluscum infections, verrucae in papilloma virus infection.. Often corneal involvement (keratitis). Very contagious.	Frequent history of recent fever, upper respiratory tract infections or pharyngitis, Enlarged preauricular lymph nodes.
Chlamydial	*Chlamydia trachomatis, psittaci and pneumoniae*	More than 3 weeks with exacerbations and remissions	Mucopurulent discharge, moderate hyperemia, follicular conjunctival reaction, pseudoptosis. Often corneal involvement (keratitis and pannus). Pronounced corneal changes and conjunctival cicatrization.	Pneumonia and otitis (in children), cervicitis and/or vaginitis (girls), symptomatic or non-symptometic urethritis (boys), enlarged preauricular lymph nodes. Examine patient and his/her parents (veneral disease).

Table 4: Blepharoconjunctivitis

Cause	Clinical features and Comments	Treatment and Comments
1. Staphyloccoccal infection 2. Meibomian gland dysfunction 3. Contact dermatitis 4. Eczema 5. Seborrheic dermatitis 6. Acne rosacea 7. Angular blepharitis—*Moraxella lacunata* 8. Unusual causes—molluscum, pediculosis	1. Lid margin edema 2. Lid crusting (scales) 3. Hyperemia of lid margins and conjunctiva 4. Small ulcerations of eyelid margin 5. Collarettes and crustings around eyelashes 6. Loss of eyelashes 7. Recurrent hordeola 8. Corneal marginal ulceration may develop (usually immune response)	1. Lid hygiene (baby shampoo lid scrubs) 2. Morning removal of crustings 3. Antibiotic ointment (tetracyclines, fluoroquinolones) to lid margin 4. Oral tetracycline for chronic or severe disease 5. Steroid ointment (selected cases)

Most common cause is underlined

Table 5: The most freqeuntly used slide stains

Stain	*What for*
Gram's stan	Bacteria, fungi
Giemsa stain	Bacteria, fungi, acanthamoeba, cytology
Gomori methamine silver stain	Acanthamoeba, fungi
Calcofluor white	Acanthamoeba
Acid-fast stain	*Mycobacteria*, *Nocardia*
Papanicolau stain	Cytology

Cultures

The conjunctival smears and corneal scrapings can be cultured on various mediums. Usually antibiotic sensitivity is simultaneously determined. The most frequently used culture mediums are presented in Table 6.

Cytology

Cytology is infrequently performed in diagnosis of infectious conjunctivitis but its results quite often can be very helpful. Previous treatment does not influence the results as in slide stains and cultures. Conjunctival smears and corneal scrapings are usually stained with Giemsa or Papanicolau method for

Table 6: The most frequently used culture media	
Culture media	*What for*
Blood agar	Most bacteria
Sabouraud's dextrose agar with cyclohexamide	Fungi
Thioglycolate broth	Aerobic and anaerobic bacteria
Chocolate agar in CO_2 jar	*Haemophilus*, *Neisseria gonorrhoeae*
Lowenstein-Jensen	*Mycobacteria*, *Nocardia*
Agar with *E. coli*	*Acanthamoeba*
Buffered charcoal-yeast extract agar	*Acanthamoeba*
Different viral cultures	Viruses

cytological examination. In patients with difficult to established and unproven diagnosis it is advisable to perform cytology and to treat according to its results.

Table 7: Interpretation of the cytology results	
Type of infection	*Cytology results*
Bacterial conjunctivitis	Polymorphonuclear leucocytes
Viral conjunctivitis	Mononuclear cells (lymphocytes and monocytes) (sometimes eosinophilic intranuclear inclusions can be found in epithelial cells in herpetic keratitis)
Chlamydial infection	Polymorphonuclear leucocytes, monocytes and perinuclear inclusions (Halberstaedter – von Provazek bodies)
Allergic conjunctivitis	Eosinophiles and basophiles
Fungal conjunctivitis	Polymorphonuclear leucocytes and giant cells with organisms
Acanthameba conjunctivitis	Corneal cysts

Immunological Tests

Immunodiagnostic tests are not routinely used diagnosis of conjunctival infections. For certain viral infections PCR tests may be used but they are not validated for ocular specimens. Herpcheck or ELISA tests for herpetic infections are also available. Suspected chlamydial infections can be confirmed by immnunofluorescent, ELISA and PCR tests.

Table 8: Neonatal and pediatric infectious conjunctivitis—main diagnostic guidelines	
Type of conjunctivitis	**Suggested diagnostic tests**
Bacterial	Diagnosed on the basis of medical history and eye examination. Diagnostic tests are indicated in neonatal bacterial conjunctivitis, difficult clinical cases, recurrent conjunctivitis and in patients not responding to medication.
Hyper-acute bacterial	It is mandatory to perform promptly slide stains, cultures and antibiotic sensitivity.
Viral	Diagnosed on the basis of medical history and eye examination. Tests (viral cultures and immunodiagnostic) are not very helpful can be performed in diagnostic difficult cases only.
Chlamydial	If diagnosis cannot been made on the clinical basis performance of cytology (Halberstaedter – von Provazek bodies), direct immunofluorescent antibody test, ELISA and PCR tests of ocular specimens may be helpful.

Toxic Conjunctivitis

Toxic conjunctivitis may develop after chronic exposure of conjunctival surface to various foreign materials. It includes eye medications (Table 9) and eye cosmetics (eyeliners and mascara). It may also occur as a reaction to proteins shed into the conjunctiva during molluscum contagiosum (see above) infections and Phthirus pubis infestations.

Toxic conjunctivitis manifests as a follicular conjunctivitis with serous discharge. In some patients trachoma-like syndrome may develop with follicles on the superior tarsus, pannus, keratitis and conjunctival scarring.

Removal of Phthirus pubis or molluscum lesions or discontinuation of eye medications cause regression of toxic conjunctivitis.

Table 9 : Ocular medications that may cause toxic conjunctivitis	
Neomycin	Dipivefrine
Gentamicin	Epinephrine
Idoxuridine	Brimonidine
Trifluorotimidine	Apraclonidine
Atropine	Pilocapine
Preservatives (thimerosal, benzalkonium chloride)	Eserine

Ligneous Conjunctivitis

Ligneous conjunctivitis is rare disorder of conjunctiva occurring primarily in children. It starts as a acute conjunctivitis with subsequent development membranes and pseudomembranes and woody (ligneous) indurations of the tarsal conjunctiva. The masses are composed of amorphous fibrous hyalinized material. Sometimes keratitis with corneal vascularization and secondary scarring can be seen in patients.Other mucous membranes, including upper respiratory tract (larynx, vocal chords, nose, trachea, bronchi), middle ear, sinuses, urinary tract, vagina, cervix and gingiva may be involved. Plasminogen deficiency has been identified as a cause of this disorder. Treatment includes surgical excision (followed by frequent recurrences), cryotherapy, chymotrypsin, hyaluronidase, topical steroids but with varying success. Other used method is combination of topical 2% cyclosporine and steroids. The most promising method of treatment to date seems to be topical plasminogen.

Folliculosis

The occurrence of multiple follicles, usually in inferior fornix, is normal in young children. Its etiology is probably similar to normal lymphoid hyperplasia which causes enlarged lymph nodes and tonsils.

Erythema Multiforme (EM), Stevens-Johnson Syndrome (SJS) and Toxic Epidermal Necrolysis (TEN)

This group of rare diseases are acute disorders of mucous membranes and skin. In 1993 a group of medical experts proposed a consensus definition and classification of EM, SJS, and TEN based on a photographic atlas and extent of body surface area involvement. According to this classification, Stevens-Johnson syndrome was classified as a separate disease from the erythema multiforme spectrum and added to toxic epidermal necrolysis. SJS and TEN are now considered as a variants of a single entity differing only in severity of clinical signs. The clinical classification is now as follows:

- EM minor – Clinical signs consists of symetrically distribiuted skin erythematous and edematous macules and papules evolving into classic "iris" or "target" lesions with bright red borders and central petechiae, vesicles or purpura. The lesions are usually self-limiting.
- EM major—Typical "target" or "iris' skin lesions with involvement of one or more mucous membranes; epidermal detachment involves less than 10% of total body surface area. Lesions may coalesce.
- SJS/TEN (Lyell's syndrome)- Widespread blisters predominant on the trunk and face, presenting with erythematous or pruritic macules and one or more mucous membrane erosions; epidermal detachment is less than 30% of total body surface area for SJS and 30% or more for TEN.

Etiology of the diseases is not completely understood but it is thought to be caused by a hypersensitivity reactions that can be triggered by a variety of stimuli, particularly bacterial, viral, protozoan fungal and food, drug and chemical products. In children most cases follow infections (usually *Mycoplasma pneumoniae* or herpes infections).

The diseases begins with the symptoms of malaise, fever headache and upper respiratory tract infections. Next symmetrical skin lesions develops on the extremities. The primary skin lesion is macula that evolve into a papule and then to a vesicles and/or bulla. Later the bullae break down and skin desquamates. In more severe cases also mucous membranes, the most frequently mouth, are involved. Sloughing of large areas or even all of the skin and mucous membranes can be observed in the most advanced cases.

Eye involvement occurs in 10% to 63% of EM patients and tends to parallel the severity of the skin and mucous membranes lesions. In EM minor it is typically mucopurulent conjunctivitis with papillary reaction of the tarsal conjunctiva. In EM major conjunctivitis is more severe with vesicles, bullae and pseudomembranes and membranes formation and symblepharon. Secondary infections may follow conjunctival changes.

In SJS and TEN eye invovement occurs approximately 85% of cases. At the beginning they are similar to EM but later there is more extensive membrane formation and conjunctival scarring. They may give rise to serious complications as lid margin deformities, punctal occlusion, metaplastic lashes, trichiasis keratinization of trasal conjunctiva and dry eye syndrome. Corneal changes such as punctate epithelial keratitis, erosions, neovascularization and eventually ulceration may be seen.

Mild cases of EM require only symptomatic treatment with topical antibiotics and steroids. Treatment should start early in the course of the disease to prevent development of secondary infections and conjunctival scarring. If synechias start to form between bulbar and tarsal conjunctiva they should be separated with a glass rod or cut with the scissors. In acute stage systemic steroids are usually necessary to control the course of the disease. In cicatricial stage artificial tears are used. In patients with advanced conjunctival scarring conjunctival, buccal mucous membrane or amniotic membrane transplantation should be considered to repair conjunctival surface. Other treatment possibilities include surface reconstruction with stem cells transplantation from other members of the family with or without use of simultaneous amniotic membrane transplantation as a carrier for proliferating stem cells. Other complications should be treated accordingly (see lid and cornea chapters).

Conjunctival Melanocytic Lesions

Melanocytic conjunctival lesions range from benign nevi and primary acquired melanosis (PAM) to malignant melanoma. Most of these lesions appear darkly-brown but in some of them the color is much less distinct or they can be even amelanotic. The melanin pigment is produced in conjunctival melanocytes and then is retained within the cytoplasm of these cells or discharged into the cytoplasm of adjacent epithelial cells or into subepithelial tissues as free particles. The melanin deposits stored within nonmelanocytic cells can induced proliferation of these cells and formation of pigmented lesions without being melanocytic in origin. So, not every melanocytic lesion is related directly with melanocytes.

Melanocytic lesions are very common. Studies performed in white population have shown that at least one patch of conjunctival melanosis in one eye can be seen in over one-third of population. The lesions can be congenital (common congenital nevus, oculodermal melanosis – nevus of Ota, blue nevus) and acquired (junctional nevus, compound nevus, subepithelial nevus, primary acquire melanosis, malignant melanoma). In children benign lesions predominate and premalignant (PAM) and malignant (melanoma) lesions occur primarily in older individuals. Some authors claim that all conjunctival nevi are congenital in origin but some of them manifest clinically later in childhood. Acquired nevi (junctional nevus, compound nevus, subepithelial nevus) share common clinical manifestations and they can be distinguished histologically. It is very unlikely that melanocytic conjunctival lesions transform to malignant melanoma in children although they can enlarge and become darker over timer. In adolescents the rate of malignant transformation is higher. Clinically conjunctival nevus presents as a slightly elevated, focal or less frequently diffuse lesions located usually in limbal or perilimbal area nasally o temporally in the interpalpebral fissure. Less common sites are extralimbal palpebral conjunctiva and semilunar folds. Their color range from dark brown to pink. They usually have associated, dilated, prominent conjunctival or episcleral vessels. Many nevi, most frequently acquired, contain microcysts. Clinical characteristics of melanotic conjunctival lesions are presented in Table 10.

Surgical excision is rarely indicated if pigmented lesions develop in childhood. Most of them could be left alone because of extremely low rate of malignant transformation. Very often they are excised because parents afraid their malignant transformation. Lesions appearing in adolescents have higher rate of malignant transformation and surgery is indicated if they enlarge.

Tumors of the Conjunctiva

Tumors of the conjunctiva may develop from epithielial cells, melanocytes (see above), lymphoid and mesenchymal tissues. Epithelial tumors are very rare in children.

Capillary Hemangioma

Conjunctival capillary hemangioma is very rare in children. Usually they are associated with lid, cutaneous or orbital hemangiomas which are very common in infancy and small children. It is hamartomatous proliferation of primitive mesenchymal tissues and is composed of endothelial-lined, anastomosing, immature blood vessels filled with blood and separated by fibrous septa.

Table 10: Differential diagnosis of pigmented lesions of the conjunctiva

Features / Type of lesion	Congenital	Location	Color	Intralesional cysts	Thickness	Movements over the globe	Boundaries	Focality	Other manifestations and remarks
Common congenital nevus	+	Bulbar and palpebral conjunctiva	Brown to nonpigmented	Rare	Often thick	Moves freely over the sclera	Distinct	Unifocal	Nevi of epsilateral upper and lower eyelids
Oculodernal melanocytosis (nevus of Ota)	+	Episclera and sclera	Bluish gray	No cysts	Does not elevate surface of the episclera	Does not move with conjunctiva	Spiculated edges, outline lymphatic and blood vessels	Diffuse	Nevi of periocular skin, uvea, optic nerve, meninges, rarely glaucoma. Primarily in dark-skinned people. In Caucasians may be correlated with conjunctival and uveal melanomas.
Blue nevus	+	Anywhere	Brown or black (blue in the skin)	No cysts	Mild thickening	Move freely over the sclera	Distinct	Unifocal	Blue colored nevi of the skin
Acquired nevus (junctional, compound, subepithelial)	–	Juxtalimbal area and epibulbar site	Brown to nonpigmented	May occur in compound and subepithelial nevi	Junctional nevi flat, compound and subepithelial nevi may be elevated	Moves freely over the sclera	Well defined	Unifocal or diffuse	Common clinical manifestations, low potential for becoming malignant
Episcleral melanosis	–	Superficial sclera	Gray	No cysts	Flat	Nonmovable	Spiculated edges	Multifocal	–
Primary acquired melanosis (PAM	–	Anywhere	Golden or chocolate brown	No cysts	Flat	Moves freely over the sclera	Nondistinct	Unifocal or multifocal	Very rare in children, usually in white persons. Malignant malanoma can develop in 50% of the patients with PAM with atypia
Malignant melanoma	–	Anywhere	Brown to nonpigmented	May be present	Elevated or nodular	Moves freely over the sclera	Nondistinct	Unifocal or multifocal	Extremely rare in children

Conjunctival lesions involve the palpebral and fornical conjunctiva and are very rarely seen in bulbar area. Often there are continous with orbital or lid or even intracranial lesions. They are small and do not cover visual axis. Usually capillary hemangiomas appear in the age of 2-5 months and increase in size during first year of life and afterwards they regress spontaneously. Treatment of conjunctival lesions is not necessary but sometimes it is indicated to treat associated lid or orbital lesions (with intralesional steroid injections, systemic steroids, radiotherapy, systemic interferon, laser or surgical excision) if their size interfere with the function of the eye. Removal is often followed by recurrences.

Lymphangioma

As capillary hemangioma also lymphangioma is very rare in children. It is also hamartomatous proliferation of vascular tissue and is composed of lymph-like channels lined of endothelial cells. Usually they appear in the first decade of life. They manifest as white, round, elevated, subconjunctival masses with clear fluid filled cystic spaces. Sometimes blood can be seen within the lymphatic spaces. Lymphangiomas can regress spontaneously. They also respond to corticosteroid therapy. Other form of therapy are cryotherapy or external beam radiation. Surgical excision is rarely indicated.

Lymphangioma should be differentiated with dilated lymphatics—lymphangiectasia. It occurs usually in the interpalpebral area and is caused by the obstruction of lymphatic drainage vessels by conjunctival anomalies like scars, tumors (neurofibromatosis) and in Turner syndrome. They are seen as translucent dilated channels under the conjunctiva and they can be easily overlooked because of intensive white color of underlying sclera. Diffuse form was also described clinically resembling chemosis. Because lymphatics have a connection with blood vessels they can be filled (usually intermittently) with blood.

Leukemic Infiltration of the Conjunctiva

Leukemic infiltrations are usually located in the fornices as a pale or pink subepithelial unilateral masses. Less frequently they can be bilateral or seen as a diffuse infiltrations. In most cases they are late signs of leukemia but rarely they can be the first manifestation of these diseases. Conjuntival leukemic infiltrations regress after chemotherapy. Radiation therapy is rarely indicated, usually in chemotherapy-resistant cases.

Choristomas

They are common congenital lesions with little growth potential composed of dermal and epithelial elements that are not normally found in the conjunctiva. Conjunctival choristomas can be divided to solid limbal dermoids, dermolipomas and complex choristomas.

Solid limbal dermoids are dense, round, elevated, smooth, yellow, unilateral tumors located at the inferotemporal limbus. Most of them are superficial but some can penetrate deeply into the sclera or cornea. Inside dermoids contain thick, gelatinous masses with hair, sweat glands, fat, sebaceous glands and sometimes teeth. They can be associated with eyelid colobomas. Surgical excision is usually performed because of cosmetic reasons. In deep lesions complete excision may require peripheral keratoplasty.

Dermolipomas are smooth, yellow, elevated tumors occurring typically on the temporal bulbar conjunctiva. They may be isolated lesions and are usually unilateral or may be part of Goldenhar's syndrome (oculoauriculovertebral dysplasia) where they are often bilateral. Dermolipomas can extend posteriorly to the orbit between superior and lateral rectus muscles. Surgical excision is indicated because of cosmetic reasons or when the tumor restricts eye movements. Usually anterior part of the tumor is excised because deep penetration into the orbit may damage rectus muscles, lacrimal gland or levator palpebrae muscle.

Complex choristomas clinically resemble dermoids or dermolipomas but often have more red and vascularized appearance. They consist of ectopic tissues such as acinar glands, cartilages, adipose tissue and smooth muscles. They can penetrate deeply into sclera or cornea. Some growth of the tumor may be seen during puberty. Surgery is usually not indicated because of deep penetration into the globe.

Other Conjunctival Lesions

Pingueculum and Pterygium

Pingueculae and pterygia are rare in children. They can found in children living in hot and dry countries. More frequent are pseudopterygia developing after corneal and conjunctival inflammatory diseases or excision of corneal lesions (dermoid).

Surgery is these lesions is rarely necessary in children. It is usually performed because of cosmetic reasons.

Papilloma

Conjunctival papillomas is common in children. They are caused by human papillomavirus. The infection usualy manifests as follicular conjunctivitis but occasionally tumor-like lesions with papillomatous surface and typical vascular pattern (hypervascularity) may develop. The lesions be removed surgically, they tend to be recurrent in children. Cryotherapy, CO_2 laser, diathermy and interferon therapy have been tried to prevent recurrences.

Xeroderma Pigmentosum

Xeroderma pigmentosum is a group of autosomal recessive diseases in which light induced damage to nuclear DNA cannot be repaired through the normal endonuclease-initiated multistep process. It causes excessive skin sensitivity to sunlight (most noticeably in exposed areas) resulting in widespread skin pigmentation, telangiectasis, keratosis, and development of basal cell and squamous cell carcinomas, malignant melanomas and other tumors. In 20% of patients may have neurological abnormalities including mental retardation, microcephaly, spasticity, ataxia, cerebellar atrophy and deafness. The most common conjunctival complications are conjunctivitis, conjunctival melanosis and dry eye syndrome. Less frequent lesions include squamous cell carcinoma, melanoma and angiosarcoma of the conjunctiva.

Management of xeroderma pigmentosum consists of protection from ultraviolet light and early excision of suspicious tumors. Survival is reduced because of possibility of malignant neoplasms development.

Epithelial Cysts

Epithelial inclusion cysts may appear in older children and can be found both in bulbar and palpebral conjunctiva. They are lined with nonkeratinized, squamous epithelium and filled with clear fluid. Usually they are symptom free and may disappear spontaneously. Treatment consists of surgical excision and is performed mainly because of concern of parents. Sometimes cysts can recur after removal.

Avitaminosis A

The disease is caused by vitamin A deficiency as well as a more generalized malnutrition. The disease is even nowadays one of the leading causes of childhood blindness worldwide. Main ocular manifestations include nyctalopia (night blindness), keratinization of corneal epithelium (xerophthalmia), pannus and progressive corneal opacification. In severe cases corneal ulcers and scars with keratomalacia (corneal necrosis) can develop. Typical conjunctival signs of avitaminosis A are Bitot's spots. They are foamy, elevated patches of the temporal, exposed areas of the conjunctiva. They consists of inflammatory cells and *Corynebacterium* xerosis. Other conjunctival changes include keratinization and thickening of the conjunctival epithelium and dry eye syndrome.

The treatment is protein, caloric and vitamin A replacement.

Conjunctival Manifestations of Systemic Diseases

Comparing with other parts of the eye conjunctiva is rarely involved in systemic diseases. Conjunctival manifestations of systemic diseases are grouped in Table 11.

Table 11: Conjunctival manifestations of systemic diseases

Disorders	*Conjunctival manifestations*	*Disorders*	*Conjunctival manifestations*
Alkaptonuria	"Oil droplet" epithelial limbal opacities, pigmentation near horizontal rectus muscles, pigmented pingueculae, pigmented granules in episclera	**Leptospirosis**	Conjunctivitis
Amyloidosis	Yellow-white, waxy, flat, nontender, subconjunctival masses, usually in the inferior fornix	**Measles**	Purulent conjunctivitis and keratitis
Ataxia telangiectasia (Louis-Bar syndrome)	Tortuous and telangiectatic conjunctival vessels	**Mucolipidosis I**	Conjunctival vessels tortuosity
Avitaminosis A	Thickening and keratinization of conjunctival epithelium, dry eye syndrome, Bitot's spots, pannus	**Riley-Day syndrome**	Tear deficiency
Cat scratch disease (Parinaud's oculo-glandular syndrome)	Unilateral follicular conjunctivitis	**Reiter syndrome**	Conjunctivitis
Cystinosis	Conjunctival cystine crystal depositions (needle-shaped, refractile, polychromatic)	**Richnert-Hanhart syndrome**	Conjunctival thickening
Erythema multiforme, Stevens-Johnson syndrome and TEN	Mucopurulent conjunctivitis with papillary reaction of the tarsal conjunctiva, erythematous and edematous macules and papules, vesicles, bullae, pseudomembranes and membranes formation, conjunctival scarring See above	**Ring D chromosome**	Epicanthal folds
Fabry disease	Conjunctival vessels tortuosity	**Sarcoidosis**	Conjunctivitis, conjunctival granulomas, symblepharon
Gaucher disease	Prominent pingueculae	**Sturge-Weber syndrome**	Tortuous, dilated conjunctival and episcleral vessels
Goldenberg syndrome	Conjunctival telangiectasis	**Trisomy 18**	Epicanthal folds
Herpetic infections (HSV 1 and 2, VZV)	Conjunctivitis with corneal involvement. See above	**Turner syndrome**	Epicanthal folds
Hyperlipoproteinemia	Conjunctival xanthomata	**13 q deletion**	Epicanthal folds
Kawasaki syndrome	Conjunctivitis	**18 q deletion**	Epicanthal folds
Klippel-Trenaunay-Weber syndrome	Conjunctival angiomas	**18 r deletion**	Epicanthal folds

Flow Chart 1: Stepwise differential diagnosis of "red eye"

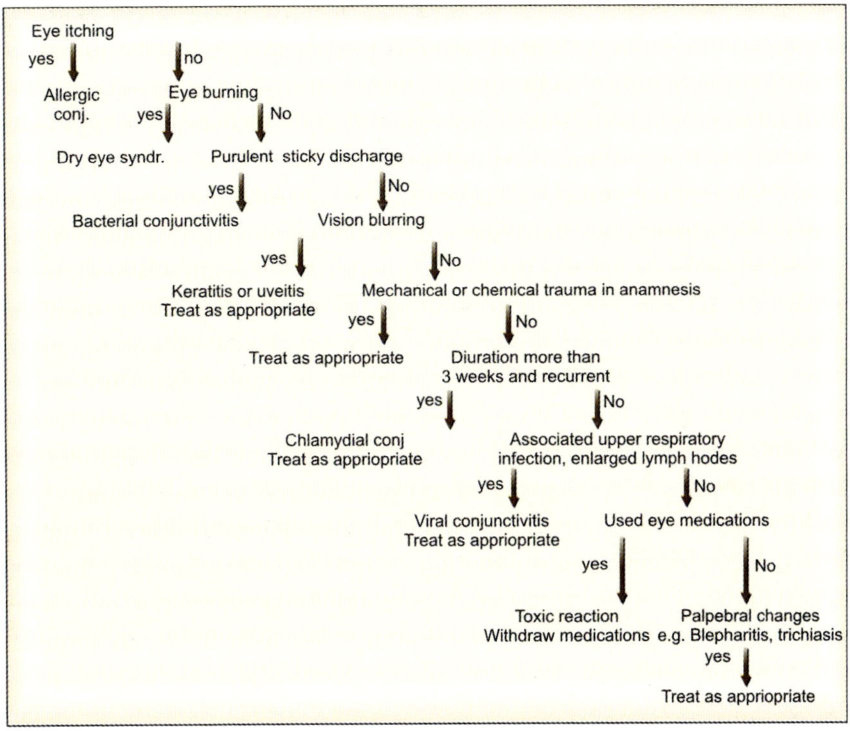

Chapter 29

Pediatric Corneal Diseases: Current Concepts and Management

Ashok Sharma (India)

Introduction

Pediatric corneal disease can be conveniently classified as congenital and acquired. In the acquired group corneal infections, eye allergy, corneal trauma, ectatic disorders, nutritional diseases and ocular surface disorder are major subgroups. Pediatric corneal disease diagnostic and management challenge. This is because of the unique presentation, non-communication of the problem and difficulties in proper examination. Majority of congenital corneal diseases may have systemic associations. Management of pediatric corneal disease requires extra effort. Immature visual system makes them susceptible to amblyopia. Decisions on surgical treatment including penetrating keratoplasty may be crucial. Although early surgery is advocated to prevent amblyopia, it is technically demanding and the outcome is less favorable than adults. In this review common pediatric corneal diseases and management is discussed.

Sclerocornea

Sclerocornea is a developmental anomaly in which the clear corneal stroma is replaced by opaque tissue simulating the sclera. The curvature of cornea is flatter, similar to sclera. The condition is nonprogressive and is known to occur bilaterally more often than unilateral. This condition is sporadic in most of the cases. However, both dominant and recessive patterns of inheritance have been reported. The autosomal recessive cases exhibit severe disease, total sclerocornea and the autosomal dominant cases, present with milder form i.e. peripheral sclerocornea. Sclerocornea has also been reported to occur due to chromosomal aberrations.

Histopathological studies of sclerocornea have demonstrated morphological features resembling sclera. The histopathological features include irregular epithelium, thickened basement membrane and fragmented or absent Bowman's layer. Elastic and collagen fibers in the stroma are of increased thickness and variable diameter. Posterior fibers are usually of smaller diameter compared to the anterior fibers. Because of irregular organization of collagen lamella, the transparency of the cornea is lost. The most common association of sclero cornea is cornea plana. Other ocular anomalies described in association with sclerocornea include, aniridia, blue sclera, cataract, closed angle glaucoma, ectopia lentis, hyperopia, micro cornea, microphthalmos, anterior segment dysgenesis, corneal opacities, retinal aplasia, retinal coloboma and uveal coloboma. Sclerocornea has been reported in association with numerous systemic anomalies including craniofacial defect, cerebellar dysfunctions, cranial dystrophies, cryptorchism, deafness, polydactyly, Hurler's syndrome, trisomy B, 18 and osteogenesis imperfecta.

The developmental abnormality for the occurrence of sclerocornea is absence of normal primitive limbal tissue at seventh to tenth gestational weeks. The normal limbal tissue at this stage allows mesenchymal cells of neural crest origin to differentiate into either sclera or cornea. The normal limbal anlarge also allows corneal curvature to exceed than that of sclera. In absence of normal

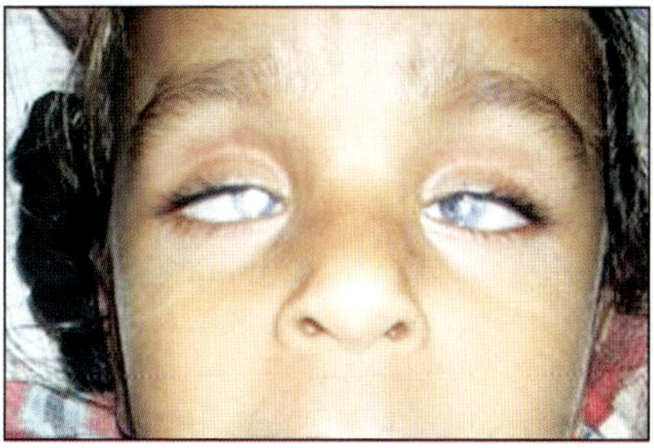

Figure 1: Bilateral sclerocornea

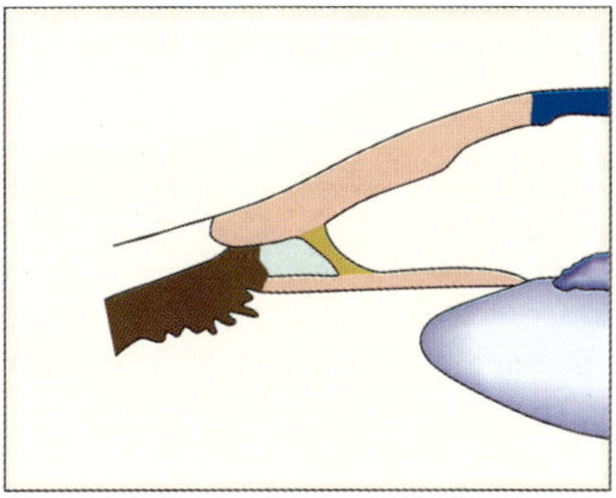

Posterior keratoconus	Peter's Anomaly	
Posterior corneal Excavation	Posterior Corneal Defect and Leukoma	Posterior corneal defect and leukoma
	Iris Adhesions to Leukoma margin	Iris adhesions to leukoma margin
		Lens appositon to leukoma

Posterior Embryotoxon	Axenfeld's Anomaly	Rieger's Anomaly
Prominent Schwalbe's line	Prominent Schwalbe's line	Prominent Schwalbe's line
	Iris Stands to Schwalbe's line	Iris Stands to Schwalbe's line
		Hypoplasia anterior Iris stroma

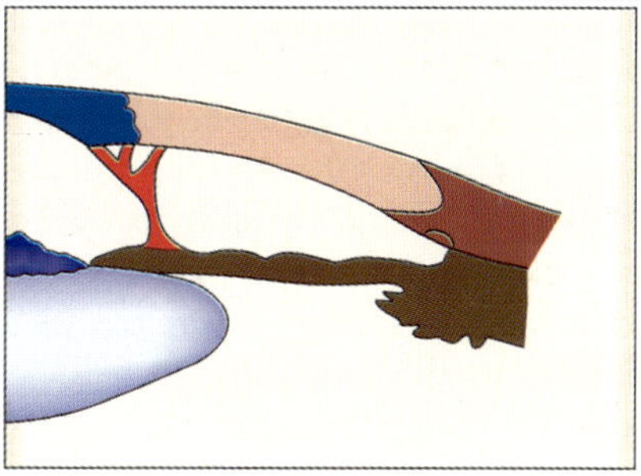

Figure 2: Clinical spectrum of congenital anomalies of anterior segment

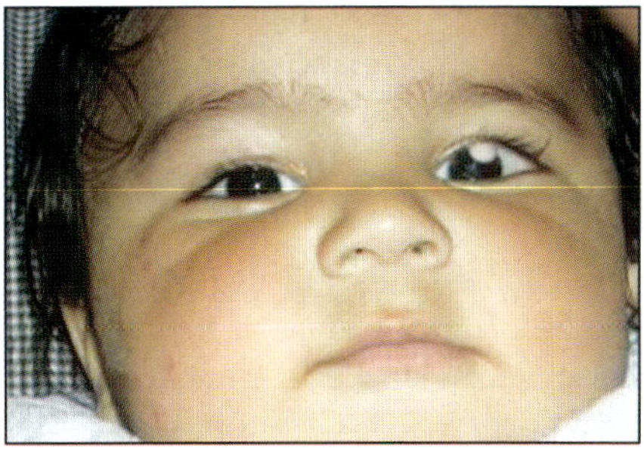

Figure 3: Limbal dermoid

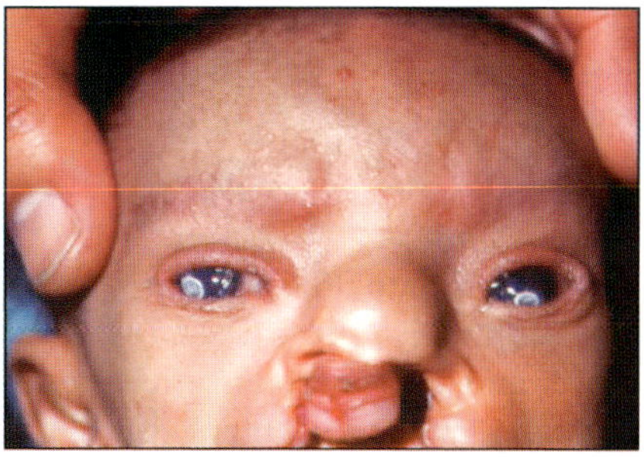

Figure 4: Bilateral corneal ulcers in a child with multiple congenital anomalies

limbal anlage cornea curvature is flattened. This may explain the close relationship between sclerocornea and cornea plana. On this basis, it has been proposed, that sclerocornea and cornea plana may be considered as a single entity.

Cycloplegic refraction and correction of refractive error at the earliest age is of paramount importance. Occlusion treatment should be initiated as soon as refractive error is detected. In cases with generalized sclerocornea with total corneal opacification early penetrating keratoplasty may considered as an attempt to improve visual acuity. However, poor visual prognosis in view of complications including allograft reaction, development of glaucoma and association with severe ocular abnormalities should be explained to the parents. In view of poor visual outcome, frequent examination of the child under general anesthesia is required. Parents should be adequately counseled before considering penetrating keratoplasty in these cases.

Development of Cornea and Anterior Segment

The corneal epithelium is formed by surface ectoderm after separation of the lens vesicle at 14 mm (6 weeks) stage. Corneal stroma and endothelium in derived from too waves of meserchyme. The first wave insulate between the surface ectoderm and detached lens vesicle at the 12 mm (6 weeks) stage and form corneal endothelium. The endothelial cells secrete collagen that form anterior banded portion of descemet's membrane during intrauterine life and post homogenous 'non-banded' layer after birth. Later at 27 mm (7 weeks) stage the second wave of mesenchyme form corneal stroma. These waves of mesenchyme are and currently believed to originate from neuroectoderm of the neural crest.

Bowman's membrane develops as modification of anterior corneal stroma at about 4 month stage. The epithelial basement membrane consists of collagen secreted by the epithelium.

Absence of the Cornea

True agenesis of the cornea as an isolated abnormality is unknown, however in association with agenesis of other ocular structures, this congenital anomaly has been described. Primary congenital aphakia with agenesis of cornea has been reported.

Cryptophthalmos

True cryptophthalmos (ablepharon) occurs when eyelids fail to form, cornea and conjunctiva are exposed. Due to the lack of appearance of lid folds the brows and lashes are absent. In addition lacrimal gland and puncta may be missing. Anterior segment of the globe is disorganized. Cryptophthalmos is usually transmitted as autosomal recessive disorder. The term cryoptophthalmos syndrome has been used to describe association of cryptophthalmos

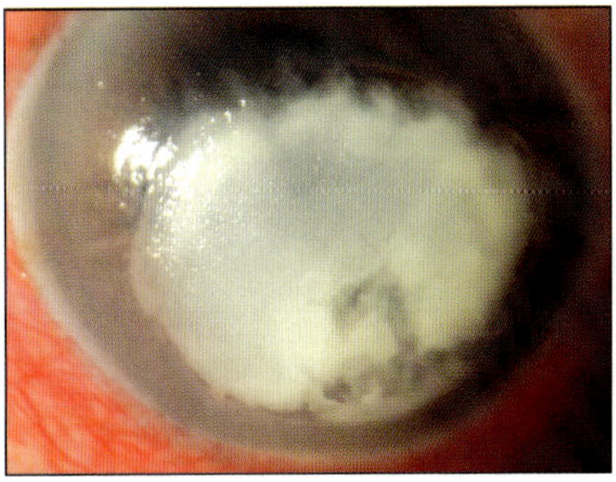

Figure 5A: Fungal corneal ulcer with hyphate margins in a child

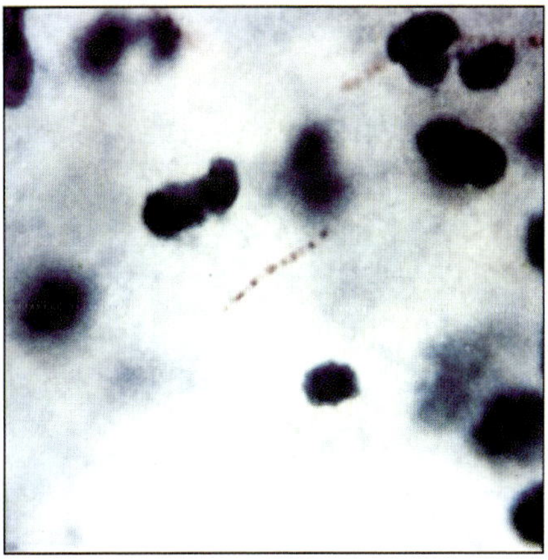

Figure 6A: Gram stain showing Streptococci viridans

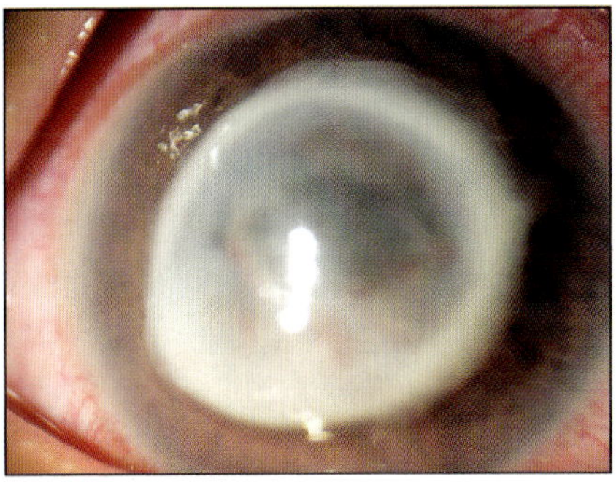

Figure 5B: Pseudomonas ulcer in a child

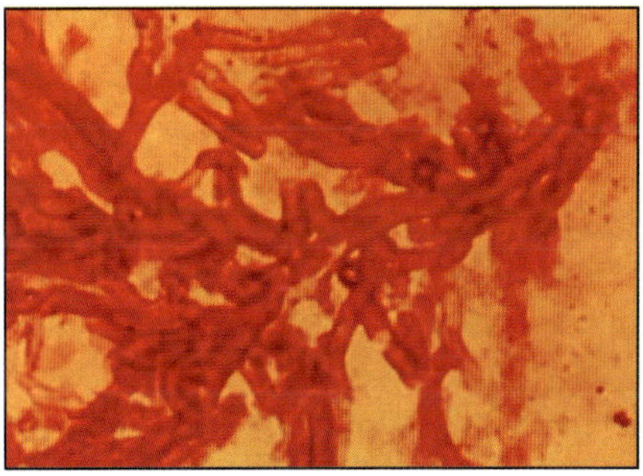

Figure 6B: KOH wet mount showing branched fungal hyphae

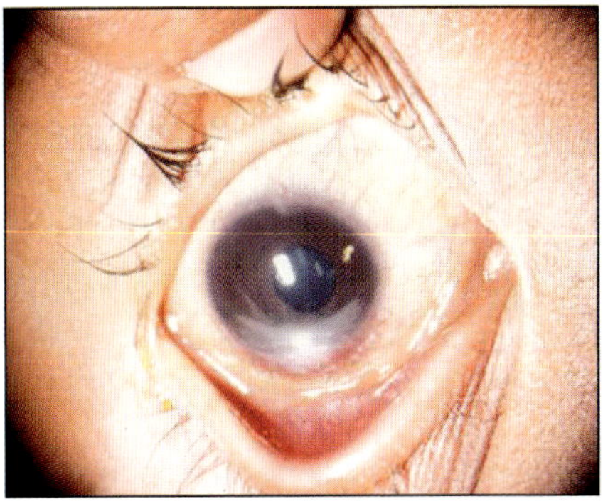

Figure 5C: Staphylococcal ulcer in a child

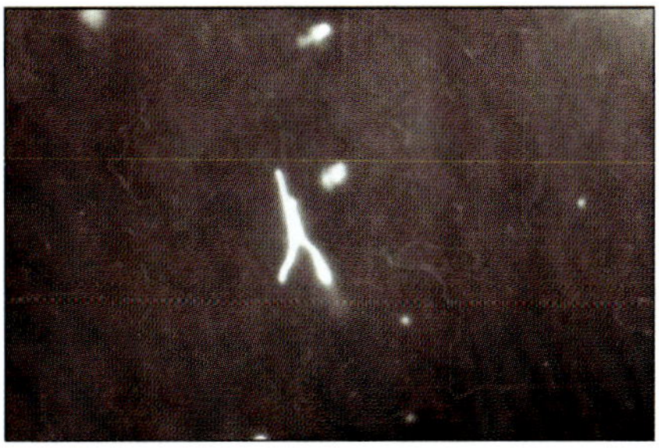

Figure 6C: Fungal hyphae on fluorescent microscopy

Table 1: Chronology and source of development of anterior segment structure

Anterior Chamber	*Differential Growth*	*Surrounding Tissue*	*20 mm (7 Week)*
Iris Stroma	Third wave mesenchyme	Neuroectoderm / neural crest	
Sphincter and dilator muscle	Third wave of mesenchyme	Neuroectoderm / neural crest	50 mm
Pigment epithelium	O??? neuroectoderm	Rim of optic cup	(3weeks)
Lens	Separation of lens vesicle	Lens vesicle	(6 weeks)
Sclera	Mesoderm	Surrounding optic cup	20 mm (7th week – 5th weeks)
Epithelium	Surface ectoderm	Lens vesicle	6 week (12 mm)
Corneal endothelium	1st wave	Surface ectoderm and lens vericle	6 week (12 mm)
Corneal stroma	2nd wave	Anterior banded I-V	7 week (27 mm)
Corneal descemet's	Secre?? By endothelium	Anterior banded I-V post non banded	After birth
Bowman membrane	Consternation of anterior stroma	Stroma	4 month
Basement membrane	Secreted by epithelium	Stroma	

with any of the extraocular abnormality. Associated systemic abnormalities include craniofacial deformities, syndactly, spina bifida, deformed ears or teeth, cleft palate and lips.

Affected patients have a layer of skin extending forehead to molar region. An incomplete form, in which nasal aspect of the lid fold is involved and the abortive form in which the upper eyelid is replaced by fold of skin adherent to upper third of cornea, the lower eyelid is normal have been recognized. In true cryptophthalmos visual prognosis is extremely poor and no treatment is indicated.

Pseudocryptophthalmos

Pseudo cryptophthalmos (total ankyloblepharon) refers to a condition in which eyelids form but fail to separate. Normal cornea and conjunctiva are covered by the skin. In contrast to true form brows and eyelashes are formed. In pseudocryptophthalmos eyeball is normal and vision may be restored surgically by creating palpebral fissure and separating the eyelids.

Abnormalities of Size

In a normal newborn, cornea is 10 mm in horizontal diameter. The normal adult cornea measures approximately 12 mm in horizontal diameter. In a child, the cornea usually reaches adult size by 2 years of age.

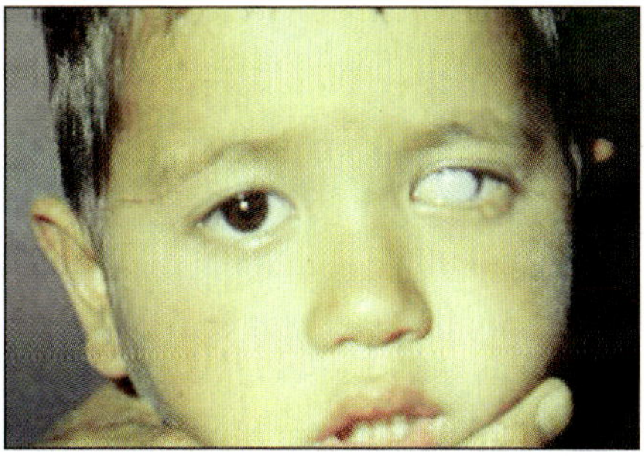

Figure 7: Opaque therapeutic graft in a child

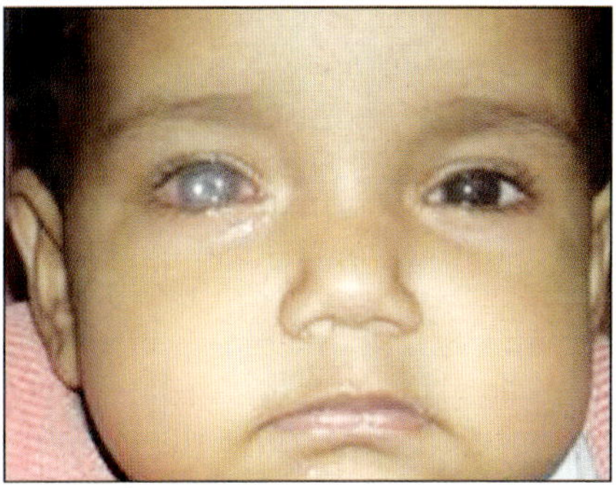

Figure 8A: Bacterial corneal ulcer in a child

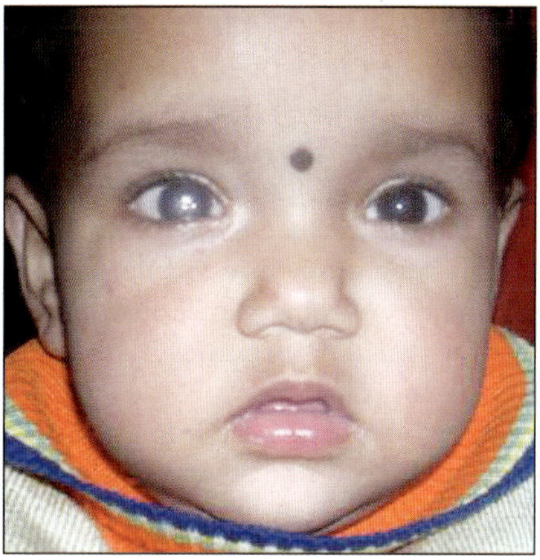

Figure 8B: Healed bacterial corneal ulcer

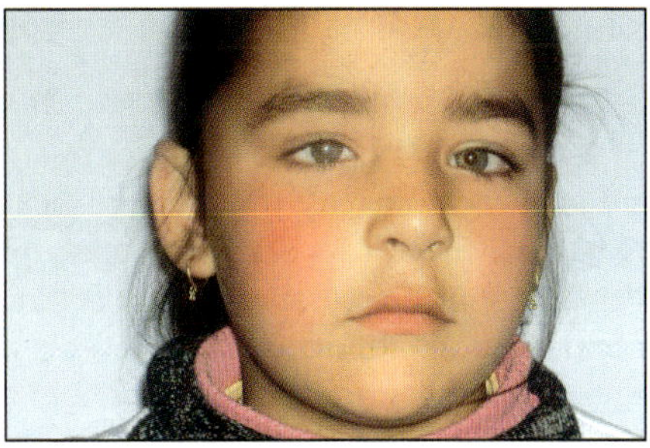

Figure 9A: Healed herpes simplex keratitis in a child (RE)

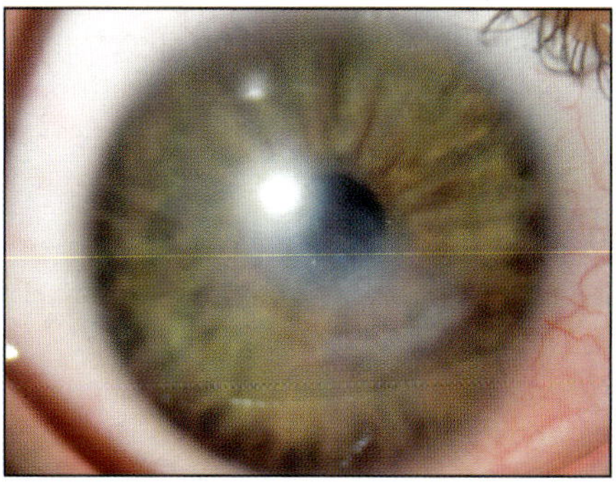

Figure 9B: Corneal opacity following herpes simplex keratitis resulting amblyopia

Megalocornea

Megalocornea is a nonprogressive condition characterized by an enlarged cornea greater than 13 mm in horizontal diameter without any evidence of glaucoma. The term anterior megalophthalmos is used to describe the condition in which the ciliary ring and the lens are enlarged. High myopia and with the rule astigmatism are frequent associations. Megalocornea is most often linked recessive and most commonly (90%) occurs in males. Complications including ectopia lentis, glaucoma secondary to associated anomalies of angle and cataract may develop in adult life. Systemic abnormalities those may be associated with megalocornea include Marfan's syndrome, craniosynostosis and Alport's syndrome. Megalocornea possibly result from failure of growth of anterior tips of optic cup.

Microcornea

Microcornea is defined as cornea that has a horizontal diameter of 10 mm or less in an otherwise normal globe. Microcornea can occur as an isolated anomaly. Anterior microphthalmos refer to a condition in which the entire anterior segment is small. The micro ophthalmic eye is usually malformed. Nanophthalmos describes an eye that is small but otherwise normal. Microcornea is non-progressive, unilateral or bilateral condition. Most of the cases are inherited as autosomal dominant or autosomal recessive. The small cornea is transparent and of normal thickness. The cornea being flatter, may cause hyperopia, depending upon the axial length. In later life 20% patients with microcornea may develop open angle glaucoma. These patients with microcornea are also predisposed to narrow angle glaucoma. Infantile glaucoma may coexist rarely. Microcornea has been reported in association with Weill-Marchesaini syndrome, Ehlers-Danlos syndrome, Rieger's syndrome, Norries Disease and rubella syndrome. Microcornea has been hypothesized to develop due to an overgrowth of anterior tips of optic cup, leaving a less than normal space for the cornea. Detailed clinical examination, including careful slitlamp biomicroscopy is performed. Ultrasonography both A and B scan may help to differentiate microcornea from other conditions. Visual prognosis in isolate microcornea is excellent with correction of refractive error. However, because of frequent associated ocular findings additional treatment may be indicated.

Peter's Anomaly

Peter's anomaly is characterized by congenital corneal opacity with iridocorneal adhesions that may extend from the iris collarette to the border of corneal opacity. The disorder is usually sporadic, however autosomal recessive and irregular dominance inheritance have been described. Ocular abnormalities including cataract, glaucoma and microcornea have been described in 50% of the patients. Peter's anomaly is bilateral in 80% off cases. Patients having systemic malformations affecting major organ system have been described as to suffer from Peter's Plus syndrome. Peter's anomaly has been classified into two types. Type I, a neuroectodermal type shows no associated lenticular changes. Type

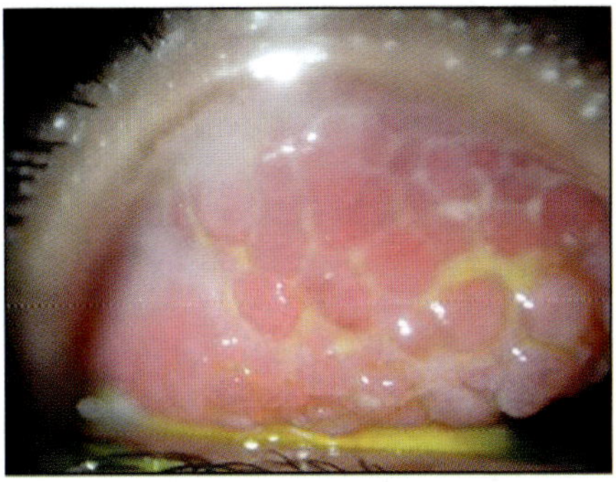

Figure 10A: Severe palpebral form of vernal conjunctivitis

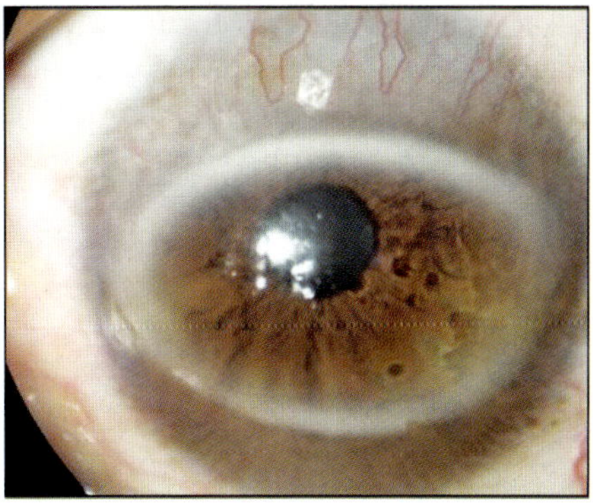

Figure 10B: Severe limbal form of vernal conjunctivitis

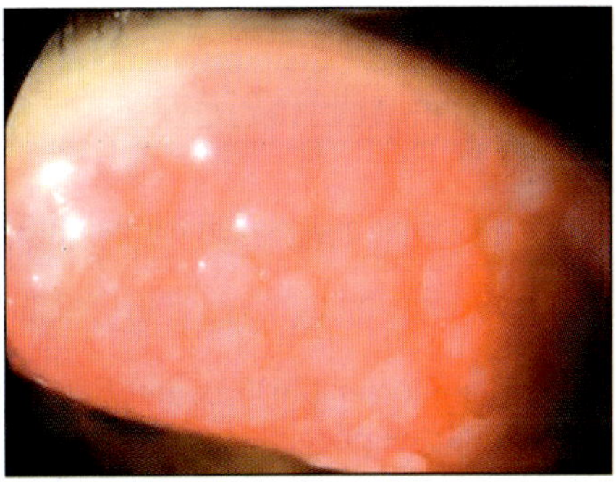

Figure 11A: Recalcitrant vernal conjunctivitis before supra tarsal injection of triamcinolone acetonide

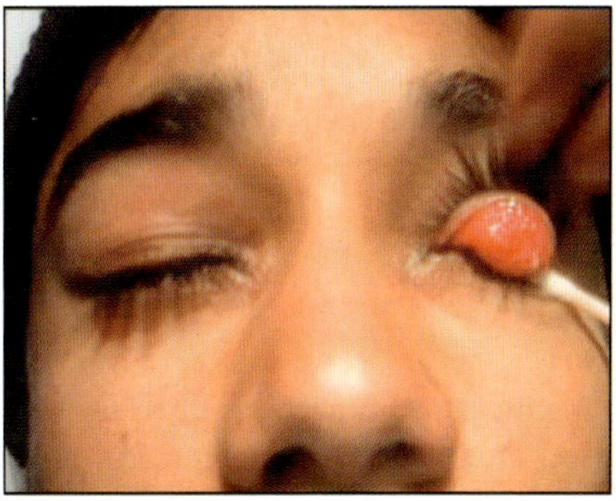

Figure 11B: Eversion of eyelid after instilling topical anesthesia

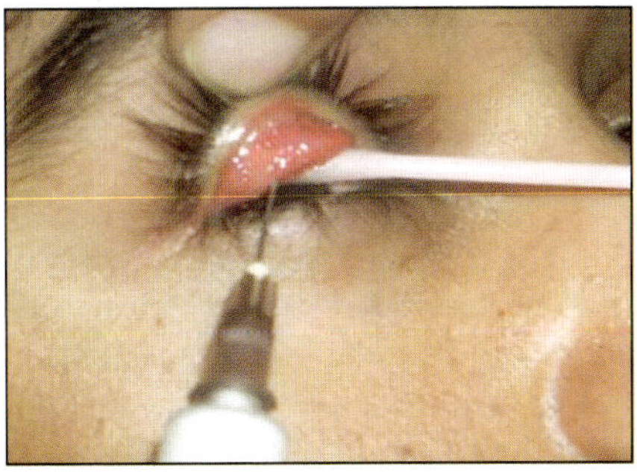

Figure 11C: Supra tarsal injection being given after lifting tarsal plate

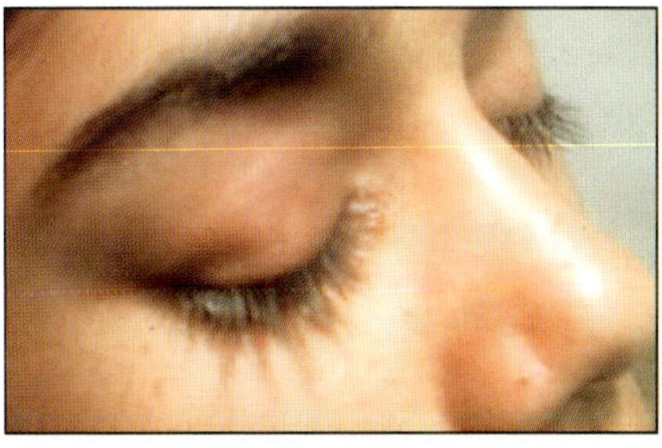

Figure 11D: Fullness, after injection above tarsal plate

II, a surface ectoderm form shows associated lens changes. Crystalline lens may lie close to the posterior corneal surface. In some cases, lens may be at normal positions but lenticular opacities may be present. Cataract may be polar subcapsular or reduplication type. Corneal opacity may be denser in Peter's anomaly type II in comparison to type I. Histopathological examination shows localized defect of posterior stroma, Descemet's membrane and corneal endothelium in area of corneal opacity. The corneal abnormalities are believed to result from incomplete migration of the neuralcrest derived mesenchymal cells during embryogenesis. It represents the spectrum of congenital anterior segment anomalies.

Corneal Involvement in Chromosomal Aberrations

Corneal Involvement in Chromosomal Disorders

Chromosomal abnormalities result in multisystem, wide spread ocular findings. The major corneal ocular and systemic associations.

Corneal Invovement in Mucopolysaccharidosis

Corneal Invovement in Mucopolysaccharidosis.
Mucopolysaccharidosis V has been reclassified as mucopolysaccharidosis I-S*

Cystinosis

Cystinosis is an autosomal recessive disorder. Gene locus 17p13 is involved. It is characterized by defect of lysosomal cystein transport system, resulting accumulation of cystine in the cornea. It is characterized by conjunctival and corneal cystine crystal deposition (needle-shaped, refractile, polychromatic crystals in full thickness of peripheral corneal and anterior central stroma band keratopathy and photophobia. Infantile and adolescent forms have been in addition patchy retinal abnormalities and occasional macular changes. Infantile form develops renal failure and ultimately death. Adolescent form also develops renal failure. In adult form there is no renal failure.

Alkaptonuria

Alkaptonuria is an autosomal recessive disorder. Genelocus 3q21-q23 is involved. It is characterized by deficiency of homogentisate-1, 2-dioxygenase resulting deposition of hemogentisic acid in the cornea. Triangular patches of intrascleral pigmentation near insertion of horizontal rectus muscles, "oil-droplet" opacities in limbal corneal epithelium and Bowman's layer, pigmented pingeculae, irregular pigmented granules in episclera are characteristic of alkaptonuria functional changes only joint pain and stiffness occurs.

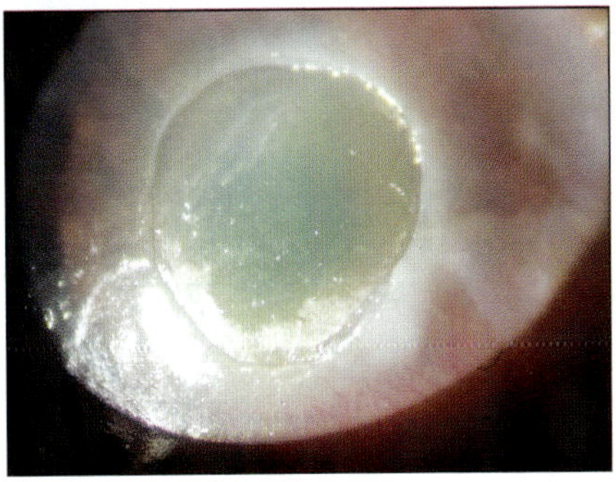

Figure 12A: Large vernal ulcer with plaque

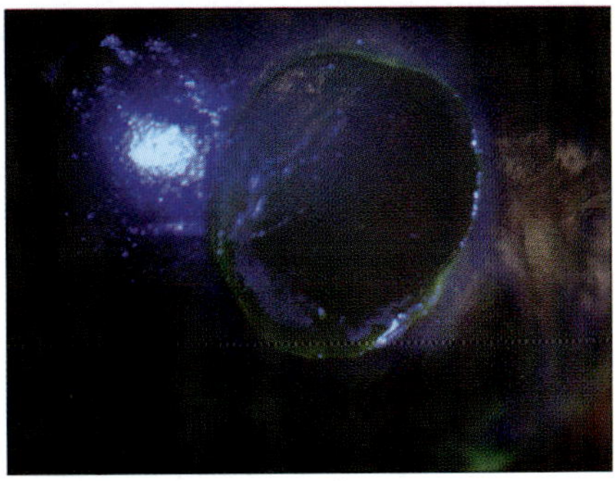

Figure 12B: Vernal plaque: staining poorly with fluorescein

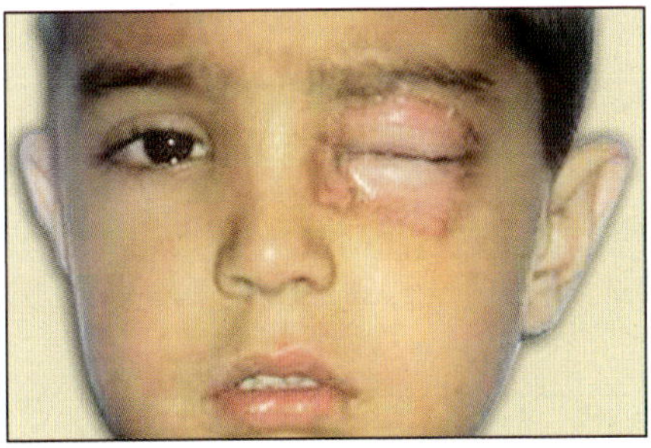

Figure 13 Cracker injury: skin burns

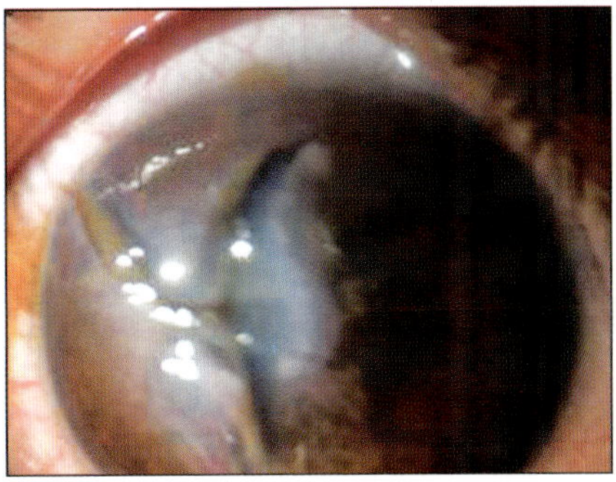

Figure 14: Corneal laceration for repair under general anesthesia

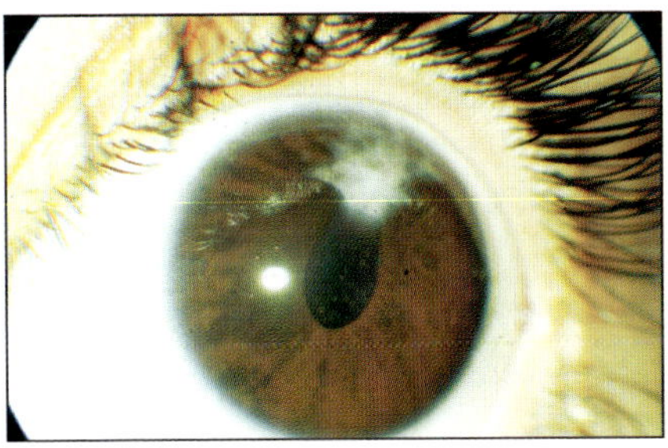

Figure 15: Repaired corneal laceration with pseudophakia following eye injury (BCVA 20/30)

Table 2: Corneal manifestations in chromosomal disorders

Sr. No.	*Genetic Finding*	*Ocular Manifestations*	*Systemic Manifestations*
1	4p deletion (Wolf-Hirschhorn syndrome)	Hypertelorism, ptosis, microphthalmos, strabismus, cataract	Growth retardation, microcephaly, micrognathia, hypotonia, seizures
2	13q deletion	Hypertelorism, ptosis, epicanthal folds, microphthalmos, retinoblastoma	Microcephaly, facial malformation, absent thumbs
3	18q deletion	Hypertelorism Ptosis, epicanthal folds, corneal opacity, keratoconus, microphthalmos	Brachycephaly, growth retardation, mental retardation
4	18q deletion	Hypertelorism, epicanthal folds, nystagmus, corneal opacity, microphthalmos, corneal staphyloma, microcornea	Growth retardation, mental retardation, facial malformation, microcephaly
5	18r deletion	Same as 10p deletion, 18q deletion	Growth retardation, mental retardation, facial malformation, microcephaly
6	Trisomy 13 (Patau syndrome)	Microphthalomos, corneal opacity, Peters' anomaly, cataract, retinal dysplasia	Microcephaly, cleft lip and palate, low set ears
7	Trisomy 18 (Edward's syndrome)	Corneal opacity, ptosis, epicanthal folds, microphthalmos, colobomas, cataract, retinal dysplasia	Low birth weight; failure to thrive; brain hypoplasia cardiac, gastrointestinal, renal and musculosketatal anomalies
8	Trisomy 21 (Down syndrome)	Shortened, slanted palpebral fissure, neonatal ectropion, later trichiasis and entropion, keratoconus, cataract	Cardiac defects, mental retardation, short stature, characteristic facies
9	Partial trisomy 22 (cat's eye syndrome)	Microphthalmos, hypertelorism, colobomas	Mental retardation, microcephaly, cardiac anomalies, ear anomalies anal atresia
10	Ring D chromosome	Ptosis, epicanthal folds, microphthalmos, strabismus, nystagmus	Mental retardation, microcephaly, facial malformation
11	Turner syndrome	Ptosis, epicanthal folds, strabismus, rarely microcornea, blue sclera, corneal opacity	Female, short stature, webbed neck

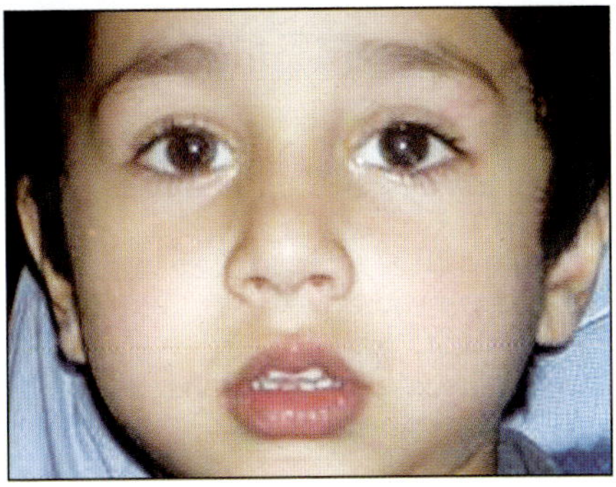

Figure 16 A: Child 1.5 years after repair of corneal laceration (LE)

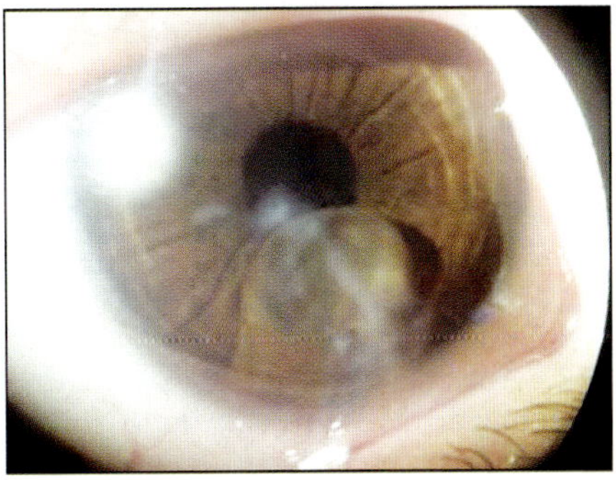

Figure 16B: Post trauma epithelial cyst from iris

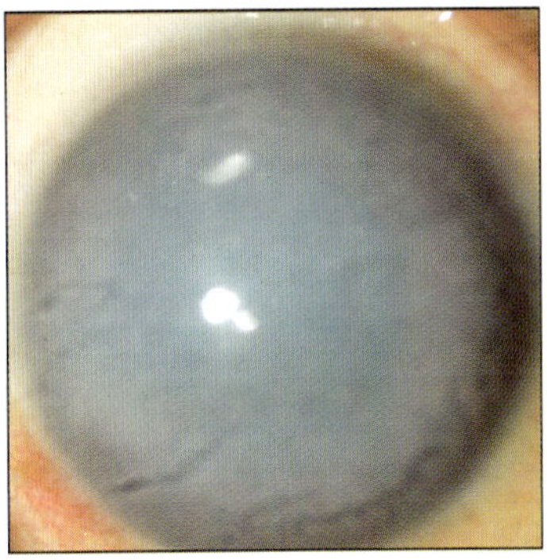

Figure 17: Corneal edema following corneal endothelia decompensation due to silicone oil following PPV and lensectomy

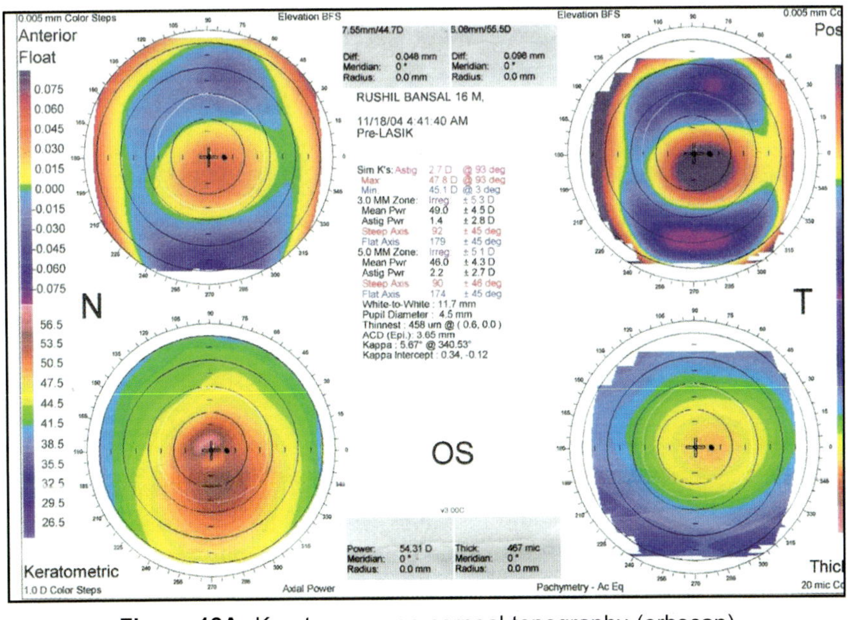

Figure 18A: Keratoconus on corneal topography (orbscan)

Table 3: Corneal opacities in association with systemic diseases (clinically not apparent at birth)

A. Biochemical deposits	*B. Non specific Opacities*
1. Mucopolysaccharidosis	1. Trisomy 13
2. Cystinosis	2. Trisomy 18
3. Mucolipidosis	3. Turner's syndrome
4. Fabry's Disease	4. Phenyl ketonuria
5. Tyrosinemia	5. Chediak-Higashi syndrome
6. Tangier disease (high density alpha-likoprotein deficiency	6. Genodermatoses
7. Refsum's syndrome	
8. Schnyder's cystalline dystrophy	

Tyrosinemia Type II (Tyrosinosis, Richner-Hanhart Syndrome)

Tyrosinemia is also an autosomal recessive disorder. Gene locus 16q22.1-22.3 is infected. It is characterized by tyrosine transaminase deficiency and it results in the deposition of tyrosine in the cornea. Dendriform corneal epithelium changes (branches or snowflake opacities), red eye, photophobia are characteristic of this disorder. Palmar — plantar hyper, keratosis, mental retardation and growth retardation occur as systemic association.

Wilson Disease

Wilson disease is an autosomal recessive disorder. The gene locus affected is 13q 14.3-q21.1. It is characterized by defective excretion of copper from hepatic lysosomes, resulting in deposition of copper. Kaiser Fleisher's ring "sun flower" cataract are it's characteristic presentation. Liver dysfunction, spasticity, behavior disturbance and nephrotic syndrome are systemic association.

Corneal Involvement in Association with Craniofacial Malformation Syndromes

Crouzon and Apert Syndrome

Crouzon and Apert syndrome is characterized by craniofacial malformation and syndactyly. Patients usually gets secondary corneal exposure as they have shallow orbits and restricted motility. The gene locus for this syndrome is 10q26.

Hallermann-Steriff Syndrome

Hallermann-Steriff syndrome is characterized by facial malformations, hypoplastic mandible, short stature and skin atrophy. Children suffering from this syndrome have microphthalmos, spontaneous resolution of cataract and macular pigmentary changes. Rarely these patients may develop Coat's disease.

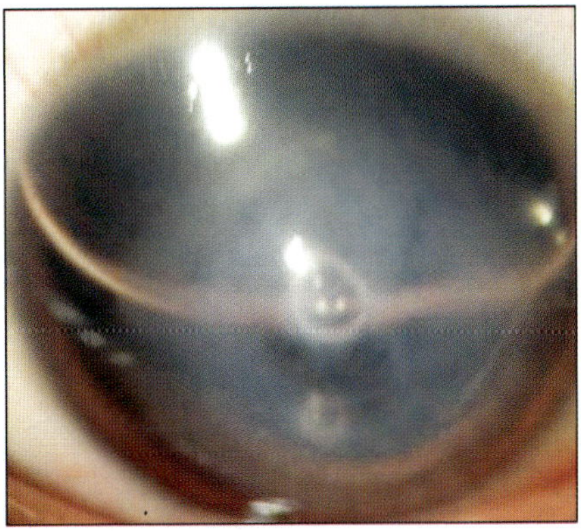

Figure 18B: Air injection for acute hydrops

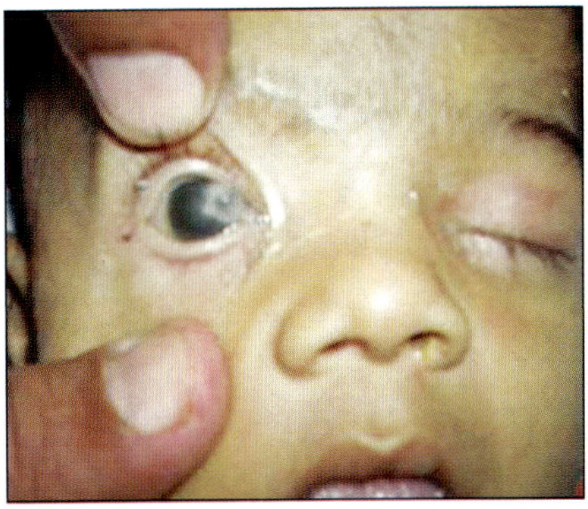

Figure 19A: Neonates (20 days old) with bilateral superadded bacterial infection following vitamin A deficiency. Active staphylococcal keratitis (RE)

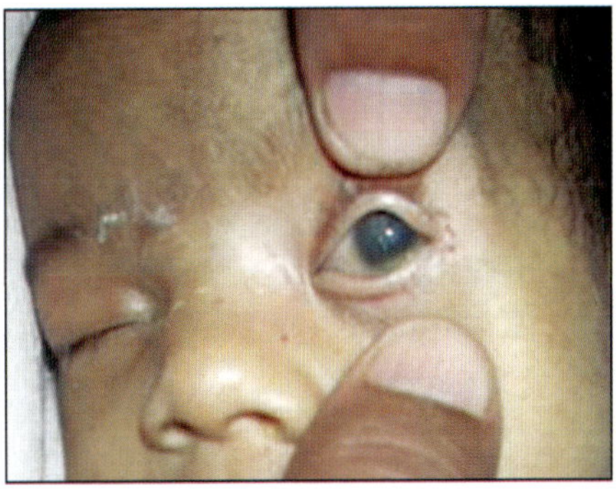

Figure 19B: Active staphylococcal keratitis (LE)

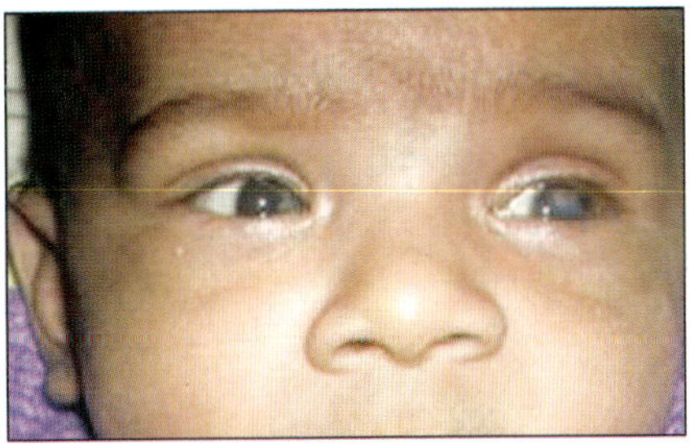

Figure 19C: Bilateral corneal opacity following healing of corneal ulcer and vitamin A deficiency

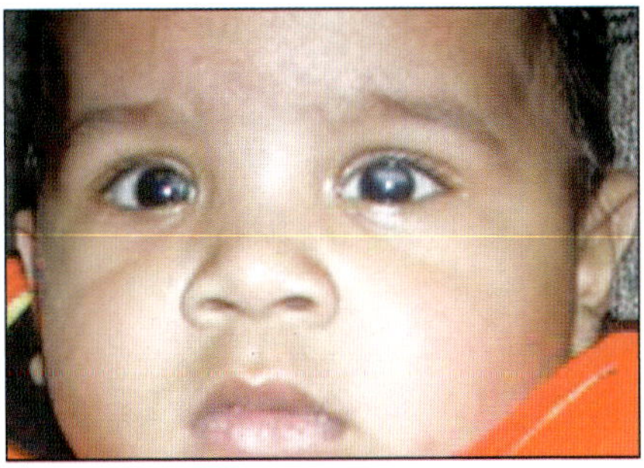

Figure 19D: Child after 2 years of follow-up

Table 4: Corneal involvement in mucopolysaccharidoses

Disorder	*Enzyme Deficiency*	*Metabolite Accumulated*	*Mode of Inheritance*	*Gene Locus*	*Ocular Manifestations*	*Systemic Manifestations*
Mucopolysaccharidosis I-H (Hurler syndrome)	L-Iduronidase	Heparan sulfate Dermatan sulfate	Autosomal recessive	4p 16.3	Corneal clouding, pigmentary retinopathy, optic atrophy, trabecular involvement	Gargoyle facies, mental retardatin, dwarfism, skeletal dysplasia
Mucopolysaccharidosis I-S (Scheie syndrome)	L-Iduronidase	Heparan sulfate Dermatan sulfate	Autosomal recessive	4p 16.3	Corneal clouding, pigmentary retinopathy, optic atrophy, glaucoma	Coarse facies, claw-like hands, aortic valve disease
Mucopolysaccharidosis I-H/S (Hurler-Scheie syndrome;	L-Iduronidase	Heparan sulfate Dermatan sulfate	Autosomal recessive	4p 16.3	Corneal clouding, pigmentary retinopathy, optic atrophy (Fig. 66-5)	More severe than I-S, less severe than I-H
Mucopolysaccharidosis II (Hunter syndrome)	Iduronate sulfate sulfatase (iduronate sulfatase)	Heparan sulfate Dermatan sulfate	X-Linked recessive	Xq28	Rare corneal clouding, pigmentary retinopathy, optic atrophy	Similar to I-H with less bony deformity

Contd...

Table 4: *Contd...*

Disorder	*Enzyme Deficiency*	*Metabolite Accumulated*	*Mode of Inheritance*	*Gene Locus*	*Ocular Manifestations*	*Systemic Manifestations*
Mucopolysaccharidosis III (Sanfilippo syndrome)	A: heparan-S-sulfaminidase (heparan sulfate N-sulfatase)	Heparan sulfate	Autosomal recessive	17q25.3 17q21.1	All forms : clinically clear cornea, occasional slit-lamp corneal opacities (mucopolysaccharide accumulation in intracytoplasmic vacuoles in keratocytes, endothelium and epithelium), pigmentary retinopathy, optic atrophy	Mild dysmorphism, progressive dementia
	B: N-acteyl D-Glucosaminidase)	Heperan sulfate	Autosomal Recessive			
	C: acetyl-CoA-glucosaminidase-N, N-acetgyltransferase	Heparan sulfate	Autosomal Recessive			
	D: N-acetylglucosamine – 6-sulfate sulfatase	Heparan sulfate	Autosomal Recessive	12q14 Chr # 14		
Mucopolysaccharidosis IV (Morquio syndrome)	A: galactose-6-sulfatase	Keratan sulfate	Autosomal recessive	16q24.3	Corneal clouding, optic atrophy	Severe bony deformity, aortic valve disease, normal intelligence
	B: galactosidase		Autosomal recessive	3p21.33		
Mucopolysaccharidosis VI (Maroteaux-Lamy syndrome)	N-acetylgalactosamine – 4-sulfatase	Dermatan sulfate	Autosomal recessive	5q11-q13	Corneal clouding, optic atrophy	Similar to I-H, but normal intellect
Mucopolysaccharidosis VII (Sly syndrome)	Glucuronidase	Dermatan sulfate Heparan sulfate	Autosomal recessive	7q21.1	Corneal clouding	Similar to I-H

Meyer-Schwickerath Syndrome (Oculodentodigital Dysplasia)

Meyer-Schwickerath syndrome is characterized by syndactyly and dysplastic tooth enamel. Children suffering from the syndrome have associated microphthalmos and microcornea. Gene locus for this syndrome is 6q22-q24.

Goldenhar Syndrome (Oculoauriculovertebral Dysplasia)

The characteristic features of Goldenhar syndrome include limbal dermoids, microphthalmos, anophthalmos, lid notching and blepharophimosis. Systemic manifestations include facial asymmetry, vertebral anomalies and ear abnormalities (accessary tragus). Fig. 3 shows isolated limbal dermoid in a child.

Ocular Involvement in Inherited Connective Tissue Disorders

Marfan Syndrome

Systemic manifestations of Marfan syndrome is characterized by long extremities, lax joints, aortic/mitral dialatation, aortic dissection. Ocular associations in Marfan's syndrome include megalocornea, lens subluxation, high myopia, retinal detachment. Biochemical defect causing clinical change is fibrillin-1 gene mutations.

Osteogenesis Imperfecta

Osteogenesis imperfect is characterized by systemic involvement including bone deformities, otosclerosis and dental anomalies. Ocular manifestation of osteogenesis imperfecta include blue sclera, keratoconus, megalocornea, optic nerve compression, corneal is brittle and ruptures with .... blue sclera, keratoconus. Biochemical defect involved in osteogenesis imperfecta is type I procollagen.

Ehlers-Danlos Syndrome Type VIA

Ehlers Danlos syndrome is characterized by skin stretching, scarring joint hypermobility and scoliosis. Ocular associations of Ehlers-Danlos syndrome type VI A include keratoglobus, lens subluxation, myopia and ocular fragility to trauma. Biochemically defect causing Ehlers-Danlos syndrome is lysyl hydroxylase. In Ehlers-Danlose syndrome type VI B lysyl hydroxylase is normal. Clinical features are same as in Ehler's Danlos VI A.

Congenital Corneal Dystrophies

Corneal dystrophies are characterized by bilateral, central, symmetrical, non-inflammatory, avascular and progressive corneal lesions. Corneal lesions are morphotogically characteristic in different corneal dystrophies and have district

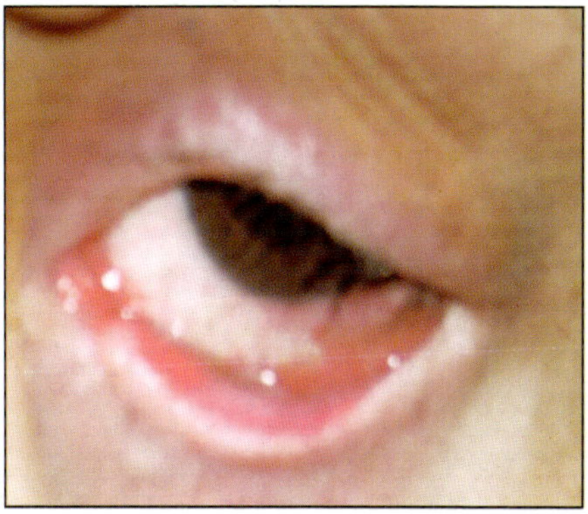

Figure 20: Stevens Johnson syndrome, Dry eye with symblepharon

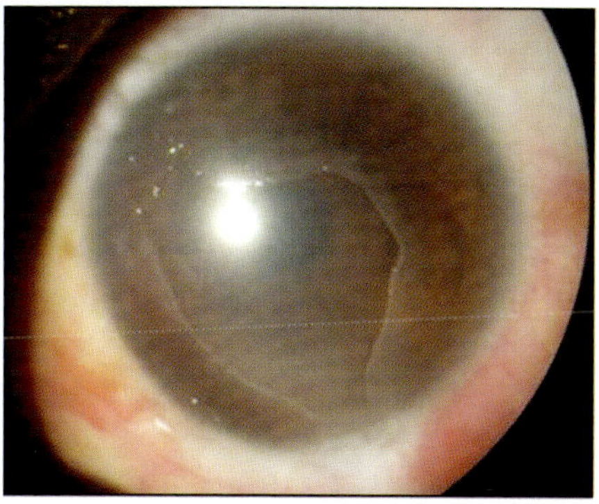

Figure 21A: Epithelial defect following severe chemical injury (Acid)

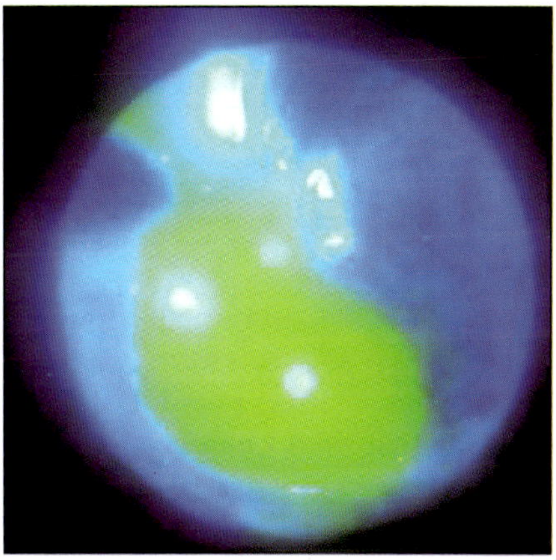

Figure 21B: Fluorescein staining showing localized limbal stem cell deficiency and scleral ulceration

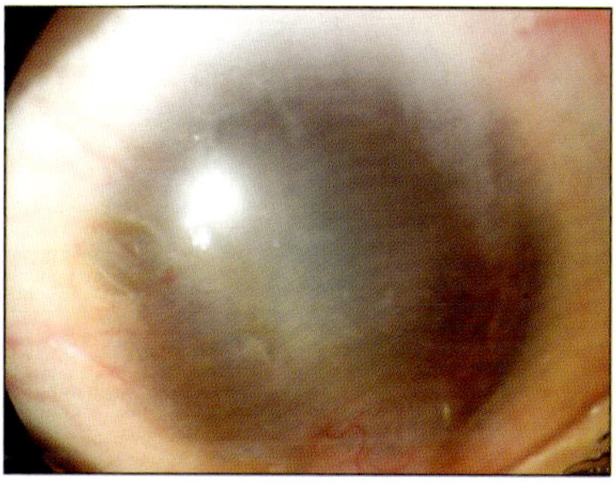

Figure 21C: Healed chemical injury following limbal stem cell transplant

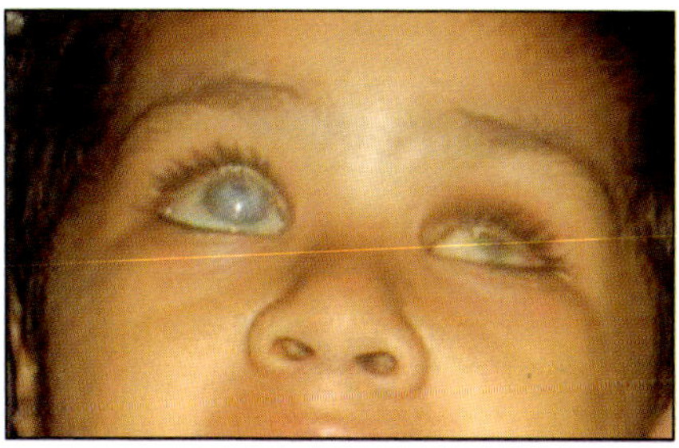

Figure 22: Bilateral corneal blind following vitamin A deficiency

features on histopathology. Although the underlying metabolic dysfunction is present congenitally but the disease may manifest later after birth. These features affect biochemical features of cornea. Dystrophies in general are hereditary in origin. Familial patterns may definite in stromal dystrophies but one unpredictable in keratoconus and Fuch's dystrophy.

Congenital corneal dystrophies include the following disorders:
- Congenital hereditary endothelial dystrophy (CHED)
- Posterior polymorphous dystrophy (PPMD)
- Congenital hereditary stromal dystrophy (CHSD)

Congenital Hereditary Endothelial Dystrophy (CHED)

Congenital hereditary endothelial dystrophy (CHED), resulting bilateral corneal clouding in a full term infant was first described by Maumenee in 1960. This dystrophy is characterized by bilateral congenital corneal edema normal IOP and normal corneal diameter. Corneal thickness increases two to three times and control corneal thickness may be move than 1.0 mm. Corneal pannus, esotropia, nystagmus and rarely glaucoma have been described in association with CHED. Clinically two forms of CHED autosomal recessive and autosomal dominant have been described.

Autosomal recessive form is characterized by presence of bilateral corneal edema since birth, nystagmus but no photophobia. The corneal edema is non-bullous diffuse.

This form of disease remains stationary throughout life. Autosomal dominant form of disease develops in the first or the scond year of life. This form of disease is gradually progressive. It is characterized by pain, watering, photophobia but absence of nystagmus. The studies have shown that the locus for autosomal dominant CHED is linked to pericentric region of chromosome. The studies for autosomal recessive form have revealed that the locus for recessive form is distinct from this region of choromosome but it has not been identified.

Clinical Features

CHED is characterized by diffuse epithelial and stromal edema. Examination under anesthesia reveals diffuse ground-glass appearance of corneal stroma. It has slight bluish grey appearance. Corneal diameter (horizontal) and intra-ocular pressure are normal. Rarely CHED may have associated glaucoma. In such a situation IOP should be controlled with medication first. After normalization of IOP if corneal edema still persists it should be labeled as CHED. This condition should be differentiated from congenital glaucoma without buphthalmos. In case of CHED, there are no breaks in the Descemet's membrane. Although rare, sensory neural deafness may occur.

Differential Diagnosis

CHED should be differentiated from other conditions resulting bilateral corneal opacification at birth. These conditions include glaucoma without buphthalmos, congenital hereditary stromal dystrophy, posterior polymorphous dystrophy, macular stromal dystrophy, mucopoly saccharidosis, birth trauma due to forceps and intrauterine infections. Of intrauterine infections congenital rubella, syndrome, toxoplasmosis, cytomegal, virus and herpes infection should be considered. The author has performed penetrating keratoplasty on a neonate having central dense lukomatous scar in one eye and the other eye having a healed lesion of congenital toxoplasma retinochoroiditis. Child had in addition central nervous abnormality resulting delayed milestones.

Pathogenesis

The primary abnormality in CHED is considered the degeneration or abnormal formation of endothelial cells during or after fifth months of gestation. CHED has been described as part of anterior segment dysgenesis, resulting from abnormal differentiation of neural crest ectoderm that forms the monolayer of corneal endothelium. Failure to complete the final differentiation blind to the prevention of dysfunctional endothelial cells. These abnormal endothelial cells may secrete posterior nonbanded (smooth) Descemet's membrane. Histopathology of corneal button shows diffuse epithelial and stromal edema with secondary changes. Spheroidal degeneration in the stroma of CHED patients helps to distinguish it from posterior polymorphous dystrophy.

Treatment

In case patient has mild edema hypertonic drops, ointment or other measures of dehydrating cornea including hair dryer may be effective. Infants and neonates having severe corneal edema require penetrating keratoplasty. However penetrating keratoplasty is neonates and infants is not only technically difficult but has poorer visual outcome compared to penetrating keratoplasty. Presence of severe amblyopia is another limiting factor even if clear graft following penetrating keratoplasty is achieved.

Posterior Polymorphous Dystrophy

Posterior polymorphous dystrophy (PPMD) was first described in 1916 by Keoppe. This rare dystrophy has a clinical spectrum that ranges from congenital corneal edema to late onset corneal edema in the middle age. Many cases are subclinical and the majority of patients have good vision. Many patients have subtle slit lamp and specular microscopic abnormalities. Posterior polymorphous dystrophy (PPMD) is a bilateral autosomal dominant disorder characterized by polymorphic posterior corneal surface irregularities with variable degrees of corneal decompensation. Characteristic feature include, vesicular, curvilinear, and placoid irregularities found on slit lamp examination. On specular microscopy rounded dark areas with central cell detail produce a doughnut-like pattern. Histopathology shows epithelial-like transformation of endothelium. Clinically these patients had reduced vision due to corneal edema. Associated features are iridocorneal adhesions, peripheral anterior synechiae and glaucoma. PPMD clinically resembles iridocorneal endothelial (ICE) syndrome, Peters' anomaly, and Axenfeld-Rieger syndrome, suggesting that PPMD may be part of a broader spectrum of disorders resulting from abnormalities of terminal neural crest cell differentiation.

Diagnosis

The majority of patients are diagnosed using the slit lamp by observing vesicular, band-like, or placoid areas on the posterior corneal surface. The diagnosis of PPMD in patients with corneal edema of unknown cause is based on light and electron microscopy of the excised buttons obtained during keratoplasty.

Differential Diagnosis

Differential diagnosis includes tears in Descemet's membrane, interstitial keratitis, Fuchs' dystrophy, and ICE syndrome. As in PPMD, endothelial cells in ICE syndrome may show epithelial characteristics, leading to speculation that they represent a spectrum of the same disease. However, unlike PPMD, ICE syndrome is unilateral, occurs sporadically, is more common in women, and is typically progressive and symptomatic. Glaucoma and iris changes can be found in PPMD but are much more prominent features of ICE syndrome. No systemic associations exist except for rare reports of PPMD associated with Alport's syndrome.

Pathology

Light microscopy of keratoplasty buttons shows pits in the posterior corneal surface, which correspond to the vesicles seen on slit-lamp examination. Descemet's membrane in these areas is attenuated, and the endothelium may be multilayered. In other areas, Descemet's membrane appears multilayered, of variable thickness, and with attenuation or loss of endothelium. Discontinuities in Descemet's membrane with anterior migration of cells to form slit-like structures or clefts in pre-Descemet's stroma have been described. Scanning electron microscopy of keratoplasty buttons may show a striking juxtaposition of normal-appearing endothelial cells adjacent to epithelial cell-like areas that show myriad surface microvilli. Transmission electron microscopy of these layers shows the cells to be multilayered and to contain numerous desmosomes and intracytoplasmic filaments. Cell culture studies of these cells demonstrate features similar to cultured epithelial cell lines.

Treatment

The majority of patients require no treatment, but those who have corneal opacification are offered keratoplasty.

Congenital Hereditary Stromal Dystrophy

Congenital hereditary stromal dystrophy (CHSD), an autosomal dominant, rare, stationary dystrophy was first described by Witschel et al (1978). The dystrophy presents at birth with bilateral, symmetrical, nonprogressive, central and superficial corneal stromal clouding. The periphery of cornea is clear. The epithelium is uneffected and the anterior stroma gives an ill-defined, flaky or feathery appearance. The child does not have any corneal edema, photophobia or tearing, but stromal opacities can be dense enough to reduce vision. Visual deprivation may lead to nystagmus and congenital esotropia.

In CHSD two types of abnormal collagen lamella constitute the entire stroma. These small collagen fibrils form alternating layers. One layer consists of compact collagen fibrils unformly arranged like normal corneal collagen. The other layer consist of irregularly arranged, loosely packed collegen fibrils.

Early penetrating keratoplasty has been reported to restore good vision. Since Descemet's membrane and endothelium is normal, LK or DALK can also be useful in restoration of vision.

Causes of Congenital Corneal Opacities

In child with congenital corneal capacity several corneal condition need to be considered. In a study Peter's anomaly (40%), Sclerocornea (18%) and dermoid (15%) were food to be the major causes.

1. Peter's anomaly
2. Sclerocornea
3. Dermoid
4. Microphthalmia
5. Congenital dystrophies
   a. Congenital hereditary endothelial dystrophy
   b. Congenital hereditary stromal dystrophy
   c. Posterior polymorphous dystrophy
6. Metabolic disorders: Mucopolysaccharidosis
7. Intrauterine infections cystinosis
   a. Intrauterine rubella syndrome
   b. Intrauterine toxoplasmosis
   c. Intrauterine cytomegalovirus
   d. Intrauterine herpes simplex keratitis
   e. Syphilis
   f. Coagan's syndrome
8. Birth trauma
9. Iodiopathic
   - Disorders cause bilateral corneal opacification.

Infections

Ophthalmia Neonatorum

Ophthalmia neonatorum refers to any conjunctivitis that occurs in the first four weeks of life. Other terms like neonatal ophthalmia, neonatal conjunctivitis and conjunctivitis of the new-born are used synonymously with ophthalmia neonatorum. The condition is characterized by swelling and redness of the eyelids, congestion of the conjunctiva and mucopurulent discharge. The infection may be gonococcal (caused by Neisseria gonorrhoeae) which is potentially blinding or nongonococcal in which risk of blindness is low. Ophthalmia neonatorum is an ocular emergency and needs early specific etiological diagnosis and prompt treatment.

Ophthalmia neonatorum affected 10-12% of children born in European countries during 1890s. Twenty percent of affected had some degree of corneal involvement. Ophthalmia neonatorum was major cause of childhood blindness during that period and accounted for 60-70% admissions in the institutions for the blind. In 1881, Carede introduced silver nitrate prophylaxis. This lead to dramatic decrease in the incidence of gonococcal ophthalmia from 10-0.3%. In developed countries the incidence of infections neonatal conjunctivitis ranges from 1-2%. High incidence of ophthalmia neonatorum still exists in developing countries. In a Nairobi hospital, the incidence of gonococcal and chlamydial conjunctivitis, 40 per 1000 and 80 per 1000 were recorded.

Sexually transmitted disease play significant role in the development of ophthalmia neonatorum. In developing countries prevalence of maternal chlamydial infection ranges from 7-29% and 3-22% of pregnant women have gonococcal infection. Ophthalmia will develop in 30-50% infants exposed to gonococci, and 33% of infants exposed to Chlamydia. Neonatal herpes simplex virus infection develops in 40-60% of newborn exposed to active genital herpes virus. Laga and colleagues reported incidence of chlamydial and gonococcal ophthalmia as 4-8 cases per 10 live births respectively. The incidence of gonococcal ophthalmia in developed countries has decreased but incidence of chlamydial diseases is on the rise. In Belgium ratio of gonococcal to chlamydial disease is 1:1000 and in United States 1:200.

Management of Ophthalmia Neonatorum

The diagnosis of ophthalmia neonatorum is made clinically. There is redness of conjunctiva, swelling of the eyelids and discharge. Neonatal ophthalmia can be of chemical, bacterial, chlamydial or viral etiology.

Chemical Conjunctivitis

Chemical conjunctivitis a reaction to prophylactic agents, most often develops following silver nitrate prophylaxis. Chemical conjunctivitis occurs within 24 hours of life and does not require any microbiological investigations. Condition is self limiting and usually resolves within 24-48 hours.

Bacterial Conjunctivitis

Bacterial conjunctivitis results from the inoculation of pathogenic bacteria into the neonate's conjunctival sac during or shortly after birth. Normal conjunctival flora has been documented within 15 minutes of vaginal delivery. In contrast conjunctiva of the babies born by cesarean section, within three hours of membrane rupture, is usually sterile. Infants born via cesarean section more than three hours after membrane rupture have intermediate bacterial isolates. Neonatal bacterial conjunctivitis is caused by streptococcus pneumoniae, pseudomonas aeruginosa or Neisseria gonorrhoeae. Differential diagnosis of bacterial ophthalmia neonatorum can be made on the basis of Gram stain. The presence of intracellular diplococci on a conjunctival smear is highly sensitive and specific for the diagnosis of gonococcal infection. Gram stain helps in establishing rapid diagnosis at places with limited laboratory facilities. As there is poor correlation between Gram stain and culture results, therapy must ultimately be modified on the basis of culture sensitivity results and clinical response.

Neonatal bacterial conjunctivitis usually responds to topical antibiotic therapy. In general gentamycin drops are appropriate for gram-negative infections whereas erythromycin ointment (0.5%) is the first choice for gram-positive conjunctivitis resistant to erythromycin has been reported, therefore antibiotic therapy need be modified on the basis of antibiotic sensitivity. Special therapeutic consideration should be given to pseudomonal and gonococcal conjunctivitis.

Pseudomonas conjunctivitis is extremely severe and carries a high risk of corneal perforation and endophthalmitis. The infant should be strictly monitored for corneal involvement. Frequent irrigation of eyes should be done to remove copious mucopurulent discharge. Fortified gentamycin (1.2%) or tobramycin (1.2%) should be administered topically every hour. Ciprofloxacin (0.3%), fluroquinolone derivative is equally effective for pseudomonas infection and has advantage of being effective for gram-positive organisms.

Until recently the standard medical therapy of gonococcal neonatal ophthalmia consisted of frequent topical aqueous penicillin G and systemically administered penicillin G 100, 000 U/Kg/day in two or for divided doses either intramuscularly or intravenously for seven days. With the emergence of β lactamase producing gonococci, currently third generation cephalosporin agents are recommended as initial therapy ceftriaxone. A single intramuscular injection of 125 mg is highly effective against gonococcal neonatal conjunctivitis and has added advantage of treating extraocular gonococcal infections. Another third generation cephalosporin, cefotaxime 100 mg I/M is also effective against gonococcal ophthalmis. A single injection of kanamycin 75 mg I/M combined with topical erytoromycin or tetracycline ointment for 10 days has also been proved effective against all stains of Neisseria gonorrhoeae. This regime is readily available and cost effective for developing countries. However inherent disadvantage of this regimen is concomitant use of topical antimicrobial agents and lower efficacy of kanamycin against nonocular gonococcal infections.

Chlamydial Conjunctivitis

Chlamydial conjunctivitis involves palpebral conjunctiva and characteristically lacks conjunctival follicles, as the infant is immunologically immature. Incubation period of Chlamydia trachomatis ranges between 5-14 days. Infant with chlamydial conjunctivitis should be systemically examined to rule out otitis media, rhinitis, proctitis, vulvitis and pneumonia. Giemsa stained conjunctival smear identifies the characteristic basophilic intracytoplasmic inclusion bodies within the epithelial cells. Currently two forms of antigen detection tests are in common use: direct fluorescent antibody assay and an enzyme immunoassay. Culture of chlamydia trachomatis is the most sensitive and specific test. Polymerase chain reaction (PCR) a newer diagnostic test has been recently used in chlamydia diagnosis.

Treatment of chlamydial conjunctivitis in addition aims at eradication of nasopharyngeal infection to eliminate the risk of subsequent development of chlamydial pneumonia. The drug of choice in infants is oral erythromycin estolate (10 mg/kg day four divided doses) combined with topical tetracycline (1%) or sulphacetamide (10%) drops or erythromycin (0.5%) ointment 4 times daily for 14-21 days. The active infection in mother should be treated with tetracycline 250 mg 4 times daily for 2-3 weeks. If the mother is breast-feeding the child, erythromycin should be substituted for tetracycline as the later is excreted in the milk.

Viral Conjunctivitis

Viral conjunctivitis is exclusively due to herpes simplex type II virus infection. Viral conjunctivitis presents with congestion of conjunctiva, lid edema and nonpurulent discharge. Isolated eye disease is extremely rare (1%). Ocular involvement occurs secondary to central nervous system involvement or disseminated infection. Central nervous system carries 50% and disseminated infection 85% mortality. Diagnosis of viral conjunctivitis is aided by inclusion bodies in the conjunctival smear and confirmed by positive viral culture. Herpes simplex conjunctivitis or blephritis should be treated with topical trifluridine or acyclovir 3% ointment five times. Neonatal herpes simplex keratitis should also be treated with topical antiviral agents. Systemic acyclovir (10 mg/KBW, IV) or vidarbine should be considered for systemic involvement.

Prophylaxis: Silver nitrate 1% solution instillation into the conjunctival sac has been routine prophylaxis over the past century. High incidence of chemical conjunctivitis and narrow antimicrobial spectrum has caused concern about the use of silver nitrate 1% as primary prophylactic agent. Silver nitrate prophylaxis is also questioned as global induce on nongonorrheal neonatal conjunctivitis is on the rise. In addition silver nitrate may present shell life problems in tropical climates. Several alternative regimens have been evaluated. Hammerschlag et al studied comparative efficacy of silver nitrate 1% solution tetracycline 1% ointment and erythromycin 0.5% ointment and found all these agents effective in preventing gonococcal ophthalmia but not chlamydial neonatal conjunctivitis. In another study, silver nitrate 1% and tetracycline 1% ointment have been shown to reduce incidence of chlamydial conjunctivitis. These prophylactic agents neither eradicate nasopharyngeal colonization nor do they prevent the chlamydia trachomatis pneumonia.

In recent studies povidone-iodine 2.5% solution has been found more effective and less toxic than silver nitrate or erythromycin as prophylactic agents. Povidone-iodine has broad antibacterial spectrum and is effective against Chlamydia, fungi and viruses. Povidone-iodine is unique as it turns the surface of the eye brown which ensures proper application of drug. Povidone-iodine is less expensive than other drugs and can be prepared locally. Thus povidone-iodine 2.5% has potential of being considered for routine prophylaxis against ophthalmia neonatorum, especially in the developing countries. In a recent study topical povidone-iodine (1.25%) solution was found safe for the neonates as it did not affect thyroid functions. No advantage was observed of two applications of povidone-iodine (2.5%) over single application, as prophylaxis for neonatal ophthalmia, the first postnatal day.

Prevention: Strategies to control neonatal ophthalmia include screening of pregnant women for gonorrhea, chlamydial infection and other sexually transmitted disease. Identified cases should be prompting treated. Those pregnant women, who are suffering from sexually transmitted disease, should also be screened for human immunodeficiency virus infection.

In view of low incidence of ophthalmia neonatorum in developed countries, routine use of prophylactic antibiotics has been discontinued in Sweden in 1982 and United Kingdom 27 years back. In Sweden, neonates born to mothers who did not receive comprehensive prenatal care require routine prophylaxis. Prophylaxis for neonatal ophthalmia is still legally mandated in the United States.

The World Health Organization (WHO) recognize that the best prophylaxis of neonatal ophthalmia is prenatal diagnosis and treatment of maternal infections. However, this method is too expensive and practically impossible on large scale basis. Hence such approach is recommended for those at high risk of contacting sexually transmitted disease. Prevention of sexually transmitted disease may reduce the risk of transferring causative agents responsible for ophthalmia neonatorum. unfortunately neonatal conjunctivitis is potentially blinding but prevention by ocular prophylaxis at birth is simple and inexpensive.

Conjunctivitis

Bacterial Conjunctivitis

Many of the bacteria can cause conjunctivitis. Gram positive organism, staphylococcal and streptococcus common organisms. Bacterial conjunctivitis should be differentiated from other causes such as nonspecific conjunctivitis, toxic conjunctivitis and allergic conjunctivitis. Allergic conjunctivitis patients complain of severe itching and have conjunctival edema. Children developing allergic conjunctivitis due to drugs have more signs in the inferior fornices. Staphylococcus aureus usually colonizes at the eyelid margins. Heavy colonization of Staphylococcus at the eyelid margin may occur without any significant symptoms. Staphylococcal blepharitis may be asymptomatic or may cause symptoms by affecting conjunctiva, cornea and limbus. Staphylococcal blepharoconjunctivitis commonly affects children. Other associated clinical conditions including meibomianitis should be looked for. Clinical signs in Staphylococcal blepharoconjunctivitis are thought to be due to inflammatory response to toxins produced by the bacteria present on the eyelid margins. Rarely other bacteria *Pseudomonas aeruginosa* and *Hemophilus influeza* may be the causative organisms. In severe cases pseudomembrane formation occurs. Bacterial cultures are helpful in isolating the organisms and determine their sensitivity but may not be necessary less the disease is chronic. Broad spectrum antibiotic drops during the day and erythromycin ointment at bed time may be used. Aminoglycosides, gentamycin and tobramycin have been used in the past. Fluroquinolone derivatives provide better coverage for gram positive organisms. Moxifloxacin fourth generation antibiotic has been recently approved by FDA for treatment of bacterial conjunctivitis in children.

Viral Conjunctivitis

Adenoviral keratoconjunctivits produces mild to moderate follicular response of short duration. Adenoviruses type 3, 7, 8 and 19 are responsible. Infection can occur as a part of epidemic or as isolated sporadic case.

Adenoviral infection causes acute, redness, watering and photophobia. Follicular response is dominant in most case. Children may present with hemorrhages. Corneal involvement early in the disease, is due to virus replication and is infective. Late involvement in the form of sub-epithelial infiltrate is a result immune response. Severe cases may develop inflammatory or pseudomembrane formation in the fornices. Preauricular lymphoide may be enlarged. The disease is self-limiting and by 2 weeks all replicating viruses are cleared by host immune response. In general there is no sight threatening sequale. Rarely adenoviral keratitis patient may develop persistent rise of IOP. Patients IOP should be monitored by noncontact tenometer. Preayrucykar ktnogiu Treatment of acute viral conjunctivitis is supportive. Topical corticosteroids reduce inflammatory response. These are avoided in the early course of disease. May be used to treat sub-epithelial infiltrates appearing later in the course of disease. Topical cyclosporin 0.5% twice daily has been used with favorable results. The major problem in treating sub-epithelial infiltrates is recurrence. However, these sub-epithelial lesions improve with minimal residual scarring.

Infective Keratitis

Infective keratitis is a major public health problem worldwide. It is a leading cause of blindness in the developing countries including India. Infective keratitis in children poses additional difficulties of compliance of frequent instillations of topical therapy and monitoring progress of the disease. Infective keratitis in children may be bacterial, fungal and viral origin. Rarely atypical mycobacterium, acanthamoeba and nocardia may be the causative organisms. Fungal corneal ulcers are usually caused by filamentous fungi Aspergillus and Fusarium. Fungal ulcers have been reported with use of contaminated contact lens solution and orthokeratology. Infective keratitis in child may also occur as secondary infection in under nourished children or those suffering from acute diarrhea or exanthematous fever including measles and chickenpox. Rarely neonates with multiple congenital anomalies eye lid coloboma, cleft lip, cleft palate had exposure, nutrition deficiency and develop bilateral infective keratitis.

Clinical Diagnosis

Clinical diagnosis and management of infective keratitis in children may be difficult as they may not complain till disease is advanced. Uncooperative children do not allow slit lamp biomicroscopy and hence detailed clinical examination may not be possible. Eye may look quiet and classical signs may be absent. Raised dry looking infiltrate should be considered characteristic of fungal keratitis due to filamentous fungi. Fungal corneal ulcers are localized with surrounding cornea clear. Patients have more signs as compared to very little symptoms. In contrast gram-negative bacterial corneal ulcers present with diffuse infiltrate, surrounding corneal edema and have rapid progression. Pseudomonas corneal ulcers belong to this category. Corneal ulcers due to gram-positive cocci, staphylococci and pneumococci usually follow corneal epithelial trauma and infiltrate progresses rapidly towards the center of the cornea. Later it may form a stromal abscess with intervening stroma relatively clear. Staphylococcal corneal ulcers are usually localized, peripheral and may be multiple. Children with bacterial corneal ulcers should be specifically examined for presence of congenital nasolacrimal duct obstruction. Fluorescein stain usually distinguishes herpes simplex keratitis form rest of the causes. Herpetic epithelial keratitis classically presents as dendritic, dentrogeographical or geographical corneal lesions. Detailed bio-microscopic examination, documentation of corneal lesions on color-coded diagrams and laboratory work-up, pre-requisites to start initial treatment may be possible in older children. Children usually require examination under anesthesia for detailed examination, performing laboratory work up including, smears (KOH and Gram Stain) and bacterial and fungal cultures and monitoring the response to the treatment. Calcofluor has higher sensitivity for diagnosing fungal corneal ulcers.

Treatment

Major consideration is to start broad spectrum, topical antibacterial agent, and frequent instillations. The combination of tobramycin (1.4%) and cefazoline (5%) every one-hour is preferred. Alternating gentamycin (1.4%) and vancomycin (5%) may be used as combination therapy. In several studies, single broad-spectrum antibacterial agent ciprofloxacin 0.3% a fluroquinolone derivative has been found effective. Single broad-spectrum antibacterial agent has several advantages over combination therapy, including less epithelial toxicity, no shelf-life problem and rapid epithelial healing. However, the treating ophthalmologist should be aware of the limitations of these drugs against gram-positive organisms including streptococcus. Reports on increasing incidence of resistance of ciprofloxacin against pseudomonas aeruginosa have been recently published. Recently gatifloxacin and moxifloxacin fourth generation flouroquinolone derivative have been reported to have lower MIC and better efficacy against gram-positive organisms as compared to ciprofloxacin. These drugs have potential for considering single broad-spectrum antibacterial treatment in bacterial corneal ulcers. These drugs have been approved by FDA in USA for treatment of bacterial conjunctivitis.

Treatment of fungal keratitis is even more challenging. It is not only because of limited options of treatment but also because of poor penetration of antifungal drugs into the deep corneal stroma and anterior chamber. Majority of mycotic keratitis (80 to 90%) in children occur due to filamentous fungi aspergillus and fusarium. Natamycin (5% suspension), a broad-spectrum antifungal agent is used every 1 hour. Other anti fungal drugs available include, amphotericin B (0.25%), miconazole (1%), fluconazole (2%), itraconazole (1%). For superficial keratomycosis natamycin suspension 5% every one-hour is started. In deep keratomycosis or superficial keratomycosis not responding to natamycin one of the above drugs is added. For deep keratomycosis systemic antifungal agents either fluconazole or itraconazole 150 mg twice daily is added to the topical therapy. Fluconazole provide higher concentration of the drug in the corneal stroma and aqueous humor. Itraconazole has a broader spectrum and is effective against filamentous fungi. Flucanazole is more specific for candida. Voriconazole has been recently introduced for clinical use in treatment of fungal corneal ulcers.

Monitoring of signs and response to the treatment is of paramount importance. Decrease in symptoms, infiltrate (size and depth) and hypopyon indicate that the patient is responding to the treatment. In fungal keratitis rounding of the hyphae margins may be one of the earliest sign of positive response. In bacterial keratitis it is the size of the infiltrate rather than corneal edema that monitored for recording the response to the treatment. One needs to distinguish between corneal edema and infiltrate on retroillumination. In case of corneal edema, cornea will be transparent where as in case of infiltrate it will be translucent. Appearance of corneal vascularization is another sign of improvement of corneal ulcer. In bacterial corneal ulcers, response is usually evident within 24 to 48 hours, whereas in mycotic keratitis response may be observed in 3 to 5 days. In uncooperative children, repeat examination under anesthesia may be required for monitoring response to the treatment.

On the basis of clinical response to the treatment, laboratory reports on the cultures and results of sensitivities of microorganism to various antibiotics initial treatment may be modified. In case positive clinical response in evident, treatment is not altered. In fungal keratitis another topical or systemic antifungal agent should be added if the patient does not show response to treatment.

Patients having nonresolving keratitis should be evaluated for a atypical mycobacterium and nocardia. Acanthamoeba keratitis may have atypical presentation closely mimicking herpes simplex keratitis. The clinical presentation may be in the form of superficial punctuate keratitis, small dendrites, superficial keratopathy or satellite lesions. Patients with resistant infiltrate may be routinely screened for acanthamoeba. Rarely nacordia infection may cause corneal perforation in a child. Patients not responding to the conventional treatment should be evaluated for rare causes infection.

In case the child shows positive response still be need to be closely monitored. Continuous collagenolysis may produce progressive corneal ulceration and thinning. The patient may develop impending or actual corneal perforation. Corneal perforation less than 3 mm may be treated with application of cyanoacrylate tissue adhesive. Use of bandage contact lens in patients with infective keratitis is avoided. A glue tarsorrhaphy may be preferred over bandage contact lens. Children having corneal perforation more than 3 mm diameter or corneal perforation not responding to cyanoacrylate tissue adhesive application are considered for therapeutic penetrating keratoplasty. Children having non-resolving keratitis or having limbal extension should also be considered for therapeutic penetrating keratoplasty. Frequent installations of topical broad spectrum antibacterial or antifungal drugs should be continued. As antifungal drugs are fungistatic, antifungal treatment should be continued for 4 to 6 weeks after resolution of infiltrate. Parents need to be counseled that even if the corneal ulcer heals successfully, there will be residual corneal opacity which may require penetrating keratoplasty at a later date.

Herpes Simplex Infection

Herpes simplex infection is very common in humans, with 90% of population showing serological evidence of exposure by the age of 16 years. Primary infection occurs in the early childhood, may present with generalized rash. Primary infection runs a clinical or sub clinical course, without circulating antibodies. Herpes simplex viruses type Iinfection causes ocular herpes, where as Herpes Simplex Virus type II causes genetic herpes. In neonates type II Herpes Simplex virus can cause ocular infection during the passage of child through birth canal at the time of delivery. Recurrent herpes simplex infective keratitis as common in children.

Recurrences and Latency

Recurrent attacks of ocular herpes are known to be triggered by stress, upper respiratory tract infection and fever. It is widely recognized that after primary infection, the virus establishes it's latency in the trigeminal ganglion. During the occurrence of recurrence, the virus travels along the trigeminal nerve and the epithelial cells of the cornea are affected. Child develops dendritic corneal ulcer, which is self-healing. Virus particles have been demonstrated in the corneal in experiment and human studies. Thus cornea has been documented as another site of herpes virus latency. T lymphocytes protect individual against herpes simplex virus infection.

Clinical Presentation

Morphological appearance of recurrent ocular herpes infection can be classified as under : Dendritic corneal ulcer, denotrogeographical corneal ulcer, geographic corneal ulcer and nurotrophic keratitis. Stromal herpes simplex keratitis can present as stromal keratitis, disciform keratitis and necrotising stromal keratitis.

Disease can also lead to keratouveits and endothelialitis. Epithetical disease including dendritic corneal ulcer, dendrogeographical and geographical forms are infective in nature. These should be treated with topical antiviral drugs. Neurtrophic epithelial defects are noninfective, have round appearance with heaped up margins. Neurotrophic ulcers are stain with fluorescein stain (2%) and the surrounding epithelium with rose bengal stain.

Clinically necrotizing stromal keratitis progresses rapidly. Disciform edema has mainly endothelial involvement and stromal edema is a consequence of endothelial dysfunction. In case of endothelitis antigen-antibody complexes deposit on the endothelial cells and cause mild stromal edema overlying the area of involvement. Virus particles have been demonstrated in the aqueous of the patients with endothelitis and disciform keratitis. In stromal keratitis immune mechanism, involving antigen antibody reaction is responsible for clinical manifestations. However, virus particles have been demonstrated an electron microscopic studies and virus cultures of the recipient buttons obtained drug penetrating keratoplasty. Herpes virus has been demonstrated in uveitis patients using the polymerase chain reaction. Limbitis and trabeculitis are other manifestations of herpes simplex keratitis.

Treatment

Topical steroids are contraindicated in the epithelial herpes simplex infection as, it aggravates the condition. Topical steroids increases the virus replication, the dendritic corneal epithelial defect ulcer may progress to dendrogeographical and finally to geographical stage. The virus may invade the deeper layers of corneal stoma and epithelial disease may progress to stromal disease. Treatment of infective forms of epithelial herpes simplex keratitis is done with the topical or systemic antiviral agents including acyclovir, vidarabine, trifluridine and iodoxuridine. Iodoxuridine being epitheliotoxic is rarely used these days.

Neurotrophic epithelial defects do not change shape with the treatment and present as persistent epithelial defect. These epithelial defect are noninfective and do not require antivirals topical or systemic as part of treatment. Topical steroids are also contraindicated as these may retard the epithelialization. In these children uses every effort should be made to promote epithelialization. Drug auditing is done and nonessential topical drops are discontinued as the preservatives present in these drops can contribute to nonhealing. Topical anti-bacterial agent preferably fluoroquinolone derivative are the least epitheliotoxic. In addition, strong cycloplegic (cyclopentolate HCl or atropine sulphate) thrice daily should be used. Frequent use of preservative free artificial teardrops promotes epithelial healing. Eyelid patenting may enhance epithelialization. In case epithelial defect is recalcitrant and is not responding, it is better to perform epithelial debridement and the fresh epithelial cells may heal the epithelial defect. The epithelial healing may be enhanced by the use of bandage contact lens. In children silicone contact lens has been found extremely useful in enhancing epithelial healing. In case the corneal sensation is absent and the tear film is inadequate one should avoid bandage contract lens. There is high risk of development of contact lens associate keratitis. In such a situation one may prefer tarsorrhaphy to the use of bandage contact lens. However in a child tarsorrhaphy may have to be performed under general anesthesia. Following tarsorrhaphy topical medication is continued and epithelial healing is monitored. Once epithelial defect heals, tarsorrhaphy can be cut at three months after the healing of epithelial defect.

Treatment of stromal herpes (stromal keratitis, necrotisug stromal keratitis and disciform edema) includes both antiviral and topical corticosteroids. In patients with epithelial disease along with stromal involvement, topical corticosteroids should be avoided. Topical corticosteroids in stromal disease along with epithelial involvement may enhance viral replication and may induce collagenolysis, causing stromal thinning. These patients should be treated with topical antiviral, cycloplegic and antibiotic. Once epithelial defect heals patient may be put on diluted topical corticosteroids to control stromal inflammation. Endothelitis and trabeculitis may be associated with raised intraocular pressure. Patients in addition to topical antiviral agents, cycloplegics, corticosteroids should also be put on topical and systemic antiglaucoma treatment.

The major problem of managing herpes simplex keratitis is recurrence. In case recurrence occurs within six month the patient is put on oral acyclovir 400 mg twice daily in adults. For children the dose may be adjusted according to the body weight. Following recurrent attacks of herpes simplex keratitis, corneal opacity results. Children with dense corneal opacity need penetrating keratoplasty otherwise they will develop amblyopia.

Herpes Simplex Zoster Ophthalmicus

Herpes zoster ophthalmicus occurs as recurrence of infection following primary infection of Varicella zoster virus. Herpes zoster ophthalmicus commonly occurs in aged and debilitating individuals. Infection in children also quite common. Herpes zoster ophthalmicus has been reported to develop following bone marrow transplantation and varicella vaccination in children. Vesicular eruption is characteristic of Herpes zoster infection. Although rare generalized cutaneous rush in herpes simplex virus infection that was mistaken for Herpes zoster has been described in a 3 year-old-girl. Herpes zoster infection involves a particular dermatome completely in contrast to incomplete involvement of dermatome in herpes simplex keratitis in herpes simplex virus infection. Herpes zoster has predilection for supraorbital nerve and is most frequently involved. Nasociliary branch that supplies cornea, conjunctiva, sclera iris, choroids, ciliary body and skin over the nose is the next common nerve affected. Once infection occurs over the tip of nose there is 85% chance that the cornea may get affected. This has been described as Hutchinson's sign. This is because of the nasociliary nerve supply both tip of nose and corneal epithelium.

Clinical Presentation

Clinically patient has prodromal symptoms in the form of fever, malaise, and pain in the distribution of trigeminal nerve, first division. After prodromal symptoms vesicles appear. These vesicles contain clear fluid and are accompanied by swelling of the skin. Patient has excruciating pain because of the inflammation of the nerves. Patients having positive Hutchinson's sign should be closely monitored for the development of corneal lesions. Patient can have conjunctivitis, mild SPK and swollen eyelids with difficulty in opening the eyes. Patients may develop corneal lesions in the form of dendritic or geographical lesion (plaque), which is different from the ulcerative lesions in epithelial Herpes simplex infection. Although diagnosis is clinical, varicella zoster virus keratitis can be confirmed using polymerase chain reaction. Here may be variable degree of loss of corneal sensitivity. Complete loss of corneal sensation is dangerous as this patient may develop neurotrophic problem later in the course of disease. Children should be specifically examined for development of iritis, cyclitis, chorioretinitis and optic neuritis. IOP should be closely monitored, as they are likely to have high intraocular pressure. These children may develop complications like scleritis, Horner's syndrome, extra ocular muscle palsies. Skin lesion usually heal with in 21 days, where as ocular involvement may take 2 to 3 months to resolve. The natural course of the disease is such that in most of the patients it heals leaving few residual problems, like post herpetic neuralgia. Some children develop chronic course of the disease, which may take longer time to resolve.

Complications

Even after the acute phase of the disease is over, children should be monitored long-term, as they are likely to develop complications. IOP should be monitored for prolonged period. Children developing complete loss of sensation and tear film in adequacy should be especially looked for development of neurotrophic keratitis. Both fluoroscein and rose bengal stain may be used to diagnose neurotrophic keratitis early. Children developing neurotrophic problem should be advised patching or the eye regularly taking care that they may not develop amblyopia. Those worsening despite full time patching or having frank corneal ulceration should undergo tarsorrhaphy. Children developing severe corneal ulceration due to neurotrophic keratitis may require amniotic membrane transplant to promote healing. In case child develops corneal perforation, cyanoacrylate tissue adhesive application may be considered. Lesions due to neurotrophic keratitis may heal resulting scar. Resolution of disciform stromal corneal keratitis has been reported to decrease myopia. Children having pain persisting one month after the resolution of the lesions in the affected dermatome in termed as post herpetic neuralgia. Patient has altered sensation and pain is severe sometimes disturbing even the sleep of the patient.

Treatment

Topical corticosteroids should be used only in severe corneal disease or in the presence of irdiocyclitis. In patients with complete loss of sensation corticosteroids should be used with great caution. Antibiotic and cycloplegics should be prescribed. Oral acyclovir (600-800 mg) adult dose 5 times for 7 days has been recommended. It should be preferably started immediately or within 3-5 days onset of infection. Oral acyclovir casue faster resolution of skin lesions, decrease incidence of host herpetic neuralgia, ocular complications including, dendriform keratitis, uveitis and scleritis. Systemic steroids should be avoided early in the course of disease. There is always a risk of developing disseminated zoster in children in whom adequate antibody response has not developed.

Interstitial Keratitis

Interstitial keratitis is nonsuppurative inflammation occurring in the corneal stroma. It consists of cellular infiltration, accompanied by dense vascularization. The most important cause of interstitial keratitis is syphilis. It can occur in both acquired and congenital form. The corneal vascularization is dense and the lesion is also known as "salmon patch". In the congenital form the inflammation is an immune response to Treponema antigen. In congenital syphilis both eyes may be involved.

Interstitial keratitis also occurs in tuberculosis and sarcoidosis. In both these diseases interstitial keratitis may be focal and affecting the periphery of the cornea. Interstitial keratitis may be mild (central peripheral) with very little vascularization. In such cases all causes of interstitial keratitis should be ruled out. Laboratory investigations should be performed to rule out both these conditions. Investigations include: VDRL, FTA-ABS, ESR, Montoux test, X-ray chest and tests for sarcoidosis and autoimmune connective tissue disorders. For inflammation topical and systemic steroids can be given. However, systemic disease syphilis should be treated with penicillin or it's alternative. Once condition resolves vascularization disappear and corneal thinning with ghost vessels remain. Antitubercular treatment should be started in case the tests for tuberculosis are positive. Cogan's syndrome is characterized by interstitial keratitis, vertigo, tinitis and hearing loss. This disorder commonly occurs in middle aged. Although rare cases of Cogan's syndrome on the children have been reported. Early diagnosis and immunosuppressive treatment to control auto-immune inflammation is key to favorable prognosis in children.

The other causes of interstitial dermatitis include herpes simplex keratitis, herpes zoster ophthalmicus, Epstein Barr Virus, mumps, rubella, lyme Boerreliosis and lymphogranuloma venerium leprosy and onrchocercosis.

Keratitis in Association with Acne Rosacea

Acne Rosacea is a common chronic skin disorder in adults. The disease is known to affect fair skinned patients but has been reported in blacks. It is characterized by malor rash, affecting cheeks, chin, nose and forehead. Ocular involvement may occur in the form of blepharoconjunctivitis, episcleritis and keratitis. Ocular involvement usually occurs between the third and fifth decade. Although rare, cases of keratitis due to acne rosacea have been described between 4 to 14 years of age. Clinical presentation of ocular involvement and treatment of the pediatric patient with this disease are not widely known.

Ocular involvement in rosacea is nonspecific and may cause inflammation of eyelids, conjunctiva and cornea. Ocular manifestation includes blephritis, meibomianitis, chalazia, hordeola, and hyperemic conjunctiva. Corneal involvement occurs in the form of peripheral corneal vascularization (lower 2/3rd) followed by subepithelial infiltrates. Resolution of infiltrates may cause peripheral corneal thinning. Significant scarring and even corneal perforation has been reported. Majority of the patients have bilateral involvement.

Treatment of rosacea includes eyelid hygiene, hot compresses and eyelid scrubs. Topical antibiotic with broad spectrum gram positive activity should be applied. Topical corticosteroids may be useful in managing keratitis and episcleritis. Extremely low concentrations of topical steroids should be used as there is a risk of keratolysis. Oxytetracycline orally is recommended as first line of treatment in rosacea. The efficacy of the drug has been reported by various authors. The exact mechanism of action of the drug is not known. Tetracycline, have been reported to improve the quality of meibomian gland secretions. It has been postulated to affect the interaction of sebaceous gland substance and bacteria without killing bacteria. The recommended dosage schedule is 100 mg a day for 1 month, then 50 mg a day for 1 month and finally 50 may every other day for 1 month. In case there is no improvement treatment regimen is switched to 250 mg of tetracycline 4 times per day.

Allergic Disorders

Allergic Conjunctivitis

Atopic Conjunctivitis

Acute atopic conjunctivitis is an allergic response to allergens such as dusts pollens, spores and animal dander. Symptoms consist of severe itching, burning, infection and chemosis. Patients may have systemic symptoms in the form of nasal and respiratory symptoms. Careful history taking usually reveals systemic allergic disorders, in the form of bronchial asthma, allergic rhinitis and allergic dermatitis. Atopic conjunctivitis is an immediate (Type 1) allergic response mediated by Ig E. Chronic form of disease is characterized by itching, burning, foreign body sensation of longer duration. Slit lamp biomicroscopy reveals conjunctival edema, papillary hypertrophy, and mucoid discharge. Giant papillae or cobblestone formation may occur.

The ideal method of prevention is avoidance of allergens. Histamine (H_z recepter specific) agonists such as levocabastine (1.05%) and emedatine hydrochloride (0.05%) may be used to control acute exacerbation of symptoms. Mast cell stabilizers including cromolyn sodium (4%), Iodoxamide tromethamine (0.1%) and nedocromil sodium (2%) are useful in chronic allergies. These drugs takes 1-2 weeks, before the effect is evident. Mild cases may respond to cold compresses, vasoconstrictors and non-specific antihistaminics. In severe cases topical NSAIDs or steroids may be used to control acute allergic symptoms. Drugs including olopatadine, ketoprofen fumarate and azelastine having both antihistamines and mast cell stabilizing effect are useful in both acute and chronic exposure of allergens.

Vernal Conjunctivitis

Vernal conjunctivitis is characterized by bilateral, recurrent inflammation of conjunctiva, occurring in children. The disease predominantly occurs in children and young adults. The onset is usually between 3 and 10 years. The disease is usually self limiting and severity decreases as the child grows. Vernal conjunctivitis is more often seen in hot climates in northern hemisphere. The peak incidence of the disease is between April and August i.e. in summer months. Most of the cases shows characteristic seasonal variation i.e. the symptoms exacerbating in the summer months and subsiding in the winder months. Inverse seasonal variation of the disease i.e. symptoms becoming worse in the winter months has been observed in 1-2% of the patients. Patients having chronic disease may also have symptoms throughout the year.

Clinical Presentation

Itching, redness, blepharospasm, and photophobia are the main symptoms of the disease. Children have mucoid, ropy discharge and difficulty in opening eyes in the morning. The disease has been described to occur in three forms : palpebral, limbal, and mixed. Palpebral form of disease is characterized by diffuse papillary hypertrophy, covered by milky layer. Papillae are localized lymphocytic proliferations with vascular tuft in the center of the cornea. Clinically presence of central vessel which branches at the surface distinguishes it from follicle, in which vessels are absent. In severe cases papillae become enlarged and more confluent. Once these papillae are tight packed they assume polygonal shape and due to the pressure from the corneal surface, their top becomes flat. In severe and chronic form of disease, papillae may become extremely enlarged, teamed as "cobblestones" or "giant papillae". White dots, termed as Horner's or Trantas, dots may occur on the papillae. Diffuse milky appearance of papillae may be due to fibrin deposit. It is described as sign. In case fluorescene stain is positive in the center of the papilla, it indicates that mast cells are degranulating and the disease is active.

Limbal form of the disease occurs more often in blacks. It is characterized by limbal hypertrophy diffuse of localized. It may be localized and limbal papilla formation may occur. Areas of chalky white pinpoint lesions Horner's or Trantas' dots may occur. These lesions should be distinguished from Herbert pits, which are flat, transparent and permanent. These occur in trachoma, caused by *Chlamydia trachomatis*. In severe limbal form of the disease micropannus may develop and encroach peripheral cornea. Superficial punctate erosions also described as micro erosions may occur, these may continue to progress to vernal or shield ulcer.

Chronic cases develop muddy discoloration of conjunctiva. Initial stages, these children develop myopic astigmatism. Some of these may progress and develop keratoconus. Later in life. Patients with chronic vernal conjunctivitis may develop fungal keratitis even if they are not exposed to topical steroids or have no vernal ulcer.

Treatment

The best method of treatment is avoidance of allergen, which is extremely difficult. Avoidance of contact with pets, exposure to dust and heat may be avoided. Cold compresses may not only provide relief from symptoms may even cut down the necessity of medicine. Mild cases may respond to cold compresses, vasoconstrictors and non-specific anti-histaminics. Moderate cases may be treated with histamine, H_2 receptor specific against (levocabastine and emedestine), most cell stabilizers (cromolyn sodium, iodoxamide and nedocromil sodium) and drugs having both antihistaminic and most cell stabilizers usually take 2 weeks to provide symptomatic relief and drugs having both antihistaminic and must all stabilizer effect provide rapid relief. Topical NSAID drugs (ketoprofen, keratorolac) and successful in controlling symptoms. Topical steroids may be used in severe cases for short duration as pulse therapy. Topical cyclosporine (0.05 to 2%) and topical MMC local application have also been reported effective in severe cases. In recalcitrant cases of vernal conjunctivitis, supratarsal injection of triamcinolone acetonide (20 mg) may be given on either side. Method of giving supratarsal injection of triamcinolone. Systemic steroids oral antihistaminic may be tried in severe cases. Long-term use of tab aspirin has also been formed helpful in resistant cases.

Vernal Keratopathy and Shield Ulcers

Arlts (1846) first described vernal disease, but corneal involvement for the first time was reported by Saemisch (1904). At that time corneal manifestations of vernal disease were considered to be extension of limbal lesions. Beigelman (1938) described epithelial changes as a specific entity and named it as dystrophy of corneal epithelium in vernal conjunctivitis. Tobgy (1935) named fine corneal epithelial disturbances as "Keratitis Epithelialis Vernalis" and reported epithelial involvement in 70% cases.

Etiology

Mechanical trauma by palpebral vegetations is considered the important cause of epithelial changes. Vigorous eye rubbing, due to severe itching aggravates epithelial damage and cause corneal epithelial changes. Chemical factors and mediators of inflammation released by degranulating mast cells, eosinophils have also been implicated in the epithelial break down.

Clinical Features

Epithelial involvement in vernal conjunctivitis almost always starts as micro-erosions. Continuous epithelial break down lead to macro-erosions or vernal/shield ulcers. Classical ulcers are transversally oral, shallow, situated in the upper half of the cornea. In case the vernal ulcer is left untreated fibrin deposition occurs and leads to plaque formation. Once plaque is formed, epithelialization of the ulcer is retarded ulcer becomes non-healing. In non-healing vernal ulcers, there is increased risk of development of infective keratitis. Bacterial and fungal corneal ulcers have been reported as secondary infection in these cases.

Treatment

Initially vernal ulcers should be treated with frequent instillations of prednisolone acetate 0.1% suspension every one hour. Topical antibiotic prophylaxis and cycloplegic are added. In case plaque formation has occurred, they do not respond to medical treatment alone. Surgical debridement and concomitant placement of bandage contact lens have been found to enhance healing of vernal ulcers. Rapid healing of vernal ulcers prevents complications including infections. Use of silicone hydrogel contact lenses have found safe and effective for continuous wear therapeutic use for vernal ulcers. In addition to bandage contact lens, amniotic membrane has been used to promote healing. Topical cyclosporine (0.05-2%) has also been used to treat shield ulcers. Supratarsal injection of tiamcinolone acetonide (20 mg) into either side may be considered as an adjuvant in recalcitrant vernal ulcers in addition to surgical debridement and bandage contact lens application. The technique of giving supratarsal injection is shown. Vernal ulcers or plaques should be treated on emergency basis as they are known to cause amblyopia in children.

Corneal Injuries

Management of Corneal Injuries

Eye injuries are common and may lead to sight threatening complications. Eye injuries can be classified as either open globe or closed globe injuries, depending upon the nature of trauma. Injuries with sharp edged objects lead to open globe injuries where as blunt trauma leads to closed globe injuries. Anatomical location of the eyes makes them less vulnerable eye injuries. Orbital walls and nasal bridge protect eyes from injuries. Most of the eye injuries occur due to the objects coming from the temporal side or from the front. In addition eyelids and eyelashes protect cornea and ocular surface from corneal epithelial trauma from the foreign bodies. Corneal sensitivity causes, watering and flushing of the injurious agents.

Epidemiology

Neonates may suffer corneal injuries at the time of birth. Most common corneal injuries occur due to forceps application. Faulty forceps application leads to Descemet's membrane rupture causing corneal edema. Severe bilateral corneal edema may be difficult to distinguish from other causes of congenital corneal clouding. Young children may get corneal injuries while playing at homes or at school. Bow and arrow injuries, crackers and wooden sticks are common objects causing corneal injuries. In contrast most of the adults suffer mechanical corneal injuries while working on high-speed drill machines. Road-side accidents, explosions and hammer chisel injuries may also cause corneal trauma. Wooden foreign bodies and injuries with vegetative material commonly occur in individuals working in the fields. Rarely children may present with self infiltrated injuries, which are usually mild. A case of bilateral self infiltrated penetrating needle injury been reported.

Clinical Examination

Infants and children may not allow eye examination to assess the severity of injury. One should not force examination as it may aggravate eye injury. Surgeon need to know whether the injury is serious and needs repair. In uncooperative children it is better to examine the eye under general anesthesia and undertake primary repair of corneal injury if required. In older children extent of eye injury is documented using slit lamp photograph or color coded diagrams. Patient is advised not to take anything orally. In case patient has corneal perforation, eye drops in an open wound are avoided. Eye drops may cause serious endothelial toxicity. If patient has not received injury tetanus toxoid during preceding six months, it is mandatory to give the injection. A pad and patch is applied. Parent's counseling is most important, as they may be anxious and have lot of questions to ask. Parents and child should be explained the nature of injury, and the importance of primary repair should be emphasized. Visual prognosis may be explained after primary repair. In case patient is having lens damage or posterior segment injury necessity of future surgeries may be explained.

Type of Anesthesia

In general open globe injuries in adults and children are repaired under general anesthesia. Patient should be kept at a deeper plane and recovery should be uneventful.

Principles of Surgical Repair

Extent of corneal injury should be measured and possible extension to the sclera should be ruled out. In case, the corneal laceration is extending up to the limbus, peritomy should be performed and the end of the corneal laceration should be identified. The extent of scleral laceration from the limbus should be measured. Wound should be thoroughly cleaned off the debris. Irrigation of the wound and removal of corneal foreign bodies is performed. Recent iris prolapse presenting within few hours should be reposited. Old iris prolaps, torn iris and iris with possible focus of infection should be abscised. In case of ciliary body prolaps, it should not be abscised. Ciliary body can be reposited. Light cautry may be applied to small portion if required.

It is good practice to divide the corneal scleral laceration into the smaller segments. One should put a suture at limbus and divide it into corneal and scleral laceration. Even scleral or corneal laceration can be further subdivided by putting sutures in between at certain landmarks. Sutures should deep up to 80-90% thickness. One should always put less number of sutures near the visual axis. Longer bites induce larger astigmatism. To close clean incised wound without any tissue incarceration continuous suture may be used. Intraoperative keratometer useful to be adjust the tension across the sutures to reduce post-operative astigmatisms. Incision of sutures used in repairing corneal laceration should be of adequate tightness. At the end of the repair of the corneal laceration anterior chamber should be reformed. A separate stab incision should be used to infect air into the anterior chamber. In the repair of corneal laceration air has advantage over ringer's lactate. In case child has an associated lid laceration, corneal repair is performed first and lid repair later. Canalicular injuries should be meticulously repaired. Continuity of the canalicular should be ensured.

Viscoelastic Materials

Viscoelastic substance should be used to deepen the anterior chamber and protect corneal endothelium. In addition one can always use air in the anterior chamber. Air gives clear view of the tissue incarcerating in the corneal wound. Mobility of the air bubble and extent of the air bubble give useful information that the anterior chamber is deep. Multiple small air bubbles indicate that there may be vitreous in the anterior chamber.

Management of Injury to Lens

In general lens extraction is avoided at the time of primary repair of corneal laceration. There is always a risk of aggravation of subclinical infection and developing endophthalmitis. However, if there is gross laceration of capsule and lose lens matter in the anterior chamber, one should aspirate the lens matter. In case there is lens matter mixed with vitreous one can perform anterior vitrectomy with lensectomy. In the exceptional case with clean incised corneal wound lens capsule laceration may be present. In since a patient one can perform aspiration of the lens matter and perform posterior chamber intraocular lens implantation. Small corneal laceration (1-2 mm) self-sealing may be left unsutured if the wound is stable and there is no tissue incarceration. Shelving wound is more stable than vertical edges of the wound. Bandage contact lens may be considered making the wound more stable. In case there is tissue incarcerations iris or capsule, corneal wound should repaired even if it is already sealed. The incarcerated tissue must be disengaged to avoid fibrous in growth and avoid fistula formation. Iris incarceration may also predispose to sympathetic ophthalmia.

Type of Sutures

Corneal laceration is repaired using 10 '0' monofilament nylon (Alcon or Ethicon) suture. Scleral ruptures are repaired using polypropylene sutures. Iridoplasty and pupiloplasty is also performed using 10(0) polypropylene sutures. Conjunctival tear should be sutured using polyglactin (vicryl 8 (0) sutures. Lid repair is done using 6 (0) silk sutures.

Corneal laceration with tissue loss require purse string suture. In case tissue apposition is not achieved with the purse string suture alone cyanoacrylate tissue adhesive should be applied. One should look for Descemet membrane detachment and repair it passing full thickness sutures and air/air gas mixture in to the anterior chamber. Birth trauma usually leads to descements membrane rupture. Extensive descemet's membrane tear will lead to flattening of corneal curvature in the meridian perpendicular to the descemet's tear. In case astigmatism is large and apply compression sutures across the descemet's tear which will act as compression sutures.

Corneal lacerations should be carefully examined for the present of eyelash. Eyelash presence in the corneal wound or intracorneal may lead to cyst formation. Cilia may also get implanted into the anterior chamber and even the traumatic cataractous lens. Patient in whom multiple cilia impacted in the capsular bag and their removal before intraocular lens implantation has been reported.

Postoperative Treatment

Following repair child is put on systemic antibiotic, systemic steroids and systemic anti-inflammatory drugs. In addition the child should be put on frequent topical antibiotic, topical steroids and cycloplegics. In the post-operative period one should monitor intraocular pressure and postoperative inflammation. Once postoperative inflammation has subsided one should perform posterior segment evaluation. In case adequate view of the retina is not obtained because of corneal edema, corneal scar or cataractous lens one should get B scan ultrasonography, to make suture that there is no retinal detachment, endophthalmitis or vitreous hemorrhage. Delayed post traumatic propionibacterium acnes endophthalmitis has been reported. Children may recover good vision after surgery for traumatic cataract despite corneal scar. In some cases of adequate posterior capsular support is not available they may need scleral fixated PCIOL.

Complications

In appropriate repair or neglected corneal lacerations may develop fibrous in growth, intraocular cysts, fistula and phthisis bulbi. Following full thickness corneal laceration epithelial cells get implanted into the corneal wound or iris tissue. This may lead to the cyst formation. Although rare it may occur even if the repair is meticulous. The management of iris cyst may be surgical enbloc removal or ablation using Nd : YAG Laser.

Corneal Abrasion

Children suffering from sharp corneal abrasions due to finger nail or paper edge corneal injury may develop basement membrane disease. This may lead duplication of basement membrane or abnormal basement membrane formation. Abnormal adhesions of basal epithelial cells to the abnormal basement membrane are weaker and result in develop recurrent erosion. Patient will have recurrent attacks of pain, redness, watering, and photophobia may be given bandage contact lens. At later stages in recalcitrant cases phototherapeutic keraectomy may be considered.

Corneal abrasions should be treated meticulously and carefully. Detailed slit lamp biomicroscopy is done to rule out infiltrate. Simple abrasions may be treated with prophylactic antibiotics alone. Topical steroids may be used only of necessary. Topical non-steroid antiinflammatory drugs should be used with caution as they have been reported to cause corneal melts.

Corneal Foreign Bodies

Corneal foreign bodies may be superficial non-metallic or impacted. Intrastromal foreign bodies wooden or metallic should be removed. Glass foreign bodies may be left as such. They are inert and the attempt to remove may cause more scarring in the cornea. Corneal foreign bodies associated with infiltrate should be subjected to KOH, Gram stain and cultures (bacterial and fungal). Children having wooden or vegetative corneal foreign bodies should be closely monitored for development of fungal keratitis. Intracorneal foreign body removed and child was treated for fungal keratitis.

Corneal Edema

Normal cornea is transparent with corneal thickness 520 to 560 µm in the centre. Corneal endothelial cells keep a cornea in a state of relative dehydration because of endothelial pump functions. In case endothelial cell count decrease below a critical value of 500 cells/mm endothelial cell function is inadequate to maintain normal transparency of cornea at corneal edema develops. Clinically corneal edema can diagnosed on slit lamp biomicroscopy which reveals increased corneal thickness. It is useful to compare corneal thickness with that in the normal eye. In case of localized corneal edema, one should compare it with corneal thickness in the area above or below the edema. Ultrasonic pachymetery is a convenient rapid and provides accurate quantitative estimation of corneal thickness. Specular microscopy is useful in providing details of endothelial cell density, polymorphism and pleomorphism. In cases with severe corneal edema and scarring confocal microscopy may delineate details of corneal endothelial cells count, shape, size and variation.

In children corneal edema may be due to congenital hereditary endothelial dystrophy, infantile glaucoma with corneal endothelial cell decompensation, following penetrating eye injuries, complicated cataract surgery and rarely toxic endothelitis due to bee sting injury. Patient suffering from congenital hereditary endothelial dystrophy may have associated raised intraocular pressure. Patients have buphthalmos with secondary corneal endothelial cell decompensation have increased corneal diameter in addition to raised intra ocular pressure. Patients suffering penetrating eye injury, under go multiple surgeries including primary repair, cataract surgery, vitreoretinal surgery for retinal detachment and secondary scleral fixated PCIOL. Patients may develop corneal endothelial cell decompensation in case he develops severe uveitis. Complicated cataract surgeries with severe intraocular inflammation, mechanical touch of the instruments and surgeries without viscoelasitc substance may cause corneal endothelial all decompensation and may lead to corneal edema. Children having undergone pars plana vitrectomy and lensectomy for retinal detachment may develop corneal decompensation and corneal edema due to silicone oil keratopathy. Rarely complication like Descemet's membrane detachment may be responsible for persistent corneal edema.

Treatment

Corneal edema of inflammatory origin, i.e. toxic endotheliatis or herpetic origin is treated with topical and systemic steroids. Patients having corneal edema due to herpes simplex virus infection need topical or oral acyclovir. Patients with non-inflammatory corneal edema are evaluated thoroughly. Retina evaluation and ultra sonography is performed to rule out retinal detachment. Patients are put on topical or systemic steroids to cut down inflammation and anti glaucoma medication to reduce IOP. Topical hyperosmatic agents, use of hair drier may provide symptomatic relief for brief period. In case patient suffering from post surgery corneal edema is improving, one should wait for 3 months before considering surgical management. Penetrating keratoplasty with IOL exchange or secondary PCIOL is the definite treatment for corneal edema.

Corneal Ectasia

Keratoconus

In this disease the central or paracentral cornea undergoes progressive thinning and ectasia. The cornea assumes the shape of a large cone. Child develops myopia, regular and irregular astigmatism. The hereditary pattern is usually unpredictable. Most of the cases are sporadic in nature. Nearly all cases are bilateral, but one eye may be affected more than the other. The disease in known to occur in chromic vernal conjunctivitis. The management of keratoconus in active vernal disease is extremely difficult. One may have to control vernal conjunctivitis before treatment of keratoconus. The disease tends to progress during the adolescent years and may stabilize later. As the progression occurs, the apical thinning of the central cornea increases, and extreme degrees of irregular astigmatism may develop.

Clinical Presentation

Most of the patients, who are not happy with the initial prescription the should be carefully examined for early keratoconus. Many of the patients are diagnosed during screening or during preoperation work up as part of laser vision correction. Scissoring of the red reflex on ophthalmoscopy or retinoscopy is considered an early sign of keratoconus. Rizzutti's sign, conical reflection on the nasal cornea as a pen light is show from the temporal side, is another early finding. Iron deposits within the epithelium around the base of the cone described a Fleischer's ring. It is best appreciated with the cobalt-blue filter. Vogt's striae or "stress lines of the stroma" can be observed. Ruptures and scars may occur in Bowman's layer. Higher magnification of slit lamp may be useful in detecting sub changes. Currently corneal topography has become the standard procedure to detect early keratoconus and monitor the progress.

Descemet's membrane rupture may results in sudden development of corneal edema, referred to as acute hydrops. The break in the Descemet's membrane may heal in six to eight weeks. The corneal edema disappears and only stromal sign may be left. Hydrops is treated conservatively with topical hypertonic agents and patching or a soft contact lens. A cycloplegic agent may be needed for ciliary pain. Air injection into the anterior chamber has been reported to enhance resolution of corneal edema.

Pathogenesis

Recent studies suggest increased expression of lysosomal enzymes and decreased levels of inhibitors of proteolytic enzymes may play an important role in corneal stromal thinning. Several investigators have suggested that abnormality in corneal collagen and its cross-linking may be the cause of keratoconus. Eye rubbing and contact lens wear have been postulated to play a role.

Treatment

In very mild cases of keratoconus vision may be improved with glasses alone. However, RGP contact lenses are helpful in mild to moderate cases. They often cause significant improvement in vision as these are able to neutralize the irregular corneal astigmatism. The majority of patients with keratoconus without central corneal scarring can be fitted contact lenses. When the routine gas permeable contract lenses do not work, one can try speciality contact lenses. Rose K contact lenses and Boston contact lenses are specially designed for keratoconus. These contact lenses provide appropriate fit when the routine contact lenses fail. When contact lenses no longer provide satisfactory vision surgical treatment is considered.

Standard surgical treatment consists of penetrating keratoplasty. Lamellar keratoplasty is also effective, but most surgeons prefer not to use this because of the technical difficulties involved and the slightly reduced visual outcome. The most preferred procedure is penetrating keratoplasty. At the time of keratoplasty, decreasing the donor/ recipient size disparity reduces post keratoplasty myopia. Intracorneal ring's have achieved some success in patients without corneal scarring in reducing the myopia and astigmatism and improving spectacle corrected visual acuity. But these patients can be fitted GP contact lenses as well.

Crosslinking treatment of keratoconus is a new method of treating keratoconus. In this procedure the photosensitizer riboflavin and ultraviolet A-light is used as an effective means for stabilizing the cornea in keratoconus. At the present stage of knowledge, the treatment should only be performed in patients with documented progression of keratoconus. To avoid serious side effects it is mandatory in each patient to perform preoperative pachymetry to exclude cases with less than 400 μ stromal thickness. The UVA irradiance should be checked using a UVA-meter, before every case.

Nutritional Deficiency Disorder

Xerophthalmia: Vitamin A Deficiency

Vitamin A deficiency is the leading cause of childhood blindness worldwide. Majority of those afflicted reside in the developing world. According to World Health Organization estimate 228 million children are affected by moderate to severe Vitamin A deficiency. In addition 500,000 cases of vitamin A deficiency with new active corneal lesions occur every year.

Vitamin A deficiency affects growth, the differentiation of epithelial cells and competency of immune system. Vitamin A deficiency mainly affects eye and may cause night blindness, xerosis of the conjunctiva and the cornea, and ultimately corneal ulcer and total corneal melt. Vitamin A deficiency may occur alone, but majority of the cases have associated generalized malnutrition. Protein energy malnutrition is common in occurrence. Severely malnourished children have typical appearance with monkey like face. These children are grossly under weight, loss of fat, listless child who responds poorly to the stimulus, usually stairs into the sky and has infrequent blinking. Specific protein deficiency leads to condition known as Kwashiorkor. Usually children taking diet rich in carbohydrates and deficient in essential aminoacids develop this condition. Due to the deficiency of essential aminoacids the body is not able to synthesize the proteins and these children develop kwashiorkor. Usually these children have edema of the extremities distension of the abdomen due to ascitis. Due to low plasma proteins the intravascular compartment is not able to hold the fluid, and patient gets edema. Malnutrition is a result of poor intake. However chronic and severe malnutrition itself can read to changes in the mucosal cells of small intestines resulting malabsorption.

Vitamin A deficiency is the single most frequent cause of blindness among the pre school children in developing countries. Vitamin A deficiency occurs when the body stores of Vitamin A are exhausted and daily intake does not meet the body requirement. The discrepancy between intake and daily requirement occurs due to dietary inadequacy, increase in daily need, faulty absorption, transport and metabolism. Neonates, who get adequate breast feed usually get protection as mothers milk provide adequate vitamin A. However children born to mothers, who have poor reserve of vitamin A and insufficient intake during pregnancy, usually develop vitamin A deficiency. Bioloigcal stressors such as diarrhea or measles precipitate Vitamin A deficiency in infants and neonates.

In vitamin A deficiency, the organs and tissue where there is rapid turn over of the cells are affected the most. These ites include skin, mucous membranes, conjunctiva and cornea.

Definition of Xerophthalmia, Keratomalacia

According to WHO classification of new signs of vitamin A deficiency have been divided into various stages. World Health Organization reclassification of xerophthalic signs.

Classification	Ocular Sign
XIA	Conjunctival xerosis
XI B	Conjunctival xerosis with Bitot's spots
X 2	Corneal xerosis
X 3A	Corneal ulceration + keratomalacia (1/3rd Cornea)
X 3B	Coreal ulceration + keratomalacia (= ½ Cornea)
X S	Cornea Scar
X N	Night blindness
X F	Xerophthalmic fundus

It is not must that the vitamin A deficiency progresses stage wise. Patient may develop keratomalacia without developing corneal or conjunctival xerosis. Secondary bacterial infections due to staphylococcus and pseudomonas aeruginosa are common. Experimental studies have shown that vitamin A deficiency increases adherence of *Pseudomonas aeruginosa* on ocular surface including cornea. Thus even subclinical vitamin A deficiency may predispose children to the development of bacterial keratitis.

Pathophysiology

Vitamin A is a fat-soluble vitamin ingested in the diet in two forms: retinal itself from animal sources such as milk, fish, meat, liver and eggs or as the provitamin, carotene from plant sources such as green leafy vegetables fruits, yellow fruits and red palm oil.

Vitamin A is absorbed in the small intestine. Within interstinal mucosa, carotene is converted to retinal along with directly ingested retinal is converted into palmitic acid through esterification. Retinal palmitate is transferred through lymphatic system to the liver, where it is stored. When required in tissues retinyl palmitate is hydrolysed and reconstituted retinal travels via blood attached to retinal-binding protein (RBP). Adequate body stores of zinc and protein are required for formation of RBP.

Vitamin A serves two important functions in the human body. As a precursor to photosensitive visual pigments it participate to initiate or neural impulses from photoreceptors. The second it is required for conjunctival epithelial cell RNA and glycoprotein synthesis which helps to maintain conjunctival mucosa and corneal stroma.

Xerophtalmia is a problem when the combined deficiency of Vitamin A and protein occurs. Xerophthalmia is common in Asia and in some parts of Africa. Xerophthalmia can affect any age group, most common affected children aged between 1 to 6 years.

Ocular Manifestation

The clinical signs of xerophthalmia were reclassified by WHO in 1982. These signs and symptoms include the following.

Night blindness: Night blindness is the earliest end the most common symptoms of Vitamin A deficiency. Electroretinography and dark adaptation studies can detect the impaired retinal function even at the stage of subclinical Vitamin A deficiency. Night blindness is the earliest sign to recover (24-48 hours) to systemic administration of Vitamin A.

Conjunctival manifestations: Xerosis (XIA) is the term used to describe dryness. Vitamin A deficiency causes loss of mucus secreting goblet cells and subsequent squamous cell metaplasia of conjunctival epithelial cells. Characteristically dry granular patch that exhibit thickening wrinkling, loss of pigmentation and transparency. It stains brilliantly with rose bengal.

Bitot's spots (X1B): Bitot's spots are triangular, grey patches of keratinized conjunctival debris overlying an area of conjunctival xerosis, in the interpablebral conjucntiva. Some times these patches appear in malnourished individuals in whom Vitamin A levels are normal. In individuals with Vitamin A deficiency these spots will disappear immediately after intiation of therapy.

Corneal manifestations: Earliest corneal manifestations of xerophthalmia include tear film instability, lack luster cornea and superficial punctate keratopathy. In case the treatment is not initiated at an appropriate tissue condition progresses to the development of corneal ulcer, stromal edema and keratinization in the inter palpebral fissure. After initiation of the treatment healing usually takes place within 1 week.

Keratomalacia is defined as full thickness liqifacative necosis of cornea clinically it appears as well defined, opaque, grayish yellow appearance. Stroma can slough leaving bare descemet's membrane or in severe cases corneal perforation. Keratomalacia may not be caused by alone Vitamin A deficiency as it is rare in Vitamin A deficient experimental animals. Often associated in the systemic stressors such as measles, diarrhea or respiratory infection or comitant severe protein energy malformation.

Xerophthalmic fundus: Xerophthlamic fundus is uncommon but it represents structural damage to the fundus in the form of yellow and while dots in retinal periphery. Fluorescein angiographs reveal these dots to be focal retinal pigment epithelial defects. Rarely patients may present with retinal scotomas. Scotoma may disappear within 1 to 2 weeks and retinal lesions fading in 1-4 month after treatment.

Diagnosis: The diagnosis of xerophthalmia is clinical and requires high index of suspicion. The most practical method of confirming the diagnosis is treatment. The biochemical definition of Vitamin A deficiency is plasma levels 35 μ mol/dl of less. Of various techniques of estimation of vitamin A high-pressure liquid chromatography (HPLC) is most reliable. Conjunctival impression cytology is a technique to detect preclinical xerophthalmia. It is a noninvasive method of obtaining superficial conjunctival layers. Microscopic examination of the stained slides reveal squamous metaplasia, enlarged irregular cells, keratinized epithelial cell, and loss of goblet cells.

Treatment

Vitamin A: The oral dose 200,000 IV of vitamin A in oil followed by 200, 000 IV of additional dose next day is given. Children with severe protein deficiency should receive an additional oral dose every 2 weeks till their protein deficiency improves. In case the child is suffering from malabsorption or severe corneal involvement 100, 000 IV water miscible vitamin A intramuscularly is preferred.

Prevention: Vitamin A prophylactic dose for new born is 50000 IV, children younger than 1 year 1100,000 IV every 4-6 month and children more than 2 years 200,000 IV every 4-6 weeks.

The most important step in the prevention of nutritional blindness due to vitamin A deficiency is to ensure that children take adequate amounts of carotene containing foods including cereals, vegetables and fruits. A comprehensive strategy designed to prevent and control vitamin A deficiency. Xerophthalmia and nutritional blindness may be taken in the short, medium and long-term. Short-term or emergency measures include administration of high doses of vitamin A to vulnerable groups. In the medium term the fortification of dietary vehicle with vitamin A may initiated. In the long-term strategy vitamin A intake is increased by dietary intake. Public education program highlighting the importance of kitchen gardening and nutrition education program may be essential.

Dry Eye and Ocular Surface Disease

Dry Eye in Children

Primary dry eye in children although relatively rare but is known to occur. Children having dry eye and congenital absence of corneal sensation develop non-healing epithelial defects. These cases in addition to standard treatment of dry eye may require prolonged eyelid patching or tarsorrhaphy. Children suffering from juvenile rheumatoid arthritis are also predisposed to develop dry eyes. In a recent study significant number of children suffering from juvenile rheumatoid arthritis were found to have dry eyes. Steroid induced dry eye is frequent in children. Diagnosis of dry eye in children requires high index of suspicion. In addition to Scirmers test, Tear Film Break up time and vital dye staining techniques, simple test a mucus ferning test has been found useful.

Preservative free artificial tear drops are the mainstay of the treatment. In addition topical cyclosporine 0.05% twice daily has been found safe and effective in children for the treatment of dry eyes. Punctal plugs may be used in moderate cases of dry eyes. Treatment of associated conditions including blepheritis and meibomianitis is essential to make child free of symptoms.

Limbal Stem Cell Deficiency in Children

Primary limbal stem cell deficiency occurring in aniridia is rare. Secondary limbal stem cell deficiency occurs in chemical injury, thermal injuries and Steven's Johnson syndrome. Iatrogenic limbal stem cell deficiency may occur following chronic medication, local application of mitomycin C and repeated surgical procedures at limbus. Prolonged contact lens wear and chronic inflammatory diseases including severe vernal conjunctivitis may also cause limbal stem cell deficiency.

Stevens Johnson Syndrome

Toxic epidermal necrolysis and Stevens-Johnson syndrome are severe cutaneous reactions, usually to drugs. Diffuse purpuric macules and epidermal detachment of less than 10% of the body surface is indicative of Stevens-Johnson syndrome, whereas epidermal detachment between 10% and 30% is called Stevens-Johnson-toxic epidermal necrolysis overlap. Epidermal detachment involving more than 30% of the total body surface is designated as toxic epidermal necrolysis. Treatment is primarily supportive care, and there are no specific therapy regimens.

Therapeutic modalities such as corticosteroids, cyclosporine, thalidomide, cyclophosphamide, and plasmapheresis, usually based on a symptomatic approach, have been tried in single patients or in small series. Intravenous immunoglobulin has recently been shown to provide rapid improvement in all three of these skin reactions. Treatment for the eye should be started immediately after the reaction to limit ocular surface damage. At later stage these patients develop severe dry eyes and limbal stem cell damage.

Aniridia Related Ocular Surface Disease

Anridic patients develop progressive corneal changes leading to opaque cornea and finally loss of sight leading to blindness. Although the major clinical finding in aniridia is the absence of iris tissue, other ocular structures may also be affected. Macular hypoplasia, nystagmus, amblyopia, cataracts, suluxation of lens, glaucoma, and corneal disease are other ocular associations of aniridia. Corneal changes in aniridia have been described as aniridia-related keratopathy (ARK). Corneal changes include corneal vascular pannus formation, conjunctival invasion of the corneal surface, corneal epithelial erosions and epithelial abnormalities, which eventually result in corneal opacity and contribute to visual loss. Progressive corneal changes in aniridia have been attributed to congenital deficiency of limbal stem cells. However, the current evidence, based on clinical observations and an animal model of aniridia suggest that the proliferative potential of the corneal limbal stem cells may not primarily be impaired. The corneal changes in aniridia may be related to an abnormality within the limbal stem cell niche. Heterozygosity for PAX6 deficiency (PAX6+/-) has been reported to cause aniridia. Mutations of the Pax 6 gene, which is important for eye development, have been identified in families with members affected by aniridia. The mechanisms underlying progressive corneal pathology in aniridia appear multi-factorial and include: (1) abnormal corneal healing responses secondary to anomalous extracellular matrix metabolism; (2) abnormal corneal epithelial differentiation leading to fragility of epithelial cells; (3) reduction in cell adhesion molecules in the PAX6 heterozygous state, rendering the cells susceptible to natural shearing forces; and (4) conjunctival and corneal changes leading to the presence of cells derived from conjunctiva on the corneal surface. Advances in surgical techniques have improved management of some of the visually disabling manifestations of aniridia, but aniridic keratopathy remains a significant source of visual loss. The management of ocular surface diseases due to limbal stem cell deficiency in aniridia is complex but has changed in recent years, as an understanding of the limbal stem cells and their microenvironment has modified the therapeutic approach. Penetrating keratoplasty alone has not been a successful treatment for severe stromal scarring, as it does not treat the underlying epithelial causes of corneal disease. However, it has been successful in corneas that have achieved stable epithelium following limbal stem cell transplantation. In addition the use of autologous serum eye drops, amniotic membrane transplantation, or cultivated limbal cell transplantation has all been reported as a treatment for several ocular surface diseases.

Chemical Eye Injury

Chemical injury is another important cause of severe limbal stem cell deficiency in children. Children usually get chemical injuries while playing inside the house and accidentally handling dangerous chemicals. Thorough irrigation of the conjunctival sac with normal saline decreases the contact time of the chemical and decreases the ocular surface damage. In acute chemical injury every effort is made to promote healing of the ocular surface. To promote epithelial healing bandage contact lens or amniotic membrane transplant may be used. Limbal stem cell transplant may be required in case the medical measures fail to achieve epithelial healing due to limbal stem cell damage. In desperate cases of progressive corneoscleral melt glued on RGP contact lens may be applied. Tectonic penetrating corneal graft is performed for tectonic reasons. These may be combined with amniotic membrane transplants.

Clinical Presentation

Conjunctivalization of the corneal surface is extreme. Conjunctival epithelium growth into the cornea vascularized pannus formation progress from the awe of limbal stem cell deficiency and finally affect the vision. Associated dry eye is due to unstable tear film. Limbal stem cell deficiency can be total or partial. In partial limbal stem cell deficiency, limbal stem cell hypo function may result in non-healing epithelial defect.

Diagnosis

Conjunctivalization of the cornea, the hallmark of limbal stem cell deficiency, needs to be documented to make diagnosis. A severe form of Conjunctivalization is usually obvious to the clinician. Whereas subtle changes in the epithelium texture, permeability, recurrent erosions may be detected on slit lamp biomicroscopy using fluorescein dye. Impression cytology of the cornea and histopathological examination of the excised fibro-vascular tissue may show the presence of goblet cells. Impression cytology can be performed by applying nitrocellulose filter paper onto corneal surface. All cytologic specimens are processed and stained with periodic Acid-Schiff reagent and a modified Harris hematoxylin-eosin stain. Under a microscope with a 40X objective, the area with the highest cell density is counted at 5 different areas with each equivalent to 5625 μm^2 , while that of goblet cell density is measured in a similar manner but at an area equivalent to 10000 μm . These data are then converted to number of cells per millimeter squared and are compared using the Student paired (match) t test.

Treatment

Once acute condition has healed and stable ocular surface has been achieve, ocular surface should be further evaluated. Effect should be made to decrease the corneal vascularization. Limbal stem cell transplants, amniotic membrane transplant may be performed to improve corneal surface and decrease corneal vascularization. Cultured limbal stem cell or corneal epithelial cell transplantation has been need to rehabilitate ocular surface. Finally visual rehabilitation occurs only after penetrating keratoplasty or lamellar keratoplasty.

Gene Therapy in Corneal Diseases

Gene therapy, the treatment or prevention of diseases by gene transfer is considered the most important recent scientific development. Several clinical condition including corneal vascularization, conjunctivalization of cornea dry eye, recurrent erosions and neurotrophic keratitis may not respond favorably to the conventional treatment modalities. For these conditions a specific drug treatment is not available. For most of these conditions treatment through gene therapy with fever side effect may be possible. In addition corneal dystrophies and modulation postoperative wound healing following refractive surgery have to potential have potential of utilizing gene therapy in future.

The eye is the most suitable organ for gene therapy. It is easily accessible, allows local application of therapeutic agents and avoid systemic effects. For gene therapy possible molecular interactions are identified and then therapeutic agent is transferred through gene delivery vehicle known as vectors. Several gene transfer techniques have been employed to alter gene expression of corneal epithelium. Both viral and nonviral have been evaluated to transfer biological active genes into the epithelial layers of the cornea. Viral vectors have the advantage of obtaining significantly higher levels of expression than nonviral vectors. But nonviral vectors are considered suffer as compared to viral redness. The use of performing the transfer *in vitro* or *ex vivo* may make gene therapy safe. In viral vector transmission viruses bind to the cell surface receptors. They infect many cell types and replicate in nonintegrating fashion. Even with topical application of viral vectors corneal abrasion expression may occur in the RPE. Thus tissue specific promoters for the corneal epithelium has been advocated. Specific promoter, keratin has been characterized in cultured cells. Transfer of this gene to neonate cornea have demonstrated expression of protein in the corneal epithelial layer.

Blindness in Childhood

Childhood blindness is a major cause of loss to the society, in terms of productive human beings. Childhood blindness is a significant contributor as number of blind years suffered by a blind child more than those suffered by a person who becomes blind in adulthood. The cumulative number of blind-person years world wide due to childhood blindness are second to only those due to cataract blindness. Thus, prevention and control of childhood blindness is of paramount importance.

Childhood blindness is defined as the best corrected visual acuity in the better eye of < 3/60 in those ≤ 15 years of age. Visual acuity of counting fingers at 3 meters is considered equivalent to 3/60. The prevalence and cause of childhood blindness may be variable throughout the world. A recent survey from India has shown that the prevalence of childhood blindness was 6.5/10000 children. The major cause of blindness included congenital eye anomalies (25%), retinal disease (22%), optic atrophy (16.7%), cataract (15.3%), corneal opacities (11.1%) and others (9.8%). Another survey from India has shown that corneal blindness contributed 26.4% of total childhood blindness.

Etiology of Childhood Blindness:

1. Congenital disease
   - Anophthalmos
   - Microphthalmos
   - Retinal dysplasia
   - Optic atrophy
2. Intrauterine cause
   - Rubella syndrome
   - Toxoplasma
   - Cytomegalovirus
3. Neonatal cause
   - ROP
   - Neonatal ophthalmia

4. Childhood
   - Vit A deficiency
   - Cataract
5. Others
   - Cataract
   - Glaucoma
   - Retinoblastoma
   - Refractive Errors.

Pediatric corneal diseases need accurate diagnosis and energetic management. Parents need to be thoroughly counseled as they have to participate actively and spare time to take care of the needs. They will be required to ensure proper follow-up and proper medication. Preventing measures also need to be emphasized. In case due to congenital or acquired disease, despite best management child develops blindness, the child should be admitted to a blind school. He will education, vocational and social training to become an active member of society.

Chapter 30

Update on Pediatric Corneal Transplant Surgery

Ashok Sharma (India)

Introduction

Visual rehabilitation of pediatric corneal blinds is a major challenge to corneal transplant surgeons. Penetrating keratoplasty is the only way to restore vision and prevent irreversible blindness due to amblyopia in children. Performing penetrating corneal grafts in children poses difficulty in evaluation, technical difficulties during surgery and problems during follow-up. Younger children do not cooperate for proper examination at slit-lamp and need to be examined under general anesthesia. In addition, the complications encountered during adult corneal transplant surgery, including allograft rejection, post penetrating keratoplasty astigmatism and post penetrating keratoplasty glaucoma are more frequent. In case the graft is successful the child will require rigorous treatment for amblyopia. Parents need to be counseled before surgery and possible visual outcome and chances of obtaining clear graft should be discussed.

Indications of Penetrating Keratoplasty

Indications of penetrating keratoplasty may be grouped into congenital corneal opacities and acquired corneal opacities. Among the congenital causes Peter's anomaly, congenital hereditary endothelial dystrophy(CHED), posterior polymorphous dystrophy, sclerocornea, dermoid and mucopolysaccharidosis are common indications for performing surgery. Of the acquired causes traumatic corneal opacities, infectious keratitis, keratoconus, postcataract surgery corneal edema, non-penetrating corneal edema, are the main indications. Corneal edema due to endothelial cell decompensation in patients with buphthalmos has been successfully treated by penetrating keratoplasty. In the acquired group it can be traumatic in nature. In case of traumatic corneal scars the visual outcome depends upon the extent of injury to the posterior segment. The occurrence of indirect optic nerve injury, choroidal rupture and retinal detachment may limit the visual prognosis after penetrating keratoplasty. In developing countries corneal opacities resulting from healed infective keratitis (bacterial, viral and fungal) constitute a major group of indications among the acquired causes. Corneal opacities following keratomalacia is another frequent indication in developing countries. Congenital corneal opacities are usually bilateral, where as acquired corneal opacities are mostly unilateral.

Age at the Time of Penetrating Keratoplasty

Recent studies have shown that penetrating keratoplasty in children should be performed at the earliest to prevent irreversible amblyopia. In neonates with congenital corneal opacities, penetrating keratoplasty is advocated as soon as the child is fit for general anesthesia. In case of acquired corneal opacities the waiting period for penetrating keratoplasty should be minimized. In case the waiting list for penetrating keratoplasty is long, the child is given priority over the adults. Penetrating keratoplasty in neonates and very young children is technically difficult and the risk of graft failure is high. In a study children

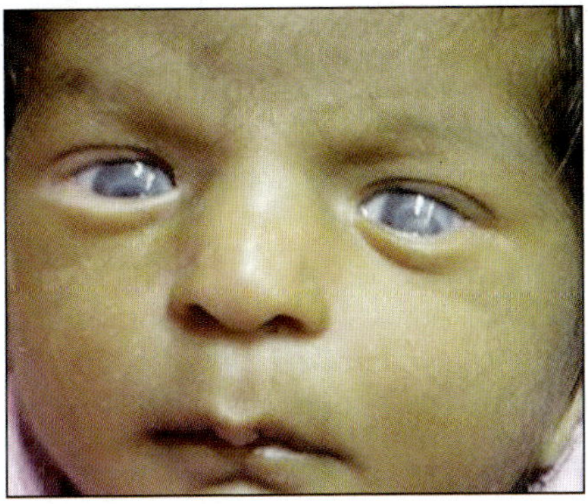

Figure 1: Bilateral congenital corneal opacity

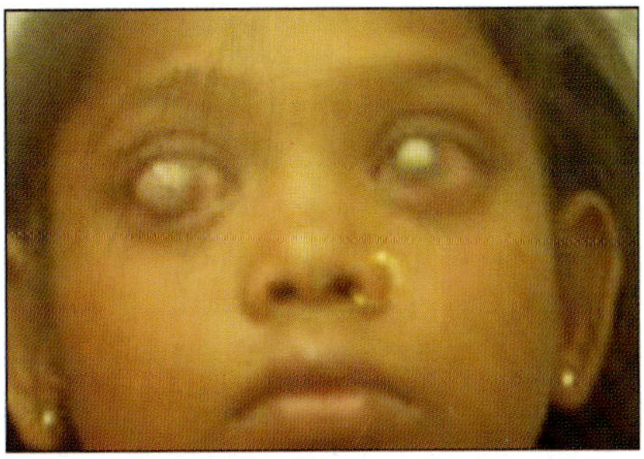

Figure 2: Bilateral acquired corneal opacities

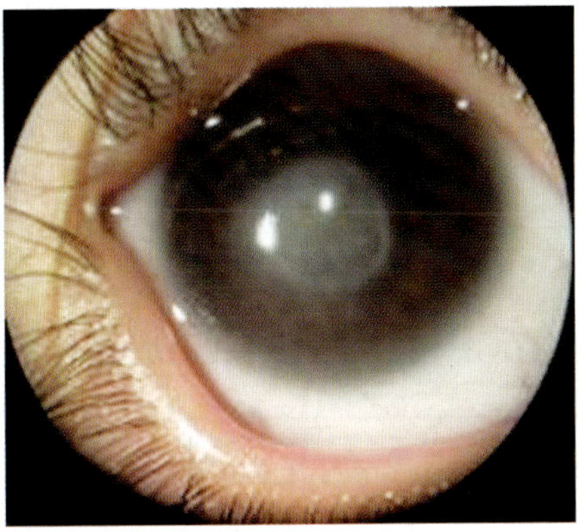

Figure 3: Unilateral acquired corneal opacity

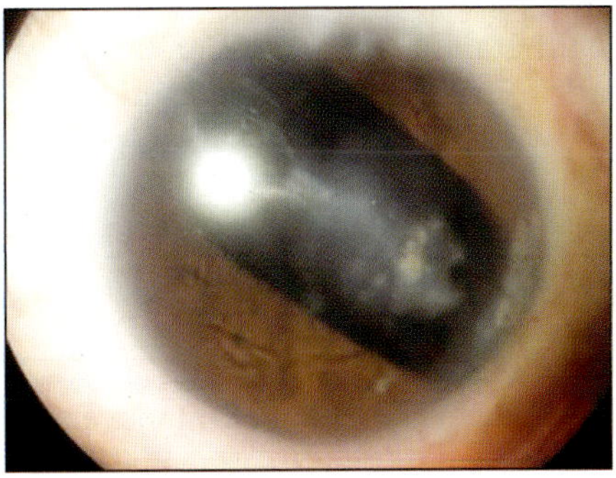

Figure 4: Healed corneal laceration for RG P contact lens fitting

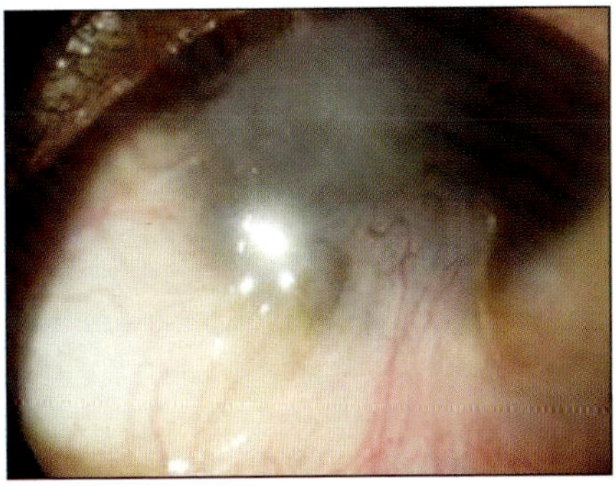

(A) Before amniotic membrane transplant

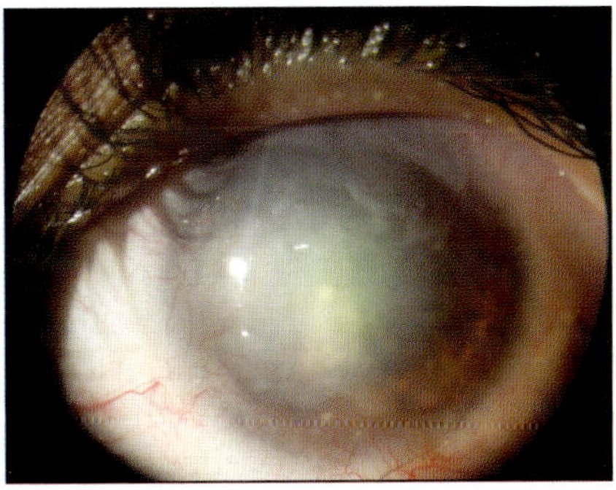

(B) After amniotic membrane transplant

Figures 5A and B: Chemical eye injury

having undergone unilateral cataract surgery before the age of four months had better visual outcome as compared to those after four months. The study indicates that penetrating keratoplasty in children should be performed early to have better visual outcome. The youngest neonate reported to have undergone successful penetrating keratoplasty for large corneal perforation is, a 34 week post conception infant weighing 1 lb.

Neonates due to immunological immaturity are less predisposed to graft rejection. The immune system in neonates develops very early in gestation and is fully developed by birth. Neonatal immune system has characteristically dominance of T-suppressor cells and qualitatively less functional B cells. It has been well documented that the anterior chamber is a privileged site for transplantation. This is mainly due to the absence of blood supply and access to lymphatic system. This makes antigen presentation, which is the part of the afferent limb of rejection, ineffective. Immunization schedules for neonates also avoid the first 4 weeks of life to avoid tolerance to the subsequent dose of antigen leading to less than optimal antibody response in future. Clinical studies have also shown that in neonates with isolated corneal opacities, corneal transplantation in the neonatal period resulted in better prognosis in terms of both graft clarity and vision improvement. The success of these grafts has been attributed both neonatal immune tolerance and clear visual axis during the most initial period of visual development.

Evaluation of Infants or Neonates with Congenital Corneal Opacities

Detailed examination of infants and neonates with congenital corneal opacities is essential to plan treatment. The visual acuity must be ascertained. Response to light stimulus, fixation at light source and following of the movement of illuminated object or light source are helpful. Responses are to be observed carefully and even parents should be demonstrated these tests. Detailed personal history, obstetric history and family history in a child with congenital corneal opacity is recorded. Detailed ocular examination may not be possible in the consultation chamber as the neonates and infants will never be steady and fixate to allow detailed slit lamp bio-microscopy. This part of the examination is better performed under general anesthesia. These days risk of general anesthesia in case of the newborns or infants is minimal. The amount of information on detailed examination we get out weigh the risk of general anesthesia. Under general anesthesia, detailed anterior segment examination, measurements of corneal diameters (both horizontal and vertical) and recording of intraocular pressure evaluation are recorded. Details of corneal opacity, whether central or peripheral, localized or diffuse, are recorded. Peripheral corneal opacities occur in partial sclerocornea and peripheral corneal ulcers. Central corneal scars may occur in Peter's anomaly. Perforated corneal ulcer may require therapeutic penetrating graft. Direct and indirect ophthalmoscopy to visualize retina is performed details of retina, macula and disc are recorded.

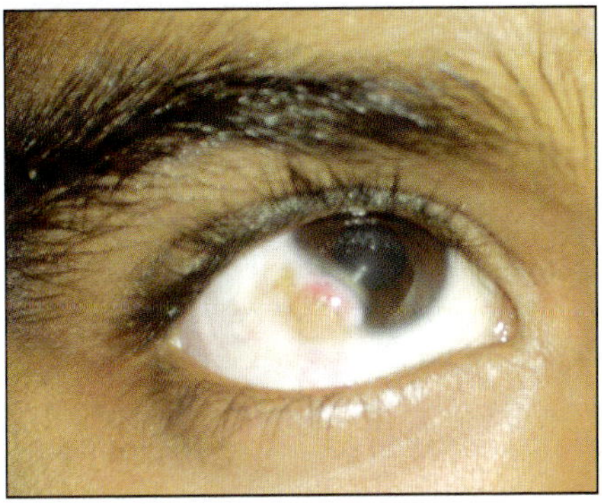

Figure 6A: Limbal dermoid pre-operative

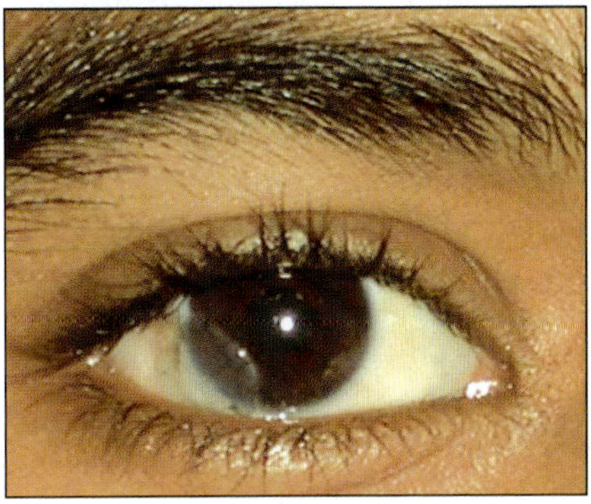

Figure 6B: Limbal dermoid post surgery, DALK

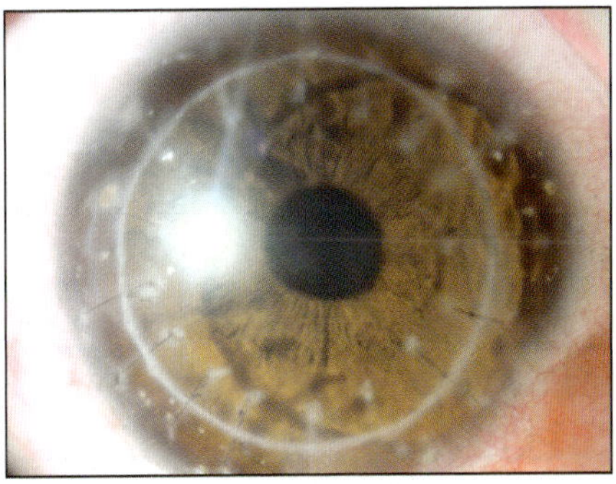

Figure 7A: (RE) DALK for multiple stromal foreign bodies

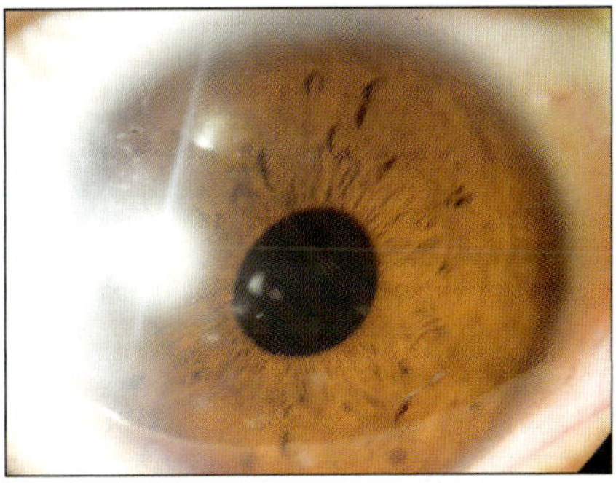

Figure 7B: (LE) Few corneal foreign bodies

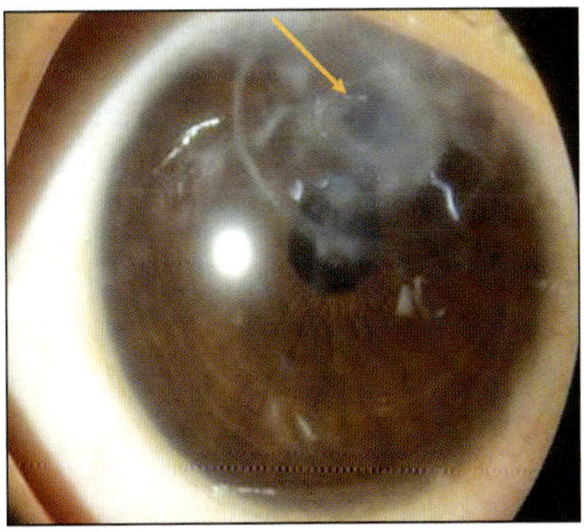

Figure 8: DALK for chronic corneal perforation with anterior staphyloma (Arrow corneal perforation)

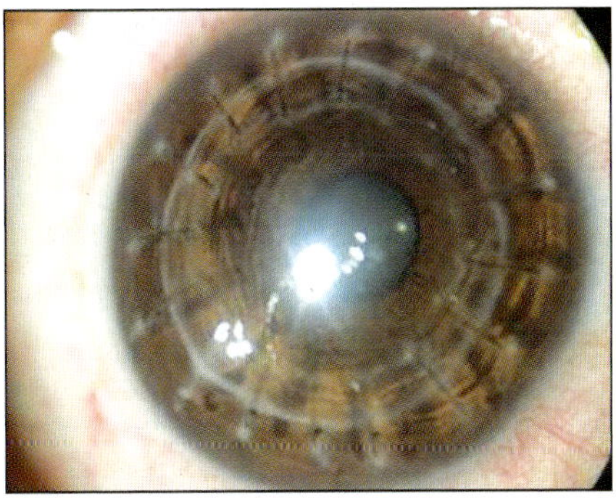

Figure 9: Penetrating keratoplasty for keratoconus

Investigations

Ultrasonography, A scan and B scan are performed to evaluate vitreous and retina status. In case eye is microphthalmic there is always possibility of associated ocular anomalies. The ultrasound biomicroscopy (UBM) give more details of intraocular pathologies. UBM is of special importance in patients with corneal opacity and associated glaucoma. Configuration of anterior chamber angle, details of angle structure and ciliary body are better delineated by UBM. In patients with anterior staphyloma, UBM may provide correct position of the iris and details of iris incarceration or iris adhesions. UBM has been of immense values on studying the structural alterations in pathological conditions including Peter's anomaly, aniridia and ocular trauma. The status of lens and the integrity of the posterior capsule should be evaluated. In case the cataract is present, an additional procedure of cataract extraction and post chamber IOL implantation along with penetrating keratoplasty should be performed.

Pediatric Keratoplasty Constraints

Pediatric penetrating keratoplasty is a challenge to corneal surgeons. The major constraints to perform corneal transplants in neonates include technical difficulties due to small eyes and positive posterior pressure. Low scleral rigidity cause extreme positive posterior pressure, resulting a forward bulge of iris lens diaphragm and make the surgery difficult. At times the positive pressure is extremely high and causes extrusion of lens, lose of vitreous. Associated ocular abnormalities i.e. cataract, glaucoma and microphthalmia make the surgical procedure complicated and increase the operating time significantly. In the immediate postoperative period severe inflammatory response is encountered. In case surgery is delayed, immaturity of the visual system leads to amblyopia.

Preparation before Corneal Transplant Surgery

The aim of the corneal surgeons is to attain clear visual axis and prevent amblyopia by performing corneal transplant at an early age. Corneal transplants have been recommended as soon as the child is fit for general anesthesia. Corneal opacification should not be considered in isolations. There is always a possibility of associated eyelid and adnexial abnormalities. These abnormalities should be first corrected so that the graft surface following surgery is well protected and the integrity is not affected. Intraocular pressure, in case it is high is controlled and brought to normal range either with medical treatment or surgical (glaucoma filtering surgery) intervention. Associated posterior segment anomalies, including retinal detachment or vitreous hemorrhage should be evaluated and treated. Child should be examined by a pediatrician before surgery and cleared for surgery under general anesthesia. Most of the children with congenital corneal opacities may be having associated cardiac abnormalities.

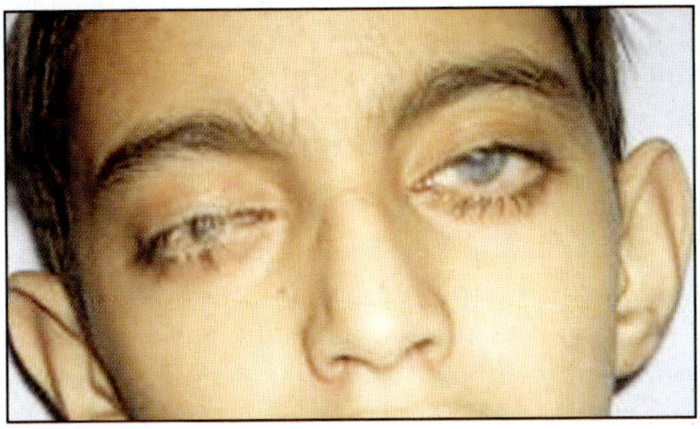

Figure 10: Regraft in a child with bilateral Peter's anomaly (LE)

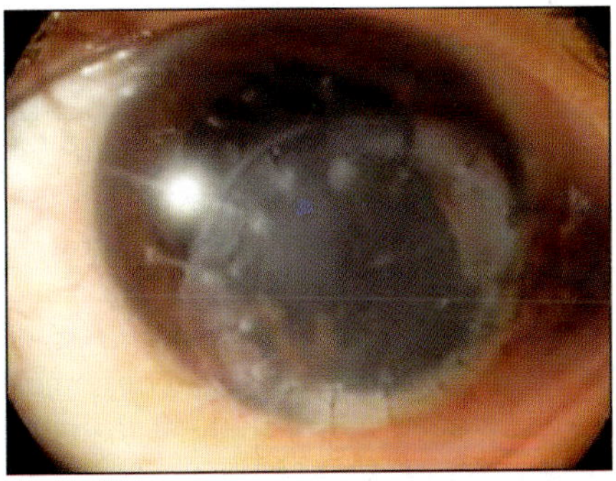

(A) Before regraft

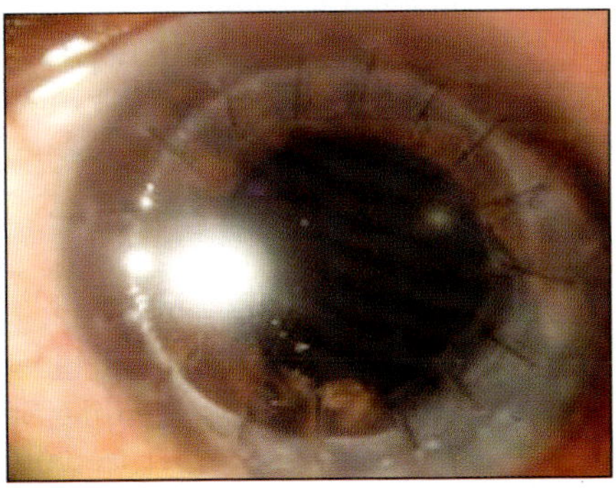

(B) After regraft

Figures 11A and B: Regraft for opaque therapeutic graft

Donor Tissue

Exact age matching between the donor and the recipient may not be possible, however excellent grades of tissue from younger donor should be used. Donor's age between 4 to 30 years is best suited for children. Donor corneas from young than 4 years are relatively difficult to handle during surgery and subsequently. Donor cornea from infants and very young children have steeper cornea and may result increase corneal curvature of the graft. In routine, oversized graft (0.5 mm) is used. Unusually high myopia (60 D) has been reported from steeper donor cornea from young donors. This makes amblyopia treatment difficult. The donor cornea for corneal transplants in children has endothelia cell count close to 3000. In published data donor age, donor cell count and death storage time did not affect grafts surgery. However, decreased death to corneal transplant surgery has been associated with better graft.

Surgery

Extremely high positive posterior pressure is a major introoperative problem encountered during corneal transplant surgery infants and neonates. Although it is impossible to eliminate the positive posterior pressure, however every effort should be make to keep it minimum. In case of smaller palpebral aperture lateral canthotomy reduce posterior pressure. Use of pre-op mitotic drops or intra cameral miotic may be useful to keep iris lens diaphragm behind. An experienced anesthetist may be asked to keep the neonate at deeper plan of anesthesia. A sudden increase in intraocular pressure have posterior pressure and may even suddenly loss the lens. A non deploarising muscle relaxant eliminates the risk of movements and contraction of extraocular muscle. Keeping head at a higher level than feet may be helpful. Anesthetist may be asked to hyperventilate child in case posterior pressure is extreme. Hyperventilation decrease posterior pressure and vitreous pressure.

Digital pressure or application of Honan's balloon is another good option to keep posterior pressure down. External pressure on the globe due to speculum should be avoided. Flieringa's ring should be applied in every case. Pre placed mattress suture is helpful in securing the graft immediately and pushing the iris lens diaphragm behind by injecting viscoelastic substance. One may use one mattress suture or two mattress sutures depending upon the requirement. These sutures if needed can also be applied after trephination of host cornea. Use of 8 '0' silk or monofilament to place cardinal sutures in case of extreme positive pressure is a good option. It secures the graft and one can inject viscoelastic substance to push iris lens diaphragm back. A cohesive viscoelastic suture i.e. healon GV or healon 5 may be used to keep positive posterior pressure down and allows suturing.

Surgical procedure should be completed in a shortest possible time. After punching the donor tissue all the instruments required for recipient trephination and donor button suturing should be kept ready. Neonates or infants may be given intravenous mannitol 20% (0.5 to 1.5 gm / KBW) to reduce the vitreous volume and thus decreasing the positive posterior pressure. At times the positive posterior pressure is extremely high and it may not be possible to suture the graft unless we reduce it. Some of the surgeons have advocated placement of flat instrument (lens spatula) over the iris to prevent lens extrusion and vitreous loss. We routinely leave the recipient corneal button attached at 3 o' clock position and do not excise it completely. We place donor button in the recipient opening and start suturing. After securing donor corneal button with 4 cardinal sutures we excise the host corneal button and continue suturing. This intact recipient bed in situation of extreme positive posterior pressure is put back on the recipient open. Few more cardinal sutures are applied and posterior pressure is reduced. Then the donor button is sutured. We have found this simple method extremely useful in combating high posterior pressure (Nirankari and Sharma, unpublished data). In case positive pressure is extreme and passing of 10 '0' nylon is difficult and it is not holding, it is wise to use 8 '0' nylon / silk suture and replace these sutures after the suturing in complete. Pars plana vitrectomy before trephination has been advocated to prevent posterior pressure for patients who are at higher risk for developing extreme positive posterior pressure during penetrating keratoplasty.

Size of the Graft

In a large multicentric study this average graft size was 7.1 mm diameter. Graft size may be determined according to the diameter of the cornea. For a normal sized cornea (10.5 mm) 7.5 mm diameter graft should suffice. However, in case of mciro-ophthalmia/microcornea graft size may be decreased according to the diameter of the cornea. Small grafts are required in the small diameter corneas because placing a normal sized graft (7.5 mm) in a small diameter cornea brings host graft junction very close to the limbus. This may predispose the graft to allograft rejection and its failure. Use of small diameter grafts in otherwise normal cornea may have several disadvantages. This may result in higher astigmatism. With the use of small grafts the number of viable endothelial cells decreases significantly. In case the graft size is reduced from the size 8 mm to 6 mm diameter the number of viable endothelial cells on the graft decreases by 44%. Thus smaller grafts will be predisposed to graft failure as the redistribution of endothelial cells will result a final cell count of the graft well below 1000 per mm. It is advisable to use over sized donor corneal button (0.5 mm) routinely. In a study 1 mm over sizing for pediatric case has been advocated to decrease incidence of peripheral anterior synechia. This option should be used with extreme caution as this may cause difficulty in suturing of the donor button. In patient with anterior staphyloma the recipient cornea is under stretch due to raised IOP. On trephination the recepient opening decreases as the tissue is relaxed and IOP is low. In such a situation 1 mm oversizing further increases and may result in malaposition of the host graft junction and difficulty in suturing. In addition if the donor happens to be young less than 2 years of age, the donor cornea is steeper and 1 mm over sizing will result in high myopia, and amblyopia therapy may be difficult.

Alternatives to Penetrating Keratoplasty

Corneal opacities partially obscuring the visual axis, gas permeable contact lens may be tried. Majority of the patients suffering from opacities resulting from traumatic corneal lacerations can be managed by fitting rigid gas permeable contact lenses. Most of the children are co-operative for fitting and monitoring the follow-up. Patients are usually apprehensive of gas permeable contact lenses. Majority of children learn quickly how to insert or take out rigid gas permeable contact lenses. They take care of contact lenses as per directions.

In case opacification is central and peripheral cornea is clearer one can evaluate the child for auto rotational keratoplasty. The significant advantage is that the risk of allograft rejection is eliminated and chance of graft success is enhanced. However, post keratoplasty astigmatism and other problem of operating up on neonates / infant remains unchased. Risk of high astigmatism is more as the disparity or defect occurs in both host cornea as well as donor cornea. In case of oval due to oblique placement of corneal trephine both host corneal bed and the donor button are oval. Placement of oval donor cornea button in an oval recipient opening with long axis at different angles result in high astigmatism.

In case corneal opacity is central and larger part of the inferior cornea is clearer, one can consider optical iridectomy. Optical iridectomy performed on the superior half of the iris do not serve any purpose as large part of it will be covered by the eyelids. Optical iridectomy is best performed in the lower nasal quadrant however one can opt for lower temporal in case opacity is extending into the lower nasal quadrant. In our experience patients are not happy with an optical iridectomy. Most of the times it does not provide an adequate vision to prevent amblyopia. Large optical iridectomies iridoplasty and pupilloplasty difficult during penetrating keratoplsty.

Infants and children with superficial corneal disease may be evaluated for superficial keratectomy. Most of the children suffering from pannus or conjunctivilization due to partial limbal stem cell deficiency can be treated with superficial keratectomy. Once a dissection plane is reached, it is extremely easy to remove the superficial corneal tissue. Children suffering from vernal ulcer and plaque formation need epithelial debridment and plaque removal in addition to medical treatment. The objective should be to achieve smooth and transparent corneal surface. To promote epithelialilzation, bandage contact lens may be applied. Children suffering from chemical eye injury and having conjunctivalization due to partial limbal stem cell deficiency need superficial keratectomy with amniotic membrane transplant.

In case of partial thickness corneal opacities or in condition where endothelium is healthy, lamellar corneal surgery, lamellar keratoplasty or deep anterior lamellar keratoplasty may be advised. In case of superficial corneal opacities due to healed bacterial or fungal corneal ulcers one should consider lamellar keratoplasty. Corneal endothelium is healthy in these cases. Depending upon the depth of involvement of cornea one may chose to perform either lamellar keratoplasty or deep anterior lamellar keratoplasty. Advantage of DALK / LK are that all the intraoperative problems (extreme positive posterior pressure, danger of extrusion of extrusion of lens and difficulties of suturing peripheral anterior synechia) may be avoided. In addition, risk of allograft rejection in DALK/LK is significantly less as compared to penetrating keratoplasty. In addition post PK astigmatism is lower and visual rehabilitation is faster. These procedures may not be suitable for children with corneal opacities and deep corneal vascularization. Patient developing corneal opacities following recurrent herpes simplex keratitis are also a not suitable candidate either LK or DALK, as they may develop recurrence of HSK infection from residual corneal tissue. Cornea has been documented as site of viral latency and recurrence may occur from corneal tissue alone. Limbal dermoids are best treated with LK/ DALK depending upon the level of involvement. We have treated a child suffering from corneal scaring due to multiple intrastromal foreign bodies in the right eye following cracker injury by performing DALK. We have also treated corneal perforation with anterior staphyloma by performing DALK.

High Risk Penetrating Keratoplasty

Presence of deep corneal vascularization in two quadrants or more predisposes the corneal grafts to higher risk of allograft rejection. Children having undergone penetrating keratoplasty for herpes simplex keratitis are at higher risk of graft rejection, recurrence of disease and failure. Children should be put on oral acyclovir prophylaxis. Children undergone regraft are at higher risk of allograft rejection due to prior sensitization. Patients having corneal opacities in association with limbal stem cell deficiency and ocular surface disease are also at higher risk of developing graft failure due to allograft rejection. Children suffering from corneal opacification and associated ocular surface disease should undergo limbal stem cell transplant and amniotic membrane transplant prior to penetrating keratoplasty. Patients with severe ocular surface disease due to chemical eye injury, Steven's Johnson Syndrome may undergo deep lamellar keratoplasty. Deep lamellar keratoplasty has lower risk of allograft rejection.

Perioperative Care

Success of corneal transplant surgery is determined by meticulous perioperative care. Thorough examination of child including slitlamp biomicroscopy should be performed. During the follow-up visits parents should be explained danger signs and should be asked to report immediately as soon as the danger signs appear. The younger children and infants do not communicate their symptoms. However, in case the child is irritable or crying without any obvious reason, he should be brought for eye check-up. The first examination is usually at 24 hours intervals. Status of the graft clarity, wound integrity, epithelial healing, intraocular inflammation and intraocular pressure every visit. Infants or children should be examined daily for one week and an alternate day for two weeks.

After that every week examination is carried out. In case child develops any problem child may be examined early to the start treatment.

Complications

Early

Delayed epithelization, disruption of host graft junction, fibrinous reaction, high intraocular pressure are the common problems encountered in the first few days. Infective keratitis although rare (5%) may occur and need intensive topical antibacterial treatment. Fibrinous exudative reaction should be treated with topical and systemic steroids. Delay in epithelization may be secondary to severe uveitis or high intraocular pressure. In these cases severe uveitis is treated with topical or systemic steroids. Once uveitis or high intraocular pressure is controlled epithelial defect heals completely. Rarely endophthalmitis following penetrating keratoplasty in children may occur.

Intermediate

Neonates and infants need to be examined under general anesthesia at around 3 weeks even if they have no visible problem. Wound healing in neonates and infants is past and sutures become lose. At 3 to 4 weeks lose suture should be removed. At 6-8 week complete healing occurs and sutures may be removed at 6-8 week period. In older children 2 to 4 years may be observed for lose suture and may be removed little later. Children above 6 years behave more or less similar to adults and selection suture removal may be performed.

Late Complications

Allograft rejection, suture related infections, recurrence of disease (HSK, keratoconus) post keratoplasty astigmatism and post keratoplasty glaucoma may occur. Suture related complications can be prevented by immediate removal of lose sutures. Lose suture may cause an epithelial defect, secondary inflammation and trigger allograft rejection due to inflammation and graft vascularization. Post keratoplasty astigmatism is higher with PKP as compare to lamellar procedure (LK/DALK). Selective suture removal can be done to reduce astigmatism in children aged 6 years of more.

Allograft Rejection

Parents should be explained that allograft rejection might occur any time after surgery. Studies have shown that 30 to 70% pediatric grafts fail within first six months and 65 to 85% within first year. Neonates and infants should be closely maintained for development of allograft rejection in the first year of life. Children are unable to complain about the symptoms and usually present late for treatment. Parents should be educated to bring the child for examination on observing any redness, discomfort, and opaqueness in the graft or decrease in vision. On every visit child should be examined at slit lamp to detect early signs of allograft rejection. Infant and children may not present with characteristic signs of allograft rejection. Graft edema even in the absence of keratic precipitates should also be treated as allograft rejection. Intraocular pressure should be monitored in these cases, they may have associated secondary glaucoma. Once allograft rejection is diagnosed, the child is put on prednisolone acetate (0.1%) eye drop every one hour and atropine ointment twice daily. In addition oral prednisolone (1 mg/kbw) should also be started. In recent studies topical cyclosporine A (2%) has been found successful in treating graft reaction. Topical cyclosporine A has also been used to prevent graft rejection in high risk cases. Cyclosporine A being lipid soluble, topical cyclosporine A (2%) need to be prepared in castor oil in the hospital pharmacy. At times young children may not tolerate it, as it causes significant ocular irritation. It has also been reported to cause persistent epithelial defects and delayed epithelial healing. Recent studies have shown that topical cyclosporine A prepared in the aqueous solution is also effective and can be prepared in preservative free artificial tear solution. Topical cyclosporine A has been reported to be equally effective in concentrations ranging from 0.05 to 1%. Topical cyclosporine A 0.05% (Restasis, Allergan) has been found effective in treatment and prevention of graft rejection in high risk cases. The formulation of the of the drug is such that it releases large number of microdroplets in the tear film.

Glaucoma

Treatment of glaucoma prior to penetrating keratoplasty or after it includes medical treatment, trabeculectomy with adjuvents and/or trabeculotomy. Treatment of refractory glaucoma is a real challenge as it will not only damage the optic nerve but also corneal graft resulting graft failure. Glaucoma drainage implant procedures have shown encouraging results in the treatment of refractory post penetrating keratoplasty glaucoma. Several authors have reported favorable results of pediatric penetrating keratoplasty following control of IOP using glaucoma drainage implant procedures. Although conventionally glaucoma is first controlled and then only penetrating keratoplasty is performed. At times due to the risk of development irreversible amblyopia glaucoma implant surgery may be combined with penetrating keratoplasty to provide early visual rehabilitation and preventing the development of amblyopia.

Treatment of Amblyopia

Amblyopia treatment should be started as early as possible following surgery. Cycloplegic refraction should be done and glasses should be prescribed. Parents should be explained that the normal eye of the child need to be patched so that he uses the operated eye. The schedule for patching may be the same as used for standard amblyopia treatment. In children upto 2 years (2:1), 2 to 3 years (3:1), 3 to 4 years (4:1), 4 to 5 years (5:1) and 6 years or above (6:1) should be used.

Outcome

Anatomical success rate following penetrating keratoplasty in childhood including infants and neonates has increased significantly. The incidence of vision restoration in children following penetrating keratoplasty is still low. Visual prognosis has been reported better in younger children and is likely determined by the incidence and severity of amblyopia. In recent study of 65 grafts on 58 eyes of 52 children (mean age 10.6 years SD 4.3 years) 38% achieved BCVA 6/9 or better and 60% had BCVA 6/18 or better. Visual acuity has been reported significantly better for the acquired as compared to congenital indications. Significant numbers of patients in this study had keratoconus as an indication for penetrating keratoplasty. Results from developing countries are less favorable. In a study from India nearly 1/3rd patients achieved > or = 20/400 vision and nearly 50% of these achieved > or = 20/50. Allograft rejection, infective keratitis and glaucoma were major causes of graft failure. The overall long term (10 years) probability of maintaining clear graft after initial penetrating keratoplasty for Peter's anomaly is 35% +/- 0.6%. Eyes with severe disease, larger donor cornea, co-existing central nervous system abnormalities and anterior synechia were reported to have significantly poorer outcome than eyes without these factors. Children with severe form of Peter's anomaly may required multiple grafts to have functional vision. One of our patient with severe Peter's anomaly had undergone four corneal transplants during 14 years and enjoyed good vision. He finally died recently due to severe CNS disease.

Repeat Corneal Graft

In case the child develops graft failure a repeat graft should be considered. Parents need to be explained that subsequent corneal grafts have less chances of success. In one of the studies, of 27 repeat grafts undergoing second graft 19% were successful and of six graft undergoing third graft none succeeded. Repeat graft may be indicated to prevent dense and irreversible amblyopia. However, in case child is having unilateral corneal capacity, parents should be explained that even if the graft may becomes opaque, later on chances of improvement of vision by performing repeat graft will be there. In adults if the grafts is fail due to the graft rejection, it is advisable to wait for 6 months before a repeat graft is performed. It is aimed to bring down the inflammation in the graft to minimum and to decrease the incidence of allograft rejection. At times it may be difficult to ascertain whether the graft failed due to allograft rejection or due to some other cause. It is better to treat it as allograft rejection. In younger children it may not be possible to wait for 6 months due to danger of development of amblyopia. In these cases the repeat graft may be performed at 3 months after the initial graft has failed. One can wait a little longer in case the child is six year old or more. Children suffering from perforated corneal ulcers need therapeutic penetrating keratoplasty and these grafts usually become opaque due to chronic inflammation. However, successful regraft can be performed for these patients at later date and both vision improvement and graft clarity can be obtained.

Keratoprosthesis

Infants and children who are at high risk of graft rejection and subsequent graft failure may be benefited with keratoprosthesis or artificial corneal transplantation. Keratoprosthesis transplantation means placing an optical device in the host cornea. It is immunologically inert and has the advantage that graft rejection does not occur. Recently, a custom made Boston type 1 keratoprosthesis is available and can be designed to correct refractive errors including aphakia. AlphaCor, a synthetic cornea made up of hydrophilic polymer poly (2-hydroxyethyl methacrylate) is another keratoprosthesis used in high risk cases for corneal transplant surgery. The alphaCor is implanted in a corneal stromal lamellar pocket in a two stage procedure. In the first stage 360 peritomy and debridement of corneal ephithelium is done. A superior 180 limbal incision at 50% of depth is extended into the corneal stroma forming an intralamellar pocket is made. A central 3.5 mm posterior corneal trephination is performed. The device is placed with in the corneal pocket and paralimbal incision is closed. After 8 to 12 weeks anterior trephination (3mm) is done to expose the optic of the device. Keratoprosthesis helps the corneal surgeon to rehabilitate those corneal blinds having visual potential, but are unlikely to be benefited by performing penetrating keratoplasty using human donor cornea.

Pediatric corneal transplant surgery is a team effort it involves combined effort of corneal surgeon assisted by glaucoma specialist pediatrician, anesthetist, counselors and rehabilitation team.

Rehabilitation of Blinds due to Corneal Disease

Children with bilateral corneal opacities either congenital, chemical burns, Stevens Johnson Syndrome may not be successfully visually rehabilitated even after performing repeated corneal grafts. The parents of these children should be counseled to get their children admitted to blind schools to provide educational and vocational training to these children. These children can lead independent life and contribute to the development of the society if proper facilities and opportunities are provided.

Summary and Conclusion

Advancement in micro-surgical techniques, quality eye banking and better anesthesia facilities have made possible to undertake corneal transplant in a neonate as soon as the diagnosis is made and corneal transplant surgery is advised. Although surgery is technically demanding but it is possible to provide clear visual axis during critical period of visual development. Treatment and prevention of development of amblyopia in neonates is extremely important even after successful penetrating keratoplasty.

Chapter 31

Pediatric Keratoplasty

Anita Panda, Geeta Behera
Abhiyan Kumar (India)

Introduction

Penetrating keratoplasty may be the necessary first step in preventing irreversible loss of visual function in a child, though the visual results of pediatric penetrating keratoplasty have been fairly disappointing. Many special difficulties encountered in the management of corneal transplantation in a child conspire to make these patients among the most challenging for the corneal surgeon.

Many aspects of an infant's or a child's preoperative, intraoperative and postoperative care differ from those of an adult undergoing a corneal transplantation. The child and the child's parents are usually very anxious when they present for preoperative evaluation. The difficulty in assessing the visual function of an infant, a child's inability to co-operate with the eye examination and the great variability in outcome all make the physicians decision regarding surgery more difficult.

Visual Assessment

Measuring vision in infants and children is a special skill. To start with, the examiner must create a rapport and gain attention of the child.

A normal child can fix and follow objects by 3 months of age, the blink response develops between 2 and 3 months, reaching out for objects begins by 6 months and binocular function develops by 3-7 months. The visual acuity of a normal child at birth is 6/120, at 6 months is 6/36, at 12 months at 6/18 and 6/6 at the age of 2 years.

WHO recommends that vision should be assessed at both distance and near with the same optotype. It should be recorded at 6, 4, 3 metres and 40 cm with a luminance of 80 and 160 candles/mm. Further, the distance and angle should be adjusted to fit the need of the child. Measuring the vision can be performed either directly or indirectly.

Direct

Up to 3 months of age by observing the baby recognize its mother's face, between 3 and 6 months by judging through colorful objects, between 6 and 12 months by its ability to differentiate details of small objects, between 12 and 36 months by Allen pictures, Lea symbols or Kay picture symbols and after 3 years and until 5 years by HOTV test, tumbling E test, Landolt broken ring test.

Indirect

Optokinetic(OKN) response, Preferential looking techniques(PLT) and Pattern evoked potentials.

Besides visual acuity, visual testing also includes assessing the pupillary reaction, fixation, ocular motility, fusion and color vision.

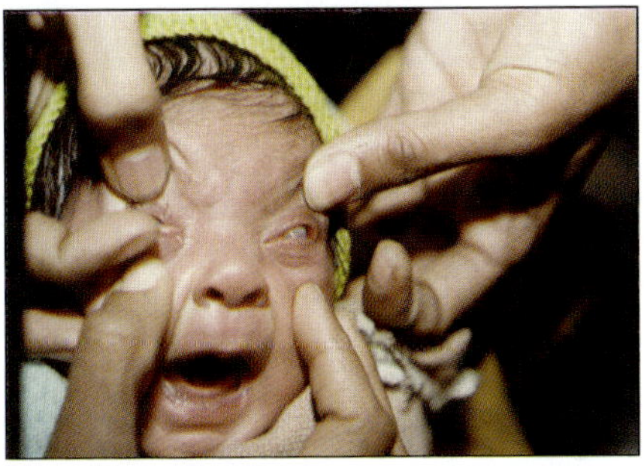

Figure 1: Bilaterally blind infant

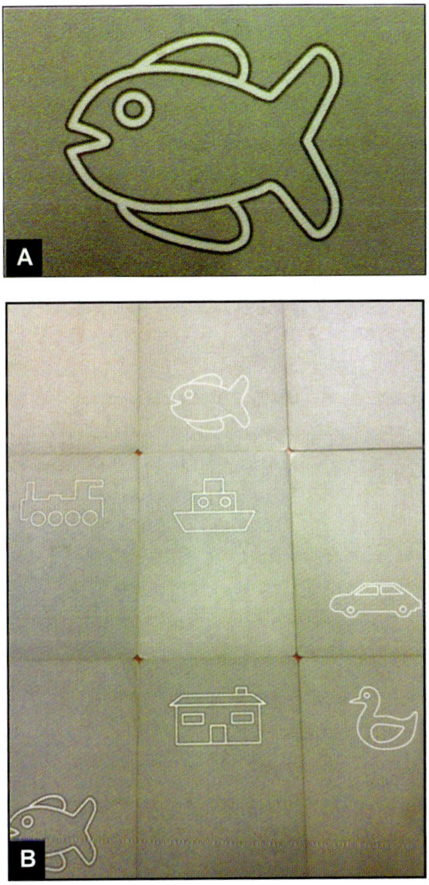

Figures 2A and B: Cardiff acuity cards

Ocular Examination

Like in adults, the ocular surface, anterior and posterior segment evaluation and adnexal examination are essential besides detailed corneal examination. A full ocular evaluation under sedation or anesthesia is necessary involving refraction, tonometry, gonioscopy and fundoscopy. Because of the difficulty in determining any associated retinal or lens pathology in an infant with an opaque cornea, ultrasound for posterior examination and a single maximum intensity bright flash Electroretinogram and visual evoked potential become essential.

Surgical Procedures

All surgery is carried out under general anesthesia. The surgery itself is technically more difficult because in infants the cornea and the anterior chamber are smaller, and the cornea is often thinner and more pliable, requiring more exacting surgical technique. Compared to an adult eye, the eye of a young keratoplasty patient is more likely to have scleral collapse and alarming posterior pressure. The iris of infants and children seems to have a greater tendency to adhere to the posterior corneal surface and the wound. Many young patients with congenital or traumatic corneal disease have significant anterior segment abnormalities, which may be difficult to anticipate but must be addressed during the surgery. In children requiring vitrectomy, the vitreous is more tenacious which makes its safe, rapid removal more difficult.

Infants and children in comparison to adults, appear to be more prone to a severe inflammatory response during the early postoperative period and more likely to have endothelial graft rejection or graft failure.

Again, the corneal wound heals more rapidly in infants and children, increasing the risks that sutures will loosen quickly, erode, vascularise and become infected. Therefore all sutures must be removed early, making selective suture removal to minimize transplant astigmatism impossible.

The graft's success may eventually decrease if parents fail to understand the important role of postoperative management and difficulties thereof. Unless the surgeon is able to communicate to them the importance of constant supervision and the need for regular medication and follow-up, it is probably wiser not to attempt such surgery.

Postoperatively, infants and young children are unable to co-operate for examinations. Therefore the examination must be either suboptimal or performed with the patients under restraint, under sedation or under anesthesia. Infants and children cannot effectively communicate that they have visual loss, pain or other symptoms that require evaluation. Therefore, compared to adults, they require more frequent examinations. Also, children are more likely to rub or traumatize their eye.

The greatest difference between the management of pediatric and adult corneal transplantation patients is that infants and young children with a visually significant corneal opacity develop visual deprivation amblyopia. The specter of amblyopia affects the decision to proceed with surgery. The timing of

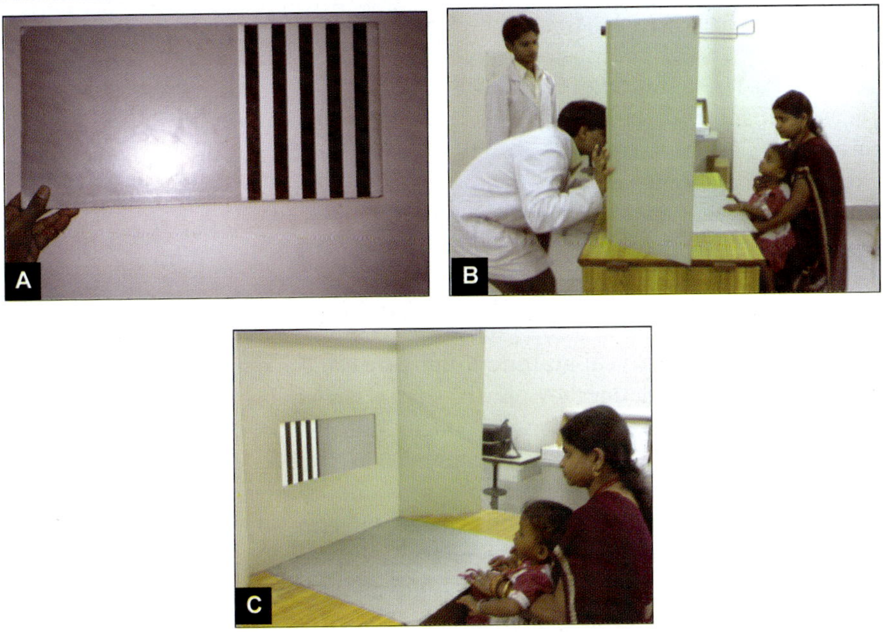

Figures 3A to C: Teller's acuity cards

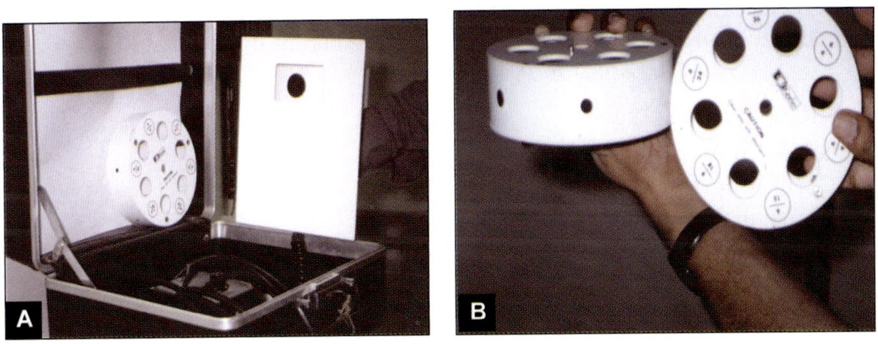

Figures 4A and B: Catford drum

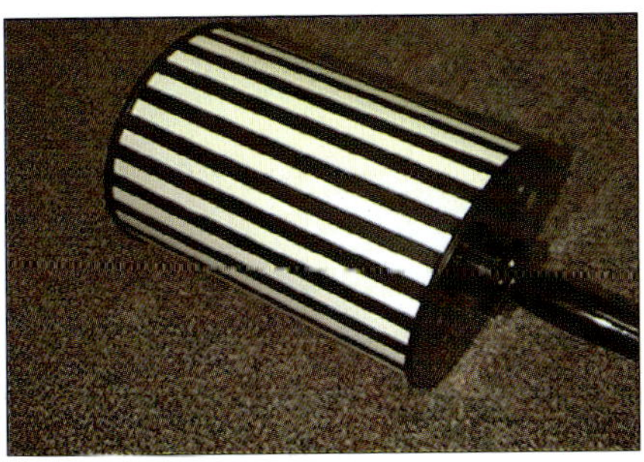

Figure 5: OKN drum

the surgery is very crucial. In fact, the fundamental goal of pediatric penetrating keratoplasty and all the postoperative care is to reverse or limit the effects of amblyopia. The duration of time the eye is capable of perceiving a clear, well-focused image and the effectiveness of amblyopia therapy during the initial years of life establish the eye's visual potential for the rest of the patient's life. Physician and parents should view the surgery itself, alike, as the first in a long series of interventions designed to treat amblyopia.

Indications

The indications for corneal grafting differ between the neonatal period and the age of 2 years. In the latter they may be somewhat similar to those for the adult. When there is a congenital corneal opacity and normal contralateral eye, the visual results following grafting are poor even in a technically successful surgery for a number of reasons. The grafting is usually done too late and there are difficulties with occlusion of the other eye. The more abnormal the cornea, the more abnormal the intraocular structure, and the use of vitreous cutters may be necessary. If there is abnormal recipient corneal tissue then a large graft may be necessary. The graft is likely to remain clear, the greater the normal tissue.

In such cases the parents are all important. If they cooperate, a vision of 3/60 may be achieved, which may provide the infant with a cosmetically acceptable spare eye. On the other hand, children with acquired corneal opacification should have surgery performed as soon as the condition has stabilized.

Congenital

- Sclerocornea
- Corneal dermoids
- Congenital hereditary endothelial dystrophy
- Peter's anomaly
- Glaucoma with corneal edema
- Posterior polymorphous dystrophy
- Mucopolysaccharidosis.

Acquired, Nontraumatic

- Ophthalmia neonatorum
- Herpes simplex keratitis
- Bacterial keratitis
- Stevens-Johnson syndrome
- Keratoconus
- Neurotrophic keratitis
- Interstitial keratitis
- Fungal keratitis
- Keratomalacia

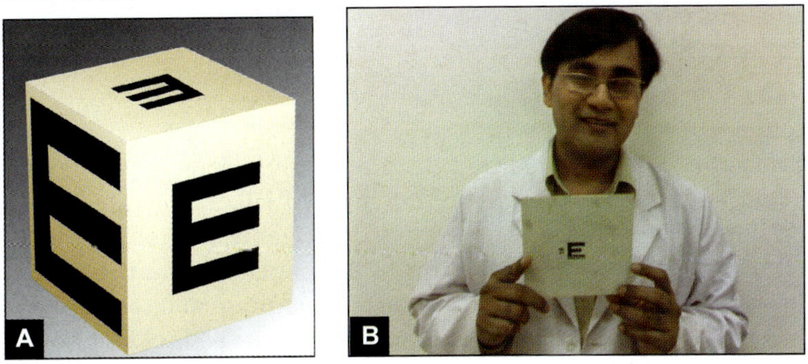

Figures 6A and B: Tumbling E

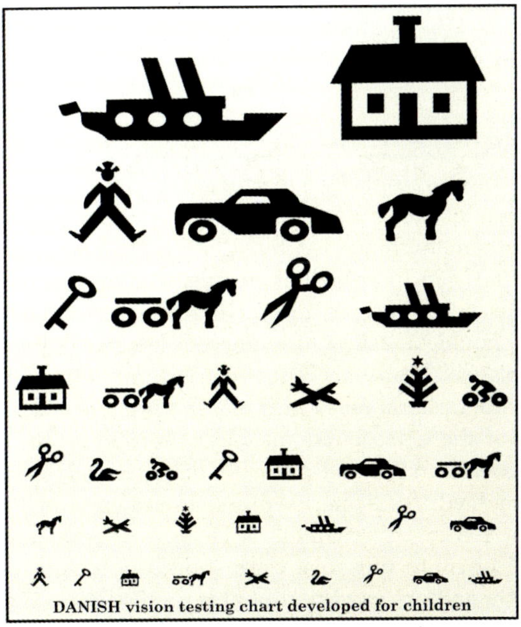

Figure 7: Allen's picture cards

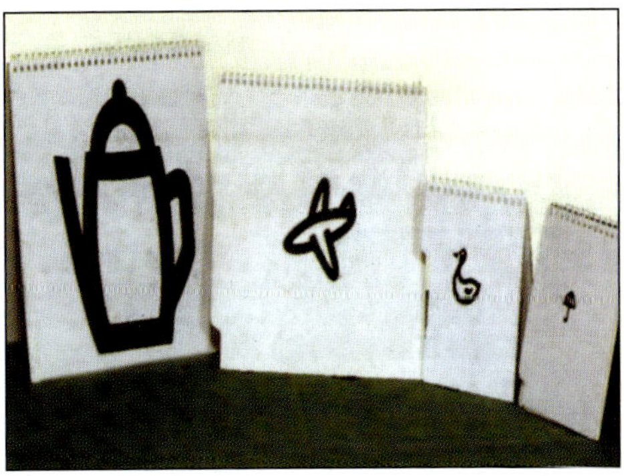

Figure 8: Kay's picture cards

Acquired, Traumatic

- Birth trauma
- Corneal or corneoscleral laceration
- Nonpenetrating injury with scar.

Of the congenital anomalies, Peter's anomaly, sclerocornea and congenital glaucoma have a particularly poor chance of success, while patients with posterior polymorphous dystrophy and congenital hereditary endothelial dystrophy fare better. Traumatic causes of congenital opacities have a better prognosis than congenital. Of the acquired, non-traumatic causes, keratoconus and herpes simplex keratitis show a good graft survival while visual outcome is poorer in the infective and nutritional causes.

Though grafts in older children tend to do better than grafts in younger ones, amblyopia occurring thereof may severely compromise visual recovery. Also, first grafts survive longer than regrafts.

Surgical Management

Pediatric penetrating keratoplasty is performed using an operating microscope, with the patient under general anesthesia. The surgery in infants and children is marked, more than anything else, by scleral collapse and alarming posterior pressure. Particularly in infants, lens expulsion often seems common. Every available maneuver to reduce posterior pressure should be used. The anesthesiologist should be asked to hyperventilate the patient, which reduces intraocular pressure. Paralysis with a nondepolarising muscle relaxant monitored with a peripheral nerve stimulator eliminates the risk of movement and contraction of the extraocular muscles. Positioning the patient with the head slightly higher than the feet probably also decreases posterior pressure.

Digital massage reduces posterior pressure and endothelial cell loss during penetrating keratoplasty. Alternatively a Honan balloon should be applied at 30 mm Hg for 5 or more minutes. Care should be taken to ensure that the speculum, surgeon and assistant do not apply pressure to the globe.

A lateral canthotomy is helpful in improving exposure in infants and may reduce posterior pressure. A Flieringa ring should be used in every pediatric penetrating keratoplasty. It should be fastened to the episclera with six to eight sutures. Four sutures should be left long so that they can be fastened to the drapes to gently support the eye.

Mannitol reduces vitreous volume as well as intraocular pressure and thus reduces posterior pressure. Because it causes systemic fluid shifts that can lead to hemodynamic instability, it should be used with care. The dose of 20% mannitol is 0.5 to 1.5 kg by slow intravenous infusion. To reduce the possibility of hemodynamic instability, each 0.5 g/kg should be given over a period no less than 20-30 minutes. The peak action is about 45 minutes after administration.

The scrub nurse should have a lens loop available so that an assistant can quickly use it to gently place pressure on the iris and lens if loss of lens seems imminent. The nurse should also have an "emergency suture (8-0 nylon/silk

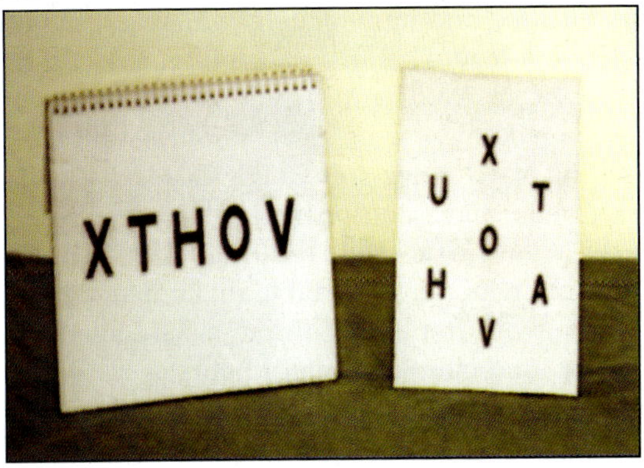

Figure 9: HOTV chart

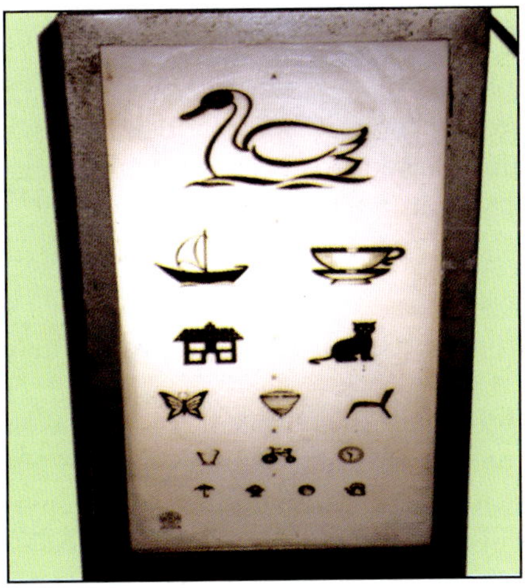

Figure 10: Snellen's picture chart

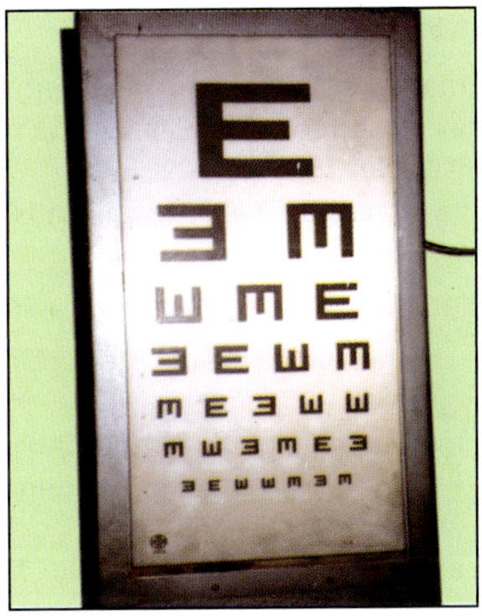

Figure 11: Snellen's E chart

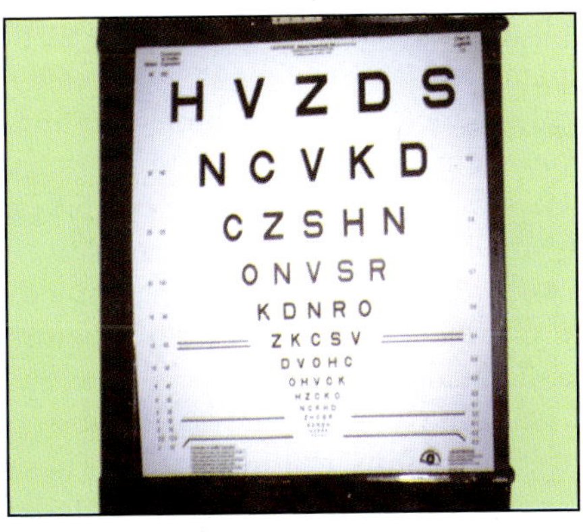

Figure 12: ETDRS chart

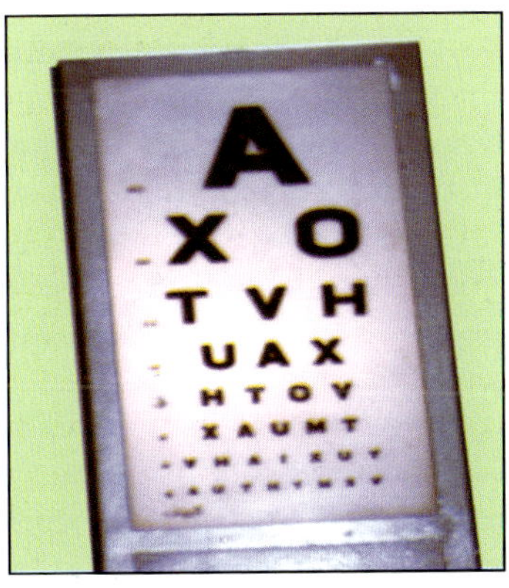

Figure 13: Snellen's letter chart

on a cutting needle) loaded and immediately available if the posterior pressure is so great that 10-0 nylon would break during placement of the cardinal sutures.

Preoperative miotic or mydriatic drops can be used depending on the procedure. If the lens is known to be clear, miotics still help protect the lens, especially in the setting of posterior pressure. If the eye has a visually significant cataract and the surgeon plans an "open sky" lensectomy, mydriatic can be used preoperatively.

A preoperative examination by a portable slit lamp and possibly pachymetry will help the surgeon avoid trephining through particularly thin areas, which would make secure wound closure more difficult.

Preoperative topical antibiotics appear to reduce the risk of postoperative endophthalmitis. If combined with preoperative irrigation of the ocular surface with dilute Povidone-Iodine, it reduces ocular surface bacterial counts even more.

Penetrating Keratoplasty

In infants, the cornea and anterior segment are smaller, and the cornea is often thinner and more pliable, making the surgery technically more difficult. Due to the smaller corneal size in an infant and marked posterior pressure, most surgeons use a smaller graft size in infants than in Adults.

Disadvantages of Smaller Graft

1. Children often have larger pupils, so a small graft may be optically less than optimal.
2. In a smaller graft, total number of endothelial cells transplanted is lower. For instance, reducing the donor diameter from 8.0 to 6.0 mm reduces the number of endothelial cells transplanted by 44%. This reduction becomes important if the recipient rim has a low density of viable endothelial cells.

Infants and children are more active postoperatively and probably are more likely than adults to stress the wound with crying, rubbing and injury. It is important to use a donor trephine 0.5 mm or more than the recipient trephine (0.5 mm over size) to facilitate secure closure of the eye.

Beveling in the corneal scissors after trephining two-third or three fourth the thickness of the cornea forms the recipient bed. This technique will create a posterior lip to help form an aqueous tight wound. In a case where the entire recipient cornea is too thin and soft to hold sutures, a total corneal or corneo-scleral graft can be performed. An alternative in this situation is to perform a large lamellar keratoplasty followed by a smaller penetrating keratoplasty.

Because the graft is often needed to push the lens and iris back, copious viscoelastic agent should used liberally on the lens iris diaphragm before bringing the graft to the wound to limit endothelial trauma.

The increased fibrin production in infants and young children, combined with posterior pressure, can produce iris adhesions to the wound. These adhesions can often be avoided by placing viscoelastic in the anterior chamber as soon as the eye is opened, before the anterior chamber collapses. If adhesions

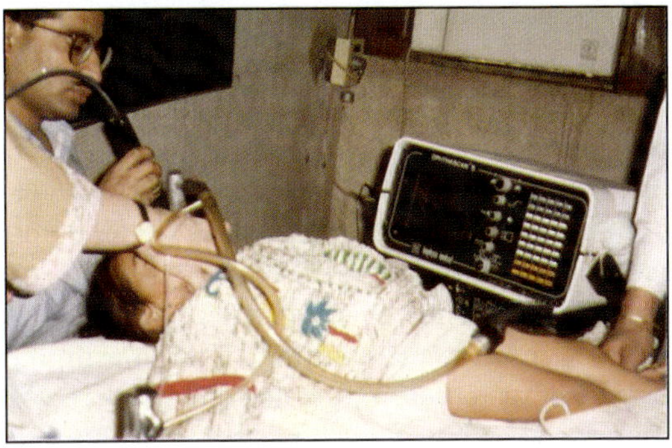

Figure 14A: Biometry under general anesthesia

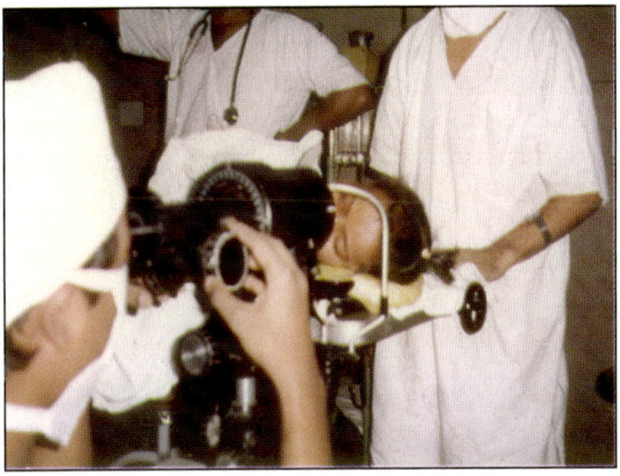

Figure 14B: Keratometry under general anesthesia

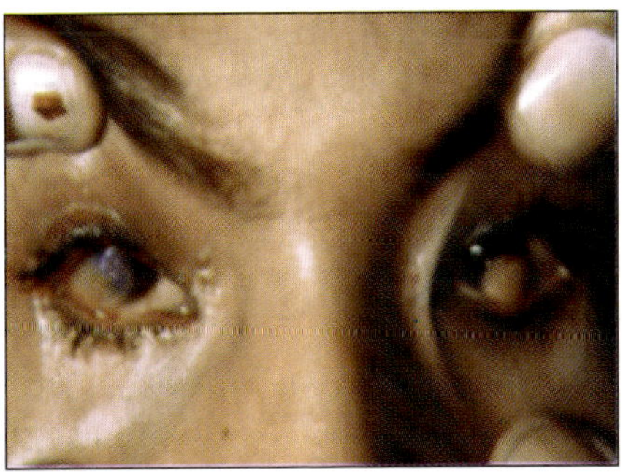

Figure 15: Bilateral dermoid

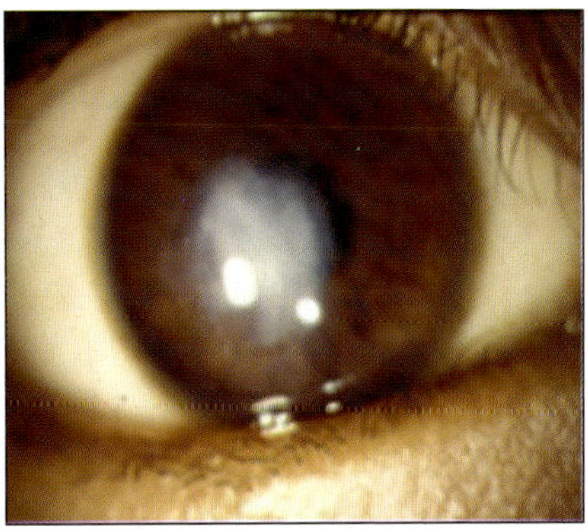

Figure 16: CHED

form, they can be lysed by placing viscoelastic in the anterior chamber after the wound is closed, entering at a distant position from the wound with a vitreous sweep, and sweeping the adherent iris out of the wound.

Blood clot can be manually removed from the anterior chamber, and tissue plasminogen activator (25 ug) can be used to lyse a fibrin clot intraoperatively.

Wound closure is achieved with three-fourths depth 10-0 nylon sutures, as in adult penetrating keratoplasty. Because the sutures can't be removed selectively in very young patients, equal distribution of the donor tissue in the recipient bed is probably important to minimize graft astigmatism. Interrupted sutures are preferred because they reduce the chance that a broken suture will result in wound dehiscence. They also allow for staged removal if some sutures begin to erode before the wound is sufficiently healed to allow removal of all sutures.

Because of the risk of postoperative trauma, a generous number of sutures, perhaps 20 to 24 on 7.0 mm transplantation, should be placed in infants and children. All suture knots should be buried to reduce the risk of ocular surface complications.

Continuous sutures may be preferred in a symmetric vascular or avascular opacity, but never in an asymmetric vascular opacity or infected case. Contraction along the vascular, scarred area leads to early loosening of sutures there and may compromise wound healing in adjacent areas if the suture is continuous.

Concomitant Procedures

Iris Procedures

Peripheral iridectomy

Indications

A. If there is posterior synechiae or persistent intraocular inflammation.

B. If associated lensectomy and vitrectomy is being performed

Anterior Synechiolysis

If there is high positive pressure and the view is sufficient, lysis can be most easily accomplished with a vitreous sweep after making a 1 mm incision at the base of the trephine groove and injecting viscoelastic into the anterior chamber.

If the view is not sufficient, synechiolysis can only be accomplished after suturing the graft into place.

In an aphakic eye, a sector iridectomy followed by creation of a smaller pupil with 10-0 prolene suture on a noncutting needle will tighten the iris diaphgram and prevent reformation of synechiae.

Pupilloplasty

If the pupil is disfigured.

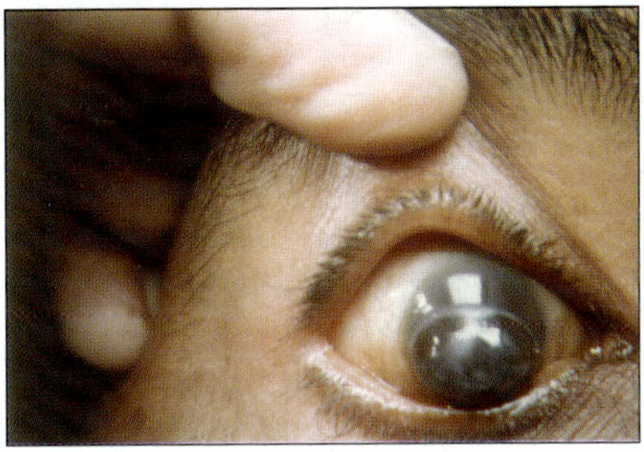

Figure 17A: Post-traumatic corneal opacity

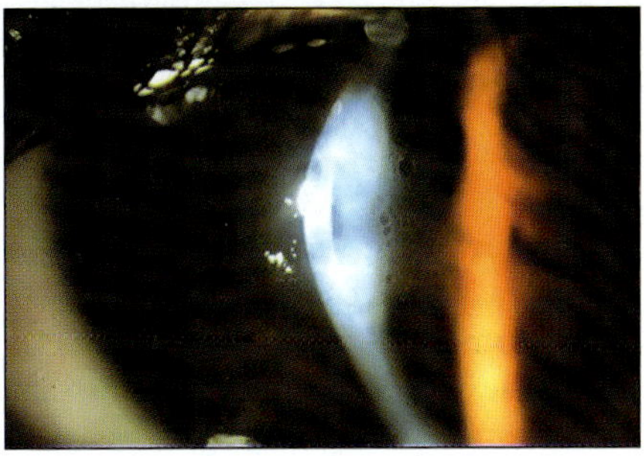

Figure 17B: Keratoconus with healed hydrops

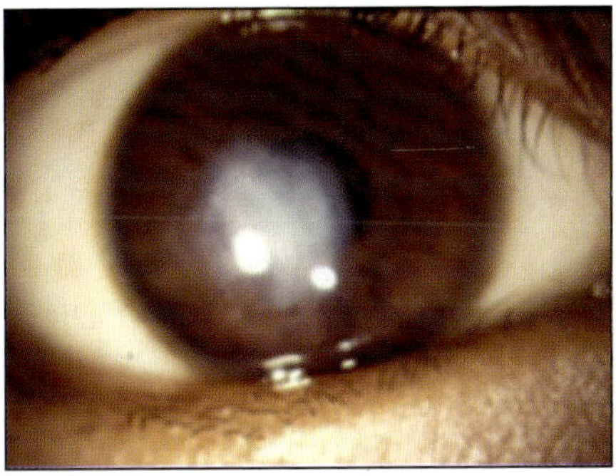

Figure 18: Healing keratitis with partial anterior staphyloma

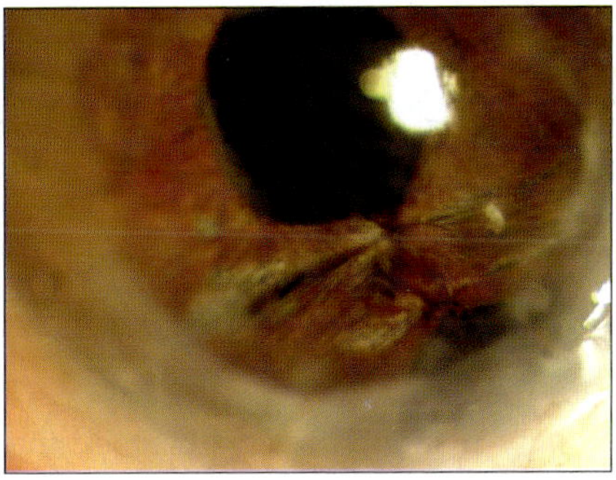

Figure 19: Postoperative therapeutic keratoplasty

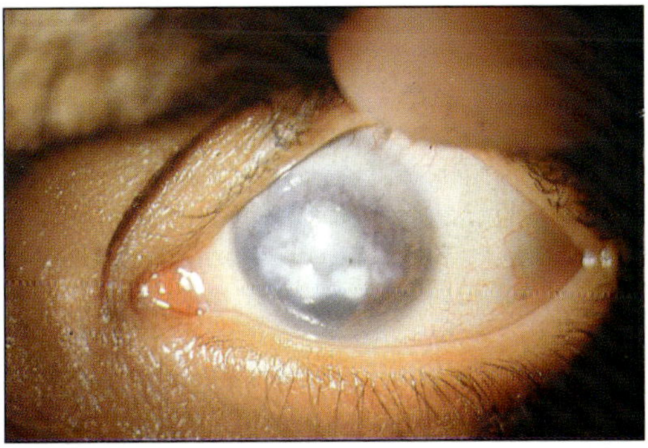

Figure 20: Corneal opacity with cataract

Lensectomy and Anterior Vitrectomy

Indications

i. If there is dense cataract associated with corneal pathology.
ii. In Peter's type II anomaly.

However, the decision to remove a lens with only a mild to moderate opacity during a pediatric penetrating keratoplasty should be made judiciously. Lensectomy and vitrectomy are statistically significant risk factors for graft failure and poor visual outcome. If lensectomy is performed at the time of penetrating keratoplasty, it is generally performed "Open sky", as in adults.

After anterior capsulotomy and expression or aspiration of the nucleus, the cortical material is removed. Removal will be difficult in the face of vitreous upthrust. An irrigation aspiration device or anterior vitrectomy instrument with its cutting action turned off can be used for cortical aspiration.

As virtually every pediatric posterior capsule will opacify, a partial posterior capsulotomy and anterior vitrectomy should be performed in infants and perhaps children. Even though older children might cooperate for an Nd:YAG capsulotomy, in the absence of a posterior chamber lens, Nd:YAG capsulotomy usually results in vitreous prolapse into the anterior chamber. This prolapse can cause pupillary block or vitreous endothelial touch, which will threaten the graft. The posterior capsulotomy and anterior vitrectomy are performed with an automated vitrector with a cut rate of about 300 to 400 cycles/minute and maximum suction setting of about 80 mm Hg. The vitrector should be used to create a circular hole of about 7 mm diameter in the posterior capsule. The capsulotomy should be this large, as the capsular remnants can contract and opacify postoperatively to block the visual axis, especially in infants. If the capsulotomy is circular, it will not tear and would provide support if a posterior chamber lens is implanted later. For immediate visual rehabilitation, majority is of view of using contact lens.

Concomitant Retinal Surgery

If the eye requires pars plana vitrectomy for retinal detachment, use of an intraoperative keratoprosthesis for the retinal surgery affords the retinal surgeon a better view than through a new transplant. After the retinal surgeon completes the retinal reattachment, the keratoprosthesis is replaced with transplantation tissue.

After the transplantation is completed, subconjunctival injections of antibiotics and steroids are generally given.

It may be useful to perform a postoperative examination while the child is still under anesthesia. A portable slit lamp is useful to confirm that there is no iris adherent to the wound and can be used to provide a cobalt blue filter to perform a siedel test of the wound.

The new transplantation may afford the surgeon the first view of the retina with an indirect ophthalmoscope. An axial eye length can be determined to help in later estimating an aphakic eye's refractive error.

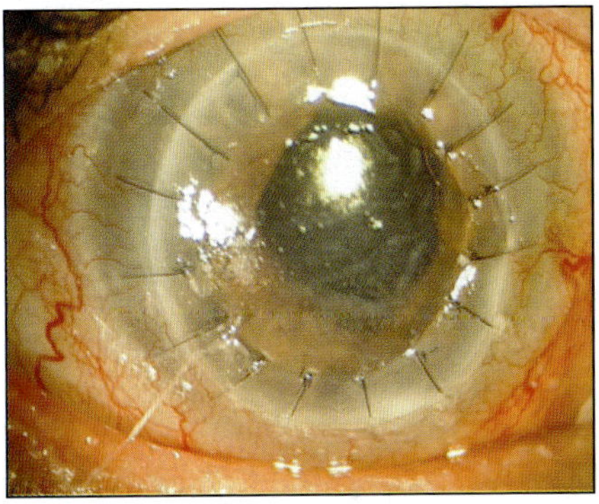

Figure 21: Pupilloplasty in penetrating keratoplasty

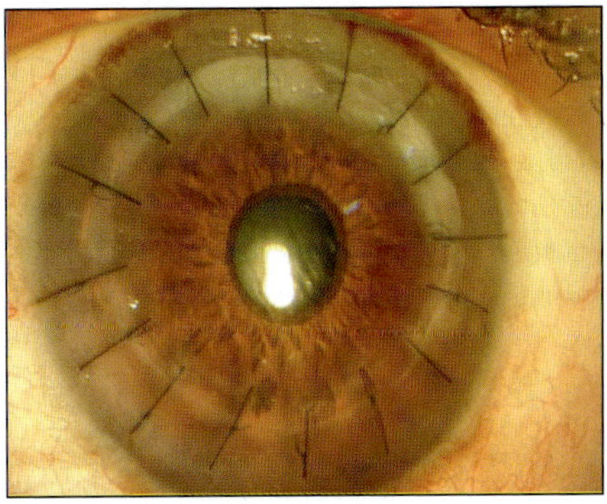

Figure 22: Clear graft following successful optical penetrating keratoplasty

Before applying a pressure patch and metal shield, a single drop of 0.5% atropine in healthy full-term infants or 1% atropine ointment in children should be applied. When seeing the family after surgery it is wise to remind them of the guarded prognosis for vision and that the transplantation is only the first step in the visual rehabilitation of the eye.

Postoperative care

1. *Immediate postoperative period:* Premature infants and infants and children with systemic diseases should be monitored carefully and the recommendations of the patient's pediatrician and anesthesiologist should be sought. The child should be discharged on the first or second postoperative day if vital signs and oral intake are normal, and the eye is epithelized.
2. *Early postoperative care:* The goals of the examination and interventions in the first few weeks after surgery are to make certain that the wound is secure and watertight, monitor and promote the decline in postoperative inflammation, monitor and control intraocular pressure. It is necessary to detect other postoperative complications and also begin amblyopia therapy.

The first postoperative examination should be within 24 hours after surgery. A reasonable schedule of routine postoperative examinations includes examinations on the first, second, fourth, seventh, tenth, and fourteenth postoperative days.

Postoperative complications are usually the same as in adults, but infants and young children are unable to communicate effectively that they have pain, visual loss or other symptoms and hence, they require frequent early postoperative examinations.

Postoperative medications: Because infants and children can have an exaggerated inflammatory response postoperatively, it seems reasonable to use more topical steroids than in adult keratoplasty patients.

A long acting topical cycloplegic, generally atropine should also be given during first two postoperative weeks to prevent formation of synechiae.

Rest of the medications is the same as in adults.

Suture removal: Typically all sutures can be removed safely according to the following schedule. During the first year of life, sutures are removed at 5 weeks after surgery; in one year olds at 6 to 7 postoperative weeks; in 2 and 3 year olds at 8 to 10 postoperative weeks, in 4 to year old at 3 months and in 7 to 10 year olds at 5 to 6 months postoperatively. Patients 10 to 20 years of age often require removal of all sutures because of rapid erosion by the sixth to eighth postoperative month.

Optical Correction and Amblyopia Therapy

Without effective optical correction and amblyopia therapy, a pediatric penetrating keratoplasty may be useless. The younger the patient, the deeper the amblyopia will be if the eye has a structural or refractive abnormality that limits vision. However, amblyopia is more easily reversed in a younger patient if it is treated promptly and appropriately.

Correction of refractive error is a vital part of amblyopia therapy. At about two postoperative weeks, the epithelium has generally healed and the graft has cleared sufficiently to perform cycloplegic retinoscopy. Retinoscopy may be difficult, and the refraction will change as the wound heals and sutures are removed; but a correction of any moderate or large refractive error should be prescribed at this time, even if it is not exact. The refraction should be repeated every 3 to 6 weeks until the sutures have been out till the age of one year. Thereafter, the refraction should be repeated at least four times a year till the age of 5 years.

Refraction of an aphakic eye may be confirmed if the axial length is known. The following formula is an approximation in an aphakic eye with a keratometry measurement of 45 diopters and a vertex distance of 10 mm

Distance spectacle power = 63.7- (2.28 × axial eye length in mm)

The results from this formula can be modified by keratometry measurements. For an aphakic eye, an infant is generally prescribed a near correction, that is +1.00 to 2.00 sphere over the distance correction. At 1 to 3 years of age, the aphakic child should be prescribed bifocal lenses with the top of the segment at the inferior border of the pupil.

Contact lens is useful in the visual rehabilitation of pediatric keratoplasty patients. Monocular aphakic silicone lenses offer the highest oxygen permeability of all lenses and are often well tolerated by aphakic patients with normal corneas.

If the contralateral eye is normal in an infant or a young child, occlusion therapy should be started as soon as the graft has partially cleared, and refractive correction is being used. Optimally this should be no later than two postoperative weeks. Occlusion during the first 6 months of life is usually limited to one-fourth to three-fourths of the infant's waking hours. If the child is older than 6 months, then vision in both eyes is monitored carefully to check for improvement of the amblyopic eye or worsening of the normal eye.

If the patient has undergone bilateral penetrating keratoplasties, he or she may still have amblyopia. If amblyopia is suspected, it should be treated as outlined previously after doing everything reasonable to correct the structural and refractive abnormalities.

In all this, the role of parents cannot be over-emphasized. They have to be appropriately counseled preoperatively of the child's condition and given a realistic view of the prognosis. Their participation and dedication to the whole procedure is what pays off in the long-term. Postoperatively they have to be trained to watch out for complications, as a child's ability to communicate is limited. They have to be told to recognize loose sutures and imminent graft rejection by redness in the eye, accumulations of mucus and loss of graft clarity. They may be trained in penlight examination.

Conclusion

Because of advances in surgical techniques and postoperative care, a clear corneal graft in an infant or a child has become commonplace over the last 20 years. Although the visual results are currently disappointing, it appears that meticulous attention to the health of the graft and the eye, correction of refractive error and adequate amblyopia therapy will yield improved visual results for eyes that are otherwise normal.

Although pediatric penetrating keratoplasty patients are among the most challenging the corneal surgeon will encounter, they can also be among the most rewarding. With a great deal of effort the vision of an infant or a child, otherwise condemned to life-long blindness, can be restored.

Chapter 32

Pediatric Iris Abnormalities

Arif Adenwala (UAE)
Mahesh Dalvi (India)

Aniridia

It represents a spectrum of disorder with iris hypoplasia. It may occur due to anomalous development of neuron ectoderm or neural crest cells. Histology: Iris is reduced to small stub and smooth muscle is usually absent. Angle may also be poorly developed.

It is defines as absence of iris tissue. But it is misnomer as at least a rudimentary tissue is present.

It is bilateral disorder.

Additional Abnormalities

- Foveal and optic nerve hypoplasia are present leading to congenital sensory nystagmus
- Decreased visual acuity is seen due to multiple risk factors like light scatter, corneal or lenticular opacities, severe glaucoma optic nerve and macular hypoplasia
- Cataract
- Glaucoma and
- Corneal opacity.

Typical Clinical Presentation

- Nystagmus
- Dilated fixed pupil
- Photophobia
- Anterior polar cataract—Persistent pupillary membrane.

Cause

- Sporadic or familial
- Defect in PAX6 gene on chromosome 11. PAX6 gene is localized to band 11p13
- Chromosome 1 and 2 plays an important role in dominant of congenital aniridia.

Familial

It is autosomal dominant with complete penetrance and variable expressivity.

Sporadic

Common association with Wilms tumor. All cases of aniridia should get chromosomal analysis for Wilms tumor gene defect.

There is also association with genitourinary abnormalities and mental retardation (ARG).

Cataract surgery in aniridia is slightly complicated. But nowadays with recent advances the success rate is good. Special aniridia intraocular lenses are used in these patients.

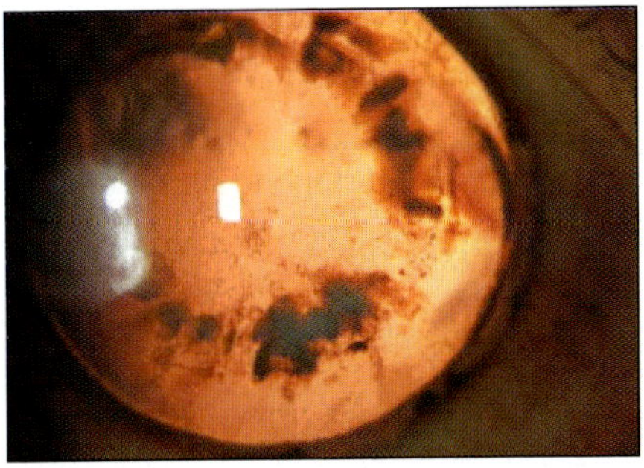

Figure 1: Aniridia (*Courtesy:* Online Journal of Ophthalmology)

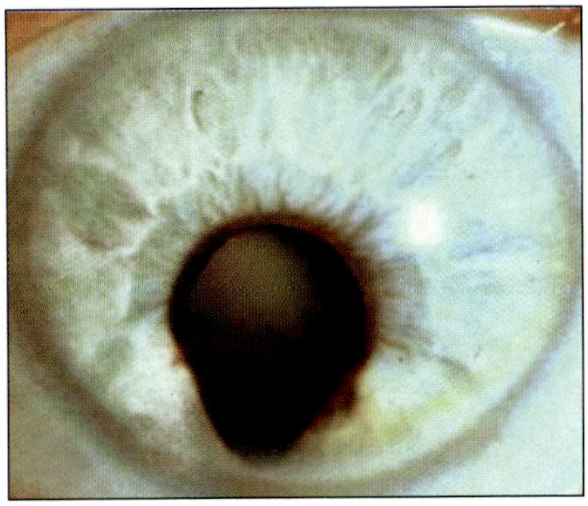

Figure 2: Coloboma of Iris (*Courtesy:* Online Journal of Ophthalmology)

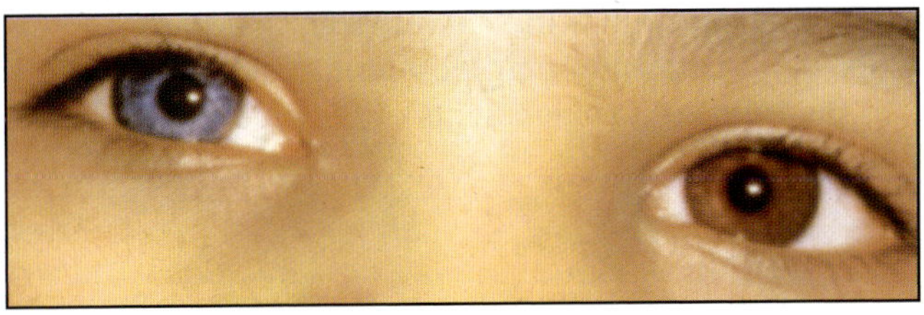

Figure 3: Heterochromia iridium

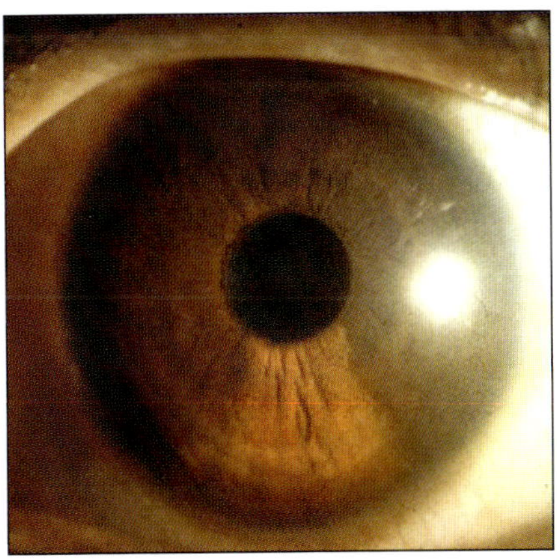

Figure 4: Ocular melanosis (*Courtesy:* Ritch, Robert, M.D, Online Journal of Ophthalmology)

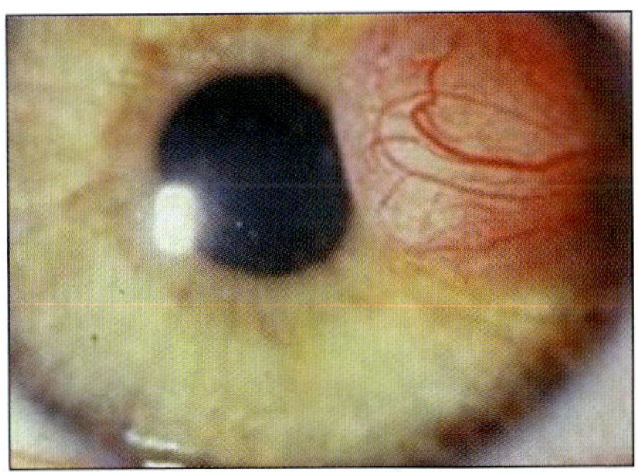

Figure 5: Juvenile xanthogranuloma (*Courtesy:* Online Journal of Ophthalmology)

Occluder contact lenses with pupillary aperture is indicated for optical correction of refractive errors.

Coloboma Iris

It is defined as partial absence of iris tissue. It is classified depending on the site of absence.

Typical

Coloboma is seen in inferonasal quadrant. It is caused by failure of closure of the embryonic fissure in 5th week.

The shape of the pupil is light bulb, keyhole or inverted tear drop.

It involves the ciliary body, choroid, retina and optic nerve.

Atypical

Coloboma is seen in areas other than inferonasal quadrant.
It is usually not associated with more posterior uveal coloboma.
It results from the fibrovascular remnants of the anterior hyaloids system and pupillary membrane.

Common Association

Iris colobomata are seen with almost any chromosomal abnormalities. The most common being, e.g. Trisomy 13, Trisomy 18, Triploidy, Klinefelter syndrome, Cat eye syndrome, etc.

Common syndromes associated are:

- CHARGE Syndrome:
  C: Ocular coloboma
  H: Heart defects
  A: Chroanal atresia.
  R: Mental retardation
  G: Genitourinary abnormalities and
  E: Ear abnormalities.
- Aicardi Syndrome
- Goldenhar Syndrome
- Rubinstein Taybi Syndrome.

Heterochromia Iridis

A difference in iris color between both the eyes is known as heterochromia iridis. It can be congenital or acquired.

An abnormal eye may be either darker/lighter than the other eye.

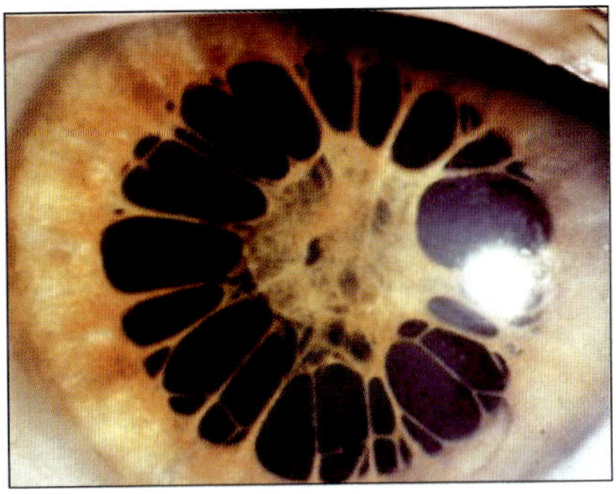

Figure 6: Persistant pupillary membrane (PPM) (*Courtesy:* Online journal of Ophthalmology)

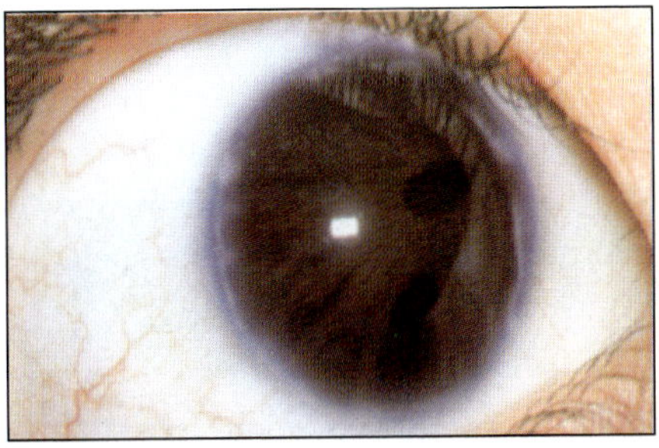

Figure 7: Reiger's anomaly with posterior embryotoxon and polycoria (*Courtesy:* John Elston: Textbook of Paediatric Ophthalmology: David Taylor)

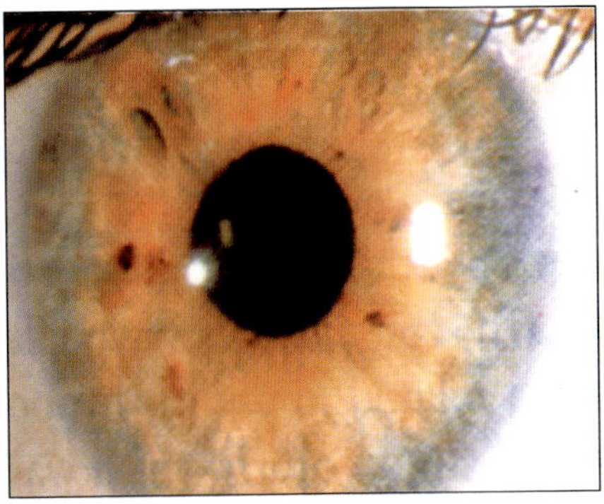

Figure 8: Reiger's anomaly with focal iris hypoplasia (*Courtesy:* John Elston: Textbook of Paediatric Ophthalmology: David Taylor)

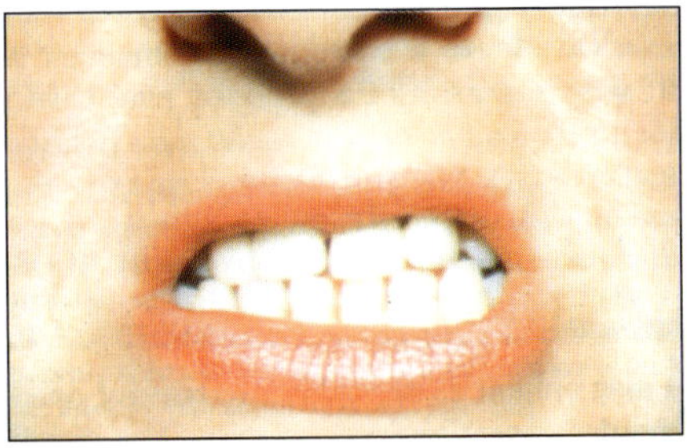

Figure 9: Reiger's syndrome showing typical teeth (Capped) (*Courtesy:* John Elston: Textbook of Paediatric Ophthalmology: David Taylor)

Congenital

Involved iris can be either dark or light in color.

Involved Iris Dark

It is seen in ocular melanocytosis or ocular dermal melanocytosis or secondary to iris hamartomas.

Involved Iris Light in Color

It is seen in Horner's syndrome and Waardenburg syndrome. Congenital Horner's syndrome includes ipsilateral hypopigmentation, miosis and ptosis.

Waardenburg Syndrome

It is autosomal syndrome inheritance. Features include lateral displacement of inner canthus, prominent root of the nose, deafness, white forelock, and heterochromia iridis.

Acquired

Involved iris dark: Usually results from infiltration process like nevus or melanomatous tumor or secondary to siderosis.

Involved iris light: It is commonly seen in Fuch's heterochromic iridocyclitis, juvenile xanthogranuloma, or metastatic malignancies.

William Syndrome

There is stellate pattern of iris. Associated features includes prominent lips, mental retardation, growth retardation, cardiac defect.

Iris Nodules

Lisch Nodule

These are neural crest hamartomas. It is seen in association with NF-1.

It is raised swelling and usually tan in color. The prevalence in NF-1 increases with age.

Juvenile Xanthogranuloma (JXG)

It is mainly cutaneous disorder. It had increase predilection for head and face.

It presents as discrete yellowish nodules/dense infiltration causing heterochromia.

Vascular iris lesion can lead to spontaneous hyphema.

Primary Iris Cysts

Primary iris cysts are rare swelling arising from pigmentary epithelium or stroma.

Iris Pigment Epithelium Cysts

These are unilateral, solitary dark brown swelling.

It occurs due to separation of two layers of epithelium anywhere between pupil and ciliary body.

It is stable condition and rarely causes any complication. It has feature of transillumination and it may dislodge and float freely in anterior chamber or vitreous.

Central Cysts (Pupillary)

Usually hereditary

It can be seen at any age group.

It is caused by the use of miotic eye drops mainly phenylepherine.

Rupture of the cyst can cause formation of iris flocculi.

Cyst Iris Stroma

It is caused by sequestration of the epithelium during embryologic development. It is seen commonly in infants and young children and usually presents in first year of life.

They are solitary swelling having smooth, translucent anterior wall filled with fluid.

These cyst may contain goblets cells and when enlarges it causes obstruction of the visual axis, glaucoma, corneal decompensation.

Preferred treatment of choice is surgical excision of the lesion although spontaneous regression may occur.

Brush Field Spots (Wofflin Nodules)

It is seen in 90% patients with Downs Syndrome.

They are areas of iris stromal hyperplasia surrounded by hypoplasia.

They are known as Brushfield spots if seen in Downs syndrome or known as Wofflins nodule.

They are non-pathologic lesion.

Persistent Pupillary Membrane (PPM)

It is common development abnormalities of the iris. It represents a complete involution of the anterior tunica vasculosa lentis.

The membrane is attached to collarette or may be free floating or span the pupil to attach to opposite side.

It may attach the anterior capsule of lens leading to formation of anterior polar cataract.

It has autosomal dominant inheritance.

It is seen in 95% of newborns.

It rarely causes impairment of visual acuity.

Treatment: In case of thick PPM, surgical excision is treatment of choice and in rest case no active treatment is advised.

Primary Iris Abnormalities

Reiger's Anomaly

It is congenital anomaly which consists of hypoplasia of the anterior iris stroma. There is presence of irido-trabecular bridge to Schwalbe's line and posterior embryotoxon.

Pupil may be abnormal in shape, size or position.

Other associated ocular anomalies seen are:

- Ectropion uveae and coloboma of the iris
- Glaucoma, depending on the extent of iris changes
- Sclerocornea
- Large corneal endothelial abnormalities
- Posterior keratoconus.

It is inherited as autosomal dominant with variable expressivity. About 30% cases are either sporadic in nature or new mutation is seen.

Reiger's Syndrome

This includes combination of Reiger's anomaly with somatic features. These include:

- Facial abnormalities like maxillary hypoplasia and short philtrum.
- Dental abnormalities which affect primary and secondary dentition with widely spaced cone shaped teeth.

Other features include umbilical hernia and hypospadias.

Reiger's syndrome is an autosomal dominant condition. Glaucoma is seen in 20-25% of affected individuals.

It is associated with abnormalities in chromosome 6 and with isolated growth hormone deficiency.

Chapter 33

Pediatric Oculoplasty: Evidence Based Update

Sunil Moreker, Milind Kirtane
Milind Navlakhe, Mayur Moreker (India)

Introduction

Medical science changes with time as more and more people submit their audits and personal experience to journals. These reports and studies make the understanding of diseases more clear. At times the natural history of diseases becomes clearer and at other times we realize that may be we as humans respond differently with time. Sometimes historical mistakes are corrected but at times we might be committing newer mistakes. This chapter is an effort at looking at present updated literature on pediatric oculoplastic procedures in a critical manner with a view to applying the recent evidence to everyday clinical practice. The commonest pediatric oculoplastic procedures are addressed here. Considering the unique problems presented by childhood oculoplastic conditions it seems appropriate to have pediatric oculoplasty as a separate speciality.

Congenital Dacryocystitis Update

The often quoted incidence of 6% was derived from a study of 200 consecutive live births in the 1940s. Actual incidences may vary from 1.2% to 30%, the disorder being commoner in children with craniofacial disorders and Down's syndrome.

Syndromes

Lacrimo-auriculo-dento-digital Syndrome (LADD)

An autosomal dominant pattern of inheritance caused by FGF10 mutations with variable expressivity including cup-shaped ears, deafness, unilateral choanal atresia, bilateral nasolacrimal duct obstruction, xerostomia, alacrima due to congenital absence of lacrimal glands, agenesis of salivary glands, chronic dacryocystitis, keratoconjunctivitis sicca, ptosis, nail dysplasia of the thumb, shortness of fifth toe, temporal bone abnormality and epilepsy. Renal and urogenital anomalies may be seen variably. In the author's experience these findings do not always occur in these clusters but if one of these is seen in association with congenital dacryocystitis then the others should be looked for as they do require a multi-specialty approach to management.

Microbiological Spectrum and Sensitivities

A recent study conducted at Madurai, India concluded that Gram-positive bacteria are the most frequent isolates with *Streptococcus pneumoniae* being the commonest. Among Gram-negative bacteria the most frequent isolate was Hemophilus influenza. Candida tropicalis has emerged as a new organism. Gram-positive bacteria are sensitive to chloramphenicol, vancomycin, and ofloxacin and Gram-negative bacteria to ofloxacin and ciprofloxacin.

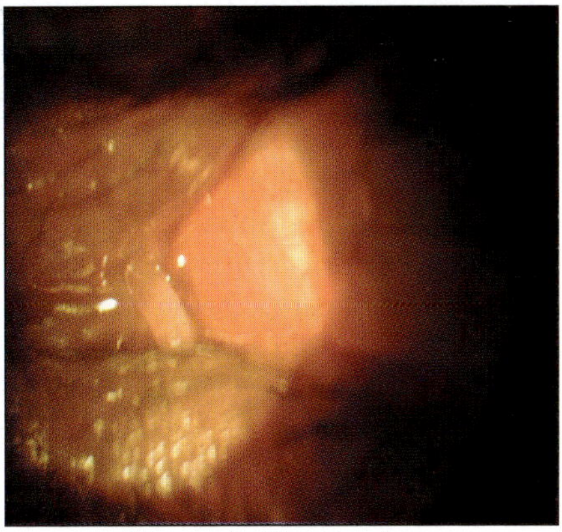

Figure 1: Stent in place

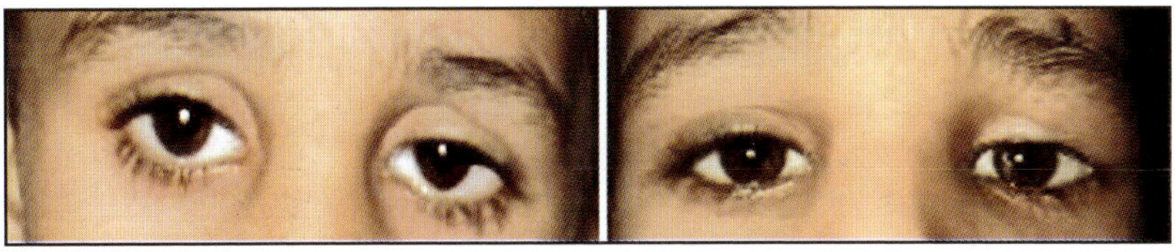

Figure 2: Pre-and post-sling

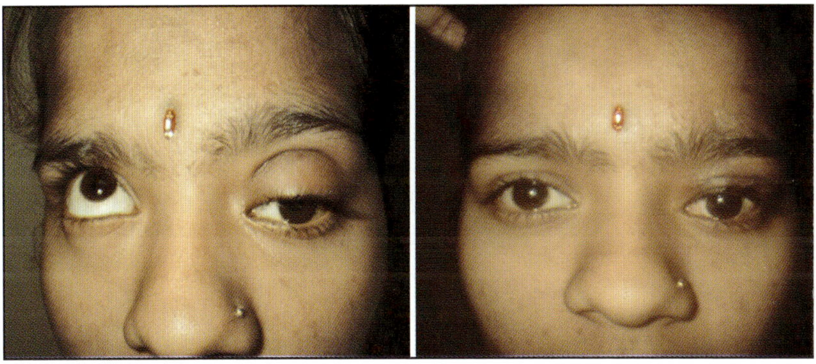

Figure 3: Ptosis with double elevator palsy—pre- and postoperatively

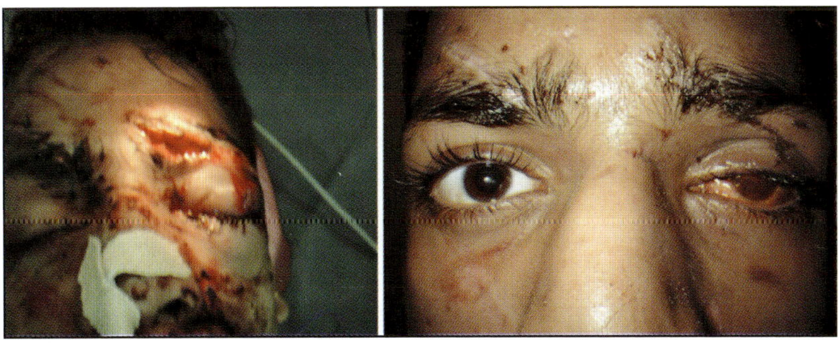

Figure 4: Traumatic globe rupture and orbital implant with cornea preserving evisceration

Treatment

Probing

Timing: In their series of 192 children with nasolacrimal duct obstruction out of 3950 children lipiec et al reported that in majority of children (77%), the nasolacrimal duct obstruction did not resolve spontaneously and early probing within first few months of child's life increased the success rate of the procedure. Becker et al on the basis of their 19 years experience have proposed that patients with congenital dacryocystocele should have probing on an urgent basis and as early in life as possible, unless the lacrimal sac decompresses into the nose at the time of the initial examination. According to them this approach reduces the incidence of dacryocystitis and cellulitis, and improves the success rate of surgery as they noticed that the initial probing was successful in 100% of lacrimal systems that did not have infection, but was successful in only 53% that had dacryocystitis with or without cellulitis. The mean age of probing in the surgical patients who did not develop infection in the Becker et al series was 5.9 days, whereas the mean age at first probing in surgical patients who developed infection was 17.3 days. The cure rate has been reported as 89% in patients 13-24 months of age and 72% after the age of 24 months by Kashkouli et al in their prospective study of 169 eyes. The more important finding was a success rate of 90.2% in the membranous and 33.3% in the complex CNLDO in both late and very late probing with a high correlation between the cure rate at 1 week and final follow-up suggesting that the outcome of the nasolacrimal duct probing at 1 week follow-up is highly indicative of the final outcome.

Endonasal Probing and Retrograde Irrigation of Lacrimal Ducts

When endonasal probing and retrograde irrigation of lacrimal ducts is performed taking into consideration the individual peculiarities of the obstruction and the anatomical accessibility of the opening of ductus nasolacrimalis in the inferior nasal passageway, it has been reported that persistent membranes in the inferior lacrimal punctum necessitates repetition of the initial dilatation. Endonasal probing and irrigation of lacrimal ducts used in the treatment of congenital stenoses has been reported to have a high effectivity (99%) by some authors. In children in whom this procedure fails endonasal dacryocystorhinostomy with balloon intubations may be tried.

Balloon Dilatation of Nasolacrimal Duct

Balloon nasolacrimal ductoplasty is performed using the LacriCATH system (Quest Medical, Inc. An Atrion Company, Allen, TX).

Becker et al in their prospective series of 61 lacrimal systems reported a 95% success rate with this procedure as early as 1996. More recently Tao et al reported that as a secondary procedure it was successful in 94% of those older than 24 months whereas the success rate was as lowas 59.1% in those younger than 24 months. Results range from 82% (Tien et al) to 95%. Yuksel et al proposed on

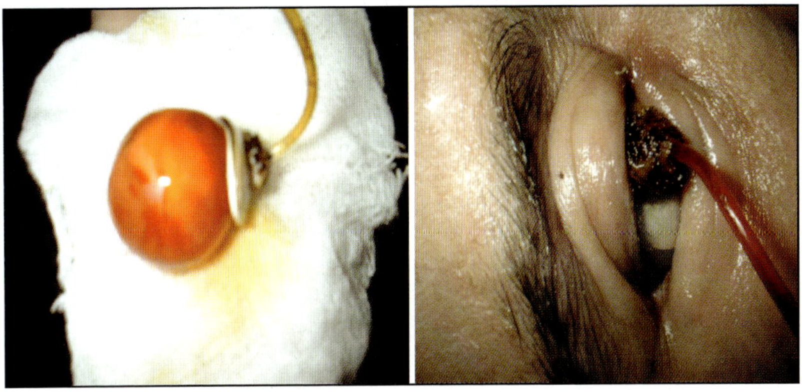

Figure 5: Moreker's expandable balloon implants

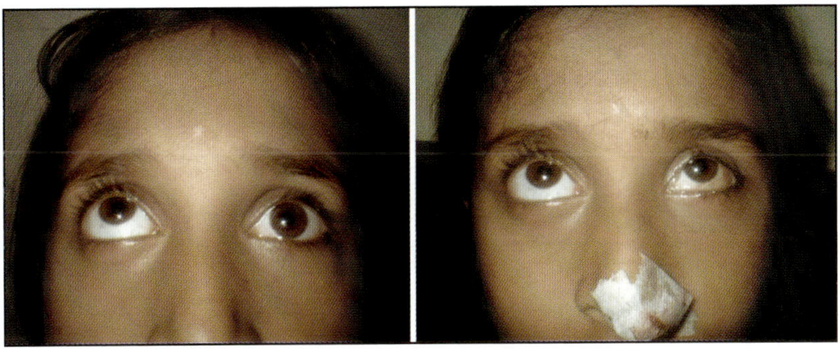

Figure 6: Pre- and post-endoscopic fracture correction (above)

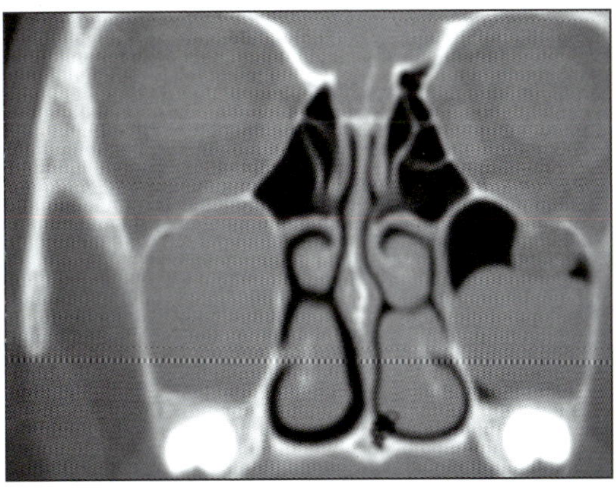

Figure 7: Trapdoor fracture of orbital floor (above)
(*Courtesy:* Dr Milind Kirtane)

the basis of their experience with endoscopic guided balloon dacryocystoplasty in children over 36 months of age that it can be an alternative treatment in older children and can be preferred to silicone intubation and dacryocystorhinostomy performed after unsuccessful probing.

Monocanalicular Stenting

Goldstein et al compared monocanalicular stenting and balloon dacryoplasty in secondary treatment of congenital nasolacrimal duct obstruction after failed primary and reported that (91%) nasolacrimal ducts responded to monocanalicular stenting, whereas 86% responded to balloon treatment. When the patient group was further stratified by age, the monocanalicular stenting was 94% successful in children younger than age 2 years and 89% successful for children older than 2 years. The balloon treatment had a success rate of 91% in the younger group and 79% in the older group.

Step wise approach: Cassady et al have proposed a treatment paradigm prescribing probing as an initial procedure regardless of age. Those who fail probing should receive balloon catheter dilation. Those who fail probing and balloon catheterization should receive silicone intubation. Dacryocystorhinostomy is reserved for patients failing the above treatments.

Congenital Ptosis

Blepharoptosis indicates the abnormal drooping of the upper lid, caused by partial or total reduction in levator muscle function. It may be caused by various pathologies, both congenital and acquired. Childhood ptosis may be congenital or acquired. An insult, acting during the second month of gestation, may affect the development of the eye, heart, and abdomen and may lead to congenital malformations. Although congenital ptosis presenting with ocular and systemic congenital malformations is a rare condition, ophthalmologists should consider the possibility of coexisting structural defects. Congenital ptosis is more challenging than adult ptosis due to these and other comorbidities like amblyopia and the difficulty of examination as well as the age at which surgery should be performed. Unilateral severe congenital ptosis and jaw-winking ptosis pose a challenge in the decision of the surgical procedure and whether surgery should be performed unilaterally or bilaterally. In congenital forms, these techniques were often associated with techniques to correct oculo-muscular imbalance (i.e. strabismus). Surgical treatment of palpebral ptosis is complex and requires precise diagnosis and indications for surgery related to clinical examination and pathogenesis. Even if these indications are strictly followed, in some cases, the outcomes are unpredictable. In view of various newer reports the author suggests the following classification.

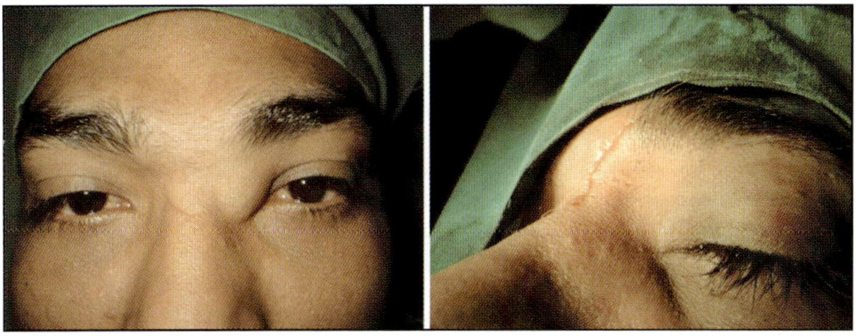

Figure 8: Dermoid — pre- and immediate postoperatively (above)

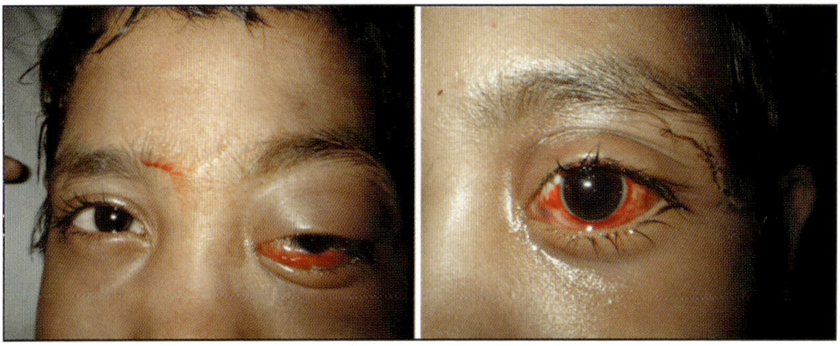

Figure 9: Lateral orbitotomy for hemangioma (intraconal) (above)

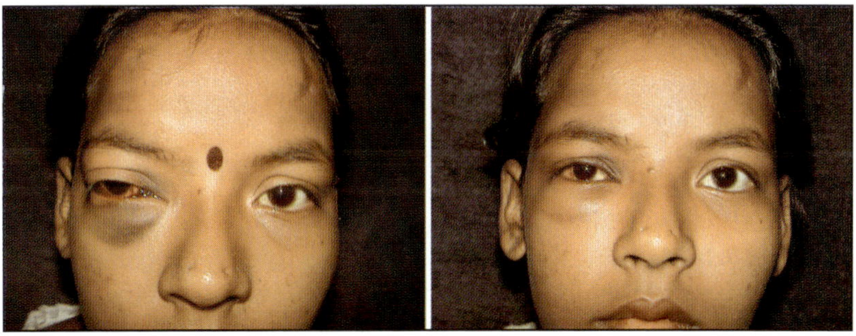

Figure 10: Complete endoscopic management of orbital tumor—hemangioma (above)(*Courtesy:* Dr Milind Navlakhe)

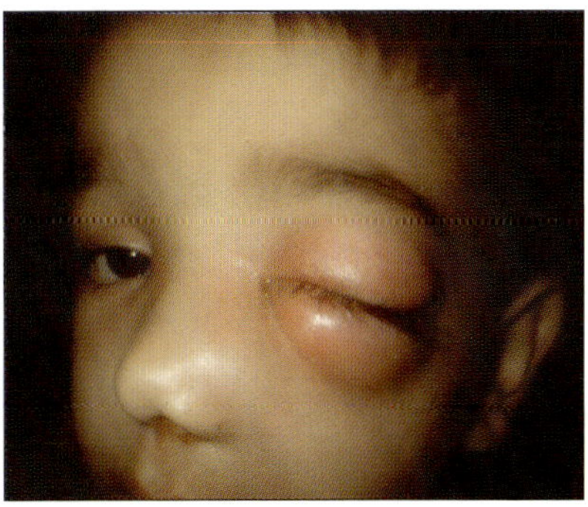

Figure 11: Orbital cellulitis (above) (*Courtesy:* Dr Milind Kirtane)

Moreker's Classification of Childhood Ptosis

A. Congenital
   1. Simple dysmyogenic ptosis
   2. Dysmyogenic ptosis with vertical strabismus
      a. Isolated superior rectus involvement
      b. Double elevator palsy
   3. Dysmyogenic ptosis with epiblepheron
   4. Childhood myasthenia
      a. Transient neonatal
      b. Congenital
      c. Juvenile
   5. Syndromic ptosis
      a. WARG,
      b. Partial trisomy
      c. Conenital fibrosis syndromes with ptosis
      d. With ocular and systemic congenital malformations including mild microphthalmia, microcornea, cataract, iris and chorioretinal coloboma, ectopic kidney, and ventricular septal defect.
   6. Ptosis with synkinesis
      a. Oculomotor abducens synkinesis-requires overcorrection
      b. Marcus Gunn jaw winking phenomenon
   7. Ptosis with muscular dystrophies.

B. Acquired
   1. Muscle infections — myocystecercosis
   2. Traumatic — aponeurotic disinsertion or dehiscence
   3. Mechanical — neurofibromatosis, lid infections.

Diagnosis—Differentiating Congenital from Aponeurotic Ptosis

Upgaze Eyelid Position

Upgaze eyelid position allows differentiation between congenital and aponeurotic blepharoptosis according to the neurophysiology of eyelid retraction. Upgaze with stretching of the mechanoreceptor of Mueller muscle increases involuntary reflex contraction of the levator slow-twitch muscle fibers. Worsening of ptosis on upgaze is common in congenital ptosis and is an abnormal differentiating sign, lacking the involuntary reflex contraction. Improvement of ptosis on upgaze is common in aponeurotic blepharoptosis and likely represents a normal physiological process, restoring the involuntary reflex contraction.

Ultrasound Biomicroscopy

The thickness of the levator aponeurosis can be measured with ultrasound biomicroscopy. The most common pathology in aponeurotic blepharoptosis is thinned-out aponeurosis. The levator aponeurosis of the ptotic eyelid is thinner than the normal eyelid in congenital ptosis. The thickness of the levator

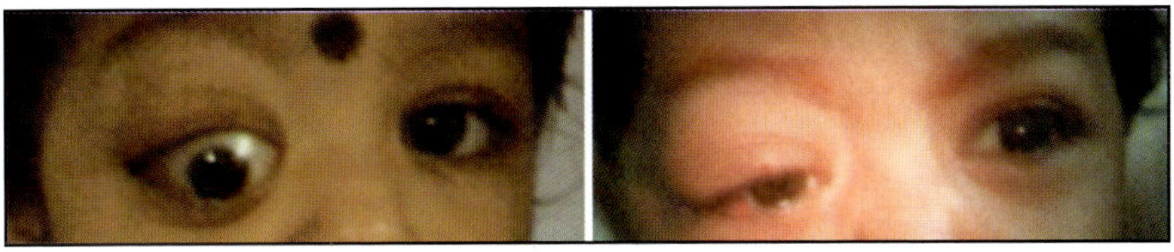

Figure 12: Pre- and post-decompression

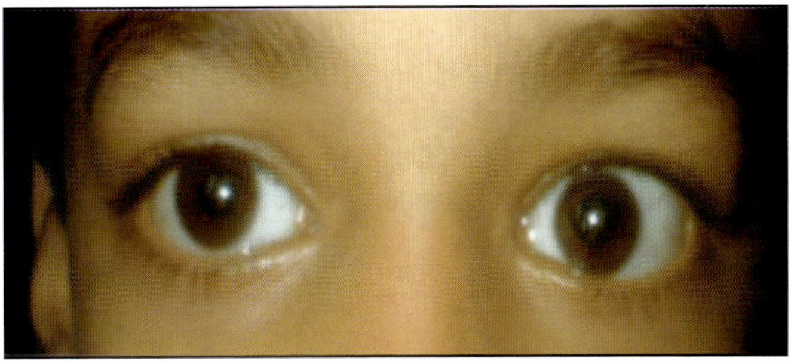

Figure 13: Congenital eyelid retraction

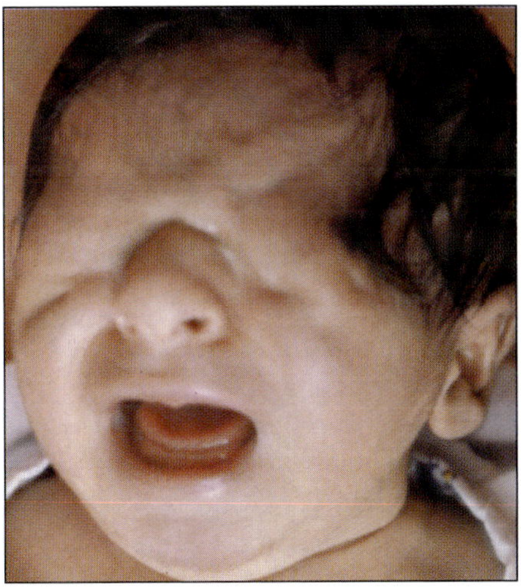

Figure 14: Cryptophthalmos

aponeurosis correlates with the levator function in congenital dysmyogenic blepharoptosis.

Unconventional Ptosis

Childhood Myasthenia

Serum acetylcholine receptor antibody may be negative frequently, girls with onset after 11 years being more likely to be Antibody positive.

Types

Three distinct groups of patients are generally reported.

Transient Neonatal Myasthenia Gravis—6.8% of childhood myasthenia. Usually do not have ocular involvement.

Congenital Myasthenia 17.2% of cases. These patients have an onset of symptoms from 1 to 12 months of age. The most frequent symptom in this group is bilateral blepharoptosis. Myasthenic crisis do not occur. Spontaneous remissions are rare.

Juvenile Myasthenia 76% of the patients. The onset of symptoms in this group ranges from 13 months to 14 years presenting purely with ocular symptoms. Myasthenic crisis may occur and spontaneous remissions are observed. Good response to anticholinesterase drugs is slightly more frequent in juvenile myasthenia.

Since patients with autoimmune myasthenia and a young age of onset are often seronegative, clinical features such as changing distribution of weakness, fluctuating severity, or response to treatment might be considered as supportive criteria for differentiating juvenile from congenital forms.

Mutations : Mutations of the acetylcholine receptor (AChR) delta subunit gene (CHRND) may lead to sporadic congenital myasthenic syndrome (CMS). Mutations in various genes encoding proteins expressed at the neuromuscular junction may cause CMS. Mutations of AChR subunit genes lead to end-plate AChR deficiency or to altered kinetic properties of the receptor. Mutations in the alpha, beta and delta subunits of the AChR are less frequent than mutations of the epsilon subunit; mutations in these subunits leading to AChR deficiency are often associated with a severe phenotype. The cytoplasmic loop of the AChR subunits is known to be essential for AChR-rapsyn co-clustering. Impairment of AChR-rapsyn co-clustering—a well-known molecular mechanism for rapsyn mutations—could also result from mutations in the delta subunit. Introduction of the same mutation in the epsilon subunit has no effect on AChR clustering indicating a special role of the delta subunit in AChR-rapsyn interactions.

Treatment: Prednisone dose is slowly increased to 50-60 mg (0.4 to 1mg/kg) and then gradually reduced to 10 mg, followed by further reduction as tolerated.

The pyridostigmine dose is begun at 180 mg daily and increased as tolerated.

WARG Syndrome and Ptosis

Lennon et al recently reiterated that ptosis may be associated with WARG syndrome which consists of Wilms tumor, aniridia, genitourinary abnormalities, and mental retardation. The aniridia and predisposition for Wilms tumor seen in WAGR are caused by haploinsufficiency for PAX 6 and WT1, respectively.

Partial Trisomy and Ptosis

Doco-Fenzy et al reported a pure de novo direct duplication dup (12)(q24.1—>q24.2). She had developmental and growth retardation, facial dysmorphism with upslanting palpebral fissures, wide downturned mouth, short neck, and Marcus Gunn phenomenon, single transverse creases, hypoplasia of the corpus callosum, and cardiac malformations consisting of a bicuspid aortic valve, multiple ventricular septal defects, and kinking of the aorta.

Management

In a recent literature review Clauser et al concluded that the most widely used surgical techniques were levator muscle recession and frontalis suspension. It is used in the repair of ptosis with poor levator function. The materials used include tissue such as autologous or banked fascia lata or permanent suture material. The procedure involves connecting the frontalis muscle and the upper eyelid. Some authors have recently reintroduced the technique of a dynamic frontalis muscle flap tunneled into the eyelid that directly attaches to the tarsal plate but its role in clinical practice remains to be defined. Some authors have reported that habituation of the pterygoid-levator synkinesis and control of the ptosis with jaw positioning can occur as early as 2 and a half months and that surgery can be delayed until a safer time in Marcus Gunn jaw winking syndrome with severe ptosis if there are no objective signs of amblyopia but the author has in his experience seen several cases with refractive changes (reduction of astigmatism) occurring with correction of ptosis which are highlighted further in the chapter.

Recent Concepts from Evidences in Terms of Management

Refractive changes: Kumar et al studied twenty-three patients between 4 and 12 years old with severe congenital blepharoptosis and poor levator function who underwent frontalis brow suspension surgery and compared them with the non-ptotic eyes and observed changes in the postoperative best corrected visual acuity, binocularity, relevant refractive parameters, lid position, lagophthalmos, lid lag, and tear break-up time for 12 weeks and found significant differences in the baseline characteristics and the postoperative changes in the eyes with and without ptosis and concluded that retinoscopy, manual keratometry, and corneal videokeratoscopy are simple and effective methods to evaluate the sequential refractive changes occurring in these eyes.

Kao SC et al published their findings of astigmatic change following congenital ptosis surgery. Their incidence of high astigmatism (>2.5 diopters, D) in congenital ptosis was 25.3% and following surgery 27.5% showed a decrease of more than 0.5 D. An average decrease of 0.18 D in astigmatism was observed.

Synkinetic ptosis-oculomotor abducens : These are extremely rare and usually require and overcorrection —a fact that has been recently highlighted by Burroughs et al. One usually needs to do excess levator correction or a two staged procedure for this extremely rare condition.

Role of steroids in childhood myasthenia: Kupersmith et al studied recently the effect of treatment of myasthenia and found that children receiving prednisone showed resolution in primary gaze diplopia, downgaze diplopia, unilateral ptosis, and bilateral ptosis in 73.5%, 75.5%, 85.7%, and 98%, respectively at 1 month. The benefit persists at 3-6, 12, and 24 months except for the bilateral ptosis. The pyridostigmine group shows resolution in primary gaze diplopia, downgaze diplopia, unilateral ptosis, and bilateral ptosis in 6.9%, 17.2%, 50%, and 76.7% of patients after 1 month of treatment. Among the prednisone responsive patients, there are recurrences suggesting that 50-60 mg daily prednisone followed by lower doses (10 mg or less) has the benefit of resolving ptosis and diplopia that lasts for at least 2 years in approximately 70% of patients.

Comparison of silastic and banked fascia lata in pediatric frontalis suspension: Hersh et al studied 131 frontalis suspension operations using either Silastic or banked fascia lata during the past 12 years at Children's Hospital at Westmead, Sydney, Australia and found that functional success rates for primary frontalis suspension procedures were not significantly different for banked fascia lata and Silastic (60% versus 67.2%, respectively). Infection and granuloma rates also were not significantly different (7.1% for banked fascia lata versus 15.2% for silastic). They however found a statistically significant difference between the two materials in ptosis recurrence (35.3% for banked fascia lata versus 13% for silastic) and concluded that silastic was significantly better than banked fascia lata in terms of ptosis recurrence. But more prospective data would be required as this study was a retrospective analysis.

Frontalis lobe suspension: A Croatian group recently reported in a retrospective study their long-term results in 146 patients operated by frontal muscle lobe shaping with or without shaping of corrugator muscle lobe attached to the tarsal plate in children with congenital dystrophic ptosis.

Their criteria of postoperative success (defined as a situation with eyes open in which upper eyelid covers the cornea at 12 o'clock position by 1-2 mm; there is a good contour of the eyelid margin; there is no lagophthalmos; and there is symmetry with the other eye) was met by 91% patients at 6 months, 85% at one year, and 83% at 5 years after resurgery for undercorrection being done in 18% of patients.

Advancement of Whitnall's ligament — conjunctival approach: Bajaj et al recently did a prospective study of ptosis correction by advancement of Whitnall's ligament by plication of the levator aponeurosis via the conjunctival route and found that good correction, i.e. within 1 mm of the normal fellow eye in primary gaze, can be obtained in 80% of patients and that patients with more than or equal to 8 mm levator function give better results. It has the advantages of shorter surgical time, minimal dissection of tissue planes and reversibility, with the conjunctival approach being cosmetically more acceptable as there is no visible scar on the lid.

Autogenous palmaris longus frontalis sling in children with congenital ptosis: Wong et al investigated the long-term outcome of using autogenous palmaris longus tendon sling for correcting congenital ptosis in children with age ranging from 2 to 7 years with a mean follow-up of 92 months (range, 80-104 months), and noted found that all eyelids were successfully corrected with good lid height. No recurrence or other postoperative complications were encountered except one patient who developed a small skin fold over the harvest site. It could be a good alternative to autogenous fascia lata, and further studies, to compare these two sling materials seem warranted.

Complication of surgery—Inverse Bell's phenomenon: Betharia et al reported three patients who underwent levator resection and showed an inversion of the Bell's phenomenon in the postoperative period, with the eye going down instead of up, during eyelid closure. This highlights the need for evaluating the bells phenomenon not only preoperatively but also postoperatively.

Orbital Implantation in Children

Orbital implants are used regularly in pediatric patients at the time of enucleation. The commonest indications for enucleation are retinoblastoma, blind eye following trauma and end stage retinopathy of prematurity. Controversy regarding the rate of complications with newer implants in the pediatric population continues to confuse clinicians.

Size of Implant

The average percent volume replaced by the implants in adult patients is 68%. The average percent volume replaced by the implants in pediatric patients is 21%. Upto seventy-one percent of pediatric patients undergo secondary implant surgery to augment volume and eliminate superior sulcus deformity and enophthalmos. The placement of an adequately sized implant in pediatric patients may obviate the need for secondary augmentation of socket volume in adulthood. Some authors suggest an implant 2 mm less in diameter than the axial length of the eye in pediatric patients.

Primary Orbital Implants in Children—Hydroxyapatite

Christmas et al studied 120 child eyes implanted and found that implant exposure rate was 0.8%, implant extrusion was not seen and implant migration rate was 2.4%. Of all patients 96% had good cosmesis and 98% had good motility and concluded that orbital implantation after enucleation is successful in the pediatric population and complications are minimal. Hydroxyapatite implants are not associated with unacceptable complications in the pediatric population.

Porous Polyethylene Implant in a Child

Iordanidou et al studied prospectively the incidence of complications of primary insertion of porous polyethylene orbital implant in the pediatric population who underwent primary placement of an anteriorly wrapped spherical porous polyethylene orbital implant with at least 17 months of follow-up weeks and found that there were no cases of implant extrusion, superior sulcus syndrome, orbital cellulitis, or significant inflammatory response.

The spherical implant size used may be 16 mm, 18 mm or 20 mm. The prosthesis is generally fitted after an interval of 5 weeks and usually the porous polyethylene orbital implant is now not drilled for peg placement. Anteriorly wrapped primary porous polyethylene orbital implant in the pediatric population appears to be well tolerated with few complications even in the author's experience. Kim et al have noted a 33% exposure rate in eyes that had conventional enucleation and porous polyethylene implantation, and none if a free orbital fat graft in addition suggesting that a free orbital fat graft is a simple, effective way to prevent orbital implant exposure in patients requiring enucleation and implantation.

Autogenous Dermis-fat graft Orbital Implant

Mitchell et al studied autogenous dermis-fat graft orbital implants and found that all implants maintained appropriate volume allowing proper prosthetic fit and facial symmetry. Some children experience excessive growth of their implants but that can be managed by surgical debulking. Some children develop a central graft ulcer, which can be managed by superficial revision and reclosure. It is indeed a promising implant for the pediatric anophthalmic socket.

Moreker's Expandable Balloon Implants

These can be used in severe anophthalmic sockets which are contracted, so as to expand them.

Orbital Fractures in Children

Inferior wall involvement is the most commonly seen, and the trapdoor type fracture is the most common with soft tissue entrapment associated with nausea/vomiting. The trapdoor fracture is described as a pure orbital-floor fracture, linear in form and hinged medially, which allows herniation of orbital contents through the fracture and then entraps these herniated contents. Management of blowout fractures involving the orbital floor has been controversial over the past several decades. One school of thought recommends conservative treatment for 4 to 6 months while another recommends a 'wait and watch' period of 2 weeks before intervention.

Baek et al suggested that early diagnosis, and prompt surgical intervention are required for patients with oculocardiac reflex. Grant et al too in their series reported that in the cases with trapdoor fracture and restricted ocular movement, early intervention was associated with better postoperative function and thus recommended that the symptomatic trapdoor orbit fracture be considered an urgent indication for surgical intervention. Cohen et al reported in their series that the positive predictive value of nausea/vomiting with a trapdoor fracture for entrapment was 83.3%. and that patients with trapdoor fractures who present with nausea/vomiting are at a high-risk of inferior rectus entrapment and poor outcome. Egbert et al reported that preoperative nausea and vomiting are immediately relieved after surgery. The median time for improvement of preoperative duction deficits and diplopia is 4 days for patients receiving surgery within 7 days and 10 days for those undergoing surgery after 14 days. Resolution of duction deficits or diplopia is not dependent on time of surgery if performed within 1 month of injury. For patients with severe limitation of ductions, early surgical repair within 7 days of injury results in more rapid improvement of ductions and diplopia than surgery performed later. Jordan et al called it the "white eyed fracture" and reported that a 2-week waiting period has been found to be of little benefit in these persons and possibly harmful to their motility. They advocated surgery within the first few days after injury as it may help to avoid permanent motility restriction.

We (authors) perform orbital wall reconstruction with Prolene/Medpor barrier sheet implantation (thickness 1mm) through transconjunctival approach under endoscopic guidance and at times whenever possible we do a **complete endoscopic correction endoscopic fracture reduction and mesh implantation with tissue glue.**

A completely endoscopic approach transnasally with reduction of the trapdoor fracture fragments with endoscopically guided mesh kept in place by fibronectin glue is done by the authors (Dr Milind Kirtane and Dr Sunil Moreker) at their institute (P.D Hinduja National Hospital and MRC, Bombay) and videos of the same were presented at the Eye Advance 2006 and the Annual conference of Asia Pacific Academy of Ophthalmology at Singapore 2006.

Lid and Orbital Tumors

Most pediatric orbital tumors are benign; developmental cysts comprise half of orbital cases, with capillary hemangioma being the second most common orbital tumor. The most common orbital malignancy is rhabdomyosarcoma. The most common intraocular malignant lesion is retinoblastoma. Choroidal melanoma, which is common in adults, is extremely rare in children. The orbit is the most common location for metastases in children, whereas the choroid is the predominant site in adults. Metastases to the orbit in childhood may be due to solid tumors such as a neuroblastoma or Ewing's tumor. Orbital cysts are quite common and varied.

Shields Classification of Orbital Cysts

The major categories in the classification include:

a. Cysts of surface epithelium,
   i. Simple epithelial cyst (epidermal, conjunctival, respiratory, and apocrine gland), and
   ii. Dermoid cyst (epidermal and conjunctival).
b. Teratomatous cysts,
c. Neural cysts—include those associated with ocular maldevelopment (congenital cystic eye and colobomatous cyst) and those associated with brain and meningeal tissue (cephalocele and optic nerve meningocele).
d. Secondary cysts—most common mucocele that can occur in children with cystic fibrosis
e. Inflammatory cysts, generally due to parasitic infestations and are more common in tropical areas of the world.
f. Noncystic lesions with cystic component—include adenoid cystic carcinoma, rhabdomyosarcoma, lymphangioma, and others.

Epidermal dermoid cyst (dermoid) is by far the most common orbital cystic lesion in children, accounting for over 40% of all orbital lesions of childhood and for 89% of all orbital cystic lesions of childhood that come to biopsy or surgical removal. Dermoid cysts are unusual neoplasms that often present in childhood, with the orbit being the area most commonly affected in the head and neck region. Imaging studies help rule out an intracranial or intraorbital extension. With complete excision, recurrence is unusual.

Capillary hemangiomas are the most common orbital tumors of childhood and can cause amblyopia secondary to occlusion of the pupil, anisometropia, or strabismus. Hemangiomas were classified based on size. Presence of aniosometropic astigmatism, ptosis, pupillary occlusion, lid margin change, proptosis, globe displacement, and strabismus need to be recorded.

Schwartz et al reported that size greater than 1 cm in largest diameter is an important predictor of amblyogenic factors and approximately half of these patients require treatment. Diffuse hemangiomas and hemangiomas in patients with PHACES syndrome cause amblyopia in the majority of cases. Periorbital hemangiomas can cause amblyopia secondary to anisometropia, induced astigmatism, strabismus or occlusion of the visual axis. Oral and intralesional steroids are considered to be the most accepted form of primary treatment. Surgery is a safe, effective treatment for selected lesions, provides a definitive early treatment, and prevents astigmatism and occlusion-related amblyopia and so some authors favor early surgery.

Preseptal cellulitis is the most common orbital disease in children older than 3 years. Awareness of orbital diseases in childhood, as a rare entity, is crucial for timely diagnosis and appropriate treatment, to save the vision and lives of affected children.

Endoscopic Management of Orbital Diseases

Both hemangiomas and orbital cellulites are amenable to treatment by endoscopy and have excellent results in the authors experience.

Nd YAG Laser and corticosteroids

Some authors have tried local Neodymium: YAG-laser therapy and in patients with large subcutaneous eyelid hemangiomas and involvement of the orbita tried with interstitial Neodymium: YAG-laser therapy in combination with systemic corticosteroids with good results.

Orbital Lymphangioma and AV Malformations

Orbital lymphangioma and AV malformations are uncommon, benign cystic appearing lesions, generally manifest in childhood. They usually present with a slowly progressive proptosis, displacement of the globe, ptosis and restriction of eye movements. Occasionally, focal lesions may remain asymptomatic. Spontaneous intraorbital hemorrhage may cause acute proptosis, compressive optic neuropathy and loss of vision. Surgical decompression of the optic nerve may be performed if there is progressive decrease in visual acuity.

Congenital Eyelid Retraction and Childhood Thyroid

Congenital eyelid retractions may affect either the lower or the upper eyelid. They make up a rare condition and most cases are associated with craniofacial syndromes such as Crouzon or Apert syndromes or childhood thyroid. Burroughs et al have proposed that thyroid eye disease may be present in children and even neonates with both mother and child being euthyroid. Upper eyelid retractions may spontaneously improve in some cases, but lower eyelid retractions do not. Treatment requires surgery, depending on the corneal consequences.

Eyelid Malpositions

Ruban's Classification

It is important to separate eyelid malpositions, which are topographical disorders, from eyelid malformations, which are constitutional morphological disorders. Eyelid malpositions can be:

A. **Static disorders**—including:
   i. epiblepharon—epiblepharon is characterized by the absence of adhesion between the lower eyelid retractors and the orbicularis-skin layer, which allows the anterior lamella to roll over.
   ii. congenital ectropion and entropion,

iii. Epicanthus—epicanthus involves a semi-lunar fold of skin extending from the upper eyelid across the medial canthal area to the margin of the lower eyelid. Four types:
  a. Supra-ciliaris,
  b. Palpebralis,
  c. Tarsalis and
  d. Inversus of epicanthus are described. Treatment requires surgery.

iv. Telecanthus—defined as an increased distance between canthi.
  a. Primary telecanthus results from attenuation of the medial canthal tendons and is usually associated with other soft tissue abnormalities such as epicanthus or blepharophimosis, or is seen after trauma.
  b. Secondary telecanthus is caused by underlying bony malpositions with an abnormal separation between the orbits because of an increased thickness of the interorbital bones such as that seen in hypertelorism or in other complex craniofacial syndromes.

v. Centurion syndrome.

B. **Dynamic disorders**—ptosis and congenital eyelid retractions. Euryblepharon is distinguished by an enlargement of the horizontal palpebral fissure associated with enlarged eyelids.

Congenital Entropion

When the eyelid margin is rolled inward against the globe, at birth, the condition is referred to as congenital entropion. Upper eyelid involvement is commonly associated with a tarsal abnormality, while lower eyelid entropion is often associated with epiblepharon. Entropion does not resolve spontaneously, and may cause corneal pathology if untreated. Serafino et al studied patients with lower bilateral congenital entropion to compare the results of incisional versus rotational surgery. The authors consider both techniques satisfactory, but the procedure of choice, considering the age of the patients and previous studies, remains rotational sutures because of its simplicity, quickness, and low risk of complication. Some authors have tried the pretarsal orbicularis muscle injection with 5 units of botulinum toxin with resolution of entropion four days after treatment and no recurrence of the entropion 7 months after botulinum toxin injection suggesting that injection of botulinum toxin may effectively treat certain cases of congenital entropion.

Surgical Correction of Entropion in Congenital Cutis Laxa

Congenital cutis laxa is a rare generalized inherited elastosis, characterized by the appearance of premature aging and skin laxity with mild to severe systemic anomalies. Ocular manifestations include excess skin in the eyelids, ptosis and lower lid ectropion. Of the hyperelasticity syndromes—Ehlers Danlos, Pseudoxanthoma elasticum and cutis laxa—only cutis laxa has normal skin wound healing. The diagnosis must therefore be established before surgical options for treatment are considered.

Congenital Ectropion

Congenital eversion of the upper eyelids is a rare condition, the exact cause of which remains unknown. It is more frequently associated with Down's syndrome and black babies. If diagnosed early and treated properly, the condition can be managed without surgery conservatively by lubricants, antibiotics and eyelid patching.

Congenital Ectropion in Congenital Ichthyosis

Congenital ectropion in congenital ichthyosis which is a generalized hyperkeratinization of the skin at birth. Depending on clinical aspects and severity, three forms of congenital ichthyosis have been defined: Mitis, tarda, and gravis. Desquamation of the parchment-like hyperkeratinized skin begins shortly after birth and may require several weeks to complete. Skin alterations in the eyelid cause shortening of the anterior lamella, subsequently resulting in ectropion. This affects the upper eyelid more often than the lower and can lead to complications such as chronic palpebral or bulbar conjunctivitis and keratinization or exposure keratopathy. In mild forms of congenital ichthyosis surgical treatment of eyelid ectropion is not required. In more severe cases a skin graft may become necessary.

Cryptophthalmos

Cryptophthalmos, a very rare congenital anomaly of the eye, is characterized by skin passing continuously from the forehead to the cheek over a malformed eye.

It is genetic disorder with systemic involvement (sometimes life threatening) and if not leaves the family devastated and unsatisfied with treatment and fearful of one more such occurrence in the family. Thoughtful and methodical approach can alleviate some aspects.

Parental Age

The average paternal age is 27 years of age and the average maternal age is 24 years of age.

Known Risk Factors

Oligohydramnios is the most frequent complication during pregnancy.

Pathogenesis

Fras1, that is specifically detected in a linear fashion underlying the epidermis and the basal surface of other epithelia in embryos. Loss of Fras1 function results in the formation of subepidermal hemorrhagic blisters as well as unilateral or bilateral renal agenesis. Homozygous Fras1 mutants have fusion of the eyelids and digits and unilateral renal agenesis or dysplasia. Modifier genes are important determinants of phenotypic variation (The pathogenesis of phenotypic modules could include disruption to a morphogenetic field or a developmental field, mutation specific effects, or malfunction of temporally distinct genes)

- Triallelic inheritance
- Autosomal recessive inheritance
- Dominant mode of inheritance.

The loss of a cytoplasmic multi-PDZ scaffolding protein, glutamate receptor interacting protein 1 (GRIP1), leads to the formation of subepidermal hemorrhagic blisters, renal agenesis, syndactyly or polydactyly and permanent fusion of eyelids (cryptophthalmos). GRIP1 can physically interact with Fras1 and is required for the localization of Fras1 to the basal side of cells. Grip1 is disrupted by a deletion of two coding exons. GRIP1 is required for normal cell-matrix interactions during early embryonic development and that inactivation of Grip1 causes cryptophthalmos.

Classification

Nouby's Classification of Congenital Upper Eyelid Coloboma and Cryptophthalmos

- Grade 1: Coloboma without cryptophthalmos.
- Grade 2: Coloboma with abortive cryptophthalmos.
- Grade 3: Coloboma with complete cryptophthalmos.
- Grade 4: Classic cryptophthalmos (absence of all eyelid structures and the eye is completely covered with skin).
- Grade 5: Severe cryptophthalmos (with severe deformity of the nose and ectropion of the upper lip).

Moreker-Agashe Classification

- Grade 1: Frasers syndrome
- Grade 2: Congenital orbito-palpebral cyst
- Grade 3: Bilateral cryptophthalmos
- Grade 4: Unilateral partial crytophthalmos
- Grade 5: Symmetrical partial lateral 'cryptophthalmos'
- Grade 6: Symmetrical medial cryptophthalmos
- Grade 7: Asymmetrical hemicryptophthalmos
- Grade 8: Congenital symblepharon associated with meningoencephalocele
- Grade 9: Bilateral abortive cryptophthalmos associated with oculocutaneous albinism
- Grade 10: Congenital symblepharon (abortive cryptophthalmos)
- Grade 11: Cryptophthalmos solum corneae
- Grade 12: Ablepheron macrostomia syndrome.

Treatment

Complete Cryptophthalmos

Weng et al described a three-stage reconstructive procedure in which a conchal cartilage 'sandwich' graft is first placed between the skin flap and the globe, mucous membrane subsequently grafted onto the inner surface of the cartilage graft, and lid level adjusted as the third stage. Ferri et al have discussed the steps in more details.

Incomplete Cryptophthalmos

Dibben et al described that incomplete cryptophthalmos can be corrected by dissection of the eyelids from the cornea, reconstruction of the conjunctival fornices with buccal mucosa, and repairing the upper lid coloboma if present in a flap reconstruction using the inferior eyelid margin is the usual procedure.

Role of Amniotic Membrane

Stewart et al reported successful creation of a superior fornix in a case of partial cryptophthalmos after an amniotic membrane graft concluding that amniotic membrane is a useful resource for fornix reconstruction in cryptophthalmos.

Prenatal Diagnosis

Ultrasound diagnosis in a prenatal state as well as genetic counseling seems to be the only way to control this condition.

Chapter 34

Amblyopia

SH Lee (Canada)

Introduction

Amblyopia, otherwise known as **lazy eye**, is a disorder of the visual system that is characterized by poor vision in an eye that is otherwise physically normal, or out of proportion to associated structural abnormalities. The problem is caused by either no transmission or poor transmission of the visual image to the brain for a sustained period of dysfunction or during early childhood.

Amblyopia normally only affects one eye, but it is possible to be amblyopic in both eyes if both are similarly deprived of a good, clear visual image. Detecting the condition in early childhood increases the chance of successful treatment.

The term functional amblyopia often is used to describe amblyopia, which is potentially reversible by occlusion therapy. Organic amblyopia refers to irreversible amblyopia.

Most vision loss from amblyopia is preventable or reversible with the right kind of intervention. The recovery of vision depends on how mature the visual connections are, the length of deprivation, and at what age the therapy is begun. It is important to rule out any organic cause of decreased vision because many diseases may not be detectable on routine examination.

Pathological Consideration

Amblyopia is a developmental problem in the brain, not an organic problem in the eye (although organic problems can induce amblyopia which persist after the organic problem has resolved). The part of the brain corresponding to the visual system from the affected eye is not stimulated properly, and develops abnormally. This has been confirmed via direct brain examination. Researchers David H. Hubel and Torsten Wiesel had won the Nobel Prize in Physiology or Medicine in 1981 for their work demonstrating the irreversible damage to ocular dominance columns produced in kittens by sufficient visual deprivation during the so-called "critical period". The maximum critical period in humans is from birth to two years old.

Although many types of amblyopia exist, it is believed that their basic mechanisms are the same even though each factor may contribute different amounts to each specific type of amblyopia. In general, amblyopia is believed to result from disuse from inadequate foveal or peripheral retinal stimulation and/or abnormal binocular interaction that causes different visual input from the foveae.

Other Important Features of Amblyopia

Prevalence of amblyopia is difficult to assess and varies in the literature, ranging from 1.0-3.5% in healthy children to 4.0-5.3% in children with ophthalmic problems. Most data show that about 2% of the general population has amblyopia.

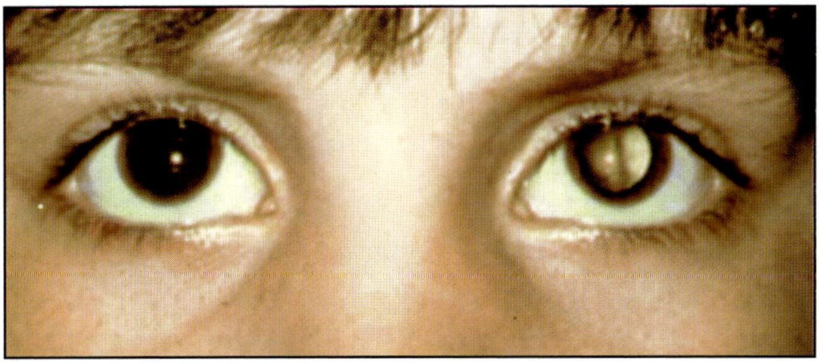

Figure 1: Child with left retinoblastoma – left organic or form deprivation amblyopia

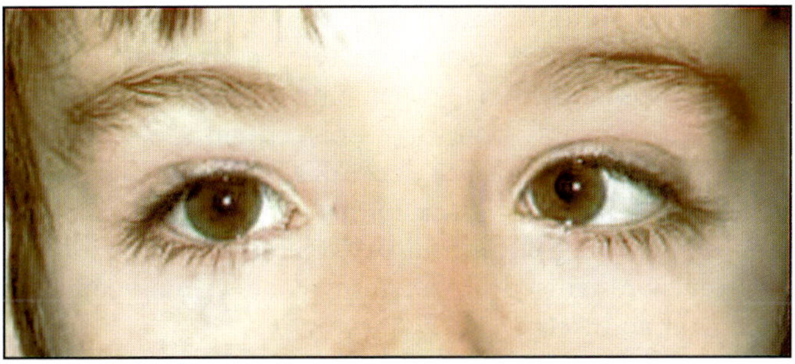

Figure 2: Child with left esotropia, left strabismic amblyopia

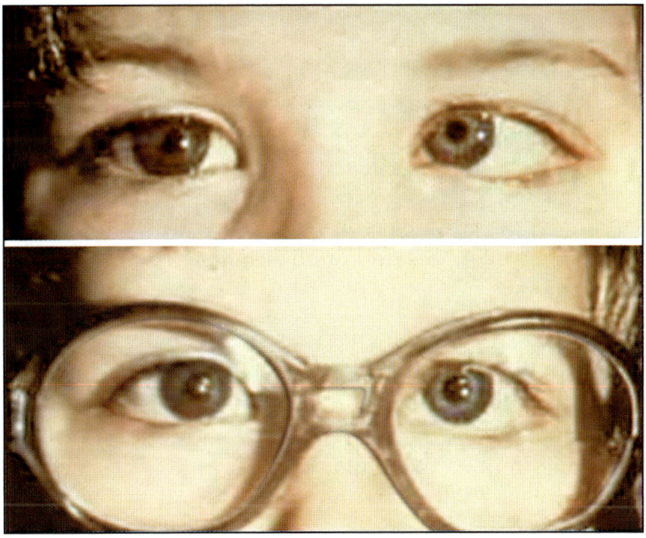

Figure 3: Child with left accommodative esotropia secondary to left eye with high hyperopia refractive error, and after optical correction, the left eye is normally aligned with the right eye, and the amblyopia is resolved

Amblyopia is an important socioeconomic problem. Studies have shown that it is the number one cause of monocular vision loss in adults. Furthermore, persons with amblyopia have a higher risk of becoming blind because of potential loss to the sound eye from other causes. No racial preference is known. No gender preference is known.

Amblyopia occurs during the critical periods of visual development. An increased risk exists in those children who are developmentally delayed, were premature, and/or have a positive family history.

Symptoms and Signs

Symptoms and signs of amblyopia are variable. Many people with amblyopia, especially those who are only mildly so, are not even aware they have the condition until tested at older ages, since the vision in their stronger eye is normal. However, people who have *severe* amblyopia may experience associated visual disorders, most notably poor depth perception.

Usually, symptoms and signs are depending upon the types of amblyopia. In general, there are three types of amblyopia –

1. Strabismic amblyopia—squinting or closing one eye while reading or watching television, crossed or turned eye and turning or tilting the head when looking at an object
2. Refractive or anisometropic amblyopia
3. Form-deprivation or visual pathway obstruction amblyopia, such as poor vision in one or both eyes.

Investigation

For Refractive or Anisometropic Amblyopia

Check Visual Acuity

Diagnosis of amblyopia usually requires a 2-line difference of visual acuity between the eyes; however, this definition is somewhat arbitrary and a smaller difference is common.

Crowding phenomenon: A common characteristic of amblyopic eyes is difficulty in distinguishing optotypes that are close together. Visual acuity often is better when the patient is presented with single letters rather than a line of letters.

Diagnosis is not an issue in children old enough to read or with use of the tumbling E. Testing in preverbal children.

If the child protests with covering of the sound eye, amblyopia can be diagnosed if it is dense.

Fixation preference may be assessed, especially when strabismus is present. Induced tropia test may be performed by holding a 10-prism diopter before one eye in cases of an orthophoria or a microtropia.

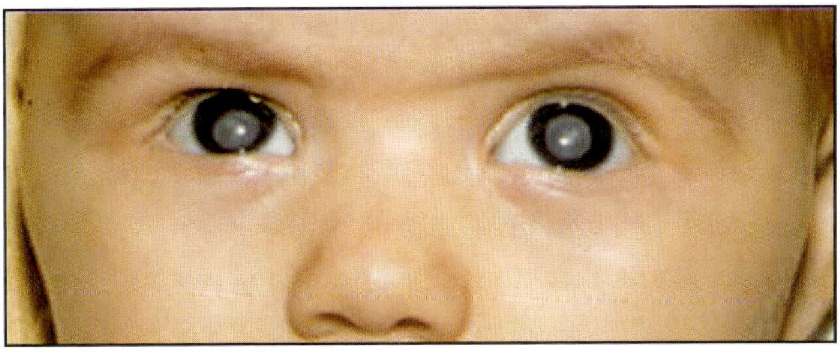

Figure 4: Child with bilateral congenital cataracts, bilateral form deprivation amblyopia

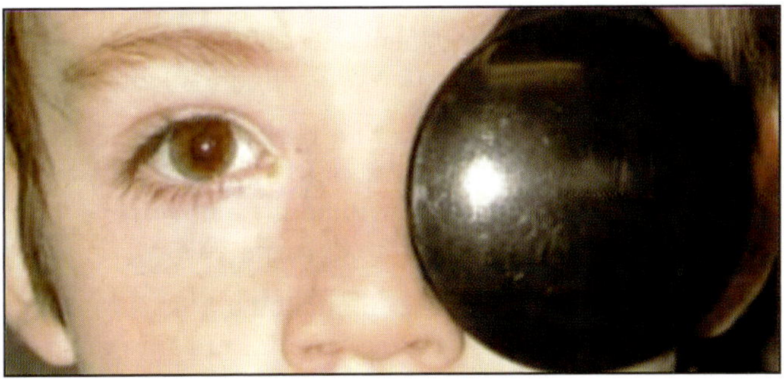

Figure 5: Cover test—Tropia-manifest

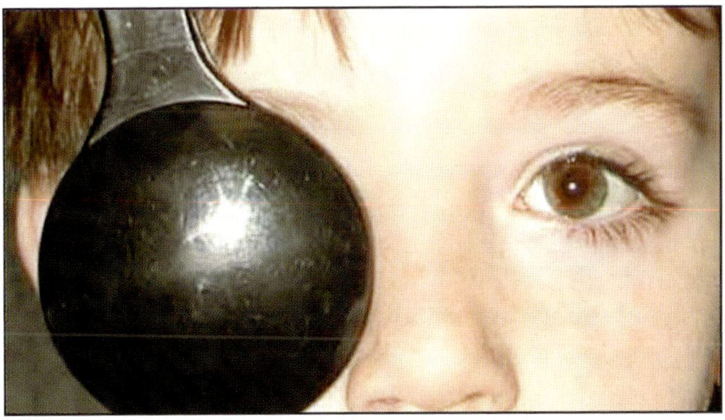

Figure 6: Alternate cover test—phoria-latent

In infants who cross-fixate, pay attention to when the fixation switch occurs; if it occurs near primary position, then visual acuity is equal in both eyes.

Contrast sensitivity: Strabismic and anisometropic amblyopic eyes have marked losses of threshold contrast sensitivity, especially at higher spatial frequencies; this loss increases with the severity of amblyopia.

Neutral density filters: Patients with strabismic amblyopia may have better visual acuity or less of a decline of visual acuity when tested with neutral density filters compared to the normal eye. This was not found to be true in patients with anisometropic amblyopia or organic disease.

Binocular function: Amblyopia usually is associated with changes in binocular function or stereopsis.

Eccentric fixation: Some patients with amblyopia may consistently fixate with a nonfoveal area of the retina under monocular use of the amblyopic eye, the mechanism of which is unknown. This can be diagnosed by holding a fixation light in the midline in front of the patient and asking them to fixate on it while the normal eye is covered. The reflection of the light will not be centered.

Refraction: Cycloplegic refraction must be performed on all patients, using retinoscopy to obtain an objective refraction. In most cases, the more hyperopic eye or the eye with more astigmatism will be the amblyopic eye. If this is not true, one needs to investigate further for ocular pathology.

Rest of examination: Perform a full eye examination to rule out ocular pathology.

In summary, Refractive amblyopia may result from anisometropia (unequal refractive indices between the two eyes).

Anisometropia exists when there is a difference in the refraction between the two eyes. The eye which provides the brain with a clearer image (closer to 20/20) typically becomes the dominant eye. The image in the other eye is blurred, which results in abnormal development of one half of the visual system.

Refractive amblyopia is usually less severe than strabismic amblyopia Frequently, amblyopia is associated with a combination of anisometropia and strabismus. Pure refractive amblyopia is treated by correcting the refractive error early with prescription lenses and patching or penalizing the good eye

For Strabismic Amblyopia

Strabismus, sometimes erroneously also called *lazy eye*, is a condition in which the eyes are misaligned. Strabismus usually results in normal vision in the preferred sighting (or "fellow") eye, but may cause abnormal vision in the deviating or strabismic eye due to the discrepancy between the images projecting to the brain from the two eyes. Adult-onset strabismus usually causes double vision (diplopia), since the two eyes are not fixated on the same object. Children's brains, however, are more neuroplastic, and therefore can more easily adapt by suppressing images from one of the eyes, eliminating the double vision. This plastic response of the brain, however, interrupts the brain's normal development, resulting in the amblyopia

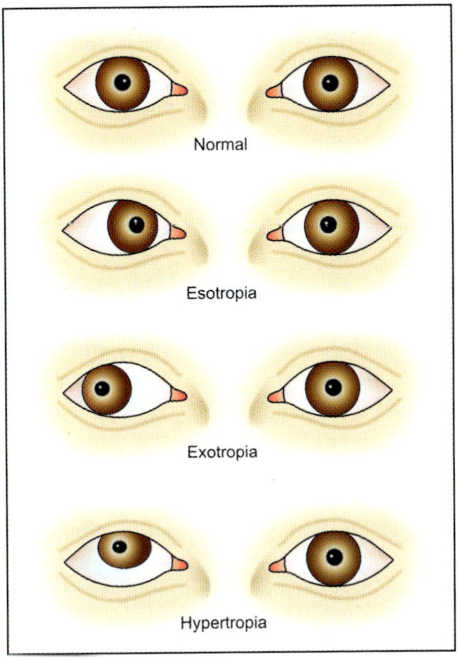

Figure 7: Types of tropia

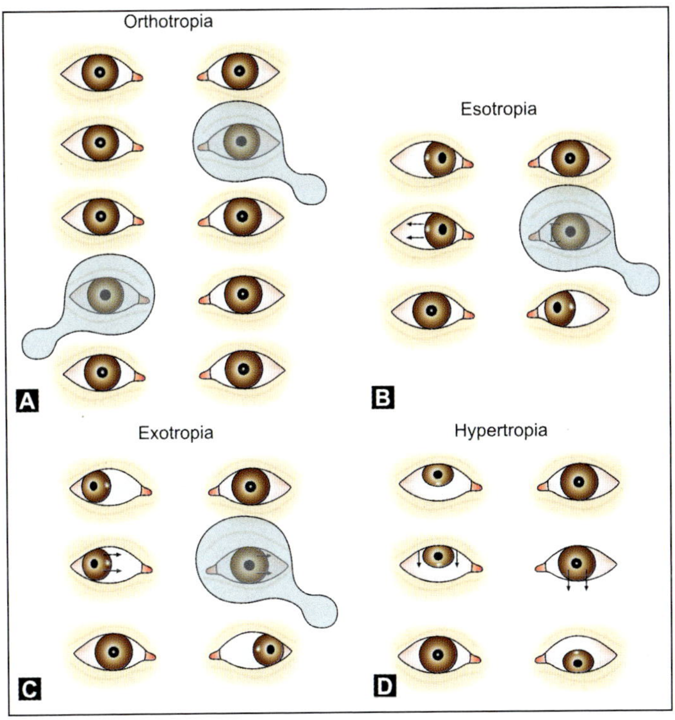

Figure 8: Cover test to detect the type of tropia

Types of Strabismus

- Esotropia and Exotropia, A-patterns
- Esotropia and Exotropia, V-patterns
- Esotropia, Accommodative
- Esotropia, Acquired
- Esotropia, Infantile
- Esotropia, with High AC/A Ratio
- Exotropia, Acquired
- Exotropia, Congenital
- Monofixation Syndrome

Any type of the above strabismus will lead to strabismus amblyopia if not treated in children after the critical time of visual pathway development.

Testing for Strabismus

Form-deprivation and Visual Pathway Obstruction Amblyopia

Form-deprivation amblyopia (*Amblyopia ex-anopsia*) results when the ocular media become opaque, such as is the case with cataracts or corneal scarring from forceps injuries during birth. These opacities prevent adequate visual input from reaching the eye, and therefore disrupt development. If not treated in a timely fashion, amblyopia may persist even after the cause of the opacity is removed. Sometimes, drooping of the eyelid (ptosis) or some other problem causes the upper eyelid to physically occlude a child's vision, which may cause amblyopia quickly. Visual pathway obstruction amblyopia may be a complication of a hemangioma that blocks some or all of the eye.

Other Problems to be Considered

Consider organic problems that may be subtle or difficult to diagnose such as optic nerve hypoplasia.

Imaging Studies

If suspicion exists of an organic cause for decreased vision and the ocular examination is normal, then further investigations into retinal or optic nerve causes should be initiated. Studies to perform include imaging of the visual system through CT scan, MRI, and fluorescein angiography to assess the retina.

Other Tests

Although differences in the electrophysiologic responses of normal versus amblyopic eyes have been reported, these techniques remain investigational and the differences are controversial.

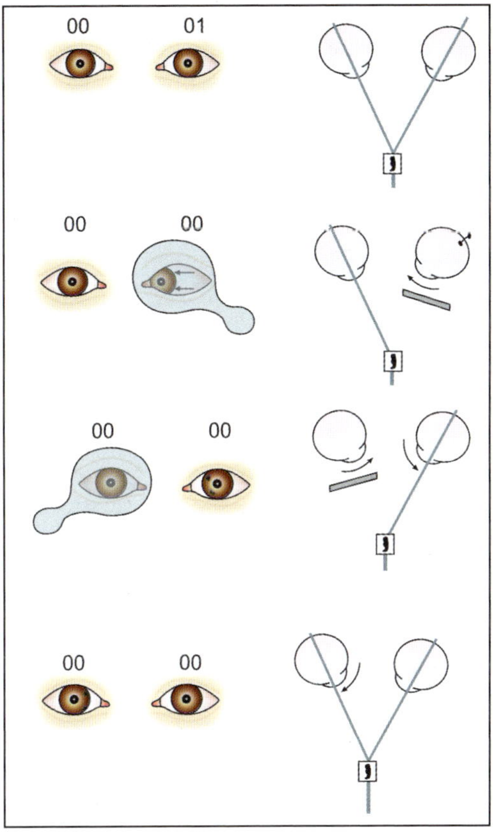

Figure 9: Alternate cover test to detect latent strabismus-phoria-strabismus Other tests for screening strabismus can be done in a large clinical center with aide of orthoptic technician at Children hospital

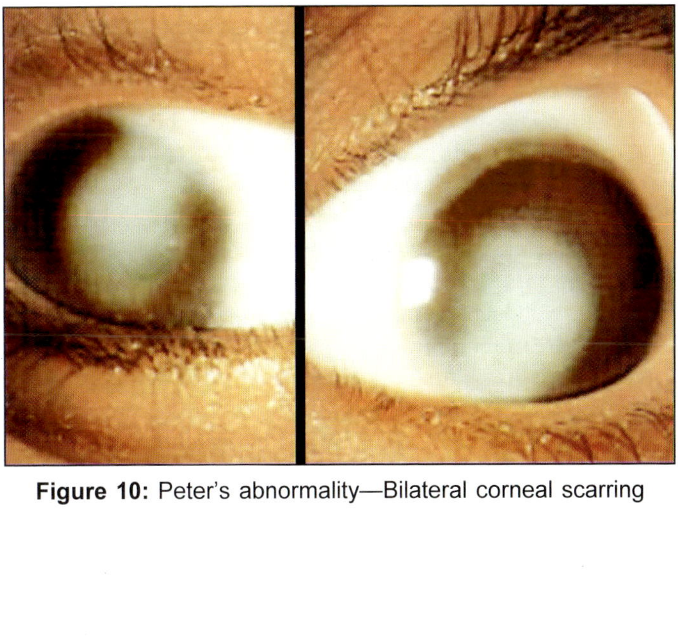

Figure 10: Peter's abnormality—Bilateral corneal scarring

Differential Diagnosis of Amblyopia

It is important to differentiate the three main different types of amblyopia, i.e. strabismus, refractive-anisometropia, and form deprivation ambylopia with the above chart. The treatment of amblyopia depends the etiology of the amblyopia.

Treatments: Medical and Surgical

Medical Care

The clinician must first rule out an organic cause and treat any obstacle to vision (e.g. cataract, occlusion of the eye from other etiologies).

Remove cataracts in the first 2 months of life, and aphakic correction must occur quickly.

Treatment of anisometropia and refractive errors must occur next.

The amblyopic eye must have the most accurate optical correction possible. This should occur prior to any occlusion therapy because vision may improve with spectacles alone.

Full cycloplegic refraction should be given to patients with accommodative esotropia and amblyopia. In other patients, a prescription less than the full plus measurement that was refracted may be prescribed given that the decrease in plus is symmetric between the two eyes. Because accommodative amplitude is believed to be decreased in amblyopic eyes, one needs to be cautious about cutting back too much on the amount of plus. Refractive correction alone can improve amblyopia in about one third of children.

The next step is forcing the use of the amblyopic eye by occlusion therapy. Occlusion therapy has been the mainstay of treatment since the 18th century. The following are general guidelines for occlusion therapy:

Patching may be full-time or part-time. Standard teaching has been that children need to be observed at intervals of 1 week per year of age, if undergoing full-time occlusion to avoid occlusion amblyopia in the sound eye. The recent and ongoing Amblyopia Treatment Studies (ATS) have helped to provide new information on the effect of various amounts of patching.

Always consider lack of compliance in a child where visual acuity is not improving. Compliance is difficult to measure but is an important factor in determining the success of this therapy.

In addition to adhesive patches, opaque contact lenses, occluders mounted on spectacles, and adhesive tape on glasses have been used.

Establishing the fact that the vision of the better eye has been degraded sufficiently with the chosen therapy is important.

The amblyopia treatment studies have helped to define the role of full-time patching versus part-time patching in patients with amblyopia. The studies have demonstrated that, in patients aged 3-7 years with severe amblyopia (visual acuity between 20/100 and 20/400), full-time patching produced a similar effect to that of 6 hours of patching per day. In a separate study, 2 hours of daily

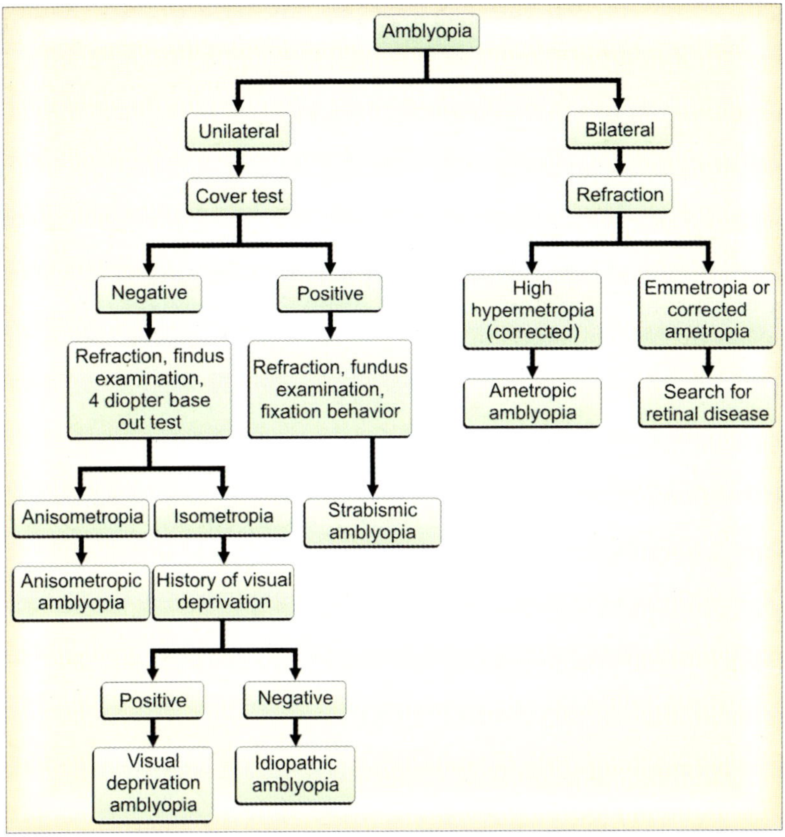

Figure 11: Flow chart of determination of differential diagnosis of amblyopia

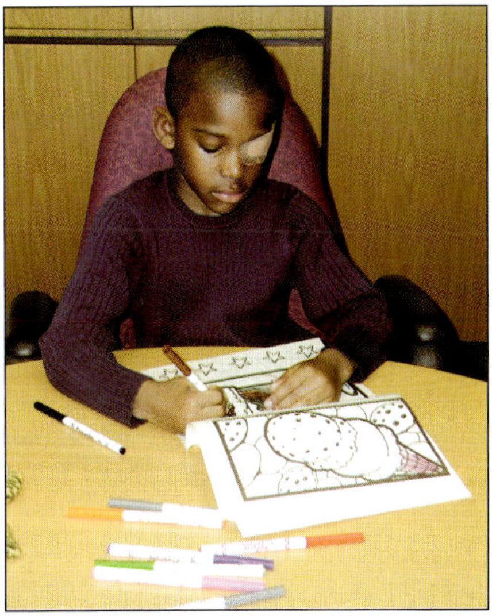

Figure 12: Child with left patching to treat the right amblyopia

patching produced an improvement in visual acuity similar to that of 6 hours of daily patching when treating moderate amblyopia (visual acuity better than 20/100) in children aged 3-7 years. In this study, patching was prescribed in combination with 1 hour of near visual activities.

Data from the Amblyopia Treatment Studies are also available for older patients. For patients aged from 7 years to younger than 13 years, the amblyopia treatment studies have suggested that prescribing 2-6 hours a day of patching can improve visual acuity even if the amblyopia has been previously treated. For patients aged from 13 years to younger than 18 years, prescribing 2-6 hours a day of patching might improve visual acuity when amblyopia has not been previously treated; however, this is likely to be of little benefit if amblyopia was previously treated with patching. Long-term results from these studies are still pending.

The amblyopia treatment studies have also found that about one fourth of children with amblyopia who were successfully treated experience a recurrence within the first year after discontinuation of treatment. Data from these studies suggest that patients treated with 6 or more hours a day of patching have a greater risk of recurrence when patching is stopped abruptly rather than when it is reduced to 2 hours a day prior to cessation of patching. Randomized studies have still yet to be performed.

Penalization Therapy

In the past, penalization therapy was reserved for children who would not wear a patch or in whom compliance was an issue. The amblyopia treatment studies, however, have demonstrated that atropine penalization in patients with moderate amblyopia (defined by the study as visual acuity better than 20/100) is as effective as patching. The amblyopia treatment studies were performed in children aged 3-7 years.

The amblyopia treatment studies have also demonstrated that weekend atropine provided an improvement in visual acuity similar to that of daily atropine when treating moderate amblyopia in children aged 3-7 years.

Atropine drops or ointment (Atropine sulfate 0.5 to 2.0%) is instilled in the nonamblyopic eye. This therapy is sometimes used in conjunction with patching or occlusion of the glasses (e.g. adhesive tape, nail-polish) by individual practitioners. In the amblyopia treatment studies that evaluated patching versus atropine penalization, atropine penalization and patching were used in conjunction with 1 hour of near visual activities.

This technique may also be used for maintenance therapy, which is useful especially in patients with mild amblyopia.

Other options include optical blurring through contact lenses or elevated bifocal segments.

The endpoint of therapy is spontaneous alternation of fixation or equal visual acuity in both eyes.

When visual acuity is stable, patching may be decreased slowly, depending on the child's tendency for the amblyopia to recur.

Because amblyopia recurs in a large number of patients (see Prognosis), maintenance therapy or tapering of therapy should be strongly considered. This tapering is controversial, so individual physicians vary in their approaches.

Treatment of strabismus generally occurs last. The endpoint of strabismic amblyopia is freely alternating fixation with equal vision. Surgery generally is performed after this endpoint has been reached.

Surgical Care

Surgical therapy for strabismus generally should occur after amblyopia is reversed. Disadvantages to surgical therapy prior to correction of amblyopia include difficulty in telling if amblyopia is present because there is no longer a strabismus to assess fixation preference and higher potential to being lost to follow-up, as the child cosmetically looks better. The improved cosmesis gives the parents a false sense of security about the vision improving.

Other surgical therapy for form deprivation amblyopia include cataract surgery for congenital cataracts, corneal transplants for bilateral corneal scarring, retinoblastoma, etc.

Activity after Treatment

Close supervision during occlusion therapy is necessary to make sure children do not peek. Various methods of preventing children from removing patches have been considered, from a reward system for older children to arm splints and mittens for infants.

Atropine penalization –Atropine sulfate 0.5-2.0% (with either ointment or drops) is an alternative method of blurring vision in the sound eye of patients who refuse patching. It may be applied once a day to patients in the preferred eye only.

Further Follow-up Care

Outpatient follow-up care needs to continue beyond the primary completion of amblyopia treatment because visual deterioration occurs in many children. In a multicenter study conducted as part of the amblyopia treatment studies, one-fourth of patients experienced recurrence of amblyopia within the first year after treatment, with the risk of recurrence greater if the treatment was stopped abruptly rather than tapered. One study by Levartovsky et al showed deterioration in 75% of children with anisometropia of 1.75 diopters or more after occlusion therapy. Recidivism can occur even several years after the initial treatment period and is as high as 53% after 3 years.

Deterrence/Prevention

Vision screening programs: Studies have shown these programs to be technically easy and that they help reduce cost as well as incidence of amblyopia because of early treatment and detection. Current programs include use of the photorefractor and school vision screening programs.

Amblyopia after Trauma

Young patients who have trauma to their eyes often are at risk for occlusion amblyopia. Possible reasons include lid edema, hyphema, occlusive dressing, vitreous hemorrhage, and traumatic cataract.

This amblyopia often is superimposed on a visual deficit caused by any structural abnormality and needs to be taken into account when treating these children.

Vision needs to be monitored closely in children after ocular trauma, especially up to 6 years and in nonverbal children. Occlusive therapy needs to be instituted if there is any suggestion of decrease vision in the injured eye.

Complications

Most cases of amblyopia are reversible if detected and treated early, so this vision loss is preventable The main complication of not treating amblyopia is long-term irreversible vision loss.

Clinical Trials and Experiments

A recent study, widely reported in the popular press, has suggested that repetitive transcranial magnetic stimulation may temporarily improve contrast sensitivity and spatial resolution in the bad eye of amblyopic adults. These results await verification by other researchers.

Virtual reality computer games where each eye receives different signals of the virtual world that the player's brain must combine in order to successfully play the game have shown some promise in improving both monocularity in the affected eye as well as binocularity.

In another recent clinical trial conducted in a hospital in China and coordinated with a research program at University of Southern California, 28 of 30 patients being treated for amblyopia showed dramatic gains with some developing 20/20 vision. The treatment involved only the use of basic computer desktop software and vision training exercises

Prognosis

After 1 year, about 73% of patients show success after their first trial of occlusion therapy. Studies have shown that the number of patients who retain their level of visual acuity decreases over time to 53% after 3 years.

Risk factors for failure in amblyopia treatment include the following:

Type of amblyopia: Patients with high anisometropia and patients with organic pathology have the worse prognosis. Patients with strabismic amblyopia have the best outcome.

Age at which therapy began: Younger patients seem to do better.

Depth of amblyopia at start of therapy: The better the initial visual acuity in the amblyopic eye, the better the prognosis.

Parents need to be educated about the importance of treatment and compliance as well as the visual implications because the treatment of amblyopia often lies in the hands of the parents.

The clinician must educate parents and patients of the implications of not treating amblyopia. Delay in treatment beyond the critical period results in irreversibility of amblyopia and could result in liability claims against the physician.

Conclusion

Early treatment and detection is the key to visual rehabilitation in amblyopic patients. Methods of identifying children at risk or who have amblyopia are needed. Further research into the mechanism of amblyopia is needed to be able to address and treat the direct etiology.

Chapter 35

Exodeviation

Ewa Oleszczynska Prost (Poland)

Pseudoexotropia

Pseudoexotropia is a condition,on which the eyes are straight ,however they appear to be outward deviation. In a very young children wide interpupillary distance are frequent. Such a state may simulate divergent strabismus. Often we observed the abnormality of the eyeballs structure (ectopia maculae in retinopathy of prematurity) or its placement in the orbits or changes in the eye protective apparatus. Pseudoexotropia present, when the visual axis (connecting fixing object with the fovea) is different (near the nose) then the optic axis (the line running through the center of cornea and pupil). The angle at which these axes crossed is called gamma angle.

Exophoria

Exophoria is a latent tendency for the eyes to deviate. Deviation of the visual axis results from the fusion interruption, which is not able to maintain binocular vision any longer.

Factors predisposing to decompensated exophoria are listed below:
- Anisometropia.
- Transient cover of one eye
- Emotional or physical shock
- Fatigue or asthenia (severe infections).

Clinical Findings

- Age of onset between 6 months and 4 years (usually at 18 months)
- Occasionally then one eye divergens patient close this eye in bright light
- Sometimes diplopia occurs
- Once suppression has been triggered by the eye drifting out
- Patients have a larger binocular peripheral visual field than normal people
- Typical cases have stereoacuity at near, this is where most patients control their deviation.

Investigations

- Cover test
- Retinoskopy with full cycloplegia
- Hirschberg's test
- Maddox rod test for distance and near
- Fusion amplitude rare is low

Differential Diagnosis

- Orthophoria
- Intermittent exotropia
- Convergens insufficiency

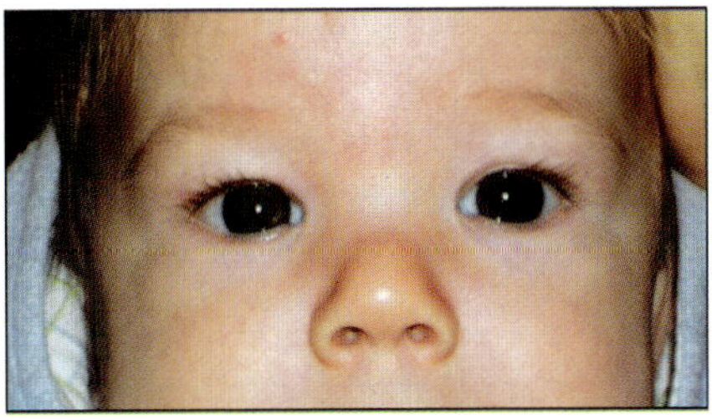

Figure 1: Pseudoexotropia in 4,5-month child with positive angle gamma

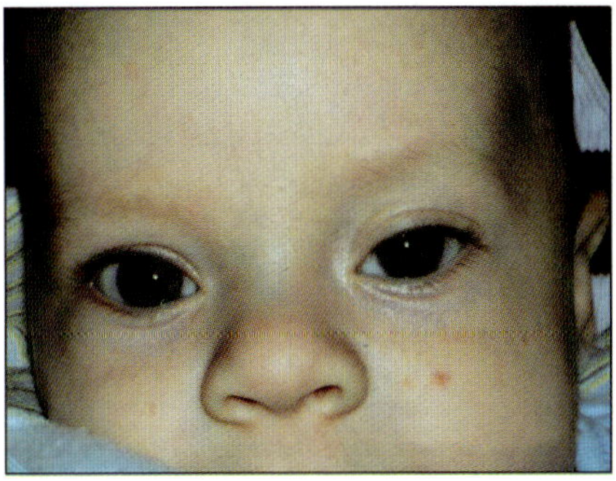

Figure 2: Two-month-old children with different appearance of palpebral fissures

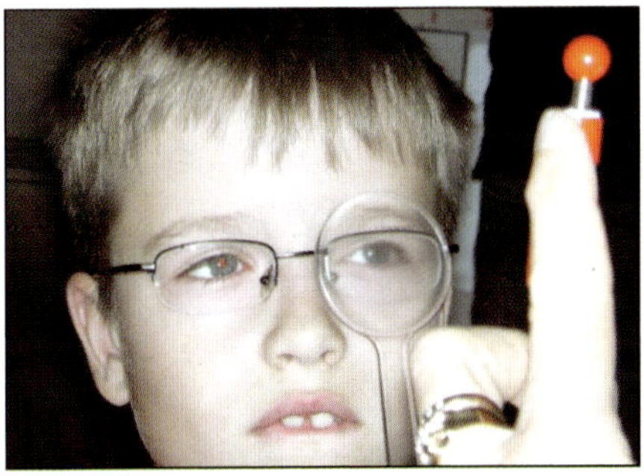

Figure 3: Exophobia. Note the deviation the left eye during cover-test

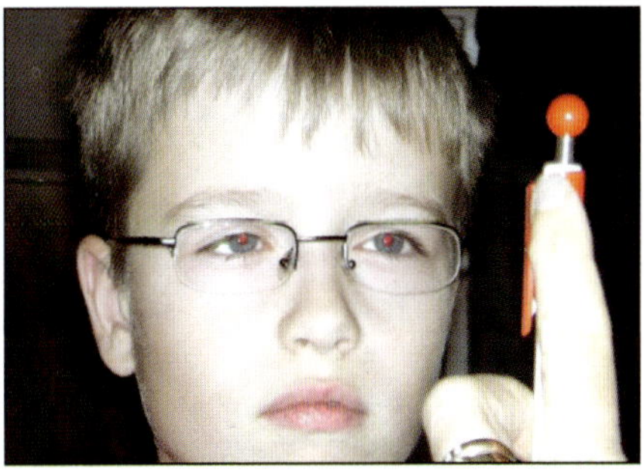

Figure 4: The same patient with exophoria. Note the straight eyes during binocular fixation

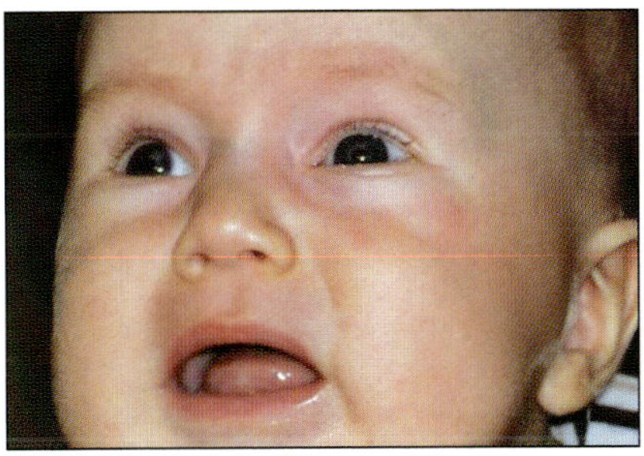

Figure 5: Congenital exotropia in 1-month child

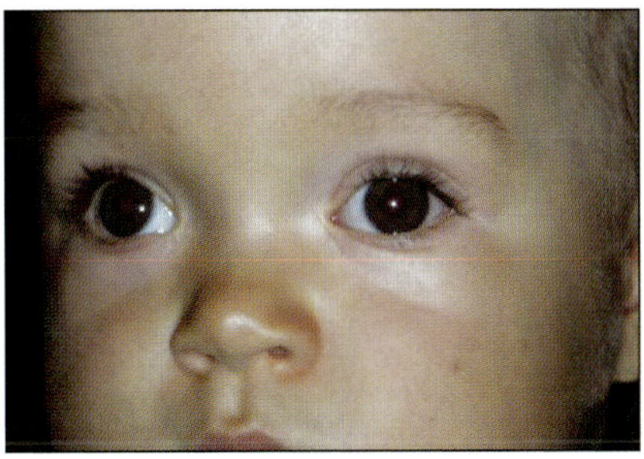

Figure 6: Eleven-year-old with congenital exotropia

Treatment

- Full correction of refractive error
- Prism base-out glasses facilitating actions of the weakened muscles
- Eye exercises strengthening binocular vision
- Sometimes botulinum toxin infection to the muscles is required
- Strabismus surgery is required only then intermittent exotropia appear.

Prognosis

- Spectacles according to the refraction with prism is the best solution
- Eye excercises improving fusion amplitude are also effective.

Congenital Exotropia

This form of strabismus is very rare present since birth. Exotropia is a manifest outward deviation of the visual axis of one or both eyes. One eye and then the fellow eye fixes alternatively in the primary position.

Clinical Findings

- Exotropia is present in all distances
- Angle of strabismus is large 35-50 PD
- The patient's fixation usually alternates
- Intermittent exotropia progress quickly to a constant status
- Good adduction is possible
- Amblyopia is not common
- If in the primary position one eye is fixing all the time, amblyopia may develop in the fellow eye
- In some cases unilateral or alternate inferior oblique muscle overaction or dissociated vertical deviation (DVD)are seen
- May occur in patients with craniofacial anomalies, cerebral palsy, neurologic disease or ocular albinism with micronystagmus.

Investigation

- Retinoscopy with full cycloplegia
- Fundus examination
- Hirschberg's and Krimsky test
- Cover-uncover test and alternate cover test
- Monocular adduction attempt
- Face turn examination.

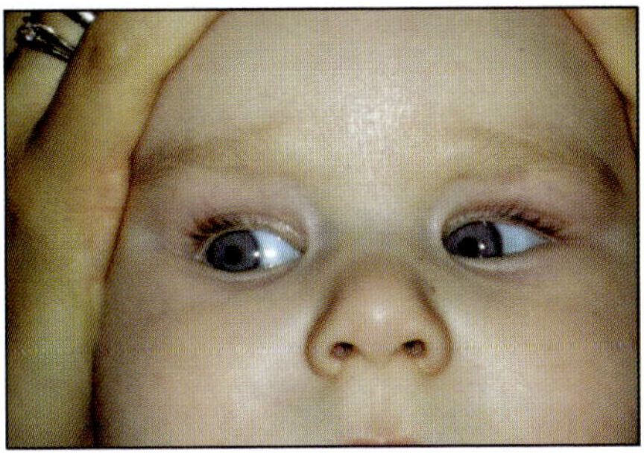

Figure 7: Intermittent exotropia in eight-month-old child during the distance fixation

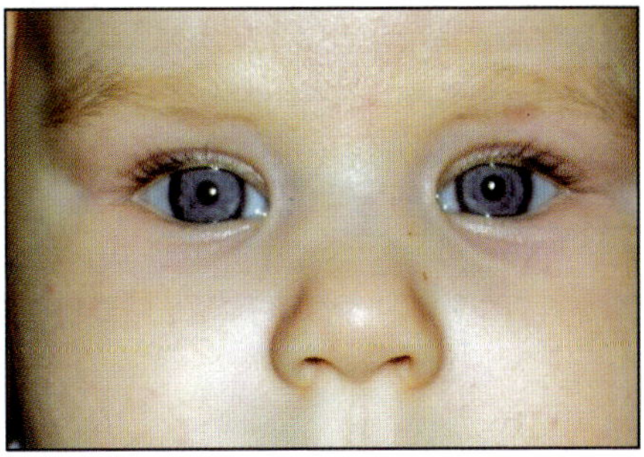

Figure 8: The eyes are straight in the same child during the near fixation

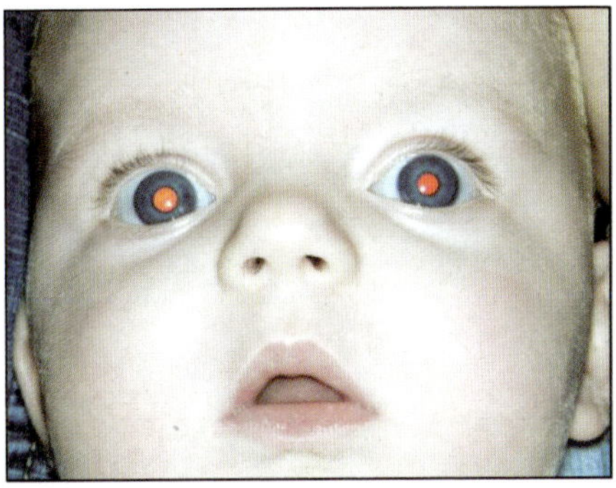

Figure 9: Convergence insufficiency. Small exotropia in the distance

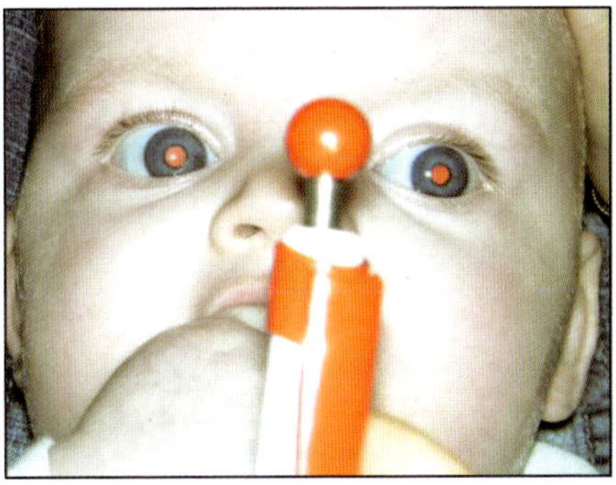

Figure 10: Convergence insufficiency when child looking at near point the exotropia appears

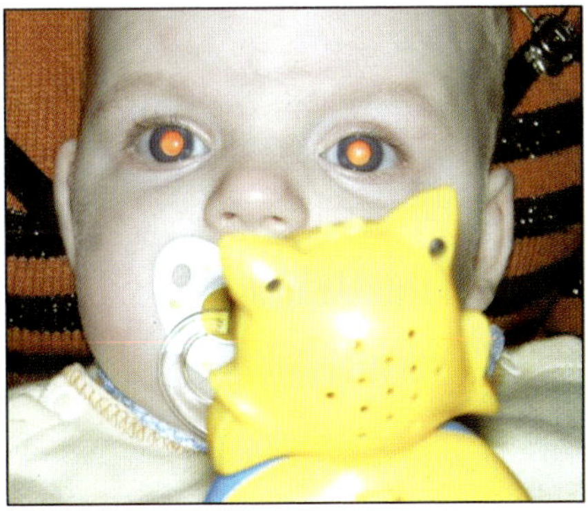

Figure 11: Convergece paralysis as a secondary status to the brain disorders

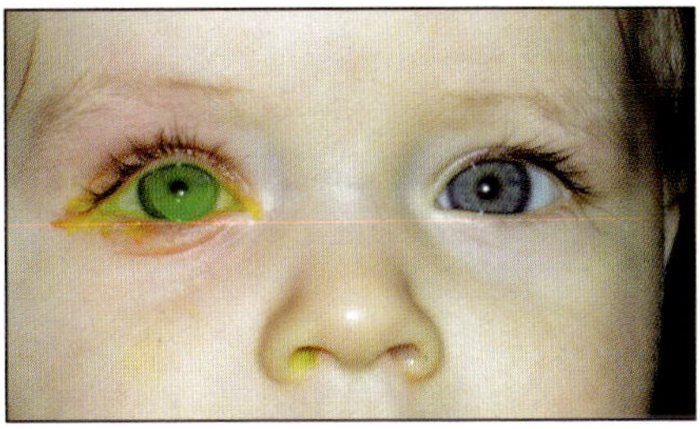

Figure 12: Deprivation exotropia.Patient after congenital cataract surgery with RGP contact lens on the right eye

Differential Diagnosis

- Intermittent exotropia
- Convergens insufficiency
- Convergens paralysis
- Deprivation (sensory) exotropia
- Consecutive exotropia.

Treatment

- Prescription of appriopriate eye-glasses or contact lenses
- Occlusion therapy if amblyopia is present
- Very early strabismus surgery should be done
- Botulinum toxin injection
- The use of prism-glasses.

Prognosis

- The goal in management is to straighten the eyes very early to achieved :
  1. Excellent visual acuity in each eye
  2. Single binocular vision in all directions of gaze
  3. Normal esthetic appearance.

Intermittent Exotropia

Intermittent exotropia is the most frequent cause of exodeviation and is often a progressive disease. Usually an exophoria decompensates to an intermittent exotropia and finally to a constant exotropia.

Clinical Findings

- Age of onset between 6 months and 4 years (usually at 18 months)
- Occasionally then one eye divergens patient close this eye in bright light
- Sometimes diplopia occurs
- Once suppression has been triggered by the eye drifting out
- Patients have a larger binocular peripheral visual field than normal people
- Typical cases have stereoacuity at near, this is where most patients control their deviation.

Investigation

- Assessment of vision, fusion and stereopsis
- Hirschberg's test at near and distance
- Cover-uncover test at near and distance
- Maddox test
- High AC/A can be diagnosed by the Patch test

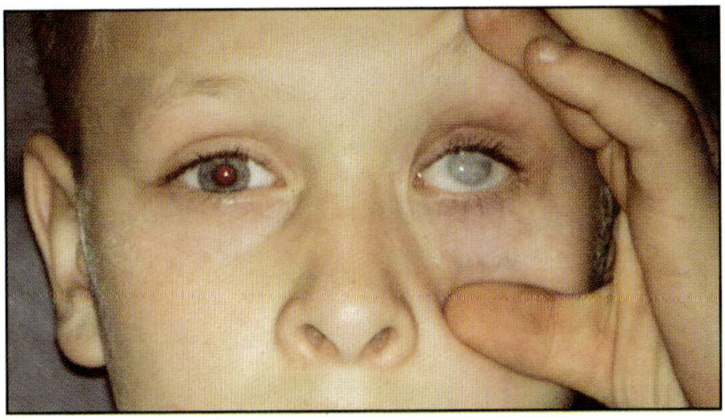

Figure 13: Deprivation exotropia. Patient with leucoma cornea on the left eye

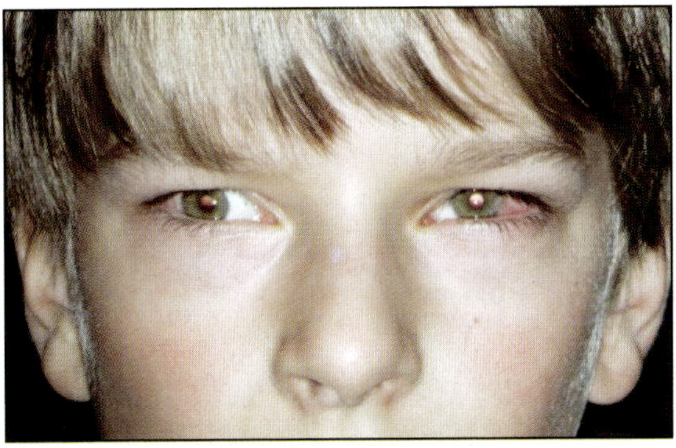

Figure 14: The child after exodeviation surgery. Consecutive exotropia

Differential Diagnosis

- Exophoria
- Congenital exotropia
- Convergens insufficiency
- Convergens paralysis
- Deprivation (sensory) exotropia
- Consecutive exotropia.

Treatment

- Correction of the refractive error especially myopia
- Myopic overcorrection should be done only for eye-exercise
- Sometimes bifocals is a good solution
- Wearing the prism-glasses
- The use of part-time occlusion
- Orthopic treatment
- Botulinum toxin A
- Strabismus surgery (bilateral recession).

Prognosis

- Cosmetic success is often defined as a deviation less than 15 PD
- Functional success is than a deviation less than 10 PD with peripheral fusion
- Some patients may miss the panoramic visual field inherent in intermittent exotropia.

Convergence Insufficiency

Convergence weakness is a type of exotropia in which the deviation is only or greater at near than at distance.

Clinical Findings

- Asthenopic symptoms usually occurs during periods of near work
- Often diplopia occurs
- Rarely convergence near point is more remote than 20-25 cm
- Patients may induced an artificial myopia
- Typical cases have stereoacuity at distance, this is where most patients control their deviation
- On repeated testing patients are easily fatigued.

Investigation

- Cover-uncover test at near and distance
- Maddox test
- Test the near point of convergence
- Test the near point of accommodation
- It is important to rule out any paretic element by testing ocular movements
- Measuring the eye alignment in all direction of gaze.

Differential Diagnosis

- Exophoria
- Convergens paralysis
- Intermittent exotropia
- Paralytic strabismus
- Accommodative problems
- Consecutive exotropia.

Treatment

- Correction of any refraction error
- Convergence exercises
- Orthopic treatment

- Wearing the base—in prisms
- Surgery is indicated in severe asthenopic symptoms
- Sometimes botulinum toxin injection is helpful.

Prognosis

- The patient be free of asthenopic symptoms
- Recognize diplopia when convergence fails
- Have a good convergence fusional amplitude.

Convergence Paralysis

Convergence paralysis is often seen as a secondary status to the brain diseases and must not be confused with convergence weakness.

Clinical Findings

- Acute beginning
- Exotropic deviation of 25-30 PD at near with straight eyes at distance
- Total and complete inability to converge the eyes
- Presence of full adduction of each eye
- Normal accommodation
- Diplopia occurs at near fixation.

Investigation

- Cover-uncover test at near and distance
- Test the near point of convergence
- Test the near point of accommodation
- Measuring the eye alignment in all direction of gaze
- Neurological investigations.

Differential Diagnosis

- Convergence insufficiency
- Intermittent exotropia
- Paralytic strabismus
- Accommodative problems.

Treatment

- Correction of any refraction error
- Convergence exercises
- Orthopic treatment
- Wearing the base— in prisms in bifocal glasses

- Surgery is not indicated
- If it is possible -treatment any neurologic disorders.

Prognosis

- Usually is not possible to have a good binocular vision
- Recognize diplopia when convergence fails.

Deprivation (Sensory) Exotropia

Sensory exotropia is a secondary to unilateral blindness.

Clinical Findings

- Unilateral eye diseases (congenital cataract, leucoma cornea, atrophia nevi toxoplasmosis, retinal tumors, foveal damage, trauma lesion)
- Anisometropia.

Investigation

- Full ophthalmology examination of anterior and posterior segment of eyes
- Visual test and checking fixation to evaluated amblyopia.

Differential Diagnosis

- Congenital exotropia
- Intermittent exotropia
- Convergence insufficiency
- Consecutive exotropia.

Treatment

- Diagnosed and treated soon after the onset
- Elimination any organic lesion, if possible
- Full correction anisometropic eye with the contact lenses
- Amblyopia treatment
- Botulinum toxin injection
- Strabismus surgery.

Prognosis

- Depends of the organic lesion of the eye
- If treated soon after the onset and patient have good anatomical condition it may be good
- Optimum optical correction and visual rehabilitation are very important.

Consecutive Exotropia

Consecutive exotropia or persistent exotropia may be present after exodeviation surgery.

Clinical Findings

- Too much exotropia surgery can provide to exodeviation
- Occasionally exotropia may increase
- Patients has learned to get rid of the diplopia.

Investigation

- Case history
- Hirschberg's and Krimsky test
- Cover-uncover test
- Hess screening
- Evaluation of exotropia angle
- Diplopia testing.

Differential Diagnosis

- Exophoria
- Congenital exotropia
- Convergence insufficiency
- Convergence paralysis
- Deprivation (sensory) exotropia
- Paralitic strabismus.

Treatment

- Prism glasses base -in over each eye
- Orthoptic exercises
- Botulinum toxin injection
- Strabismus surgery on the nonoperated muscles.

Prognosis

- Sometimes patients are able to hold their eye straight after a few months nonsurgical treatment
- Patients with good fusional potential and normal duction can be successfully treated with injection of botulinum toxin
- Reoperation of persistent exotropia are also satisfactory.

Chapter 36

Esodeviations

Ewa Oleszczynska Prost (Poland)

Pseudoesotropia

Pseudoesotropia is a condition, which only simulates squint. The eyes are straight, however they appear to be crossed. In very young children wide, flat bridge of the nose and small folds of the eyelid skin or narrow interpupillary distance are frequent. Such a state may simulate convergent strabismus. Often we observed the abnormality of the eyeballs structure or its placement in the orbits or changes in the eye protective apparatus. Pseudoesotropia present, when the visual axis (connecting fixing object with the fovea) is different then the optic axis (the line running through the center of cornea and pupil). The angle at which these axes crossed is called gamma angle.

Esophoria

Esophoria is a latent tendency for the eyes to deviate. This latent deviation is normally controlled by fusional mechanisms which provide binocular vision. Deviation of the visual axis results from the fusion interruption, which is not able to maintain binocular vision any longer.

Factors predisposing to decompensated esophoria are listed below:
- Uncorrected refraction error
- Anisometropia
- Transient cover of one eye
- Emotional or physical strock
- Fatigue or asthenia (severe infections).

Clinical Findings

- Feeling of the eyes fatigue
- Sometimes headache
- Blurred near vision, especially with prolonged reading
- Sometimes diplopia
- Normal retinal correspondence
- Lack of the symptoms of extraocular muscles paralysis.

Investigations

- Retinoscopy with full cycloplegia
- Hirschberg test
- Alternate cover test
- Maddox rod test for distance and near
- Fusion amplitude rate is low.

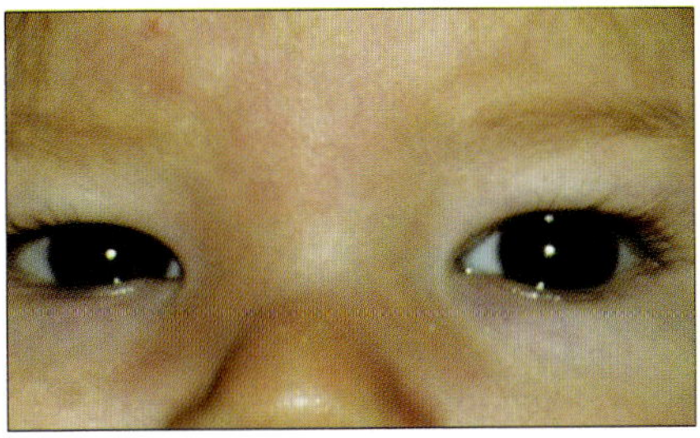

Figure 1: Pseudoesotropia

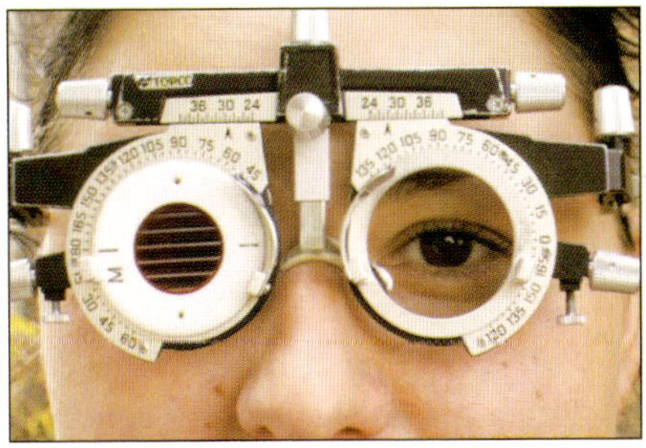

Figure 2: Red Maddox rod test

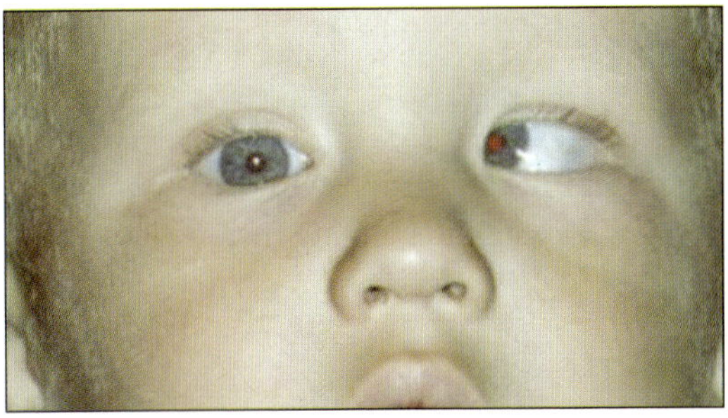

Figure 3: Congenital esotropia in 4-month-old boy

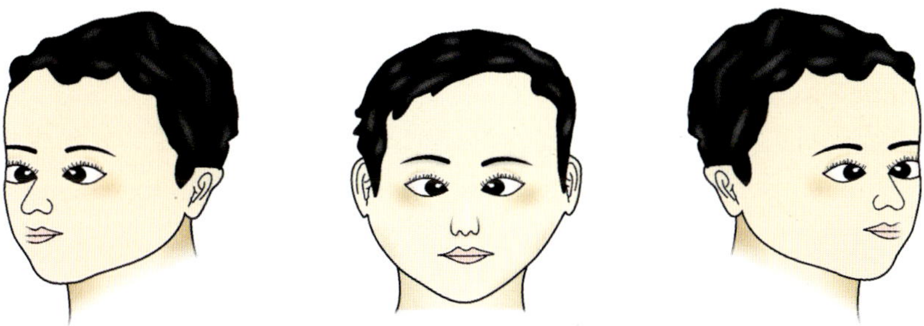

Figure 4: Infantile esotropia showing alternating fixation

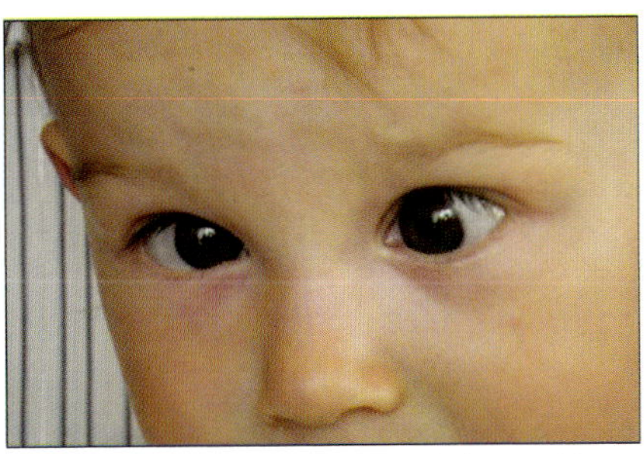

Figure 5: The 3, 5-month-boy with nystagmus blockade syndrome

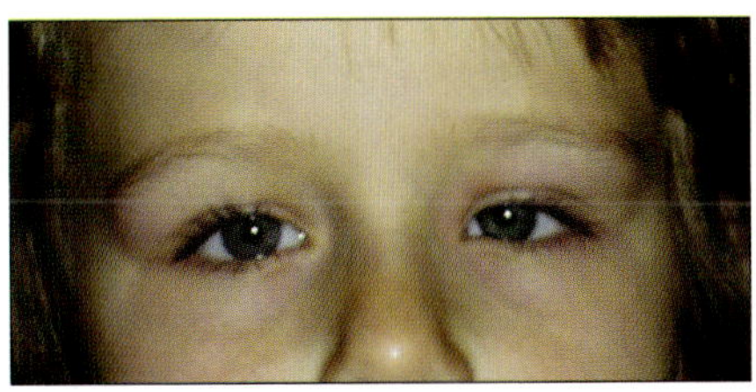

Figure 6: Accommodative esotropia without glasses

Differential Diagnosis

- Orthophoria
- Cyclic esotropia
- Accommodative esotropia.

Treatment

- Full correction of refractive error
- Prism glasses facilitating actions of the weakened muscles
- Eye exercises strengthening binocular vision
- In rare cases botulinum toxin injection to the muscles is required
- Very rare strabismus surgery is required.

Prognosis

- Spectacles according to the refraction with prism is the best solution
- In young children eye exercise improving fusion amplitude are also effective.

Congenital Esotropia

This form of strabismus is present since birth. It is characterized by the large and constant angle of strabismus. One eye and then the fellow eye fixes alternatively in the primary position.

Clinical Findings

- At side viewing cross fixation is present
- The right eye is used in left gaze and the left eye is used in right gaze
- Patients show limited abduction of both eyes
- Angle of strabismus is large 30-70 PD
- If in the primary position one eye is fixing all the time, amblyopia may develop in the fellow eye
- In 75% of cases unilateral or alternate inferior oblique muscle overaction or dissociated vertical deviation (DVD) are seen.

Investigation

- Retinoscopy with full cycloplegia
- Fundus examination
- Hirschberg and Krimsky test
- Cover-uncover test and alternate cover test
- Monocular abduction attempt
- Face turn examination.

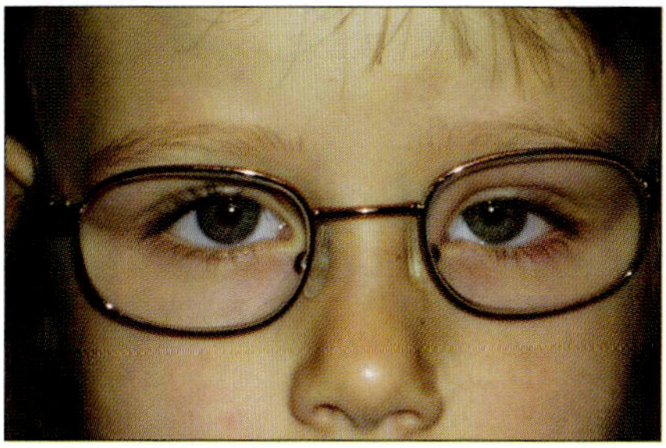

Figure 7: Accommodative esotropia is reduced with the hyperopic glasses

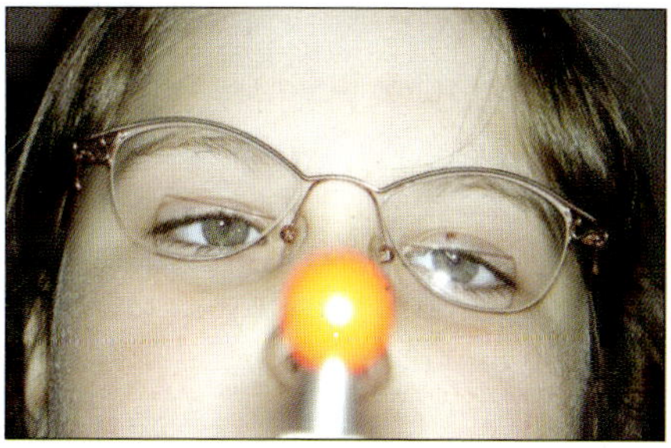

Figure 8: Bifocal glasses with +3 Dsph addition at near reduced convergence excess

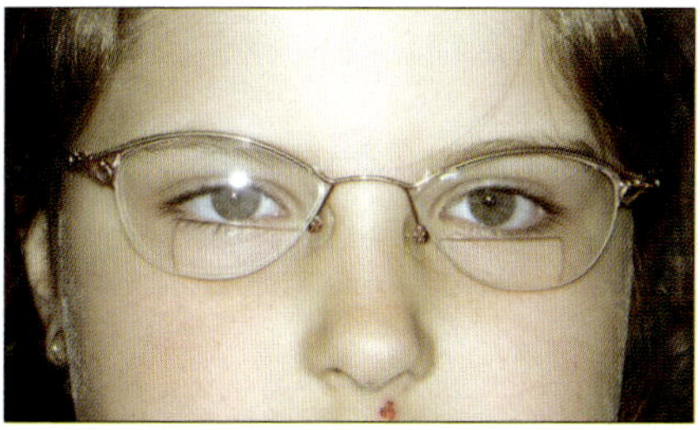

Figure 9: Full correction of squint with glasses at distant

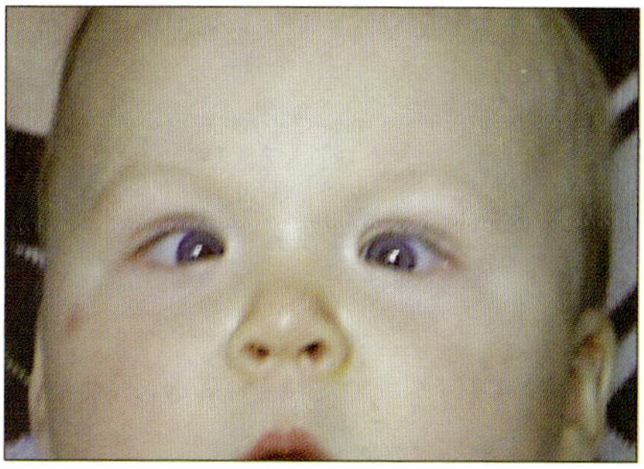

Figure 10: Small angle deviation on the 4-month-old child with cyclic esotropia

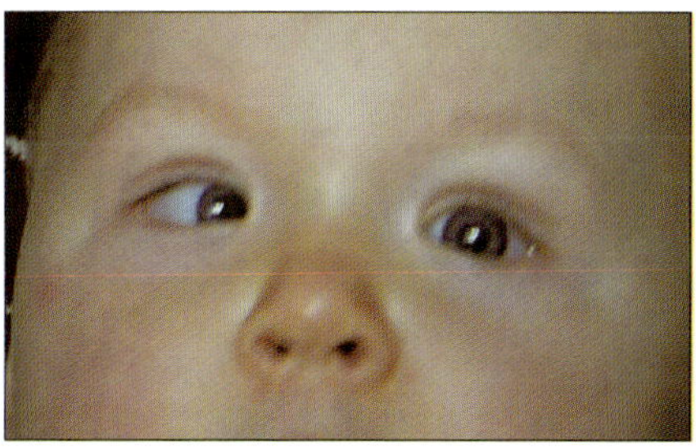

Figure 11: The same patient on alternating day with cyclic esotropia in the right eye

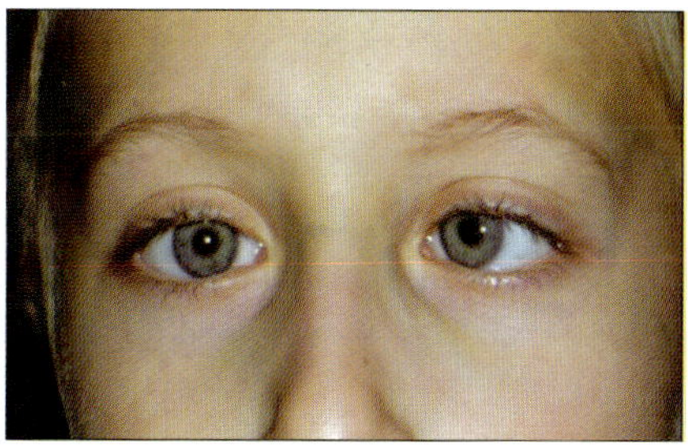

Figure 12: A 10-year-old girl with acute acquired esotropia in the left eye

Differential Diagnosis

- Nystagmus blockage syndrome
- Infantile accommodative esotropia
- Cyclic esotropia
- Sixth nerve palsy
- Congenital fibrosis syndrome (fixed strabismus)
- Congenital myasthenia
- Congenital six nerve palsy
- Moebius' syndrome
- Duane's syndrome.

Treatment

- Prescription of appriopriate eye-glasses or contact lenses
- Occlusion therapy if amblyopia is present
- Very early strabismus surgery should be done
- Botulinum toxin injection
- The use of prism-glasses.

Prognosis

Only an early treatment of the congenital esotropia excellent visual acuity in each eye, single binocular vision in all directions of gaze and normal esthetic appearance may be achieved.

Nystagmus Blockade Syndrome

Then nystagmus begins in early infancy and associated with esotropia it is called nystagmus blockade syndrome.

Clinical Findings

- Convergence is used to dampen nystagmus
- Both eyes are frequently esotropic at the same time
- Large angle deviation is present (80-90 PD)
- Limited abduction bilaterally
- In abduction the nystagmus increases
- Face turn to the side of the fixing eye.

Investigation

- Refraction and fundus examination
- Hirschberg light reflex test
- Cover-uncover test
- Monocular abduction attempt
- Face turn examination

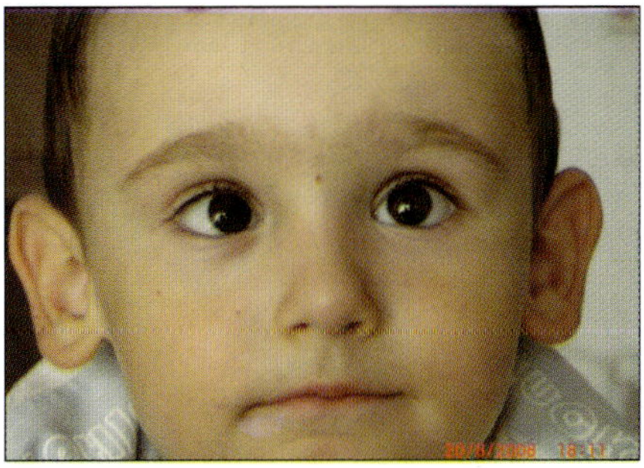

Figure 13: Esotropia greater in the distance

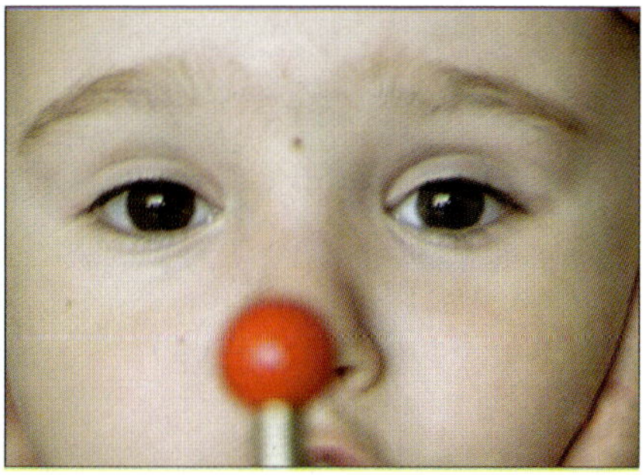

Figure 14: At near fixation only small angle of esodeviation

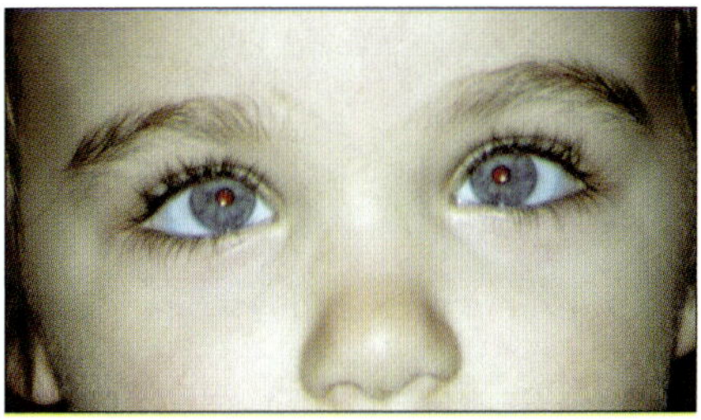

Figure 15A: The child aged 1,8-year-old with spasm of the near reflex

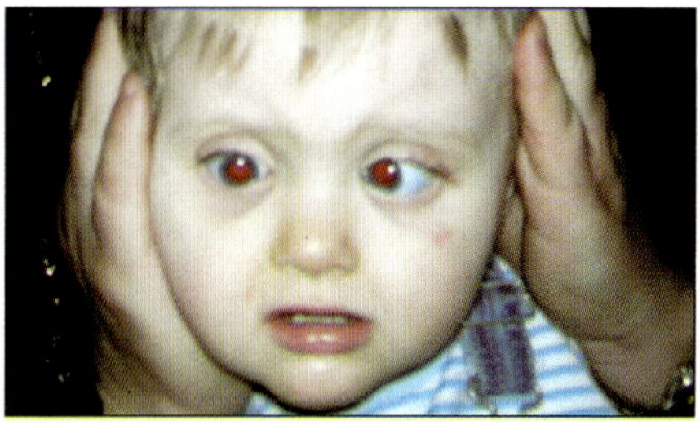

Figure 15B: Spasm of the near reflex on 7-month-old child

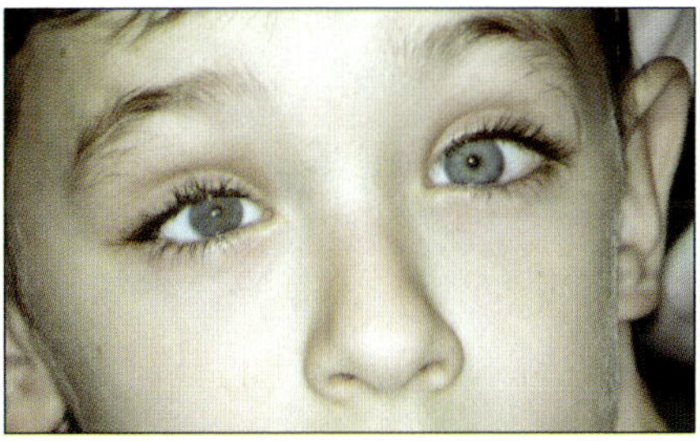

Figure 16: A 7-year-old patient with congenital cataract in the right eye. Note sensory esotropia and torticollis ocularis

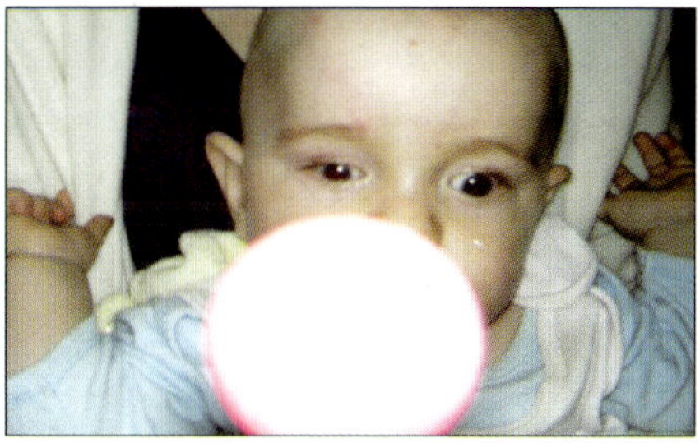

Figure 17: A 7-month–old patients with congenital exotropia before strabismus surgery

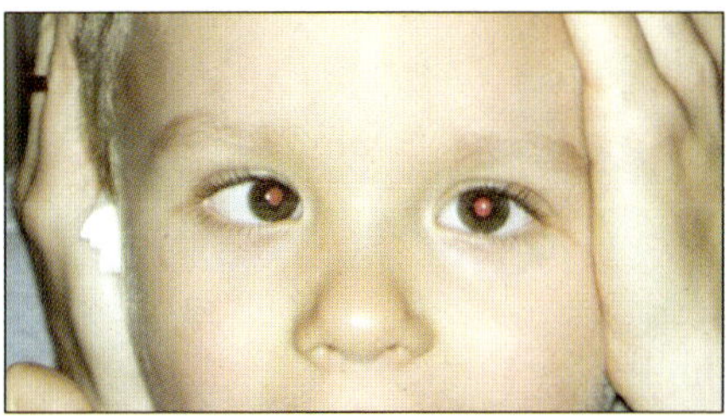

Figure 18: Consecutive esotropia. The same patient—4 years after exotropia surgery

Differential Diagnosis

- Congenital esotropia
- Infantile accommodative esotropia
- Cyclic esotropia
- Congenital fibrosis syndrome (fixed strabismus)
- Congenital myasthenia
- Congenital six nerve palsy
- Moebius' syndrome.

Treatment

- Appropriate eye-glasses or contact lenses
- Botulinum toxin injection
- Large amount of surgery are required; recession of both medials (6-8 mm) and resection of one lateral rectus muscle (8-10 mm).

Prognosis

- If residual esotropia persists (about 15 PD) surgery on the unoperated lateral muscle shoud be done
- Sometimes adduction may be lower after surgery.

Accommodative Esotropia

Accommodative esotropia is a deviation of the eyes associated with activation of the accommodative reflex. Related to accommodative effort may be divided into 3 categories:i) refractive ii) nonrefractive iii) partial or decompensated.

Refractive Accommodative Esotropia (Fully Accommodative Esotropia)

Clinical Findings

- Age of onset between 2-3 years old
- Intermittent at onset then becoming constant
- Average esotropia 20-40 PD nearly the same to distance and near fixation
- Refraction range of +3, 0 to +10.0D
- Amblyopia is common
- Low accommodative convergens to accommodation ratio (AC/A).

Investigation

- Full cycloplegic retinoscopy with atropine (3-4 days)
- Hirschberg or Krimsky light reflex test
- Cover test
- Visual test and checking fixation to evaluated amblyopia

Differential Diagnosis

- Congenital esoptropia
- Nonrefractive accommodative esotropia
- Partial accommodative esotropia
- Divergence insufficiency
- Persistent esotropia
- Non-comitant strabismus.

Treatment

- Full correction of the refractive error
- Constant wearing of the glasses
- Cure the amblyopia
- Monitor the vision and fixation to make sure the amblyopia does not return
- Anticholinesterase drops shoul be used if non-compliant with glasses
- Orthoptic exercises.

Prognosis

The complete cure with bifoveal fusion will be achieved in patients unless:

- Diagnosed and treated soon after the onset
- Amblyopia and suppression can be eliminated
- Fusion and stereopsis strongly estabilished than the onset is over 3-years-old
- Adults have a chance to give up the glasess.

Nonrefractive Accommodative Esotropia (High AC/A Ratio, Convergence Excess)

This condition is characterized by overconvergence associated with accommodation.

Clinical Findings

- Age of onset between 2 month-5 years old
- Esodeviation is greater at near than at distance
- Refraction is over +2, 0 D or myopic
- Amblyopia is common
- High accommodative convergens to accommodation ratio (AC/A).

Investigation

- Full cycloplegic retinoscopy with atropine (3-4 days)
- Hirschberg or Krimsky light reflex test
- Cover test
- Visual test and checking fixation to evaluated amblyopia

- Clinical evaluation of distance and near deviation
- Binocular vision tests.

Differential Diagnosis

- Congenital esotropia
- Refractive accommodative esotropia
- Partial accommodative esotropia
- Divergence insufficiency
- Persistent esotropia
- Non-comitant strabismus.

Treatment

- Full correction of the refractive error
- Constant wearing of the bifocal glasses
- Eliminate amblyopia
- Miotics are not as effective as bifocals
- Orthoptic treatment
- Sometimes prism glasses are necessary
- Botox injection sometimes is required
- Bimedial recession on teenagers.

Prognosis

- Amblyopia and suppression can be eliminated
- Try to wean off bifocals after 8-years-old patients
- Good fusion in distance with straight eyes or small angle esotropia.

Partial Accommodative Esotropia

Clinical Findings

- Hypermetropia
- High accommodative convergence to accommodation ratio (AC/A)
- Great esotropia at near and small esotropia at distance.

Differential Diagnosis

- Congenital esotropia
- Refractive accommodative esotropia
- Nonrefactive accommodative esotropia
- Divergens insufficiency
- Persistent esotropia
- Non-comitant strabismus.

Investigation, treatment and prognosis : similar like other accommodative esotropias.

Cyclic Esotropia

Cyclic strabismus is a rare type of esodeviation and classically a large-angle esotropia alternating with ortophoria or small–angle deviation on 48-hour cycle.

Clinical Findings

- Frequently affects older child
- Diplopia and lack of fusion appear only when strabismus is present
- Squint appeared every 24-48 hours cycle.

Investigation

- Good anamnesis
- Full cycloplegic retinoscopy
- Clinical observation for a few days
- Evaluation of angle deviation during the strabismic cycle
- Stereopsis testing

Differential Diagnosis

- All types of accommodative esotropia
- Acute acquired esotropia
- Secondary esotropia (after occlusion, organic lesion, following recover nerve VI palsy, consecutive esotropia).

Treatment

- Full correction of the refractive error
- Surgical correction of the total esodeviation.

Prognosis

- Surgery eliminates the whole strabismic problem.

Acute Acquired Esotropia

This is the rare condition occurs in older children or adults which characterized by the dramatic onset of the large angle esotropia with diplopia.

Clinical Findings

- Mild hyperopic or myopic refractive error (from-5,5 to +3,0)
- Diplopia
- Concomitant strabismus in all direction of gaze
- Strabismus is usually large 30-60 PD

- Patients can fuse if the angle is eliminated with prism
- Absence of any neurologic disease.

Investigation

- Cycloplegic refraction
- Cover test
- Evaluation of angle deviation in all direction of gaze
- Hess chart
- Family history of strabismus
- Complete neurologic examination.

Differential Diagnosis

- Strabismus paralytic
- Secondary esotropia (after occlusion, organic lesion)
- Spasm of near reflex
- Cyclic esotropia
- Refractive accommodative esotropia
- Nonrefactive accommodative esotropia
- Partial accommodative esotropia
- Divergence insufficiency
- Following recovered nerve VI palsy
- Consecutive esotropia.

Treatment

- Strabismus surgery
- Wearing glasses.

Prognosis

- The results are excellent in the absence of any neurologic disease.

Divergence Insufficiency Esotropia

Divergence insufficiency causes the esotropia that is greater in the distance than the near.

Clinical Findings

- Esotropia on distance fixation 10-20 PD
- Orthophoria at near
- Normal ductions and versions
- Sometimes mild bilateral sixth nerve paresis.

Investigation

- Cover test at near and distance
- Eye movements exam
- No fusion divergence
- Neurologic examination to evaluate any neurological syndrome, intracranial tumor or head trauma
- Cycloplegic refraction
- Eye fundus evaluation.

Differential Diagnosis

- Congenital esotropia
- Acute acquired esotropia
- Following recovered nerve VI palsy
- Bilateral sixth nerve paresis
- Incomitant (paralytic) strabismus.

Treatment

- Neurological treatment
- Prismatic glasses
- Very rare bilateral muscle resection
- Orthoptic training.

Prognosis

- Some patients get better spontaneously
- Results of neurological treatment are not so good.

Spasm of the Near Reflex

This condition appear periodically and is characterized by an overconvergence associated with accommodation and miosis.

Clinical Findings

- Present from early age
- Large angle esotropia at near
- Good ductions with bad versions
- Sensitive individuals in whom emotions can be seen to play a large part in the severity of esotropia
- Miosis.

Investigation

- Refraction before and after cycloplegia
- Eye movement exam
- Cover test at near and distant
- Complete neurologic examination.

Differential Diagnosis

- Congenital esotropia
- Cyclic esotropia
- Nystagmus blockage syndrome
- Accommodative esotropia
- Moebius' syndrome.

Treatment

- Cycloplegic drops should be used (atropine, homatropine)
- Patiens with great hyperopia should wear full correction glasses sometimes bifocals
- Exercises to relax accommodation.

Prognosis

- Overconvergence associated with accommodation tend to lessen as the child grows older and may disapper in adults.

Deprivation (Sensory) Esotropia

This condition is an esotropia secondary to unilateral blindness.

Clinical Findings

- Unilateral eye diseases (congenital cataract, leucoma cornea, atrophia nevi optici, toxoplasmosis, retinal tumors, foveal damage, trauma lesion)
- Anisometropia

Investigation

- Full ophthalmology examination of anterior and posterior segment of eyes
- Visual test and checking fixation to evaluated amblyopia.

Differential Diagnosis

- Congenital esotropia
- Acute acquired esotropia
- Consecutive esotropia

Treatment

- Diagnosed and treated soon after the onset
- Elimination any organic lesion, if possible
- Full correction anisometropic eye with the contact lenses
- Amblyopia treatment
- Botulinum toxin injection
- Strabismus surgery.

Prognosis

- Depends of the organic lesion of the eye
- If treated soon after the onset and patient have good anatomical condition it may be good
- Optimum optical correction and visual rehabilitation are very important.

Consecutive Esotropia

Consecutive esotropia or persistent esotropia may be present after exodeviation surgery.

Clinical Findings

- **After exotropia surgery** 15-30 PD esotropia can appeared
- Status post exodeviation surgery
- Occasionally esotropia may increase
- Patients has learned to get rid of the diplopia.

Investigation

- Case history
- Hirschberg and Krimsky test
- Cover test
- Hess screening
- Cycloplegic refaction
- Evaluation of angle esotropia
- Diplopia testing.

Differential Diagnosis

- Accommodative esotropias
- Divergence insufficiency
- Spasm of the near reflex
- Acute acquired esotropia
- Noncomitant strabismus.

Treatment

- Prism glasses base out over each eye
- Full hyperopia correction
- Orthoptic exercises
- Botulinum toxin injection
- Strabismus surgery on the nonoperated muscles.

Prognosis

- Sometimes patients are able to hold their eye straight after a few months nonsurgical treatment
- Patients with good fusional potential and normal duction can be successfully treated with injection of botulinum toxin
- Reoperation of persistent esotropia are also satisfactory.

Chapter 37

Cranial Nerve Palsies and their Management

Rohit Saxena, Ankur Sinha
Swati Phuljhele (India)

Incomitant Strabismus

Definition

Incomitant strabismus refers to varying degrees of misalignment between the two eyes in different positions of gaze.

Types

Incomitance can occur due to due to restrictive, paralytic or spastic causes.

Clinical Features

The characteristic features of incomitant squint are as follows:

Difference between Primary Deviation and Secondary Deviation

The secondary deviation is more than the primary deviation in paralytic as well as restrictive squint, but in spastic deviation the primary deviation is more than secondary deviation.

Limitation of Movement

The movement of the eye is limited in the field of action of the involved extraocular muscle. The forced duction test differentiates between restrictive and paralytic squint. The active forced generation test can also differentiate whether the restriction is the primary pathology of the incomitance or because of development of contracture in the antagonist muscle consequent to paralysis. The movements can be charted on Hess/Lees charts which help in finding the involved muscle.

Incomitance

The ocular deviation is variable in different positions of gaze. The deviation is maximum in the field of action of the muscle.

Other Clinical Features

- Diplopia: diplopia charting allows identifying the gaze with maximum deviation.
- Head posture: to compensate for the loss of action of the paralysed muscle.
- Associated neurological findings may be present depending on the location of lesion.

Classification Paralytic Squint

1. Neurogenic
    - Supranuclear
    - Nuclear
    - Infranuclear
      e.g oculomotor, trochlear and abducent nerve palsies

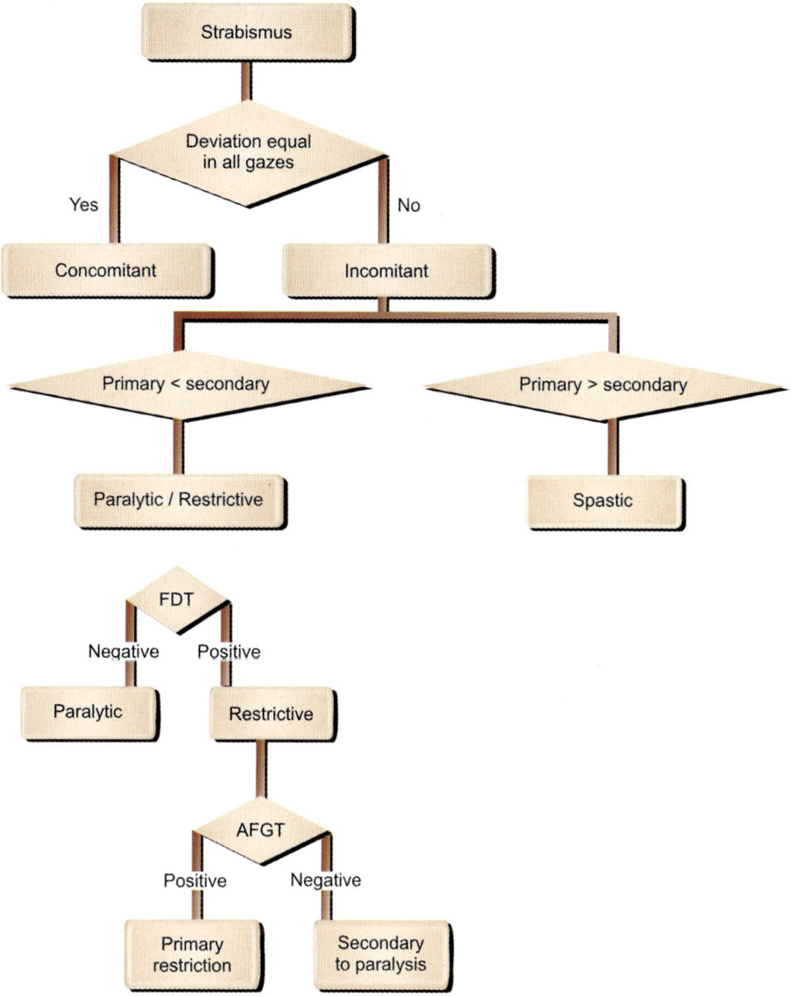

Figure 1: Flow chart of strabismus

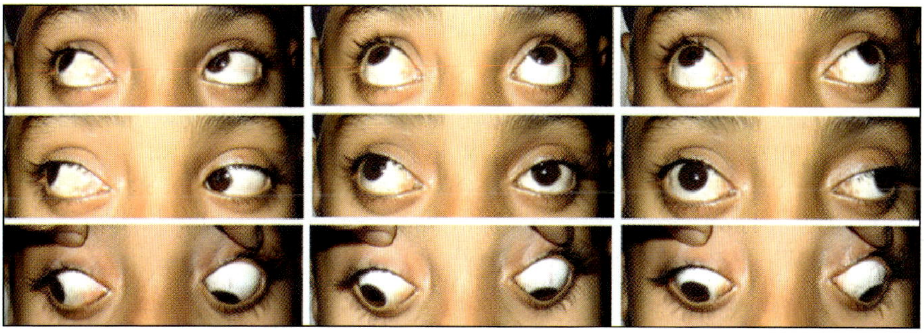

Figure 2: Case of right congenital partial third nerve palsy

2. Myogenic- e.g myotonic dystrophy, CPEO, myositis, Graves disease
3. Neuromuscular junction disease- e.g Myasthenia gravis.

Third Nerve Palsy

Anatomy

Third nerve nucleus is the complex, which supplies the superior rectus-levator complex, medial rectus, inferior rectus and inferior oblique, and provides parasympathetic innervation to the pupillary sphincter. This nucleus is located beneath the gray matter of the dorsal mid-brain. The Edinger-Westphal subnuclei provide the parasympathetic motor innervation to the pupillary sphincter. The fibers supplying to the superior rectus decussate to provide the innervation to the contralateral superior rectus. The nerve then passes through the red nucleus and the medial aspect of the cerebral peduncles. The nerve then travels in the subarachnoid space to the cavernous sinus. The pupillomotor fibers travel superolaterally in the periphery of the nerve making them more susceptible to external compressive lesions. The nerve travels in the sheath of cavernous sinus. Before entering into the orbit the nerve divides into the superior and inferior division. The nerve then enters in to the orbit through the superior orbital fissure. The superior division supplies superior rectus and levator while the rest of the muscles and pupil is supplied by the inferior division.

Etiology

Third nerve palsy may be congenital or acquired. Birth trauma and neonatal hypoxia are the leading causes of congenital third nerve palsy. In acquired cases the causes are ischemic mono-neuropathy, PCA aneurysm, trauma, brain-stem tumors, infarction, Cavernous sinus thrombosis and migraine.

Congenital Third Nerve Palsy

Congenital third nerve palsy is a rare entity. They are presumed to be secondary to maldevelopment of the nucleus, intrauterine injury, or birth trauma. The palsy is usually unilateral and isolated.

Acquired Third Nerve Palsy

Lesions of nucleus: The most common cause for nuclear third nerve palsy is infarction due to thrombotic occlusion of vessels. The other causes are hemorrhage, neoplasm and tumors. Lesions of the nerve nucleus can present with bilateral ptosis along with ipsilateral ophthalmoplegia. If the lesion is rostral pupillary involvement is likely and lid may be spared while if the lesion is caudal, bilateral ptosis may be prominent.

Lesions of oculomotor fascicle: fascicular lesions may produce complete or partial third nerve palsy. Although pupillary involvement is common it may the spared occasionally. The fascicular lesions are associated with other neurological

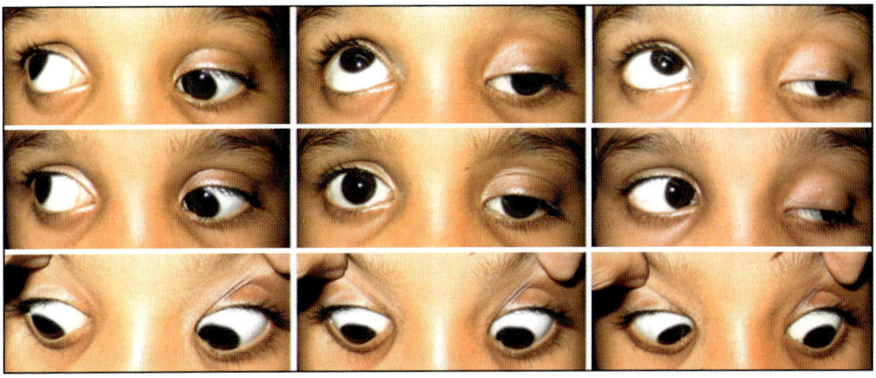

Figure 3: Case of left congenital third nerve palsy with aberrant regeneration, note the elevation of lid on adduction

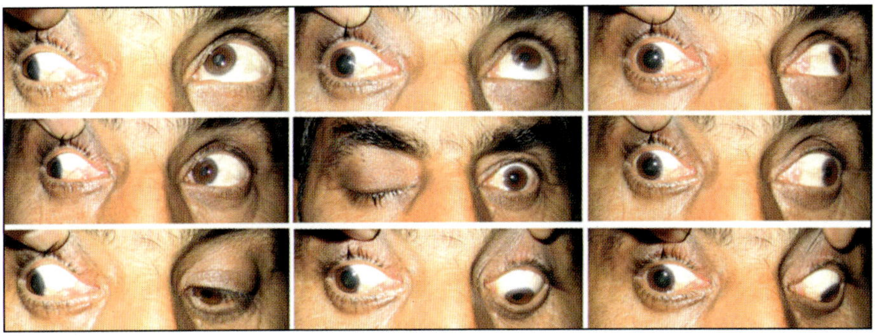

Figure 4: Case of right complete third nerve palsy with pupillary involvement due to herpes zoster

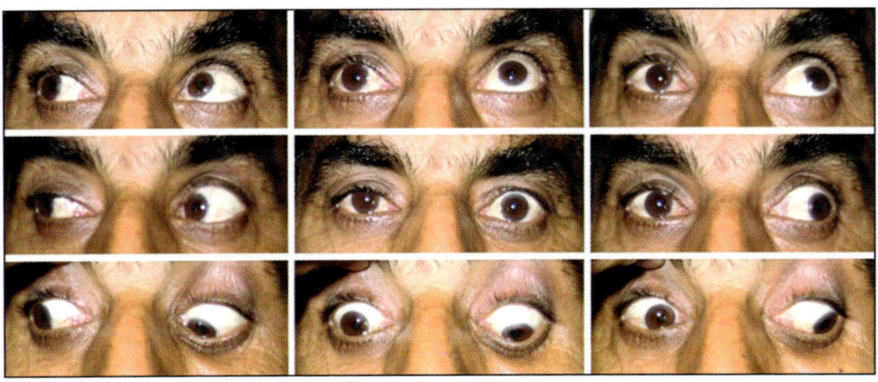

Figure 5: Same patient as shown in figure 3, partial recovery after 3 months of follow up

manifestation and syndromes. Lesion in the area of brachium may produce ipsilateral oculomotor palsy and cerebellar ataxia known as "**Nothnagel's syndrome**". Third nerve palsy with contralateral involuntary movements is known as "**Benedikt's syndrome**". Weber's syndrome, characterized by contralateral hemiplegia along with the ipsilateral third nerve palsy, is caused by the involvement of cerebral peduncles. The causes of fascicular lesions are ischemia, hemorrhage, infection, infiltration, neoplasm and demyelination.

Lesions in the subarachnoid space: This region is the most likely site of injury in cases of isolated third nerve palsy. Involvement may be complete or partial. Pupillary fibers are present peripherally and therefore pupillary involvement may be the first sign of compression in this region. The most common cause of isolated third nerve palsy with pupil involvement is the compression due to aneurysm of the Posterior Communicating Artery (PCA). Ischemic neuropathy due to diabetes is the most common cause of third nerve palsy where pupil is spared. Other causes include infiltrating lesions, infection, inflammation, tumors, and trauma and raised ICT. Third nerve palsy may also present as a component of Guillain Barre syndrome. Third nerve is particularly vulnerable to stretch and contusion where it is firmly attached to the dura mater adjacent to the posterior clinoid process just posterior to the cavernous sinus. Herniation of hippocampal gyrus compresses the nerve where it passes over the ridge of the dura associated with the attachment of the free edge of tentorium to the clivus.

Lesions in cavernous sinus and superior orbital fissure: Lesions of the cavernous sinus, like thrombosis, carotid-cavernous fistula, pituitary tumors, craniopharyngioma, menigioma, metastasis, infection and inflammation usually present as involvement of multiple nerves i.e. third, fourth, fifth, sixth etc. The granulomatous inflammation at the orbital apex involving third, fourth, sixth and sympathetic fibers along with the involvement of optic nerve, is known as Tolosa-Hunt syndrome.

Lesions in the orbit often cause partial or isolated muscle palsies though this divisional palsy may also be present in cases of cavernous and subarachnoid lesions. The processes within the orbit that can cause third nerve palsy are inflammation, ischemia, infiltration, compression and trauma. Other signs of orbital disease include loss of vision, proptosis, and other ocular motor nerve palsy.

Clinical Presentation

Clinically the third nerve palsy may present as complete, partial, isolated or with aberrant regeneration.

Complete Third Nerve Palsy

Total third nerve paresis may be with pupil sparing or pupil involving depending upon the site and the cause of lesion. Pupillary fibers are located in the peripheral

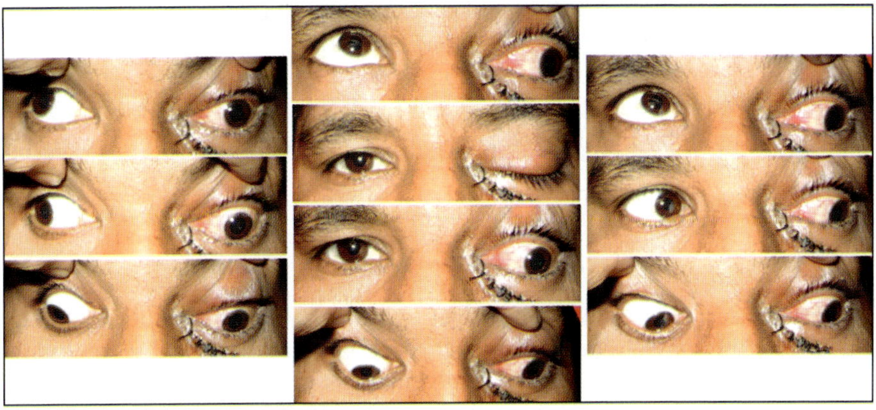

Figure 6: A case of left post-traumatic complete third nerve palsy

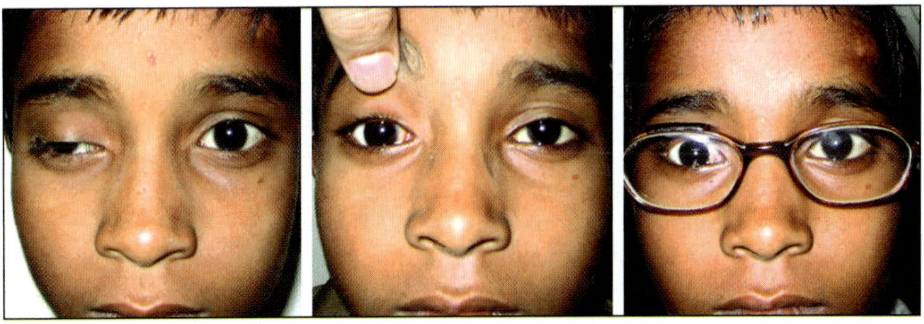

Figure 7: Case of right congenital third nerve palsy, before treatment, after surgery and with crutch glasses

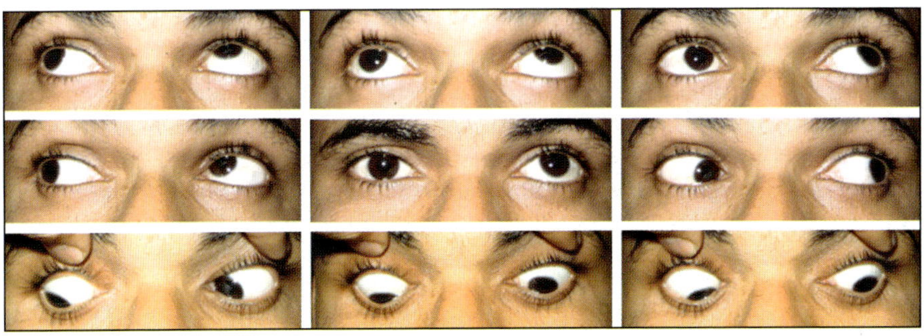

Figure 8: Case of left superior oblique palsy

part of the nerve so they are usually spared in vascular causes and first one to be involved in compressive lesions. The common causes of total third nerve palsy are ischemic neuropathy, aneurysm, and brainstem tumors. The patient presents as large angle exotropia with hypotropia along with ptosis, which masks the diplopia. Pupil is fixed and dilated; neither direct nor consensual reaction is present. On attempted adduction the eye intorts indicating the normal function of the fourth nerve.

Partial Third Nerve Palsy

The partial third nerve palsy is due to involvement of either superior or inferior division of the nerve in the region of cavernous sinus where the nerve divides into two. The superior division involvement is often associated with other cranial nerve involvement. The patients presents with hypotropia and ptosis.

Inferior division is more common to be involved in isolation. Direct trauma to orbit, neoplasm is the common cause. This presents as internal ophthalmoplegia of the eye and involvement of the inferior rectus, medial rectus and inferior oblique.

Isolated Muscle Palsy

Superior rectus palsy: An isolated palsy of superior rectus is usually congenital. Acquired cases may occur from direct trauma or post cataract surgery. The involved eye is hypotropic in primary position. The upgaze is limited in primary and abduction while it may be normal in adduction for a recent onset paralysis. However in long standing cases elevation in adduction is also affected. Head posture may be present in form of chin elevation. There may be presence of true or pseudoptosis. It is associated with poor Bell's phenomenon.

Inferior rectus palsy: is commonly seen following orbital trauma (blow out fracture), or post peribulbar and retrobulbar injections. The paretic eye is hypertropic with maximum deviation in down gaze.

Medial rectus palsy: an isolated MR palsy is a rare phenomenon. It presents as large angle exotropia with face turn toward the uninvolved side. It important to differentiate the isolated medial rectus palsy with internuclear ophthalmoplegia where the convergence is normal in spite of limitation of adduction. Other differential diagnoses include DRS, congenital aplasia of MR, medial orbital wall trauma.

Inferior Oblique palsy: This is the rarest of all isolated extraocular muscle palsies. The onset is almost always congenital. The eye may be hypotropic in primary position. It can be diagnosed by using Parks three step test. Bielschowsky head tilt is positive on tilting the head on the normal side.

Evaluation

Evaluation of systemic conditions like diabetes, hypertension, hyperlipidiemia is important particularly in cases of pupil sparing palsy. Neuroimaging should

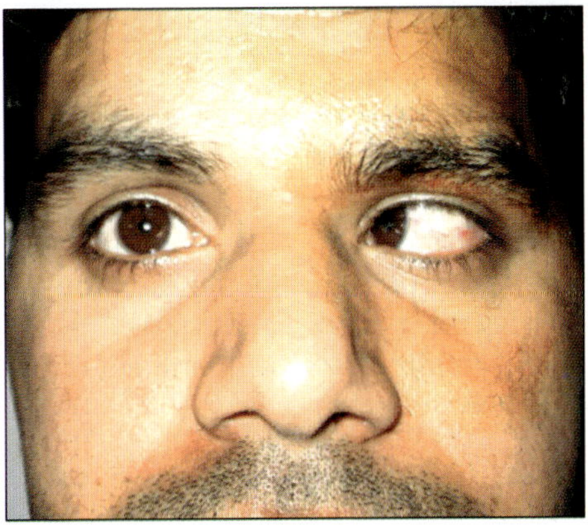

Figure 9: Case of left sixth nerve palsy

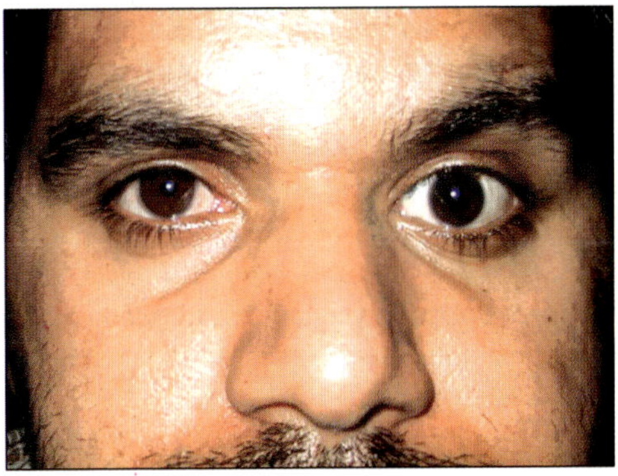

Figure 10: Same case as in figure 8, after left supramaximal medial rectus recession along with half thickness vertical muscles transposition to lateral rectus

be carried out in all cases suspected with a compressive cause of third nerve palsy. Clinical localization of the lesion is important so as not to miss the lesion on neuroimaging. Ophthalmic examination includes Prism Bar Cover Test in all nine gazes for fixation with each eye. Evaluation of fourth nerve function is done by examining for incyclotorsion. FDT is done to note for the restriction of lateral rectus and vertical muscles.

Differential Diagnosis

Third nerve involvement, particularly isolated muscle palsy should be differentiated from local restrictive conditions like blow out fracture, thyroid disease, local anesthetic injections, post cataract/sinus surgery. Systemic conditions like myasthenia gravis and CPEO which can produce isolated muscle palsy should be differentiated.

Management of Third Nerve Palsy

In cases of acquired paralytic strabismus, the management can be divided into two parts, i.e. during the acute phase of the disease, to overcome the problem of diplopia and later on, after 6 months of the definitive management, in the form of ocular alignment and maximizing the binocular single field of vision.

In cases of congenital third nerve paralysis, the patient may not have diplopia as the patient may have suppression of the deviating eye and in cases of complete third nerve palsy there may be amblyopia due to complete ptosis. The presence of amblyopia in children calls for treatment of amblyopia in the form of patching or penalization.

During the Acute Phase

During the acute phase of the disease, it is important to rule out a life threatening intracranial lesion, which may be presenting initially as a third nerve paralysis. After the cause of third nerve is established the acute phase treatment is aimed at eliminating the diplopia and making the patient comfortable for his/her routine daily life. Cases with medical causes of IIIrd nerve paralysis will show improvement over time. In the waiting period, overcome the diplopia and prevent complications like ipsilateral antagonist contracture. In case of complete third nerve, due to ptosis there is no diplopia, however as the recovery begins and the ptosis improves the patient has a troublesome diplopia. Diplopia is of concern in cases of partial third nerve paralysis and may need intervention in the form of one of the following modalities. In cases of traumatic third nerve paralysis there can be a troublesome intractable diplopia due to central fusion disruption and this diplopia would not be treated even with perfect alignment of the eyes.

Occlusion: Occlusion is required in acute cases. In cases where the images are very much far apart the patient may be able to ignore one of the images and may not complain of diplopia, however as the deviation decreases and the images come closer it is not easy to ignore and the problem of diplopia starts.

Patching, use of frosted gasses in spectacles, occluder patches for spectacles, pirate patches, occluder contact lenses etc are the various methods employed for patching depending upon the patient's demands and comfort.

Prisms: The use of prisms may provide benefit as it shifts the image to the desired direction depending upon the orientation and the power of the prism used. However, the role of prism is limited in cases where both the vertical and horizontal components of diplopia are present and in cases of complete third nerve palsies.

Fresnel prism can be used in cases with residual medial rectus function and may be added on to the glasses temporarily. The prisms may also find a role in post-operative cases where there is small amount of deviation left and patient complains of diplopia.

Botulinum Toxin: In the acute phase of the palsy, Botulinum injection toxin injection of the lateral rectus may be performed; this would cause paralysis of the lateral rectus and would prevent development of contracture.

It is not recommended to use toxin injection for the superior rectus muscle as it may aggravate the ptosis, however, inferior rectus injection can be performed in case of severe hypotropia.

Definitive/Surgical Management

Definitive management of a case of third nerve palsy is meant to achieve, alignment in the primary gaze and maximizing the binocular single field of vision. In cases of congenital third nerve palsy one may have to wait for the amblyopia therapy. If there is no associated amblyopia or there is dense amblyopia in the form of eccentric fixation, one may plan a reconstructive surgery early. However, in cases of acquired third nerve palsy, one should wait for at least six months for the deviations to stabilize and the surgical option should be thought only after there is stabilization of deviation for six months. Management requires careful assessment of each muscle function and aimed at avoiding diplopia at least in the primary and the downgaze.

Isolated Muscle Paralysis

Superior rectus palsy: Most cases of superior rectus palsy are congenital and may have associated ptosis. If the hypotropia is not significant and the downgaze is not having any diplopia, it would not be advisable to go for a surgical intervention. If there is significant hypotropia in the primary gaze and which persists even in the down gaze surgical intervention may be required. A forced duction test is a must to rule out associated inferior rectus contracture. If there is presence of inferior rectus contracture then inferior rectus recession may be required.

In cases where forced duction test for inferior rectus is free, one can opt for a Knapp's procedure where both the horizontal muscles are disinserted and a full tendon transposition to the superior rectus is done.

Inferior rectus palsy: In cases where the inferior rectus muscle paralysis is because of muscle entrapment the blow out fracture, the management is very challenging. Surgical plan is to explore the inferior rectus area. To attain the alignment of the primary gaze ipsilateral superior rectus recession can be performed after the muscle is free of adhesions. For the management of diplopia in downgaze contralateral faden operation of inferior rectus may be an option.

Medial rectus palsy: The management in cases of isolated medial rectus palsy depends upon the amount of adduction and the muscle power regained by the medial rectus. If the adduction is good (eyeball crossed the midline) and there is no contracture of the lateral rectus, then conventional recession-resection procedure on the horizontal recti can be performed. However the amount of recession and resection would be larger than what is required for a comitant exotropia and supra-maximal recession-resection may be a good option. In cases with residual exotropia, contralateral eye surgery in the form of lateral rectus recession may be required.

In cases with very poor medial rectus function where the eye does not cross the midline or there is contracture of lateral rectus recession, supramaximal recession of the lateral rectus along with conjunctival recession may be required along with periosteal anchoring of the medial rectus may be an viable option.

Inferior oblique palsy: The management of inferior oblique palsy is indicated in cases with marked vertical deviation and in cases with significant head posture. If there is associated superior oblique overaction, a superior oblique weakening procedure may be the first choice to be considered. If even after the weakening of superior oblique the adequate alignment is not achieved then one may consider inferior oblique tuck or resection and advancement of the inferior oblique.
Inferior oblique strengthening procedure as a primary surgery is indicated in cases, where there is marked inferior oblique underaction without associated superior oblique overaction.

Complete third nerve paralysis: Complete third nerve is a big challenge to a strabismologist as there is involvement of four (medial rectus, superior rectus, inferior rectus and inferior oblique) of six extra-ocular muscles, this leaves the eye in fixed hypotropic and exotropic position. Secondary contractures of the lateral rectus may develop. For the management of a case of horizontal supramaximal recession-resection procedure may work in cases having some function of medial rectus; however there is always a risk of exotropic drift of the eye due to unopposed pull of the lateral rectus muscle.

The only muscle which can be utilized to counteract the force of lateral rectus is superior oblique. Superior oblique tendon transposition has been described as a viable alternative and has been shown to provide cosmetically acceptable results, however it is technically difficult as it requires skin incision at upper eyelid to fracture trochlea and disinsert tendon and carries a risk of severe orbital hemorrhage. Scott procedure is a relatively simple modified transposition technique of above mentioned procedure. However it often leads to inadequate horizontal alignment and postoperative hypertropia in adduction, or paradoxical ocular movements.

Anchoring of the medial rectus to periosteum of medial orbital wall using different materials (Superior oblique tendon, silicon bands, non-absorbable sutures and facia lata) has been used to provide cosmetically acceptable results. Most of the above mentioned procedures utilize skin approach for the exposure of medial canthal ligament of the medial wall periosteum. Most of the anchoring procedures are associated with moderate restriction of the motility of the globe. However, due to paralysis of four of the six muscles there is not much possibility to restore the motility in such cases.

Authors recommend use of non-absorbable sutures for the anchoring of the globe as there is no problem of harvesting fascia lata or superior oblique tendon. Authors have devised a new technique of periosteal anchor using non-absorbable (5-0 ethibond) suture, through a precarancular approach. This technique obviates the need for a skin incision and proves effective and cosmetically better as compared to other available techniques.

Fourth Nerve Palsy

Superior oblique muscle palsy is the most common extraocular muscle palsy.

Anatomy

The fourth nerve nucleus lies in the preacqueductal gray matter of the mid brain at the level of inferior colliculus. It is the only cranial nerve, which arises from the dorsal aspect of the brain and to decussate to supply the contralateral superior oblique muscle. It emerges from the dorsal aspect of the brainstem curving around the brainstem and lies in the free edge of the tentorium, penetrates the tentorial dura to enter the cavernous sinus. In cavernous sinus it travels in the lateral wall and enters the orbit through the superior orbital fissure outside the annulus of Zinn. It's long intracranial course and dorsal exit makes it most susceptible to trauma.

Etiology

Congenital Fourth Nerve Palsy

Congenital fourth nerve palsy is the most common cause of superior oblique palsy. Most of the cases are sporadic but autosomal dominant transmission has also been reported. It has been observed that, in congenital superior oblique palsy, the tendon is usually lax, long and posteriorly inserted or even may be absent.

Acquired Fourth Nerve Palsy

Lesions of nerve nucleus: The damage to the trochlear nerve nucleus may occur as result of compression of the dorsal mesencephalon and lesions involving tegmentum at the junction of pons and mesencephalon. The lesions that can damage nerve nucleus are hemorrhage dure to trauma, tumor, aneurysms, ischemia. Perinaud's syndrome from penial tumors, aqueductal stenosis and hydrocephalus is associated with unilateral and bilateral fourth nerve palsy.

Lesions of nerve fascicle are compression, infiltration, ischemia, hemorrhage, trauma, inflammation and demyelination. The most important association in this region is central Horner's syndrome due to involvement of descending sympathetic fibers, and RAPD unassociated with evidence of optic nerve involvement due to damage to afferent pupillary fibers in the brachium of superior colliculus. Bilateral fascicular damage at the level of the superior medullary velum is the site of damage of fourth nerve fascicle secondary to trauma or hydrocephalus. Trauma is the most common cause of bilateral fourth nerve palsy.

Lesions in the subarachnoid space: The fourth nerve emerges from the dorsal surface and has long intracranial course which makes is susceptible to trauma, neurosurgical manipulation or any kind of stretching due to hemorrhage or raised ICT. This portion of nerve may also be damaged by posterior fossa aneurysm and infections like basal meningitis.

Lesions of nerve in cavernous sinus and superior orbital fissure: Fourth nerve palsy in this region is rarely isolated. Associated palsy of other cranial nerves like; sixth nerve, third nerve or trigeminal nerve is often present and helps in localization of lesion. Disease processes like neoplasm, inflammation, infiltration, and fistula are the common causes of fourth nerve palsy in this region.

Lesions in the orbit: Neoplasms, trauma, inflammation, ischemia are again the common conditions that may affect the nerve, the SO muscle, or the trochlea.

Clinical Presentation

The patient may complain of asthenopia, vertical diplopia, tilting images and head posture. Congenital palsy is usually compensated; therefore the torsional diplopia may not be present in these cases. Examination of family album may also help to differentiate between the congenital and acquired cases.

On examination the patient will show presence of compensatory head posture, with head tilted away from the affected side and chin down position. There will be hypertropia in the affected side more marked on adduction, along with overaction of IO muscle. Patients with congenital SO palsy have larger vertical fusional amplitude. Park's three step test is a useful method for determination of the involved extraocular muscle. In case of superior oblique palsy the hypertropia in the involved eye increases on contralateral gaze and ipsilateral head tilt. Torsion is measured subjectively with double Maddox rod test and on synaptophore while objectively by ophthalmoscopy. Torsion is frequently absent in congenital cases and when greater than 10 degrees suggests bilateral palsy.

Bilateral SO Palsy

Traumatic cases usually involve both the eyes. The severity of the paralysis is asymmetrical, and may not be unmasked until the eye with more severity gets operated, so it's important to look for bilateral involvement preoperatively. The important features of bilateral SO palsy are increase in hypertropia in both lateral gazes, positive Bielschowsky head tilt test on either side, subjective complains of torsion, objective excyclotropia of both eyes on fundus examination, V pattern esotropia and chin depression.

Evaluation of systemic condition is necessary in acquired cases especially that are associated with other neurological signs.

Differential Diagnosis

Primary IO Overaction

Absence of primary position hypertropia, lack of subjective torsion, and negative three step test distinguishes primary IO overaction from SO palsy.

Brown Syndrome

There's underaction ipsilateral IO owing to restriction of SO in cases of Brown Syndrome.

Pseudoparalysis

Plagiocephaly may cause pseudoparalysis of SO muscle. The retroplacement of trochlea due to early fusion of coronal sutures increases the angle between the SO tendon and AP axis of eye reducing the vertical effect of SO muscle while increasing its incyclotorsional effect.

Myasthenia Gravis

Should be considered as differential in any acquired muscle palsy. Tensilon test differentiates it from the rest of myogenic causes.

Management of Fourth Nerve Palsy

Superior oblique palsy usually presents with an abnormal head posture in the form of a head tilt to the opposite side or "ocular torticollis". An incident finding in the absence of abnormal head posture is rarely an indication for surgery.

Nonsurgical Management

The non-surgical management in fourth nerve is similar to what has been described for the third nerve palsy. The management of fourth nerve with prisms is difficult as the vertical deviation is incomitant and there may be associated "V" in cases of bilateral fourth nerve palsy.

In children, presence of fourth nerve palsy may be noticed due to the anomalous head posture. They keep a head tilt as they enjoy the advantage of binocularity. In such cases parents may be advised to allow the child to have a head posture, till it is surgically corrected.

In adults, with acquired fourth nerve palsy having diplopia, patching may be the only mean of relieving symptoms as other forms of management in the form of prisms and botulinum toxin may not be feasible to use.

Surgical Management

This is the definitive management of the fourth nerve palsy when the deviations are stable for a period of six months or more. Knapp's classification and management protocol is one of the important landmarks in management of cases of fourth nerve palsy. The Knapp's management strategy depends upon the maximum deviation in different gazes. This has been summarized in Table.

Table 1: Management of IVth nerve palsy (Von Noorden modification of Knapp's Classification): For a case of Left Superior Oblique palsy

Class	*Maximum deviation in gaze*	*Management*
1	Dextro-elevation (L/R maximum in this gaze)	Left inferior oblique recession
2	Dextro-depression	Left superior oblique tuck or Harada Ito's procedure + Right inferior rectus recession
3	All right gazes	If Hypertropia < 25 PD then left inferior oblique recession If hypertropia > 25 then add left superior oblique tuck
4	All down and right gazes	Treatment plan as in 3 with right inferior rectus recession or left superior rectus recession
5	All down gazes	Left superior oblique tuck with Right inferior rectus recession
6	Bilateral with a "V" pattern	Bilateral surgery as in class 5
7	All downgazes, primary gaze and dextroversion	Explore trochlea

Another classification and management strategy was proposed by Scott and Kraft:

1. Type 1—Overacting inferior oblique (1+ to 2+) with no underaction of superior oblique resulting in less than 15 prism Dioptres of hypertropia in primary gaze, in such cases any ipsilateral inferior oblique weakening procedure may be chosen depending upon its overaction.
2. Type 2—Overacting inferior oblique (3+ to 4+), with underaction of superior oblique (3- to 4-) resulting in less than 15 prism Dioptres of hypertropia in primary gaze, inferior oblique weakening procedure may suffice.. According to Knapp's classification in such cases a tuck of superior oblique (if torsional symptoms significant) or recession of contralateral inferior rectus may be required.
3. Type 3-
   a. 3A—Unilateral superior oblique palsy with less than 15 prism Diopters of hypertropia in primary gaze, inferior oblique overaction is very little and superior oblique has significant underaction then weakening of contralateral inferior rectus or ipsilateral superior oblique tucking may be done.
   b. 3B—Similar to 3A except much more underaction of superior oblique is present superior oblique strengthening procedure in the form of Harada-Ito with recession of contralateral inferior rectus may be required.

4. Type 4—Overacting inferior oblique with underaction of superior oblique with less than 15 Prism Dioptres of hypertropia in primary gaze, the deviation is greater in upgaze than downgaze; in such cases the weakening of ipsilateral inferior oblique along with ipsilateral superior rectus recession may be planned.
5. Type 5—More than 15 prism Dioptres of hypertropia in primary gaze along with mild to moderate inferior oblique overaction and mild to moderate superior oblique underaction, and deviation greater in downgaze than upgaze, ipsilateral inferior oblique weakening along with contralateral inferior rectus recession may be done (Knapp-SO tuck)
6. Type 6—More than 30 prism Dioptres of hypertropia in primary gaze along with marked overaction of inferior oblique with marked superior oblique underaction and mild contralateral superior rectus underaction, the surgical plan in such cases would be weakening of inferior oblique along with ipsilateral superior rectus recession and inferior rectus resection (Knapp-IO recession+ SO tuck)
7. Type 7—Concomitant hypertropia and mild inferior oblique overaction and less then 15 prism Dioptres of hypertropia, in such cases ipsilateral superior rectus recession may be planned. In cases with more than 15 prism Dioptres of hypertropia in primary gaze ipsilateral superior rectus recession along with ipsilateral inferior rectus resection or contralateral inferior rectus recession may be planned.
8. Type 8—Fallen Eye Syndrome-contralateral eye drops as the patient moves his eyes across the horizontal towards contralateral eye, this is because of overacting inferior oblique and less innervation is supplied to its yoke muscle that is the superior rectus, in such cases contralateral inferior rectus may becomes tightened and a recession of contralateral inferior rectus may be needed.

Sixth Nerve Palsy

Abducens nerve palsy is the most common ocular cranial nerve palsy. The long course and position of the nerve in brain make it susceptible to various disorders like trauma, meningitis, raised ICT etc.

Anatomy

The paired sixth nerve nuclei are located in the brainstem at the level of the pons and fourth ventricle. It supplies ipsilateral lateral rectus and contralateral medial rectus through median longitudinal fasciculus. The seventh nerve nucleus lies ventrally with fascicles that loop around the sixth nerve nucleus forming facial colliculus. The nerve then travels ventrally through the pontine tegmentum towards pontomedullary junction. The nerve exits the brainstem at pontomedullary junction and enters the subarachnoid space within the cerebellopontine angle where it lies in relation with seventh and eighth nerve. The nerve pierces the dura shortly after exiting and run in the dura of the clivus and passes beneath the petroclinoid ligament and over the petrous apex to enter the cavernous sinus. In the cavernous sinus the nerve runs through the substance of the sinus, thus is extremely vulnerable to the lesion of the cavernous sinus. The nerve enters orbit through superior orbital fissure inside the annulus of Zinn and innervates the lateral rectus muscle.

Etiology

The paralysis of abducens nerve can be congenital or acquired.

Congenital Sixth Nerve Palsy

A unilateral isolated, congenital deficit of abduction is a rare finding and most likely related to birth trauma.

Mobius syndrome is facial diplegia associated with defective horizontal gaze. The patients have mask like facies with unilateral or bilateral limitation of abduction. Other congenital associated congenital defects are deafness, webbed fingers or toes, supernumerary digits, and atrophy of tongue muscles, aplasia of hands, feet, fingers, or toes.

Duane's retraction syndrome, characterized by unilateral or bilateral abduction limitation, is due to congenital absence of abducens neurons with innervation of the lateral rectus muscle by branches of the oculomotor nerve.

Acquired Sixth Nerve Palsy

Nucleus lesions: Damage to the sixth nerve nucleus leads to ipsilateral gaze palsy. It is often accompanied by the ipsilateral seventh nerve palsy because of proximity of the facial colliculus to the sixth nerve nucleus. The causes of lesions of sixth nerve palsy are infarction, infiltration, hemorrhage, trauma, infections, inflammation and tumors.

Lesions of the sixth nerve fascicle: The involvement of sixth nerve fascicle can be recognized by the presence of associated clinical syndromes. Foville's syndrome presents as abduction deficit or horizontal gaze palsy along with the ipsilateral facial weakness, ipsilateral loss of taste, ipsilateral central Horner's syndrome, ipsilateral analgesia of face, ipsilateral peripheral deafness. The structures affected by the lesion in tegmentum of pons are sixth and seventh nerve fascicles, nucleus of tractus solitarius, superior olivary nucleus, and spinal tract of trigeminal nerve. When the lesion is ventral it produces ipsilateral sixth nerve palsy and contralateral hemiplegia (Raymond's syndrome) and associated ipsilateral seventh nerve palsy along with contralateral hemiplegia (Millard Guber syndrome). Fascicular lesions of sixth nerve are produced by ischemia, tumour compression, demyelination, infection and inflammation.

Lesions in the subarachnoid space: The location and long course of the sixth nerve are the major factors that make it susceptible to various pontine, posterior fossa and basal lesions. Meningitis, trauma, neurosurgical manipulation, neoplasms of the base of the brain are the common lesions that affect the sixth nerve in this region. Raised intracranial pressure, due to any cause, results in unilateral or bilateral stretching of sixth nerve along their course between the pons and petrous apex. Other causes include aneurysms of anterior inferior cerebellar attery, acoustic neuromas, trigeminal schwannoma, and lumbar puncture.

Lesions at petrous apex: The nerve in this region lies close to the mastoid antrum and thus is involved in patients with mastoiditis known as Gradengio's syndrome. Other lesions in this region include tumors, aneurysm of internal carotid artery, and lateral sinus thrombosis with inferior petrosal involvement.

Lesions at cavernous sinus at orbital apex: The sixth nerve lies in the substance of cavernous sinus and is often the first one to get involve in the lesions of cavernous sinus, like certico-cavernous fistula, cavernous sinus thrombosis, aneurysm of internal carotid artery. There can be associated involvement of other cranial nerves, third, fourth and fifth that lie in the dural sheath of cavernous sinus.

Inflammation of orbital apex leads to the paresis of nerve is associated with the involvement of third, fourth, and fifth cranial nerve known as Tolosa- Hunt syndrome.

Isolated sixth nerve palsy may occur in diabetes mellitus, hypertension, Giant cell arteritis or migraine.

Clinical Presentation

Patients usually complain of horizontal diplopia more in the lateral gaze of the involved side. On examination there is esotropia and limitation of abduction of the involved eye. A compensatory face turn to the same side may be present to maintain binocular vision. Medial rectus contracture may be present in prolonged cases and can be confirmed on forced duction test. There may be presence of associated cranial nerve palsies and neurological features depending upon etiology. Laboratory investigations and systemic evaluation for the cause of isolated sixth nerve palsy; like blood glucose level, hemogram, ESR etc should be done.

Differential Diagnosis

Myasthenia Gravis

Myasthenia gravis can mimic any cranial nerve palsy supplying the eye. Associated signs such as ptosis, diurnal variation and tensilon test can differentiate it from sixth nerve palsy.

Graves Ophthalmopathy

Graves ophthalmopathy involving the medial rectus may give rise to limitation of abduction but presence of associated features will differentiate it.

Duane Retraction Syndrome

Duane retraction syndrome especially type I is another important differential diagnosis. It is associated with globe retraction and narrowing of lid fissures on adduction. The magnitude of the esotropia in primary position is small compared with what may be expected from LR palsy.

Infantile Esotropia

Infantile esotropia with cross fixation may be confused with bilateral sixth nerve palsy. Doll's head movements will show abduction and saccadic velocity analysis will show normally rapid abducting saccades.

Management of Sixth Nerve Palsy

As with other cranial nerves supplying the extraocular muscles, the treatment of sixth nerve can also be divided into two i.e. non-surgical or the acute phase management and the definitive or the surgical management.

Non-surgical Management

In children in the amblyogenic age group, the immediate treatment is aimed at prevention of amblyopia. In order to prevent amblyopia alternate occlusion may be advised, which also helps in preventing diplopia. For small deviation, where the diplopia may be controlled by head posture, the parents should be in told to permit head posture. Another option for small deviations is use of fresnel prism.

In adults, for smaller deviation anomalous head posture or use of patching or prisms can be advised avoid diplopia. The patient is advised to occlude the better eye for as long as possible. For larger deviations due to a complete paralysis one can opt for use of patching or Botulinum toxin injection at the site of medial rectus to prevent its contracture.

Surgical Management

One should allow approximately six months time for a spontaneous recovery of a case of sixth nerve, as sometimes there may be a total recovery of sixth nerve. Once the deviations are stable for six months, one can plan a definitive treatment in the form of surgical intervention.

The surgical decision is based upon the amount of abduction possible, amount of deviation in the primary gaze, muscle power of lateral rectus on active force generation test and contracture of medial rectus as on forced duction test.

In cases where there is moderate recovery of lateral rectus functions, horizontal muscle surgery in the form of medial rectus recession and lateral rectus resections may be an effective plan.

In cases, where there is total sixth nerve palsy, recession-resection procedure may not work, and one may have to opt for, large recession of medial rectus along with a full or partial vertical rectus muscle transposition. While operating on three of the recti one has to keep in mind the risk of anterior segment ischemia and vessel sparing surgery may be needed. There is low risk of anterior segment ischemia if medial rectus recession is combined with half tendon transposition of vertical muscles.

Hummelsheim procedure: Lateral halves of the superior and inferior rectus muscles are disinserted and reattached to the superior and inferior margins of the lateral rectus. This is preceded by a large recession of medial rectus. To decrease the risk of anterior segment ischemia, one vessel of both the vertical recti must be preserved at the original insertion. One can also replace the large recession of medial rectus by chemodenervation of the medial rectus but in a long-standing case with fibrotic tight medial rectus the effect may not be significant. The effect of the transposition can be enhanced by placing a non-absorbable posterior suture 8 mm behind the new insertion of the transposed muscle. This suture changes the direction of vector of the action of transposed muscle towards the new insertion site and thus augmenting the effect brought about by transposition.

Jenson's procedure: Lateral halves of superior and inferior recti are tied with upper and lower halves of lateral rectus respectively. The lateral rectus is dissected free for about 14mm from their insertion and both the muscles are then tied with a non absorbable suture at around the equator. Although this procedure claims to have less chance of anterior segment ischemia there is always a possibility of strangulation of vessels by the sutures.

The primary aim of all surgeries for paralytic strabismus is to increase the area of binocular single vision and reduce diplopia, particularly so in primary and down gazes, although the complete motility of the eye may not be restored in most cases of long standing paralytic squints.

Chapter 38

Paralytic Strabismus

Kali Cole Bliss (USA)

Introduction

The evaluation and treatment of paralytic strabismus is challenging. The patients typically suffer from diplopia, abnormal head position, and multiple eye muscle surgeries. Because paralytic strabismus causes an incomitant strabismus, surgical correction is difficult. The challenge of surgical correction is to improve diplopia and expand the field of single vision while maintaining good ocular alignment in primary position. In this chapter, third, fourth, and sixth nerve palsies and the associated surgical interventions will be discussed.

Third Nerve Palsy

Etiology

Congenital third nerve palsy is a rare condition. Of those children born with a third nerve palsy, approximately half other neurological or physical signs. The most common associations are cerebral palsy, ipsi- or contralateral hemiparesis/plegia, and developmental delay. More commonly, third nerve palsy is seen following head trauma associated with a loss of consciousness. In children, other causes of third nerve palsy include inflammation, viral infection, migraine, and neoplastic lesions. In adults, causes include intracranial aneurysm, diabetes, inflammation/infection, trauma, or tumor. Most of adults referred for surgical treatment have palsy due to trauma.

Clinical Signs and Symptoms

Congenital third nerve palsy presents with ptosis, exotropia, and hypotropia of the involved eye. This is because there is a limitation of adduction, elevation, and depression against an unopposed lateral rectus muscle and superior oblique muscle. Aberrant regeneration of the damaged nerve may complicate the clinical findings with characteristic features including elevation of the ptotic lid on attempted adduction and downgaze and pupil constriction on adduction and upgaze.

Differential Diagnosis

Differential diagnosis includes midbrain lesions, meningeal tumor or infection, cavernous sinus disease, intraorbital structural lesions that restrict ocular motility, ocular myopathies, and myasthenia gravis.

Treatment and Prognosis

Amblyopia is a common finding the pediatric population. Amblyopia treatment should be aggressive and started as early as possible. Anisometropia and astigmatism are common findings but, surprisingly, accommodation is often well preserved. Before surgical correction is performed in acquired cases, it is advisable to wait 6-12 months to allow for any spontaneous recovery. Those

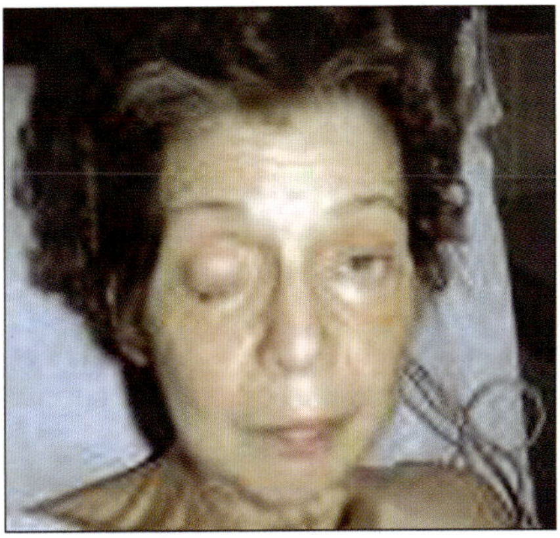

Figure 1: Third nerve palsy 1

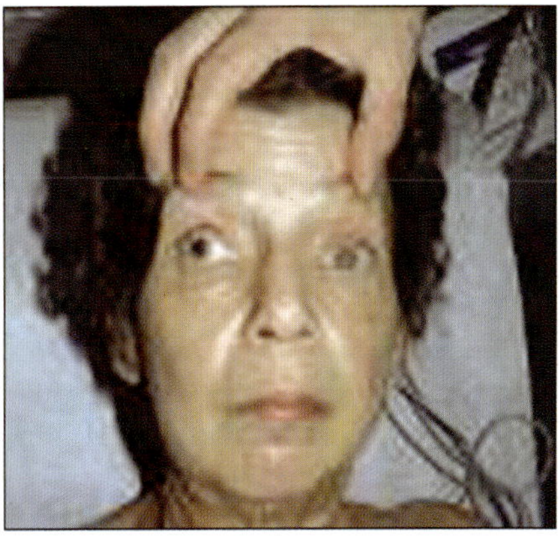

Figure 2: Third nerve palsy 2

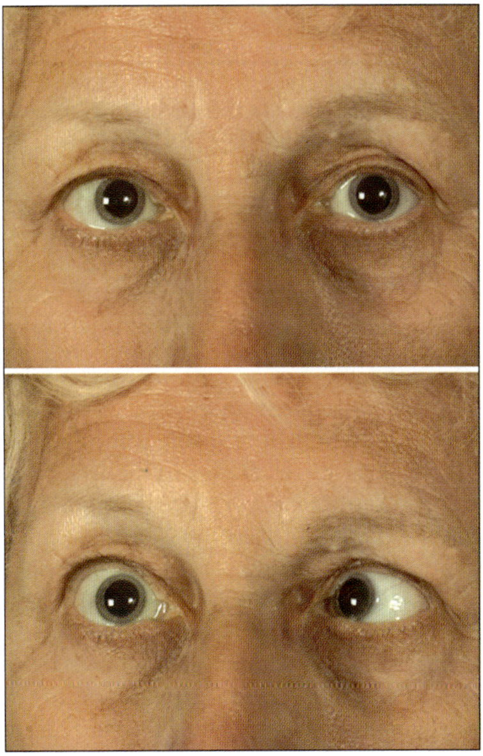

Figure 3: Sixth nerve palsy

patients who obtain at least partial function are better candidates for a good functional and cosmetic result. Because multiple extraocular muscles as well as the levator may be involved, adequate alignment for binocular function in primary position and in slight downgaze for reading may be all that can be expected. Frequently, a large resection of the paralytic medial rectus muscle combined with a large recession of the antagonist lateral rectus muscle is performed to correct the exodeviation, with supraplacement of both to correct the hypotropia. Standard transposition procedures generally are not effective because the adjacent rectus muscles are often paretic. Most surgeons reserve correction of ptosis for a subsequent procedure to allow for a more accurate assessment of lid position.

The use of botulinum toxin in treating strabismus has generally been reserved for sixth nerve palsies. However, Talebnejad et al have reported success in using botulinum toxin injection in the lateral rectus muscle in patients with acute traumatic partial third-nerve palsy. The patients showed marked recovery when injection was performed within 2 months of the onset of palsy. This suggests that botulinum toxin injection may provide temporary relief of symptoms.

Fourth Nerve Palsy

Etiology

Fourth nerve palsy is the most common form of paralytic vertical strabismus. It is also the most common of all congenital ocular motor palsies. Acquired cases are usually the result of closed head trauma. Other acquired etiologies include central nervous system vascular problems, diabetes, or brain tumors. Congenital cases are usually unilateral and acquired cases are more often bilateral.

Clinical Signs and Symptoms

Unilateral cases almost always present with torticollis with a head tilt away from the affected side, where bilateral cases may or may not have a head tilt. Diagnostic criteria include hypertropia of the affected eye that increases on adduction and ipsilateral head tilt, as shown in the 3-step test.Versions usually reveal underaction of the involved superior oblique muscle and overaction of its antagonist inferior oblique muscle. Torsional imbalance should be measured using the double Maddox rod. Unilateral cases may show little if any V pattern and less than 5 degrees of excyclotorsion. Large vertical amplitudes as well as facial asymmetry from a long-standing head tilt may be present. In addition, a phenomenon known as "spread of comitance" occurs in long standing superior oblique paresis as a result from ipsilateral superior rectus muscle contracture. This results in a vertical deviation that is equal or nearly so in all fields of gaze. In bilateral cases, a V pattern esotropia is typically seen. Excyclotorsion is at least 5 degrees and is highly diagnostic when 10 degrees or more. The Bielschowsky head-tilt test shows a positive result to each side with a right hypertropia on right head tilt and a left hypertropia on left head tilt.

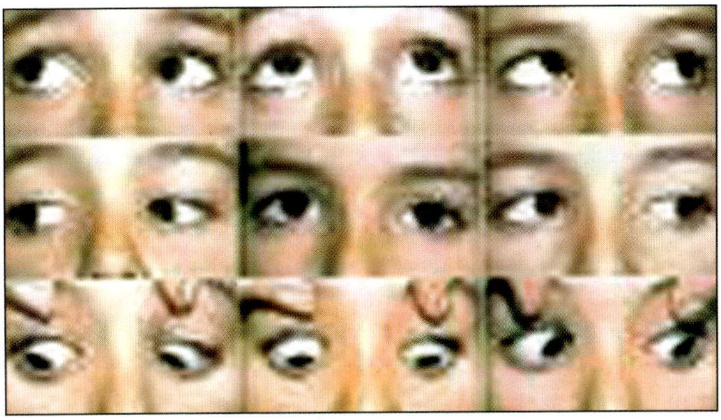

Figure 4: Superior oblique palsy motility

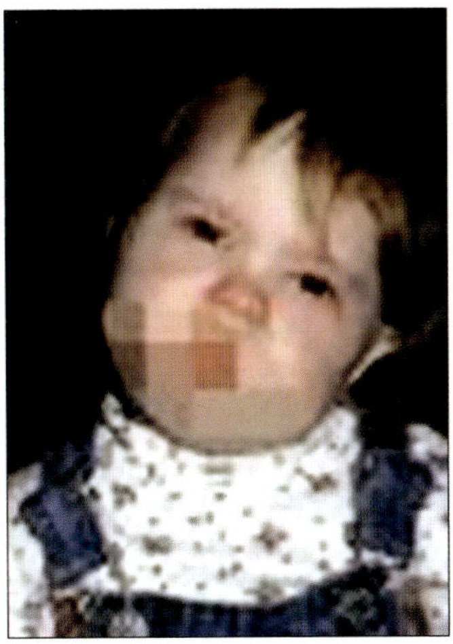

Figure 5: superior oblique palsy head tilt

Differential Diagnosis

The differential diagnosis for binocular vertical diplopia includes restrictive etiologies, partial third nerve palsy, myasthenia gravis, and skew deviation.

Treatment and Prognosis

Amblyopia may be present in congenital palsies and should be treated aggressively. In adults, prisms may be used to overcome diplopia if the deviation is small, nearly comitant, and not predominantly torsional. Surgery is indicated in most cases of superior oblique palsy. The indications include abnormal head position, significant vertical deviation, diplopia, or asthenopia. Measuring the ocular deviation in all diagnostic gaze positions, as well as with right and left head tilt, will guide surgical planning. Typically the first surgical approach with a unilateral fourth nerve palsy is to weaken the antagonist inferior oblique muscle. This should be done when the hypertropia is no more than 15 prism diopters in primary gaze and there is overaction of the inferior oblique muscle. The degree of overaction seen in the inferior oblique muscle will be proportional to the amount of correction that can be achieved with a weakening procedure. If the hypertropia in primary position is greater than 15 prism diopters, a second muscle should be added to the procedure. Options for the second muscle include recessing the contralateral inferior rectus muscle, tucking the palsied superior oblique muscle, or recessing the ipsilateral superior rectus muscle, as dictated by forced duction testing. If the hypertropia is greater than 35 prism diopters in the primary position, three-muscle surgery may be indicated. For bilateral cases, bilateral inferior oblique muscle weakening is appropriate but may not be sufficient. Other options included inferior rectus muscle recession, superior oblique tendon tuck, and the Harada-Ito procedure. In bilateral cases where the patient has torsional complaints, the Harada-Ito is preferred. This involves displacing the anterior fibers of the superior oblique tendons to the lower edge of the lateral rectus muscle several millimeters posterior to that muscle's insertion. This procedure can correct the extorsion as well as the abducting weakness in downgaze. If a vertical rectus muscle is recessed, one millimeter of recession will correct approximately 3 prism diopters of vertical correction. In tucking the superior oblique tendon, one should tuck the tendon until a positive forced duction test result is created. This occurs when tightness is felt when the eye is placed in adduction and as the inferior limbus crosses an imaginary line drawn between the medial and lateral canthi.

Stager et al described a new surgical procedure for patients with a cranial nerve IV palsy consisting of anterior and nasal transposition of the inferior oblique muscle, converting it from an extorter and elevator of the globe to an intorter and depressor. They describe success in using this procedure on a 3 year old patient with no superior oblique tendon. Further indications of this new procedure remain to be determined.

Sixth Nerve Palsy

Etiology

The most common cause of sixth nerve palsy in childhood is trauma. Congenital sixth nerve paralysis is uncommon and may be due to increased intracranial pressure secondary to the birth process and usually resolves spontaneously. In adults, the most common cause of sixth nerve palsy is vasculopathic. Other causes for adults and children include intracranial lesions, infection, and immunologic processes involving cranial nerve VI. Spontaneous benign lesions usually resolve over several months.

Clinical Signs and Symptoms

Paralysis of the lateral rectus muscle causes an incomitant esodeviation with an ipsilateral horizontal gaze palsy. In gaze toward the paretic muscle, the esotropia increases. As a result, patients may complain of double vision and often have a face turn toward the side of the paretic sixth nerve. Strabismic amblyopia is uncommon in sixth nerve palsies. Versions demonstrate limited or no abduction ability of the affected eye and active force generation tests document the weakness of that muscle.The possibility of previous trauma, infection, or neurologic insult should be explored and computed tomography (CT) or magnetic resonance imaging (MRI) are indicated when neurologic sign or symptoms are present.

Differential Diagnosis

Differential diagnosis for sixth nerve palsy includes infantile esotropia, Duane's syndrome, ocular myasthenia gravis, and thyroid-associated orbitopathy.

Treatment and Prognosis

If a child is unable to maintain binocular fusion with a face turn, patching may be required to prevent amblyopia. Treatment options to improve the strabismus include injection of botulinum toxin, muscle surgery, or both. Botulinum toxin can be injected into the antagonist medial rectus muscle. This will align the eye by temporarily paralyzing the medial rectus muscle. Quah et al retrospectively analyzed the use of botulinum toxin for the treatment of cranial nerve VI palsy at the Singapore National Eye Center. Six out of 19 patients treated with botulinum toxin achieved fusion in the primary gaze position without strabismus surgery. Patients with a smaller deviation and a shorter interval between onset of strabismus and botulinum toxin injection tended to achieve a better outcome.

Surgery is indicated when spontaneous resolution does not take place after 6 months or more of follow-up. In patients with some lateral rectus function, a large recession of the antagonist medial rectus muscle with resection of the lateral rectus muscle is often a successful first operation. In cases of total paralysis, muscle transposition procedures may be required. A standard

Hummelsheim procedure in patients with cranial nerve VI palsy involves transposition of the temporal halves of the vertical rectus muscles to the insertion of the lateral rectus muscle. Often, this is combined with a recession of the antagonist medial rectus muscle. Brooks et al described an augmented Hummelsheim procedure in which the temporal halves of the vertical rectus muscles are resected 4-8 mm before transposition to the lateral rectus muscle. They combined this procedure with a recession of the ipsilateral medial rectus muscle and found they were able to correct large angles of strabismus in all eight of their patients.

Chapter 39

Strabismus Syndromes

Ewa Oleszczynska Prost (Poland)

Duane's Retraction Syndrome

The etiologic factors of this syndrome are: Structural anomalies (abnormal posterior insertion of the medial rectus, nonelastic lateral rectus, fibrosis and contracture of the muscle) and abnormal innervations (hypoplasia of sixth nerve nucleus, paradoxical innervations lateral, superior rectus or inferior oblique).

Duane's syndrome is classified into three types:

1. *Type I:* Characterized by limitation or absence of abduction with widening of the palpebral fissure , normal adduction with narrowing of the palpebral fissure and retraction. The patients usually have esotropia.
2. *Type II:* Limitation or absence of adduction with narrowing of the palpebral fissure and retraction. Normal or slightly limited abduction. This may be associated exotropia.
3. *Type III:* Limitation or absence of both abduction and adduction with narrowing of the palpebral fissure and retraction of the globe on attempted adduction.

Clinical Findings

- See above: types I,II,III
- Usually vision is full
- Stereopsis is good
- Diplopia occur when the patient attempts to abduct the affected eye
- The face turn to have normal binocular vision.

Investigation

- Ocular movements exam
- Hirschberg's test
- Electromyographic studies

Differential Diagnosis

- Congenital esotropia
- Accommodative esotropia
- Divergens insufficiency
- Deprivation (sensory) esotropia
- Congenital exotropia
- Deprivation (sensory) exotropia
- Noncomitant strabismus
- Moebius' syndrome

Treatment

Surgery is only indicated when functional and cosmetic aspects can be evaluated.

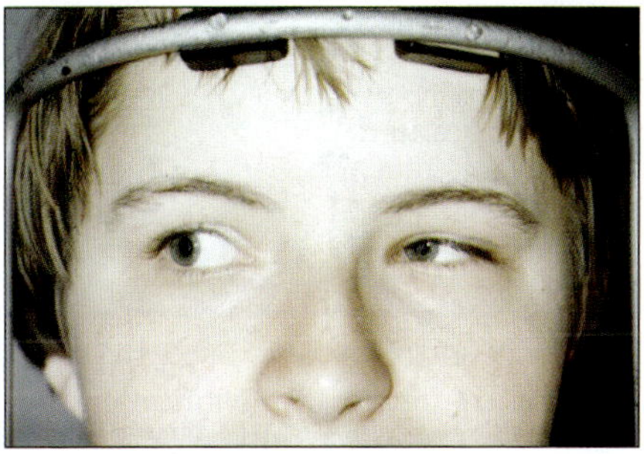

Figure 1: Duane's syndrome type I in the left eye-adduction with narrowing of the palpebral fissure and retraction. *(Courtesy: Prof K Krzystkowa, Cracow, Poland)*

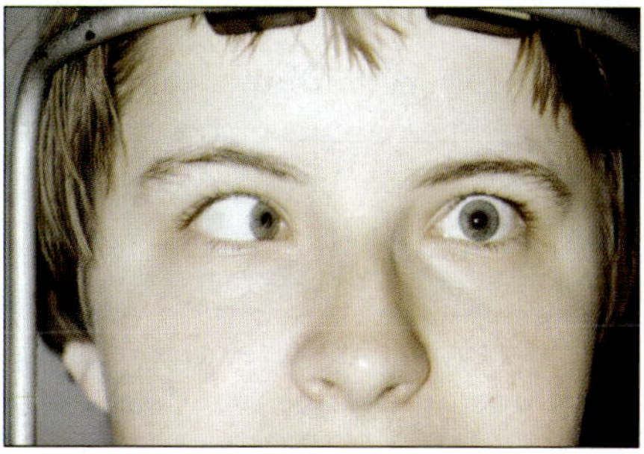

Figure 2: Duane's syndrome type I in the left eye-absence abduction with widening of the palpebral fissure. *(Courtesy: Prof K Krzystkowa, Cracow, Poland)*

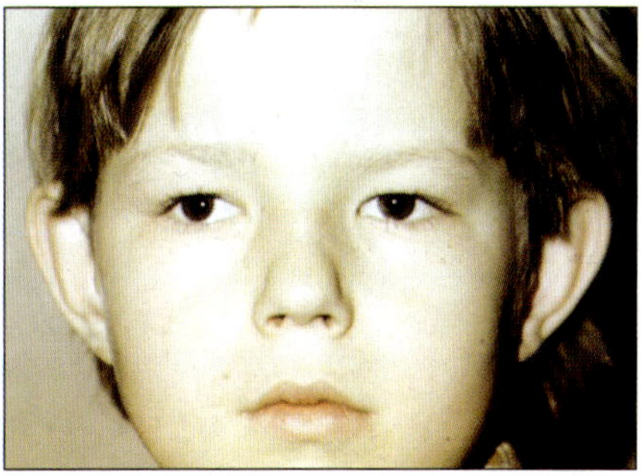

Figure 3: Duane's syndrome type II in the right eye. Note the exotropia in the primary position *(Courtesy: Prof K Krzystkowa, Cracow, Poland)*

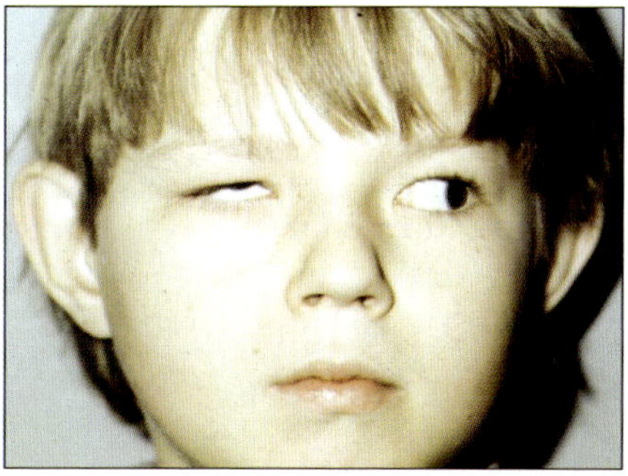

Figure 4: The same patient with Duane's type II syndrome. Note absence of adduction with narrowing of the palpebral. *(Courtesy: Prof K Krzystkowa, Cracow, Poland)*

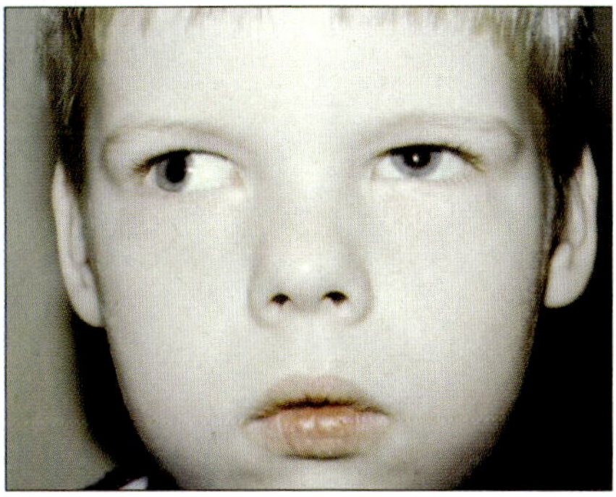

Figure 5: Duane's syndrome type III-absence of adduction in the left eye *(Courtesy: Prof K Krzystkowa, Cracow, Poland)*

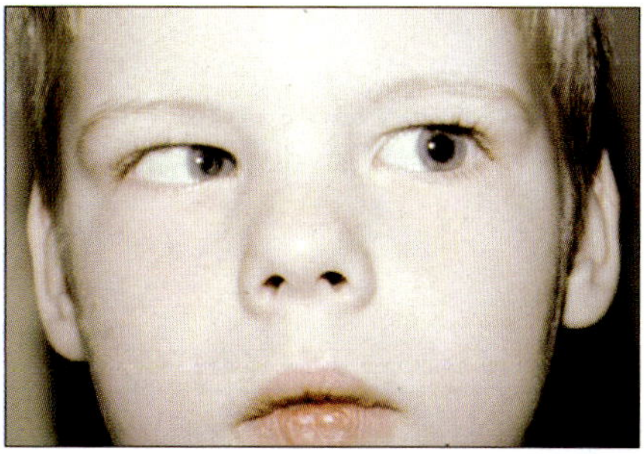

Figure 6: The same patient–limitation of abduction in the left eye *(Courtesy: Prof K Krzystkowa, Cracow, Poland)*

Prognosis

- Face turn or strabismus after the surgery can be smaller
- Sometimes results of the surgery can be disappointed.

Brown's Syndrome

Brown's syndrome or superior oblique tendon syndrome is caused by short tight superior oblique tendon and characterized by deficit in elevation during adduction. This syndrome could be congenital or acquired.

Clinical Findings

- Active elevation is limited
- Also passive elevation on forced duction test is limited
- Presence of head posture.

Investigation

- Ocular movements exam
- Hirschberg's test
- Forced duction test.

Differential Diagnosis

- Inferior oblique palsy
- Superior oblique overaction
- Double elevator palsy.

Treatment

Surgery is only indicated to attempt to restor binocular function in primary position.

Prognosis

- Face turn after the surgery can be smaller
- Sometimes results of the surgery can be disappointed
- Elevating the involved eye in adduction after surgery of the superior oblique is often poor.

Moebius Syndrome

Moebius syndrome is a rare congenital disturbance with bilateral abducens and facial nerve paralysis.

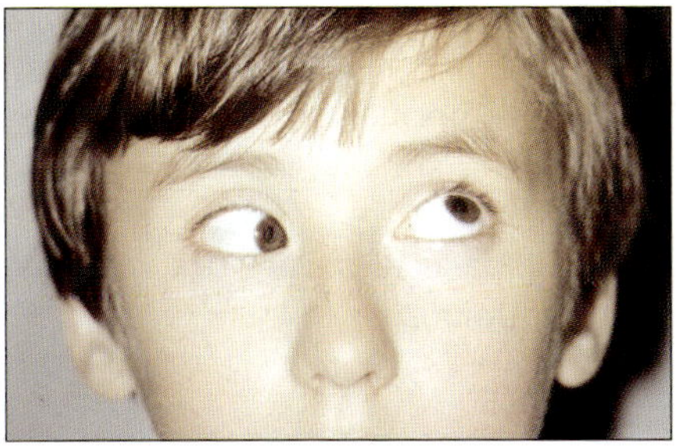

Figure 7: Brown's syndrome. Note the restriction of the elevation on adduction of the right eye. *(Courtesy: Prof K Krzystkowa, Cracow, Poland)*

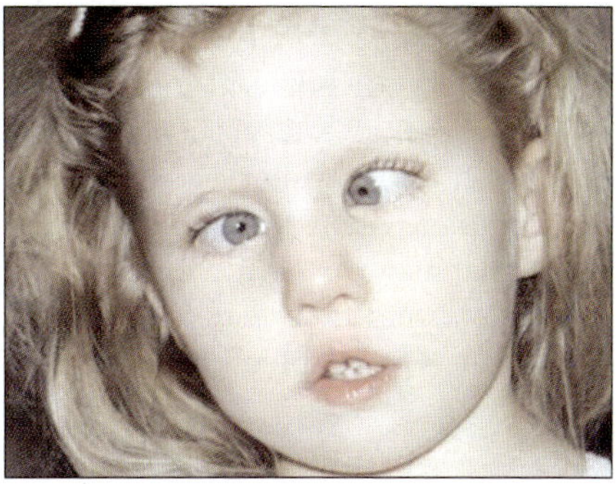

Figure 8: Moebius syndrome. *(Courtesy: Prof K Krzystkowa, Cracow, Poland)*

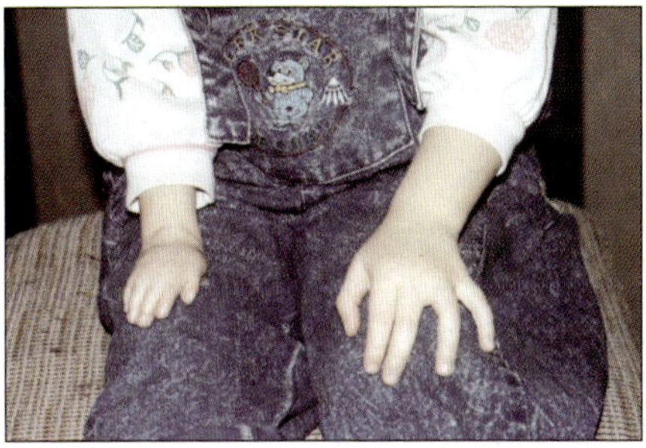

Figure 9: The syndactyly in patients with Moebius syndrome *(Courtesy: Prof K Krzystkowa, Cracow, Poland)*

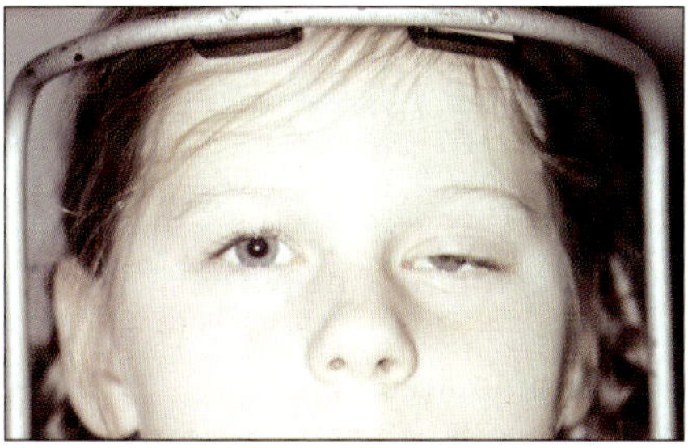

Figure 10: Marcus-Gunn syndrome in a 7 years old girl *(Courtesy: Prof K Krzystkowa, Cracow, Poland)*

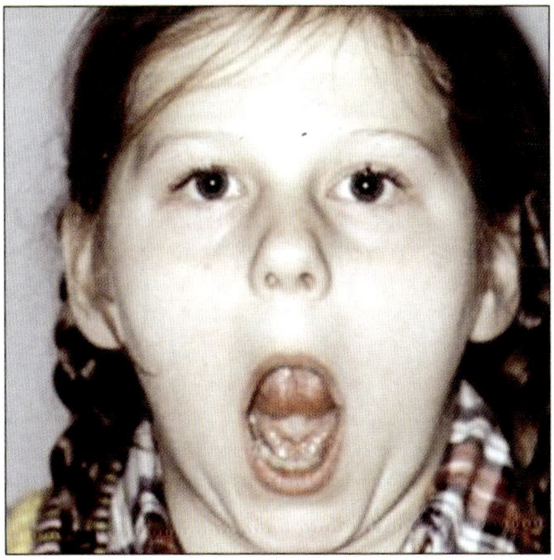

Figure 11: The girl opens the mouth and the eyelid elevates *(Courtesy: Prof K Krzystkowa, Cracow, Poland)*

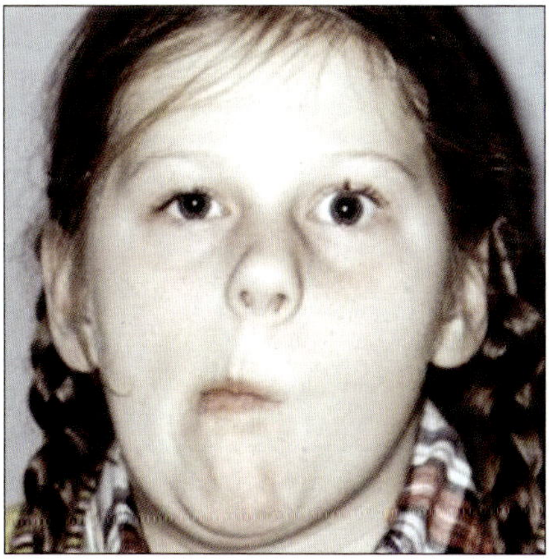

Figure 12: The same patient with Marcus-Gunn syndrome-tried to jaw from side to side we see the elevation of the eyelid. *(Courtesy: Prof K Krzystkowa, Cracow, Poland)*

Clinical Findings

- Unilateral or bilateral inability to abduct the eyes
- Convergence and vertical movement are intact
- Vision and papillary constriction are generally normal
- Complete or incomplete facial palsy
- Partial atrophy of the tongue
- Skeletal and muscle defects are common (hypoplasia of the pectoral muscles, syndactyly, clubfeet, congenital limb amputations).

Investigation

- Hirschberg's test
- Esotropia about 50 PD
- Forced duction test are positive to both adduction and abduction
- Horizontal muscles are often thickened and fibrotic
- Electromyographic studies have shown waxing and waning of electrical activity
- NMR and CT examination.

Differential Diagnosis

- Congenital esotropia
- Nystagmus blockage syndrome
- Infantile accommodative esotropia
- Congenital fibrosis syndrome (fixed strabismus)
- Congenital myasthenia
- Congenital six nerve palsy
- Duane's syndrome.

Treatment

Surgery for the esotropia consisting of recession of the medial rectus muscles.

Prognosis

- Usually patients have a little horizontal movements after surgery
- Reduction of squint is visible.

Marcus Gunn's Syndrome

Marcus Gunn jaw-winking is a synkinesis between the nerve supply to the muscles of masticacion and the levator palpebrae superiosis.

Clinical Findings

When the patient opens or close the mouth or jaw from side to side we see the elevation of the affected lid above its ptotic level.

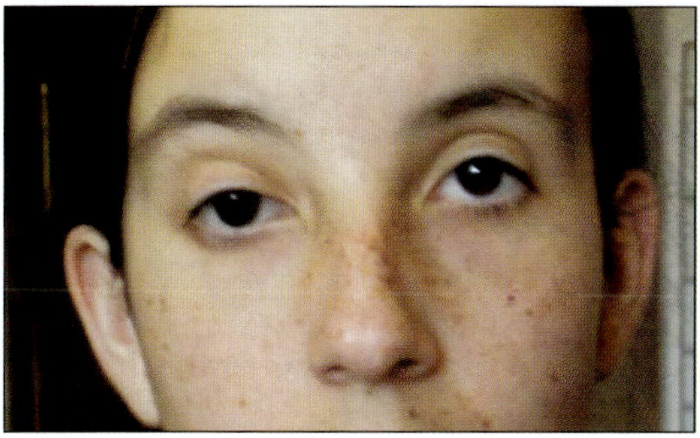

Figure 13: Double elevator palsy. Note the ptosis of the right eye

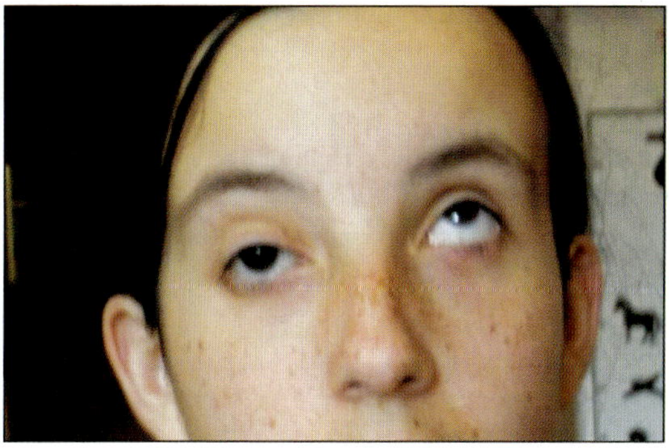

Figure 14: The same patient with restricted the elevation of the right eye

Investigation

Observation the eyes asocciated with mouth's movements.

Differential Diagnosis

- Congenital ptosis
- Congenital blepharoptosis
- Telecanthus
- Epiblepharon
- Euryblepharon
- Paresis of III or V cranial nerves.

Treatment

If significant lid retraction with ptosis is present -directed towards disinserting the levator muscle and suspending the lid.

Prognosis

Treatment result are only partially satisfactory.

Double Elevator Palsy

Congenital or acquired double elevator palsy is the paralysis of both the elevators: superior rectus and levator palpebrae.

Clinical Findings

- Inability or reduced ability to elevate the eye
- Paretic eye have the hypotropia with ptosis when fixates nonparetic eye
- When fixates paretic eye no hypotropia in the primary position and no ptosis
- The lid may become ptotic
- Patient with chin-up position to maintain binocularity
- Diplopia may usually occured in upward gaze
- Sometimes the pupillary anomalies can occured.

Investigation

- Hirschberg's test
- Ocular movements exam
- Observation the eyes during alternate fixation
- Forced duction test
- Observation the head posture
- Pupillary exam on the light.

Differential Diagnosis

- Congenital ptosis
- Congenital myasthenia
- Congenital fibrosis of inferior rectus
- Blow-out syndrome
- Brown's syndrome.

Treatment

- Surgery is not indicated if a patient is ortoptic in primary position
- If the forced duction test is negative on the paretic eye, the Knapp's surgery is indicated
- If the paralyzed eye fixates then weakening procedure of the elevators of the nonparetic eye is done
- Lid surgery also be required if the ptosis not disappear.

Prognosis

- Only a modest increase in elevation is usually observed after surgery
- Often surgery give satisfactory results and head posture disappears.

Chapter 40

Dissociated Deviations

M Edward Wilson, Berdine M Burger (USA)

Introduction

Dissociated movements and misalignments of the eyes are grouped into what is known as the dissociated strabismus complex (DSC). Dissociated ocular deviations can be vertical (DVD), horizontal (DHD), or torsional (DTD). DSC obviates the semantic confusion that occurs when referring to a dissociated deviation as a DVD when, in some patients, the most prominent movement is horizontal or torsional. The DSC is commonly associated with congenital esotropia, but it may also be seen in association with other forms of strabismus. In addition, it can be seen to develop whenever a child suffers from a permanent unilateral vision loss or in association with acquired tropias. All conditions have in common an absence of high-grade stereopsis (bifixation or macular binocular vision).

Clinical Signs and Symptoms

The classic DSC pattern is of a nonfixating eye slowly elevating, extorting, and abducting upon the spontaneous loss of binocular function or with cover testing. A reversal of these movements is seen with recovery and refixation. Latent nystagmus is also often seen on exam, but macular binocular vision with high-grade stereopsis is never present.

The DSC is nearly always bilateral but asymmetric. Dissociated deviations may be controlled by binocular fusion mechanisms and remain latent, or the deviation may manifest spontaneously. When DSC becomes manifest, it does so intermittently, changing as the state of attention of the individual changes and variability is the rule. Although dissociated horizontal and torsional movements are being recognized with greater frequency, DVD remains the predominant manifestation in most cases of DSC.

Investigations

Placing base-down prisms before the higher eye or base-up prisms before the lower eye until all refixation movements are neutralized can quantitate a true hypertropia. The alternate cover test reveals these refixation movements to be upward in one eye and downward in the other eye. The absence of upward refixation movements in either eye on alternate cover testing usually distinguishes DVD from true vertical tropia. In addition, the upward deviation is very slow (2-40°/s) in DVD compared with true hypertropia (200-400°/s).

When one is attempting to quantify DVD or DHD, each eye must be measured separately. Prisms are placed before the eye to be measured until it no longer drifts behind cover; this is the endpoint. A true neutralization is not reached. Manifestations of DSC vary and tend to decrease with prolonged occlusion. For these reasons a subjective 1+ to 4+ scale is sometimes used instead of an exact prism diopters measurement to describe each component of DSC and the largest deviation seen during the exam is usually the one graded. For a DVD < 10 prism

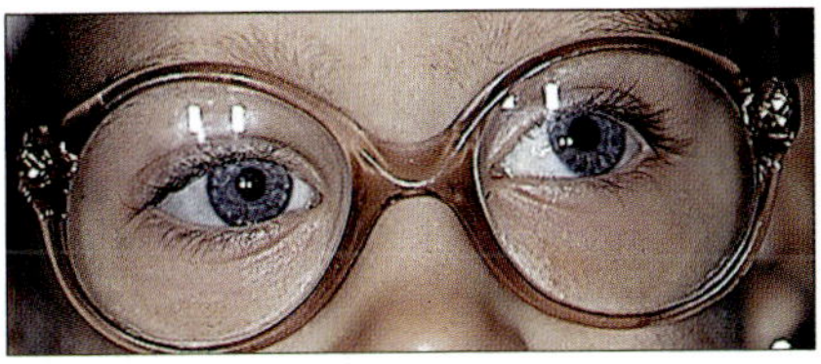

Figure 1: DVD left eye with glasses

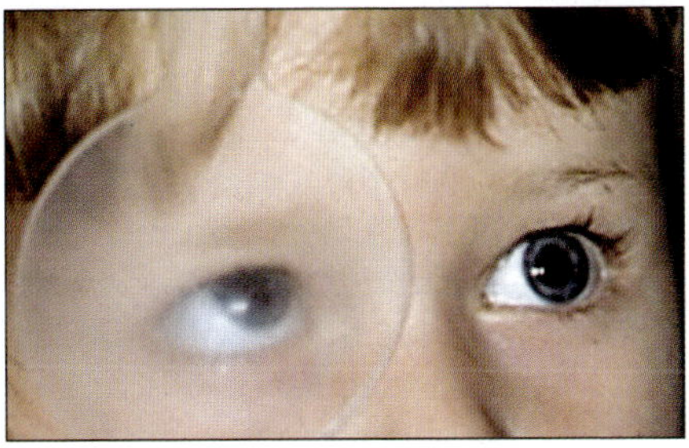

Figure 2: DVD right eye with translucent occluder

diopters (PD), a 1+ designation is used. Deviations between 10 and 15 PD are labeled as 2+, 15-20 as 3+, and > 20 PD as 4+. If a true hypertropia and DVD coexist, prism and alternate cover test neutralization of the hypertropia should be made first. Use a rapid alternate cover test to measure the true hypertropia, not allowing the hypotropic eye time to dissociate behind the cover. The true hypertropia and the more marked DVD usually are present on the same side.

The Bielschowsky phenomenon is unique to DSC. It can be demonstrated most easily when DVD and amblyopia are present. Downward movement of the elevated occluded nonfixating eye occurs when filters of increasing density are placed before the fixating eye.

Differential Diagnosis

DHD is distinguished from intermittent exotropia by the slow speed of the abducting movement, the association of DTD, and the absence of true neutralization with prisms. Close inspection also reveals that the DHD does not begin to drift until the formerly covered eye has returned to the primary position and picked up fixation. In contrast, exotropia produces simultaneous movement of one eye (as it is uncovered) toward fixation and the other eye (as it is covered) away from fixation. Many patients with DHD will reveal a micro-esotropia on rapid alternate cover testing, but slow alternate cover testing (allowing the eye with DHD to fully dissociate) reveals the exodeviated posture behind cover.

DSC can coexist with oblique muscle dysfunction. In addition, it is well known that in adduction the nose may act as an occluder, allowing DVD to simulate inferior oblique muscle overaction (IOOA). A true hypertropia present in side gaze but absent in primary gaze is evidence that oblique muscle dysfunction exists. The adducted eye would manifest a hypotropia when superior oblique muscle overaction (SOOA) is present and a hypertropia when IOOA exists. Oblique muscle dysfunction causes the DVD to appear incomitant. The IOOA reduces DVD in abduction, and SOOA reduces DVD in adduction. In other words, if DVD is evident in primary gaze but much less elevation is present behind cover when either eye is in abduction, bilateral IOOA should be suspected and a V pattern sought to confirm the diagnosis. If elevation behind cover is much less in adduction, SOOA should be suspected and an A pattern sought to verify the diagnosis.

Torticollis has been documented in up to 35% of patients with DVD when an ocular fixation preference is present. When present, the head tilt usually is toward the side of the nonfixating eye with the more manifest DVD; thus, the DVD usually increases with forced tilt away from the eye with the more severe DVD and decreases on tilt toward the eye with more severe DVD. This tilting pattern is opposite from that seen in superior oblique muscle palsy, in which the hypertropia increases on ipsilateral tilt and decreases on contralateral tilt.

Treatment and Prognosis

Despite its ability to be disfiguring, most patients with DSC do not need treatment. If a DSC drift is seen only rarely, with fatigue, reassurance and observation is the best course of therapy. Available treatments are imperfect and none of them can eliminate DSC totally. Successful treatment merely reduces the frequency and magnitude of spontaneously manifest DSC so that it is rarely seen at home. Despite treatment, dissociated strabismus can almost always still be detected during alternate cover testing. No patient is cured of DSC and recurrence of manifest deviations is common even after aggressive treatment.

Nonsurgical treatment options to reduce the frequency of manifest DSC have met with limited success. Because DSC is usually asymmetric, switching the fixation preference to the eye that deviates most often may improve the patient's control of DSC and reduce how often the eyes are seen to drift. The Worth four-dot test can be used to verify this fixation switch.

DVD, when manifest frequently, can be treated surgically by several different approaches including superior rectus muscle recession, inferior oblique muscle anterior transposition, and inferior rectus muscle resection. DHD is not treated effectively by DVD surgery alone. When prominent, DHD requires a special surgical strategy that usually involves recession of the lateral rectus muscle on the side of the manifest DHD. The DTD is not treated surgically. Latent nystagmus can become manifest in patients with poorly controlled DSC. Treatment that restores DSC control and gross binocularity may also result in a manifest-latent nystagmus converting back to its latent status.

In conclusion, DSC should be used to refer to the entire complex of dissociated deviations, and subdivided into its vertical (DVD), horizontal (DHD), and torsional (DTD) axes when patient examination data are recorded. Latent nystagmus should be included as part of the complex. DSC does not occur in patients with macular binocular vision and high-grade stereopsis.

Chapter 41

Botulinum Toxin in Strabismus

Eric Crouch (USA)

Introduction

Botulinum toxin (Botox) has been used in a variety of conditions since 1989. The first report of extraocular muscle paralysis using botox was reported by Scott in 1973. Botox is a neurotoxin derived from the gram-negative anaerobic bacteria, Clostridium botulinum. Over the past 30 years, botox has been investigated in horizontal and vertical strabismus, nystagmus and dissociated vertical deviation. There have also been investigations regarding the management of patients with external ophthalmoloplegia and paradoxical diplopia. Botox administration is a treatment option in a variety of strabismus cases. In general, current clinical recommendations regarding botox should be considered in the context of few available comparative studies. In select cases, botox is a reasonable and at times preferable alternative to surgery. Few reports provide direct comparison of botox versus strndard strabismus surgery.

Clinical Signs and Symptoms

Botox has been utilized in a number of different clinical scenarios, with varying success. In cases of chronic cranial nerve palsy, optimal return of function can be difficult. In some cases, botox can prevent muscle contracture prior to deviation stabilization or improvement. In the acute phase, particularly for cranial nerve VI palsies, botox injection may restore fusion and prevent medial rectus contracture. Cranial nerve III palsies may also be managed with botox injections. As with cranial nerve VI palsies, the goal is to prevent muscle contracture of the antagonist muscle while waiting for spontaneous recovery of the affected muscle. The best indication of botox injection is when the paresis persists or progresses over a 4-week period.

Botox has also been utilized in cases of horizontal strabismus. Some surgeons offer botox injections as another option for surgical correction. In cases of consecutive strabismus following initial strabismus surgery, botox has been used to improve ocular alignment, though success rates are generally lower than traditional surgery. Botox has also been performed for both esotropia and exotropia.

There have even been studies using botox for vertical strabismus. For hypertropia, the superior rectus may be injected, though maximal effect is usually accomplished by also injecting the inferior oblique. Superior rectus injection should be avoided in the amblyogenic period due to the risk of deprivation amblyopia.

Botox has also been attempted in cases of paradoxical diplopia, sensory strabismus, dissociated vertical deviation, and nystagmus. In general, most cases have limited long-term success compared to traditional strabismus surgery. However, there are few comparative studies between botox applications and traditional strabismus surgery.

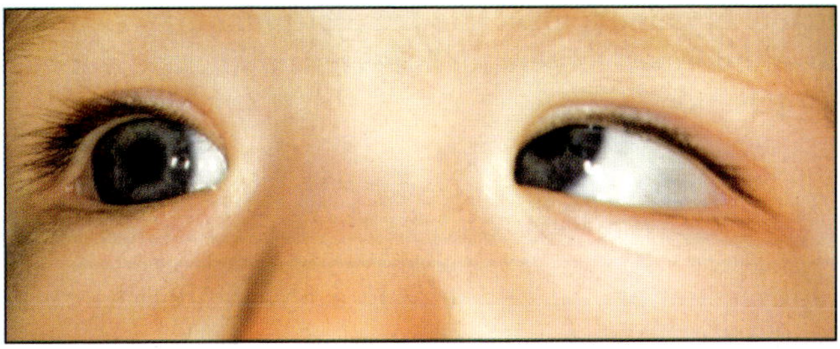

Figure 1: Child with acute cranial VI palsy following upper respiratory infection with amblyopia in the left eye and loss of stereopsis

Investigations

In general, botox has limited benefit for large angle-strabismus or dissociated vertical strabismus. Additionally, there is generally no significant benefit for most cases of ophthalmoplegia, whether external or internal ophthalmoplegia. In paradoxical diplopia, botox can sometimes be beneficial. Most cases of paradoxical diplopia achieve only temporary improvement in diplopia. The same temporary benefit applies to select cases of nystagmus. In cases undergoing strabismus surgery, some surgeons will temporarily augment the surgical dose through the application of botox. Surgical augmentation can be provided a temporal period during which stereopsis may develop as the paralytic effect diminishes.

Treatment

Botulinum injection can be performed as an outpatient procedure in adults and has the potential to reduce misalignment. Botox may be performed on cases unable to undergo general anesthesia, paralytic strabismus, strabismus angles of less than 40 prism diopters, postoperative consecutive strabismus, and difficult strabismus cases with multiple prior surgeries. Botox can also prove useful in patients with active thyroid orbitopathy. Botox is less successful in cases of the vertical strabismus as listed previously.

Precautions

The risk profile for botulinum is generally low. Some of the disadvantages to botox treatments include multiple repeat injections, temporary improvement, diplopia, sensory disorientation, and temporary overcorrection due to underaction of the paralyzed muscle. Periocular injection carries the risk of globe trauma, globe perforation, extraocular muscle damage, chronic pupillary dilation from damaged pupillary fibers, retrobulbar hemorrhage, changes in eyelid position, and injection-site reaction. There may also be inadvertent administration of botulinum toxin into the orbicularis and levator muscle with resultant ptosis. Informed consent for botox should include discussion of these potential complications.

Prognosis

Botulinum administration can be useful in a few strabismus cases. Surgeons may wish to discuss botox treatment alternatives with some patients. Many strabismus cases will remain surgically managed because botulinum generally requires more interventions than traditional surgery. Currently, based on available literature, the best treatment modality for congenital esotropia remains surgical correction. With respect to sixth nerve palsies, cases of acquired palsy are generally conservatively managed with observation for 6 months. However, in patients with loss of stereopsis or development of amblyopia, botulinum may be used to temporarily correct the misalignment without muscle surgery. Botox may also provide symptomatic relief of double vision for older patients with cranial nerve VI palsies. For patients with nystagmus, botulinum administration may be offered as a trial or ongoing treatment to improve visual acuity when other treatment options fail. Select cases such as postoperative overcorrection and augmentation of strabismus surgery can also sometimes benefit from botox treatments. Overall, most surgeons continue to employ traditional strabismus surgery rather than botox injections. The disadvantages associated with botulinum, especially ptosis, should be carefully considered particularly during the amblyogenic period.

Section 2

Posterior Segment

Chapter 42

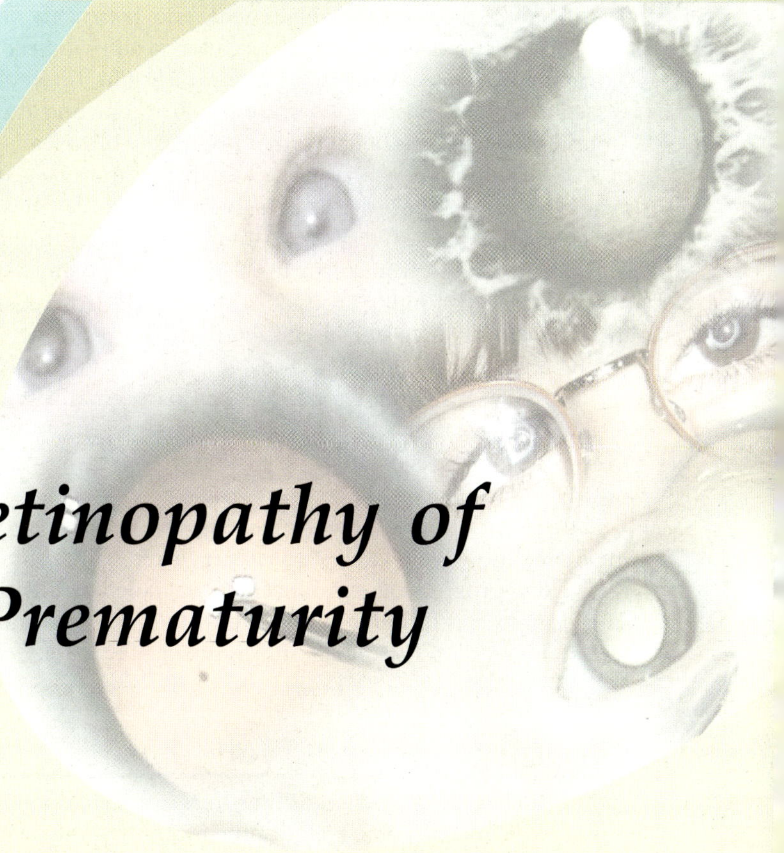

Retinopathy of Prematurity

Ronald GW Teed (USA)

Introduction

Terry first described in 1942 the end-stage sequelae of a disease process that would later be called retinopathy of prematurity (ROP). Over the following half-century, the clinical characteristics and pathophysiology of ROP were elucidated. Recently, the International Classification of Retinopathy of Prematurity and two large multi-centered clinical trials have defined the classification, diagnosis, management, and prognosis of ROP.

ROP is caused by abnormal vascular proliferation in response to hypoxia. Normal retinal vasculogenesis begins around 16 weeks gestation, and the vessels reach the nasal ora serrata by 36 weeks and the temporal ora serrata around 40 weeks. It is believed that premature birth leads to the clinical changes of ROP through a two-phase process. In the first phase, the developing retinal vasculature is exposed to excessive ex-utero oxygen levels. This relative hyperoxia suppresses vascular growth factors and results in vaso-obliteration. This phase occurs from birth to 30-32 weeks postmenstrual age (PMA). The second phase, beginning around 32-34 weeks PMA, is characterized by hypoxia-induced proliferative neovascularization. The resulting vascular abnormalities can be observed by the clinician.

The major risk factor for acute ROP is prematurity, as measured by birth weight and gestational age. In the developed world, ROP is usually observed in premature infants with a birth weight less than 1000 grams and/or a postmenstrual age of 31 weeks or less.

Supplemental oxygen exposure was early on shown to increase ROP incidence; however, later studies suggested that supplemental oxygen may retard ROP progression. A multicenter trial failed to fully support this conclusion. The dynamic relationship between oxygen supplementation and ROP is uncertain, as both hyperoxia and hypoxia play a role in ROP pathogenesis.

Clinical Signs and Symptoms

Acute ROP is described according to the international classification of ROP. The classification scheme includes the location of the disease, the severity of the disease, the extent of disease, and the presence or absence of plus disease. The location is determined by dividing the retina into three zones centered on the optic disk. Zone I consists of a circle with a radius twice the distance between the optic disk and fovea. Zone II consists of the surrounding area with a radius from the optic disk to the nasal ora serrata. The remaining crescent is Zone III.

ROP disease severity is described by five stages. ROP generally progresses sequentially through these stages; however, severe posterior (Zone I) disease may proceed directly to an advanced stage from immature retina. Stage 1 describes a flat, thin demarcation line separating vascular from avascular retina. Stage 2 consists of a ridge of fibrous tissue with width and height. Stage 3 is characterized by extraretinal neovascularization extending from the ridge into the vitreous. Stage 4 disease is a partial retinal detachment, either extrafoveal (4A) or foveal (4B). Total retinal detachment, which can be open or narrow,

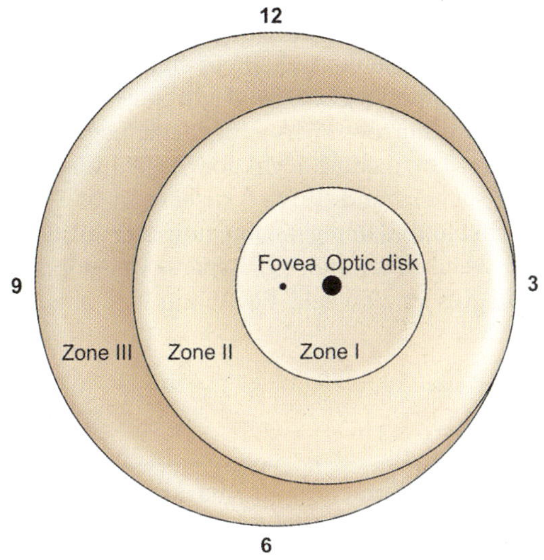

Figure 1: Zone diagram of the retina of the right eye, based on the ICROP guidelines

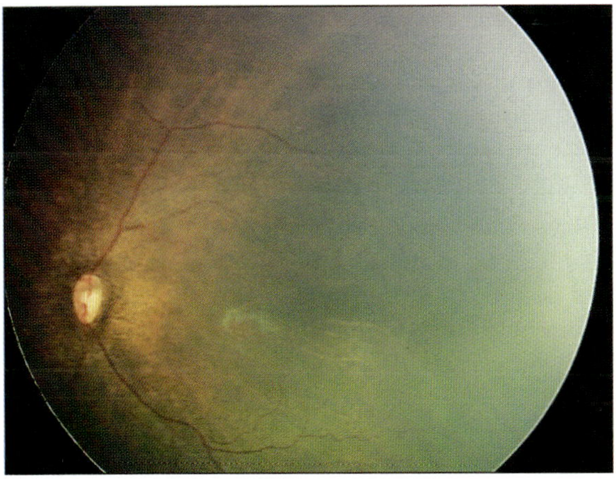

Figure 2: Stage 1 ROP. A demarcation line can be appreciated in at the vascular-avascular interface in zone I

defines Stage 5 ROP. The extent of acute ROP is noted as the number of clock hours of involvement.

Plus disease is a measure of vascular activity. Venous dilatation and arteriolar tortuosity of the posterior pole vessels of sufficient severity in at least two quadrants are classified as plus disease. Other signs of plus disease are vascular engorgement of the iris, pupil rigidity, and vitreous haze.

ROP develops over a narrow PMA range, and usually progresses through the stages sequentially. The median PMA for Stage 1 disease is 34 weeks, with Stage 2 disease at 35 weeks and Stage 3 disease at 36 weeks. Stage 1 and 2 diseases have a high likelihood of regression; however, around 20% of premature infants with a birth weight less than 1251 grams develop severe disease. ROP regression usually begins by 39 weeks PMA, and 90% of cases show involution before 44 weeks PMA.

Investigations

Our knowledge of ROP risk factors and natural history allow us to define appropriate screening guidelines to evaluate premature infants. ROP examinations require skill with indirect ophthalmoscopy and 360 degrees of scleral depression to fully examine the retina.

In the United States, premature infants less than 1500 grams or born at less than 31 weeks PMA should be screened for ROP. Premature infants with a birth weight 1500-2000 grams, or born after 31 weeks PMA may also be examined if they have had an unstable clinical course. A review of natural history data from two large multicenter clinical trials of ROP recommended that eye examinations begin at 31 weeks PMA or 4 weeks chronological age, whichever is later. Examinations should continue until the retinal vasculature is fully developed or the risk of severe ROP is negligible. This occurs when the infant has reached 45 weeks PMA without prethreshold ROP or when the retinal vessels have reached zone III without previous zone II ROP. Examinations should occur every two weeks, except in cases at high risk for progression. This includes zone I disease or zone II stage 3 disease.

Screening guidelines vary by location, as medical systems have different neonatal care that impacts ROP risk. The guidelines in the United Kingdom roughly correspond to those in the United States; however, they suggest expanding the criteria to include infants born less than 32 weeks PMA. Guidelines for low- and middle-income countries are not developed fully as ROP incidence and severity varies widely.

The standard of care for ROP examination is a complete anterior segment and retinal examination by an ophthalmologist trained in ROP diagnosis and management. National and regional shortages in qualified ophthalmologists have led to the development of remote digital imaging as an alternative. Remote diagnosis has been shown to be useful and cost-effective in the diagnosis of ROP but the routine use of telemedicine in ROP management currently is not recommended.

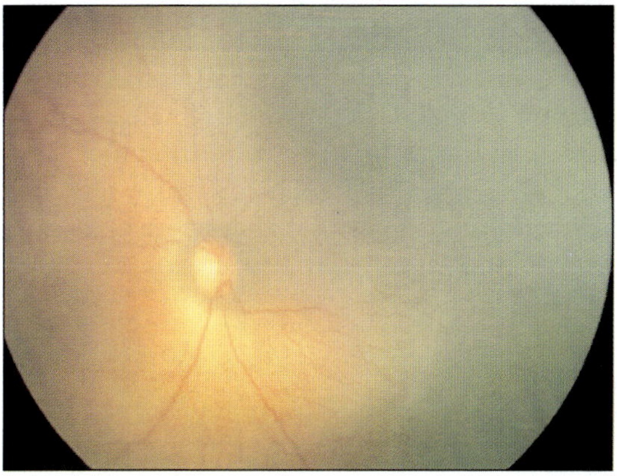

Figure 3: Stage 2 ROP. A thickened ridge can be appreciated in zone I

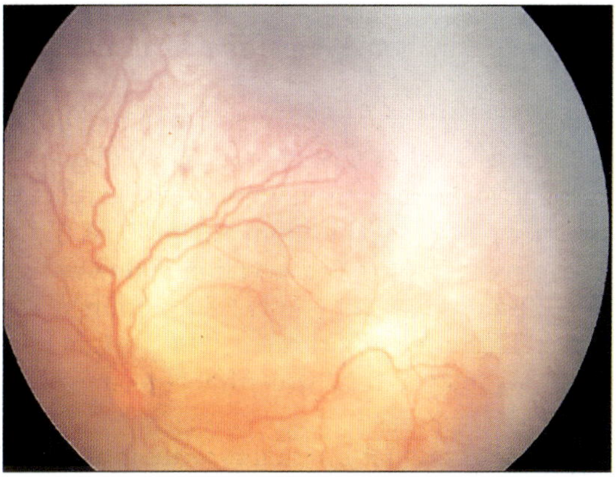

Figure 4: Stage 3 ROP. Florid neovascularization is present

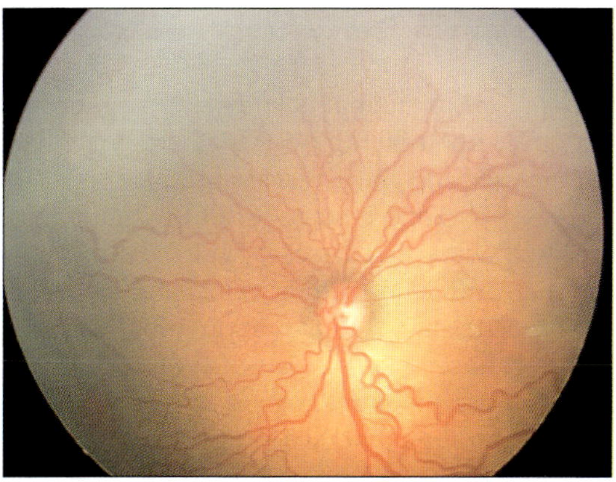

Figure 5: Severe plus disease in a patient with aggressive posterior ROP

Differential Diagnosis

Acute ROP is rarely confused with other retinal vascular diseases, particularly in the premature infant. Familial exudative vitreoretinopathy can present with areas of peripheral avascular retina, vascular dilatation and tortuosity, and vitreoretinal traction. Incontenti pigmenti can cause retinal vascular changes and vitreoretinal traction; however, the characteristic skin lesions make the diagnosis clear. Norrie disease can cause severe vitreoretinal dysplasia, but is rarely confused with ROP.

Prognosis

The outcome of premature infants with ROP depends on the severity of disease. Mild disease tends to regress spontaneously with little sequelae. Rarely, ROP can progress to advanced stages and cause retinal detachment, retinal folds, macular ectopia, and severe vision loss. In cases of severe retinopathy, significant structural and functional impairment can occur even if therapy is initiated.

Two large multicenter trials were conducted to determine timing of therapy for ROP. The Multicenter Trial of Cryotherapy for Retinopathy (CRYO-ROP) prospectively determined whether cryotherapy to the peripheral avascular retina was effective in limiting poor outcomes in infants with ROP. Infants in this trial were randomized to cryotherapy or observation if they achieved "threshold" ROP, defined as 5 continuous or 8 cumulative clock hours of stage 3 in zone I or II with plus disease. This trial determined that peripheral retinal ablation effectively reduced unfavorable retinal structural outcomes and improved visual outcomes.

A significant number of premature infants without threshold may progress to have severe ROP sequelae. Therefore, the Early Treatment for Retinopathy of Prematurity Randomized Trial (ETROP) investigated the efficacy of retinal ablative therapy on less severe disease. Predominately using laser therapy, ETROP showed the benefit of earlier treatment in select cases with prethreshold disease.

The current indications for retinal ablation therapy for ROP are defined by the ETROP study. Laser phototherapy or cryotherapy should be administered when ROP has progressed to type 1 disease, defined as: (1) zone I, any stage ROP with plus disease; (2) zone I, stage 3 ROP without plus disease; and (3) zone II, stage 2 or 3 ROP with plus disease. Type 2 disease should be monitored closely for progression, and is defined as: (1) zone I, stage 1 or 2 ROP without plus disease and (2) zone II, stage 3 ROP without plus disease. Treatment should be conducted within 72 hours of diagnosis of type 1 ROP.

The standard of care for the management of severe ROP is retinal ablation. Early evidence is demonstrating that medical treatment of severe ROP, designed to mediate the hypoxia-induced neovascular response, may be useful. A multicenter clinical trial is underway to investigate this approach.

Chapter 43

Pediatric Retinal Diseases

Anjli Hussain, Nazimul Hussain
S Natarajan (India)

Best's Disease or Best's Vitelliform Macular Dystrophy

Introduction

Best's disease is inherited as an autosomal dominant disease. The true prevalence of Best's disease is unknown. It is a bilateral macular dystrophy characterized by subretinal accumulation of yellowish material in the macular area. It is slowly progressive and eventually results in retinal pigment epithelial (RPE) and photoreceptors atrophy. At the end stage, impairs severely the central vision.

Classification and Clinical Features

Stage 1: This is characterized by normal fundus finding but associated by abnormal electro-oculogram.

Stage 2 or Pre-vitelliform stage: The lesions appear as yellow subfoveal pigment disturbance associated with RPE mottling with small yellow spot.

Stage 3 or Vitellifrom stage: This is characterized by a yellow orange slightly elevated lesion. Visual acuity is maintained at this stage. This appears like a "egg yolk".

Stage 4 or Scrambled egg stage: Here, the vitelliform appearance gets ruptured and appears granular. This gives a scrambled egg appearance. Visual acuity starts reducing at this stage.

Stage 5 or Pseudohypopyon stage: Here the yellowish subretinal material collects in the inferior part of the cyst giving a pseudohypopyon appearance.

Stage 6 or Atrophic stage: Eventually the subretinal material gets absorbed and RPE atrophy occurs with minimal scarring. Visual acuity (VA) is impaired significantly at this stage.

Each patient may not follow each stage and may skip one or the other stage. Mutation in VMD 2 gene is associated with Best's disease. Most patients have VA of 20/40 or better. Despite better VA, patients complain of metamorphopsia and lacunar scotoma causing difficult reading ability. Choroidal neovascularization (CNV) may occur as a complication.

Investigations

Best's disease is characterized by normal electroretinogram (ERG) and abnormal electro-oculogram (EOG). The Arden ratio is usually greater than 1.7 on exposure to light. However, this response is blunted by changes in illumination where the ratio falls below 1.5. Dark adaptation is normal in Best's disease. In general, EOG is distinctly abnormal with complete absence of light induced rise.

Fundus fluorescein angiographic (FFA) finding depends on the stage of the disease. FFA is useful in detecting the extent RPE abnormality and presence of CNV.

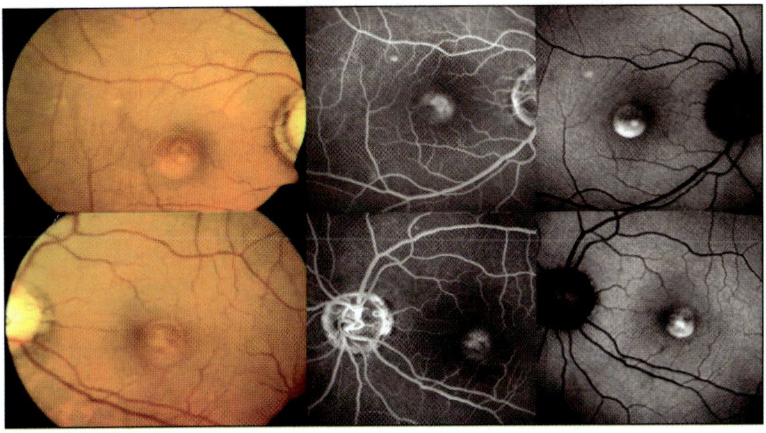

Figure 1: Shows pseudohypopyon stage in the right eye and later stage in the left eye

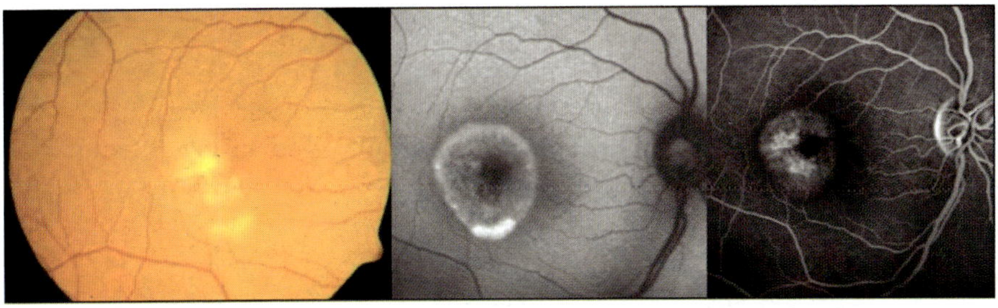

Figure 2: Shows late showing RPE atrophy and minimal scarring

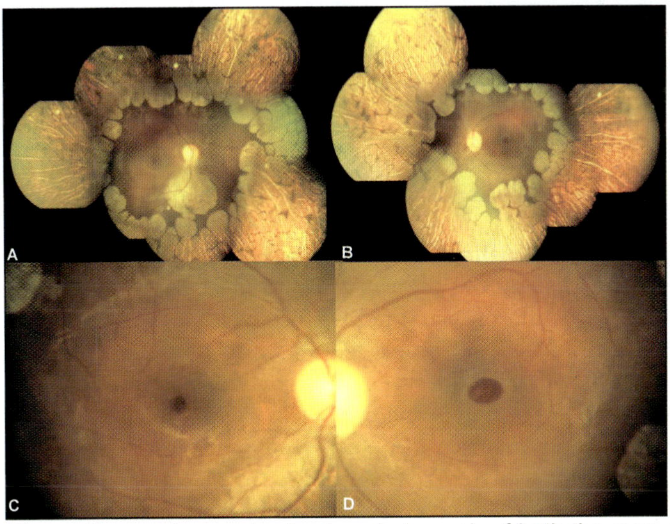

Figure 3: Shows the montage color fundus photograph of both the eyes (A and B) multiple coalescent areas of choroidal atrophy with scalloped edges. Magnified photograph of the macula shows a thin foveal roof with pseudo appearance of macular hole (C) in the right eye. The left eye showed appearance of full thickness macular hole (D)

Differential Diagnosis

1. Pattern dystrophy: They appear almost similar to Best's disease as there is a phenotypic overlap. Molecular diagnostic testing may help to differentiate between the two.
2. Stargardt's disease: They can have poor VA at early stage and usually worse in comparison to the fundus lesion. Has dark choroid or masked appearance in FFA.
3. Age-related macular degeneration (AMD): In the late stage with atrophic scar, CNV or RPE abnormality, Best's disease may simulate AMD.
4. Traumatic maculopathy.

Management

There is no definite treatment for this disorder. The management mainly includes genetic counseling and support services to improve the quality of life. When VA is impaired, low vision services is a definite advantage.

Inference

Best's disease is a abnormality of the RPE associated with accumulation of yellowish lipofuschin like material in the macula. Known genetic mutation occurs at VMD2 gene. Genetic counseling and Low vision services are essential when needed.

Gyrate Atrophy

Introduction

Gyrate atrophy of the choroid and retina is a rare autosomal recessive disorder associated with hyperornithinemia. Hyperornithinemia is due to the deficiency of ornithine aminotransferase. The precise pathomechanism is unknown.

Clinical Features

It usually presents in the first decade with night blindness and high myopia, subsequent development of posterior subcapsular cataracts by second decade, progressive constriction of visual fields, and eventual loss of central acuity in the fourth to fifth decades. Clinical features also follow a slowly progressive time course. One usually observes circular, well circumscribed regions of chorioretinal atrophy with hyperpigmented margins in the midperiphery. These regions enlarge and coalesce in a scalloped pattern, spread anteriorly and posteriorly and eventually encroach on the macula, threatening central vision.

Natural history study of gyrate atrophy has shown that central visual loss can begin at any age. Visual acuity decreased rapidly in phakic eyes within less than ten years. Even after cataract extraction, there was transient improvement of vision especially in young patients; subsequently visual loss was slow until macula was involved. The study also quotes that macular involvement is often

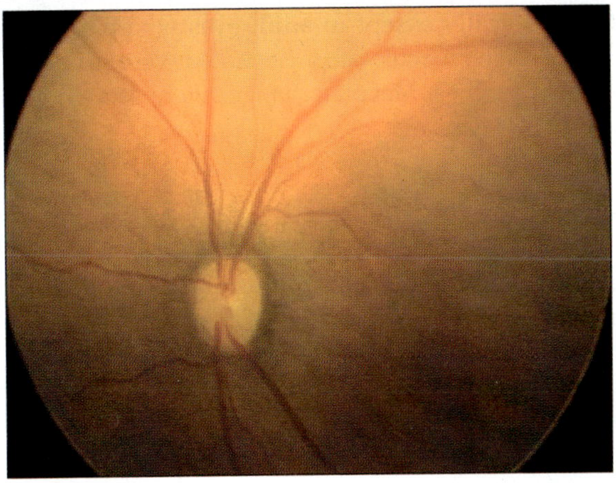

Figure 4: Showing a mature retina in a neonate *(Courtesy: Anjli Hussain, Ex. Consultant, L.V. Prasad Eye Institute, Hyderabad)*

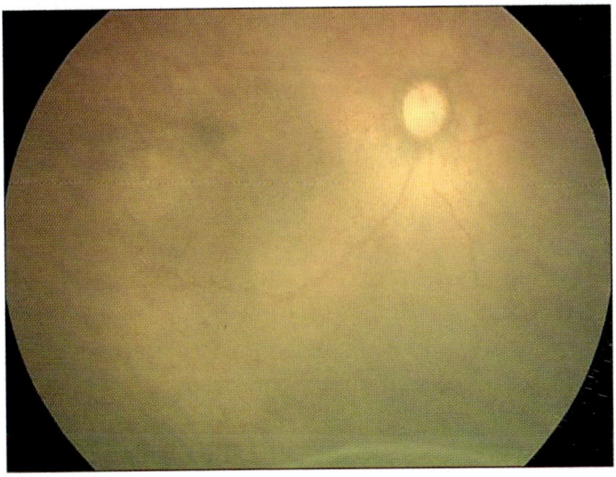

Figure 5: Showing Zone 1 immature retina *(Courtesy: Anjli Hussain, Ex. Consultant, L.V. Prasad Eye Institute, Hyderabad)*

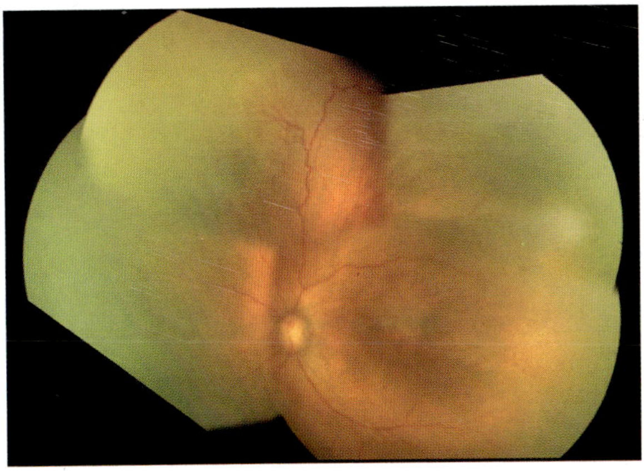

Figure 6: Showing Zone II stage 1 disease *(Courtesy: Anjli Hussain, Ex. Consultant, L.V. Prasad Eye Institute, Hyderabad)*

difficult to perceive ophthalmoscopically except in adult eyes where obvious chorioretinal atrophy could be seen. The macular changes noted were primarily pigmentary dystrophy or atrophic patches. Macular changes were seen in 30% at 20 years and 60% at the age of 30 years.

Investigations

On fundus fluorescein angiography, one may observe leakage at the margins of healthy and affected tissue, with hyperfluorescence within the gyrate lesions. Besides atrophic or pigmentary macular changes, fundus fluorescein angiography and optical coherence tomography study showed additional changes like epiretinal membranes, cystoid macular edema and macular hole. Sparsely available anecdotal reports suggest that cystoid macular edema may precede macular hole formation in eyes with gyrate atrophy. Since recent literature shows that such macular changes are seen in the younger age, it can be speculated that the atrophic changes in the macula may be a late sequelae of the same. A macular complication of foveal atrophy has also been reported. Natural history of gyrate atrophy suggests 43% macular involvement.

An electrophysiological test usually reveals early impaired scotopic and photopic responses, which becomes extinguished as the disease progresses.

Biochemical test for amino acid analysis will show increase plasma ornithine level.

Treatment

Therapeutic regimen is directed towards reducing the plasma ornithine level. In majority of the patients, a diet low in arginine results in lower plama ornithine level. In pyridoxine responsive individuals, vitamin B_6 may be tried.

Differential Diagnosis

1. Retinitis pigmentosa
2. Other causes of night blindness

Inference

Gyrate atrophy is a rare autosomal recessive disorder associated with hyperornithinemia. Amino acid analysis for plasma ornithine level is essential to restrict arginine free diet.

Retinopathy of Prematurity

Introduction

Retinopathy of prematurity (ROP) is a potentially blinding eye disorder that primarily affects premature infants weighing 1250 grams or less, that are born before 31 weeks of gestation (A full-term pregnancy has a gestation of 38–42 weeks). The smaller an infant is at birth, the more likely that infant will develop

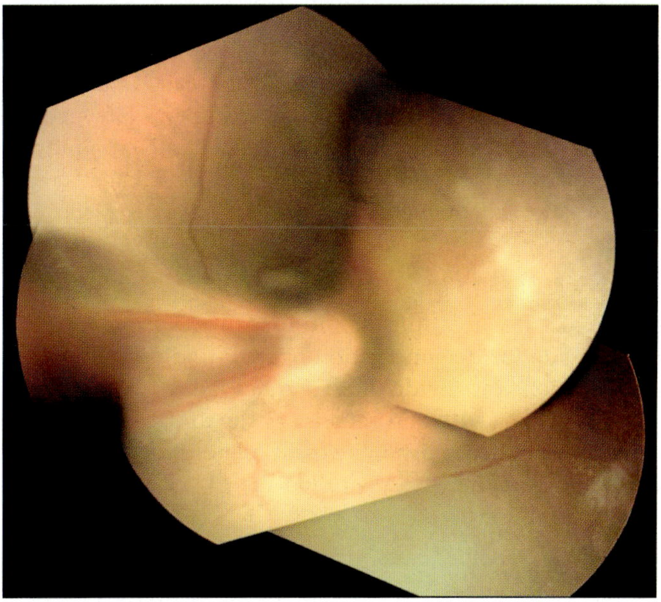

Figure 7: Showing Stage 4b ROP. Note the macular detachment and the falciform fold. *(Courtesy: Anjli Hussain, Ex. Consultant, L.V. Prasad Eye Institute, Hyderabad)*

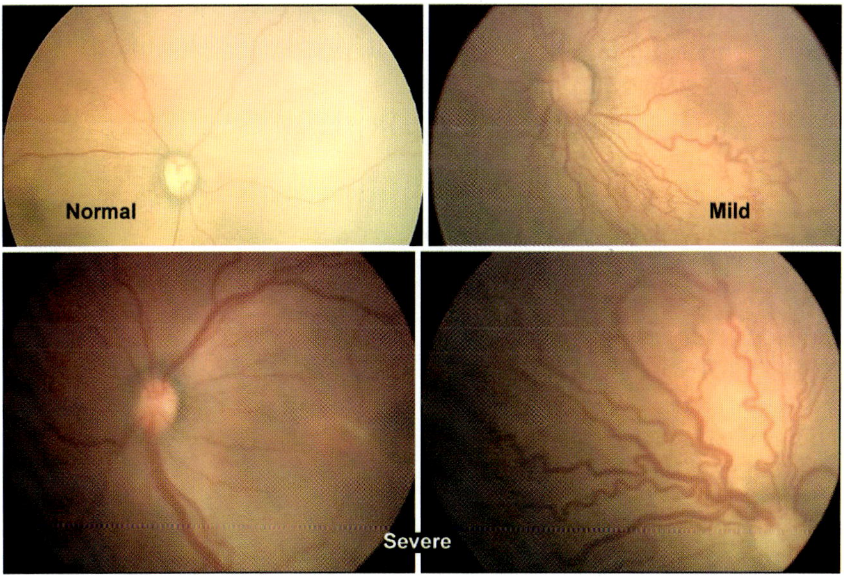

Figure 8: Showing various grades of Plus disease. *(Courtesy: Anjli Hussain, Ex. Consultant, L.V. Prasad Eye Institute, Hyderabad)*

ROP. The incidence of ROP worldwide ranges from 21.3 to 64.5%, and the estimated incidence in India is 38 - 42.3%. The disease improves and leaves no permanent damage in milder cases of ROP. About 90% of all infants with ROP are in the milder category and do not need treatment. However, infants with more severe disease can develop impaired vision or even blindness. ROP is a multifactorial disease. Low birth weight, low gestational age and supplemental oxygen therapy following delivery have been consistently associated with ROP.

Classification and Clinical Signs

An International Classification of Retinopathy of Prematurity (ICROP) is followed worldwide for documentation of ROP findings. The antero-posterior extent or the location was divided into 3 zones (zones 1-3), the circumferential extent into clock hours (1-12) and severity of the disease in 5 stages (stage 1-5). The presence of dilated and tortuous vessels denotes an aggressive, potentially sight threatening component and is called the **PLUS** disease.

Location of the Disease (Zones)

The normal blood vessels of the retina progress from optic nerve posteriorly to the edge of the ora serrata anteriorly. The location of ROP is a measure of how far this normal progression of blood vessels has reached before the disease takes over. Three circular zones are defined with the optic disk at the center.

Zone I: This is the area around the optic nerve and the macula. The radius of zone I is equal to two times the distance between the disk and the fovea.

Zone II: This is up to ora serrata on the nasal side and up to the equator temporally.

Zone III: This is the remaining crescent of retina from the equator to the ora serrata temporally.

Extent of the Disease (clock hours)

The extent of ROP is defined by how many clock hours of the eye circumference is diseased.

Plus Disease

Plus disease is characterized by abnormal dilated vessels on the iris and/or engorgement and tortuosity of the blood vessels in the retina. Additional findings include retinal hemorrhages, poorly dilating pupil and hazy media.

Stages of the Disease (Severity)

A white line separating the clear normal red retina from the sharply contrasting underdeveloped gray retina characterizes **stage 1** ROP.

Stage 2 ROP shows a rolled ridge of scar tissue, which may be limited to a small area or encircle the entire inside of the eye, around the middle of the eye.

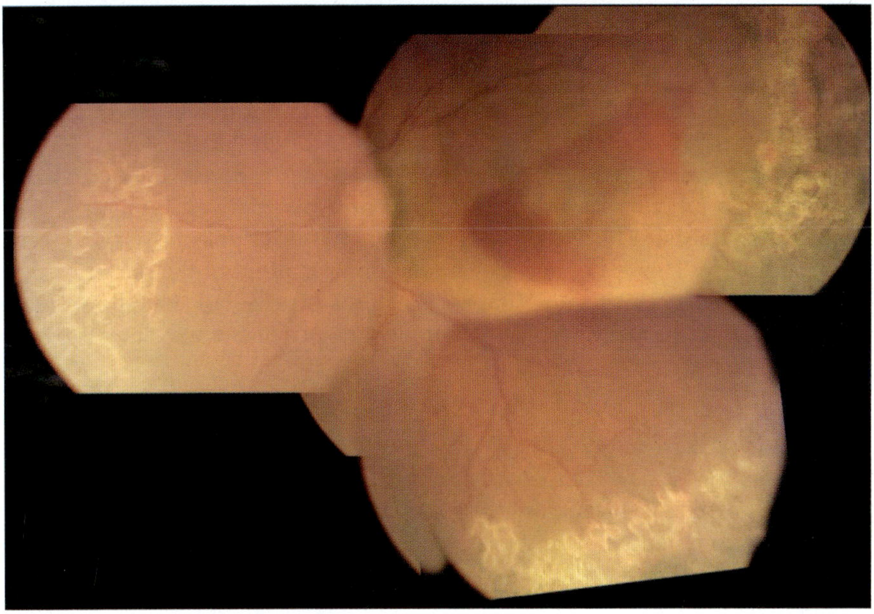

Figure 9: Showing regress ROP following laser. Note the preretinal hemorrhage. *(Courtesy: Anjli Hussain, Ex. Consultant, L.V. Prasad Eye Institute, Hyderabad)*

Stage 3 ROP is characterized by the development of abnormal new blood vessels and fibrous scar tissue on the edge of the ridge seen in stage 2. These vessels are lifted off from the surface and project into the vitreous cavity.

Stage 4 ROP occurs due to pulling of the retina by the scar tissue. As a result retina separates from the wall of the eyeball. Depending on the extent of RD stage 4 is further subdivided into Stage 4A (sparing macula) and 4B (involving macula).

Stage 5 ROP involves complete RD with the retina assuming a partial or closed funnel configuration. The infants usually develop a white reflex in the eye (leucokoria).

Rush Disease

This is zone1 ROP with plus disease. In this the progression is rapid and fulminant. In this new vessels are initially flat and in groups and later tend to get elevated into the vitreous cavity and may rapidly progress in nasal retina. This is also termed ***Fulminant ROP/Type II ROP or Posterior Zone I ROP***.

Threshold ROP is defined as zone I or II ROP stage 3 more than 5 contiguous or 8 cumulative clock hours with plus disease present. **Pre-threshold ROP** is defined as any stage of ROP in zone I with plus disease or ROP stage 3 with plus disease with 3 contiguous or 5 interrupted clock hours of retinal involvement in zone II but less than threshold.

A. **Aggressive posterior ROP:** This is most virulent form of ROP observed in the tiniest of babies. This is new terminology for Rush disease or type 2 fulminant ROP where posterior pole vessels show increased dilatation and tortousity in all 4 quadrants out of proportion to peripheral retinopathy. It progresses rapidly and does not progress through classic stages 1-3 and may appear only as a flat network of neovascularization at the deceptively featureless junction of vascularized and non-vascularized retina.
B. **Pre-plus disease:** This is in between normal posterior pole vessels and frank plus disease. This is defined as vascular abnormalities of the posterior pole that are insufficient for the diagnosis of plus disease but that shows more arterial tortuosity and venous dilatation than normal and may later progress to plus disease.

Screening for ROP (Investigations)

Proper planning is a key component of efficient screening in a neonatal intensive care unit (NICU). The screening protocol at each NICU should be based on published recommendation and preferences of screening ophthalmologists and neonatologists.

In Indian population, significant number of infants fall outside the screening criteria than the high income group countries, so screening criteria suiting Indian population were proposed as follows:

1. Birth weight of less than or equal to 1700 grams.
2. Gestational age at birth of less than or equal to 34-35 weeks.
3. Exposed to oxygen for more than 30 days.
4. infants weighing less than 1200 grams at birth and those born at 24-30 weeks gestational age are at particular high risk of not only developing ROP but also developing it earlier, in more aggressive form. Hence, definite need to screen these babies at the earliest
5. Other factors that can increase the risk of ROP and where the screening should be considered are other premature babies (<37 weeks and/or <2000 grams) with:
   - Respiratory distress syndrome
   - Sepsis
   - Multiple blood transfusions
   - Multiple birth (twins/triplets)
   - Apneic episodes
   - Intraventricular hemorrhage
   - Pediatricians has index of concerns for ROP.

Time for Screening the Infants at Risk

Screen all eligible babies at:

- 31 weeks PCA or 3-4 weeks after birth, whichever is earlier.
- Infants weighing less than 1200 grams at birth and those born at 24-30 weeks gestational age are screened early, usually not later than 2-3 weeks after birth.

- No examination needed in first 2 weeks of birth
- Next date of examination to be decided by the ophthalmologist based on initial findings
- Complete one screening session definitely before **Day 30** of life

Ideally, a fixed time should be arranged for screening. Dilatation can be started by the NICU staff, 15-20 minutes before arrival of the Ophthalmologist. Babies, should be evaluated in an appropriate temperature controlled, clean environment where risk of hypothermia, infections and apnea are minimum. For in-patients in NICU, the screening can be done in temperature-controlled environment of the incubator. The room illumination should be low to avoid glare and annoying reflexes during examination with the indirect ophthalmoscope and viewing lens.

The child should be fed and burped preferably an hour before examination so as to minimize the risk of vomiting after instillation of drops. The pupils are dilated using 0.5-1% tropicamide and 2.5% phenylephrine instilled twice 10 minutes apart, about 15-20 minutes before the due time of evaluation. Due to small size of the palpebral fissure, detailed examination may require use of a self-retaining pediatric size wire speculum. A wire vectis or a pediatric depressor is useful to stabilize the globe and visualize the periphery.

Differential Diagnosis

1. Familial Exudative Vitreoretinopathy (FEVR)
   - Mostly autosomal dominant and observed in full term infant
   - Avascular peripheral retina with associated changes with progression of the disease. They are vascular buds at the junction of the vascular and avascular retina, dragging of vessels in the posterior pole and retina folds
   - Often associated with subretinal exudates and advanced disease can lead to total retina detachment.
2. Congenital Falciform fold
3. Incontinentia pigmenti
   - 33% have ocular defects
   - Associated with retinal hypopigmentation, peripheral nonperfusion with intravitreal neovascularization (important finding), retinal detachment, microphthalmia, cataracts and strabismus
   - Systemic affections: Cutaneous (100%), CNS and structural.
4. Toxocara canis infection
   - Parasitic infection of the eye and are mostly unilateral
   - Posterior segment findings: Peripheral granuloma, posterior pole granuloma, chronic endophthalmitis.
   - Peripheral retinal locations is most common
5. Causes of leukocoria: this represents Stage 5 ROP

Treatment

The indications for treatment of threshold ROP (5 or more contiguous or 8 cumulative clock hours of stage 3+ ROP either in Zone I or Zone II) were initially proposed by the CRYO-ROP study for those stages of the disease that are likely to result in adverse visual outcomes. The ETROP study proposes newer criteria for early treatment of eyes that have more than 15% risk of adverse outcomes. Retinal ablation should be considered for any eye with type 1 ROP that includes the following:

1. Zone I, any stage ROP with plus disease.
2. Zone I, stage 3 ROP with or without plus disease
3. Zone II, Stage 2 or 3 ROP with plus disease.

Plus disease is defined in this case as at least 2 quadrants of dilation and tortuosity of the posterior retinal blood vessels. The treatment should be done at the earliest, preferably within 24 hours and not later than 72 hours. The aim of treatment is to ablate the whole of the avascular retina as rapidly and completely as possible with minimum side effects. Treatment for acute ROP can be done either by laser photoablation or cryotherapy. Laser effect is usually apparent within one week of adequate laser therapy. An alternate to cryotherapy and LIO ablation is to use a transconjunctivo-scleral laser diopexy. The main indication for the use of TCSDL is for initial management of severe cases of threshold ROP in situations where LIO is difficult or unavailable. Disadvantages of cryotherapy can be circumvented.

Signs that indicate disease has reached a quiescent phase of acute ROP after retinal ablation include:

- *Pupil dilates well*
- *There is no rubeosis*
- *Media is clear*
- *Vascular dilatation and tortuosity are absent*
- *Feeder vessels to proliferation/ hemorrhages are 'silent' and not dilated or tortuous*
- *No increase in traction*
- *All elevated focal areas have an avascular base with no feeder vessels.*

Lens sparing vitrectomy and scleral buckle have been used to manage stage 4A ROP. Lens sparing vitreous surgery can interrupt progression of ROP from Stage 4A to stages 4B or 5 by directly addressing transvitreous traction resulting from fibrous proliferation. The surgical goal for stage 5 ROP is to reattach as much as retina as possible. Form vision can be preserved following vitrectomy for stage 5 ROP.

Inferences

Start screening for ROP between 20 to 30 days of life, earlier (20 days) for smaller babies (less than 30 weeks gestational age and 1500 grams birth weight). One screening session should be completed before Day 30 of life. The critical factor to ensure better outcomes are to screen early, follow-up weekly or more closely, watch out for Plus and/or new vessels and treat such eyes vigorously for full retinal ablation of avascular retina. ROP is a continuous race against time with a very small window of opportunity of 7-10 days where optimum treatment outcomes with least complications can be achieved. Surgical interventions offer the potential for preservation of vision for eyes with ROP related retinal detachment; especially if it is directed prior to macular distortion.

Chapter 44

Pediatric Retinal Detachment

Rajvardhan Azad, Bhuvan Chanana (India)

Introduction

Pediatric retinal detachment is a rare entity but an important cause of visual loss in children. Trauma is the most common cause of retinal detachment in this age group. Apart from trauma, there are several causes but prominent among them are persistent hyperplastic primary vitreous (PHPV), iridofundal coloboma, retinopathy of prematurity, hereditary familial vitreoretinopathies etc.

Classification of Pediatric Retinal Detachment

1. Retinal detachment without systemic associations.
2. Retinal detachment with systemic associations.
3. Retinal detachment associated with optic nerve anomalies.
4. Miscellaneous syndromes.

Retinal Detachment without Systemic Associations

Persistent Hyperplastic Primary Vitreous (PHPV)

PHPV is a sporadic, usually unilateral disorder characterized by abnormal regression of the primary vitreous and fetal vascular system encasing the posterior surface of the lens. This gives rise to a fibrovascular stalk originating from the optic disk and joining the posterior lens capsule. PHPV is not associated with systemic manifestations. Typically the child presents with leukocoria, microphthalmous or both.

Both an anterior and posterior variant exist. The purely posterior form exists in only 10 to 20% of cases. Manifestations of either variant are highly varied, and overlap between them occurs.

Anterior PHPV: Anterior manifestations include persistent pupillary membrane, tunica vasculosa lentis and iridohyaloid blood vessels. Clinically, it appears as a pinkish-white retrolental fibrovascular membrane of variable size found centered just nasal to the central axis of the lens. The ciliary processes are drawn towards the retrolenticular membrane. Over time the membrane contracts, which pushes the iris-lens diaphragm anteriorly, thus shallowing the anterior chamber and may lead to angle closure glaucoma. An associated dehiscence of the posterior lens capsule may lead to cataract.

Posterior PHPV: Posterior manifestations include persistence of the hyaloid artery, Bergmeister papilla, macular and optic nerve head hypoplasia. In the pure posterior form the lens is clear and ciliary processes are normal. The hallmark is a white opaque membrane or a non-opaque retinal fold, extending from the optic disk to the peripheral retina or retrolental area. The traction causes progressive detachment of the retina.

Anterior segment surgery involving lensectomy prevents the development of angle closure glaucoma and improves visual prognosis. The prognosis is poor in cases of significant retinal detachment. It is technically difficult to release the retinal traction and flatten the retina. Iatrogenic breaks may occur leading to

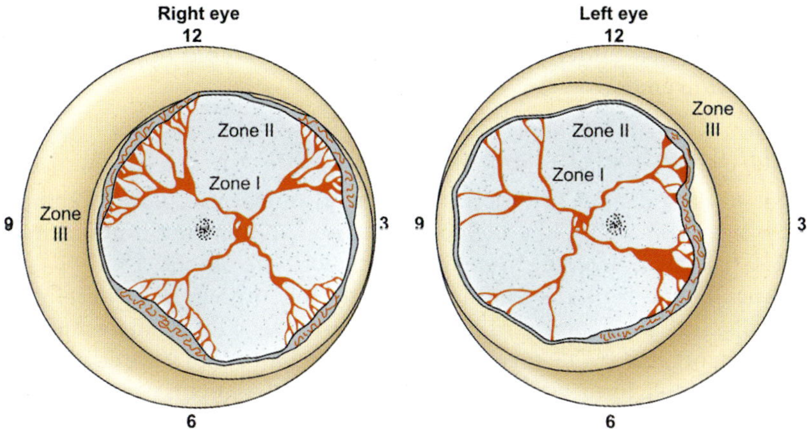

Figure 1: Three zones of ROP

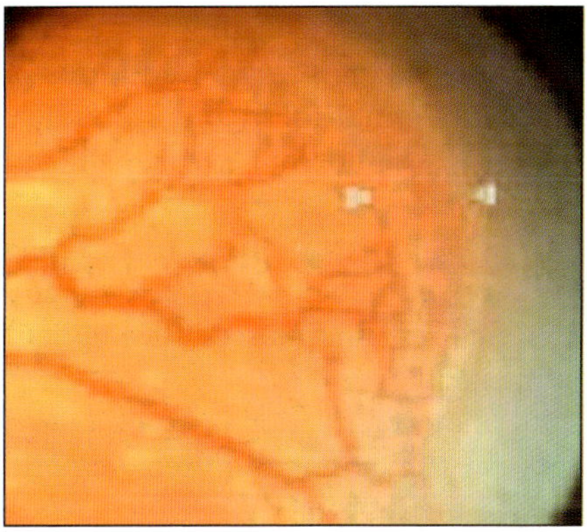

Figure 2: Stage 3 ROP

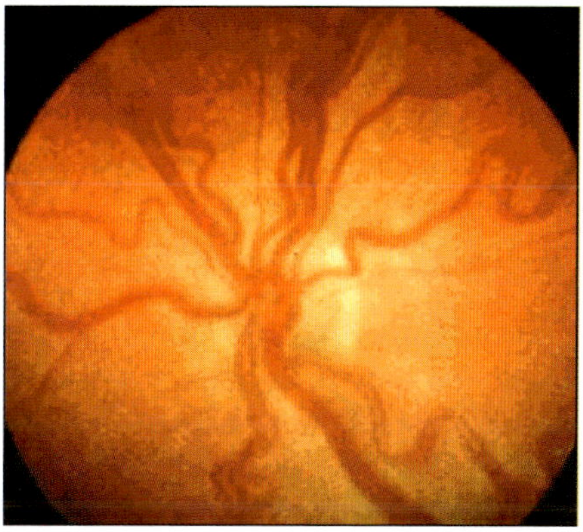

Figure 3: Plus disease in ROP

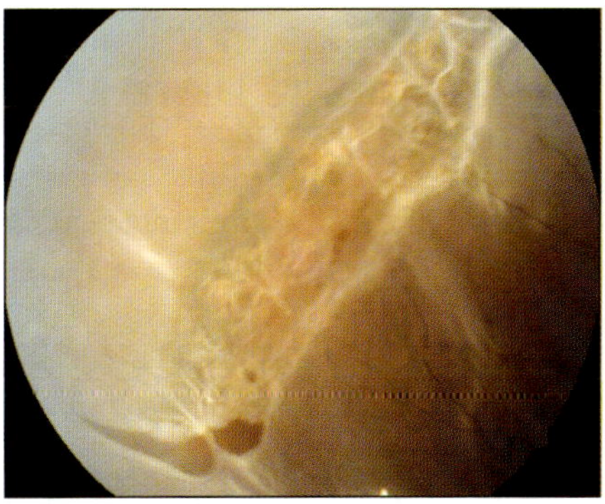

Figure 4: Fundus photograph showing lattice degeneration with break at the edge

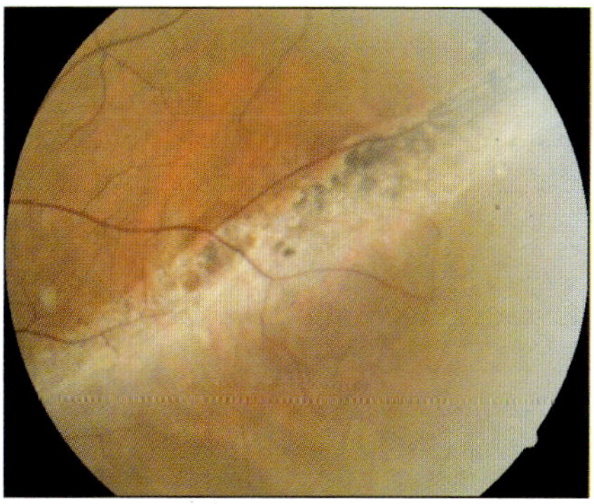

Figure 5: Fundus photograph showing lattice degeneration with atrophic holes

rhegmatogenous RD and hypotony further complicating the disease. Hence, surgery should be undertaken only in cases with simple retinal traction or bilateral involvement.

Familial Exudative Vitreoretinopathy (FEVR)

FEVR is a rare bilateral disorder of peripheral retinal vascular development. FEVR is most commonly inherited as an autosomal dominant trait or rarely as X-linked recessive disorder. Systemic associations are absent .

Clinically the retina is characterized by incomplete peripheral retinal vascularization, particularly of the temporal retina with telangiectasias and vascular engorgement. The severity of FEVR is classified into three stages. *Stage 1* includes the mild form which reveals a peripheral avascular retina, adjacent telangiectatic vessels, arteriovenous shunts and peripheral vitreoretinal degenerations. Many cases show intraretinal crystal-like deposits in the avascular retina. *Stage 2* includes more advanced forms of FEVR showing neovascularization and vascular exudation in the subretinal and intraretinal spaces. Peripheral fibrovascular mass and tractional RD with dragging of the macula and optic disk may occur. *Stage 3* includes the most advanced forms of FEVR with frank tractional RD associated with retinal folds and secondary rhegmatogenous RD. Other features are vitreous hemorrhage, rubeosis and neovascular glaucoma.

The retinal manifestations are similar to ROP, however, the course differs and also there is no history of premature birth or supplemental oxygen therapy in neonatal period. The retinal vasculopathy may remain quiescent throughout childhood only to become active during adulthood.

Early stages of the disease are treated with photocoagulation or cryotherapy. Retinal detachments are difficult to treat. Scleral buckling with vitrectomy and removal of the membranes is required to attach the retina.

Coat's Disease

Coat's disease (Leber's miliary aneurysms or congenital retinal telangiectasias) is a developmental anomaly of the retinal vasculature consisting of telangiectatic leaking vessels associated with subretinal lipid exudation. Etiology of the disease is unknown with no genetic, familial or racial predisposition. The disease affects males 3 times more than females and is unilateral in over 80% of cases. Two-thirds of patients present in the 1st decade of life with complaints of poor vision, strabismus or leukocoria. However, cases have been reported in patients as young as 4 months and also in patients in the 7th decade of life.

The hallmarks of the disease are aneurysms and telangiectasias involving the retinal arteries, capillaries and veins. These abnormal vessels are incompetent and leaky giving rise to lipid-rich yellow subretinal exudation. Intraretinal and vitreous hemorrhages also may be present. Usually the vascular abnormalities are in the retinal periphery with the exudates forming some distant away. The clinical course is variable, but generally progressive if untreated. Spontaneous remissions have been reported.

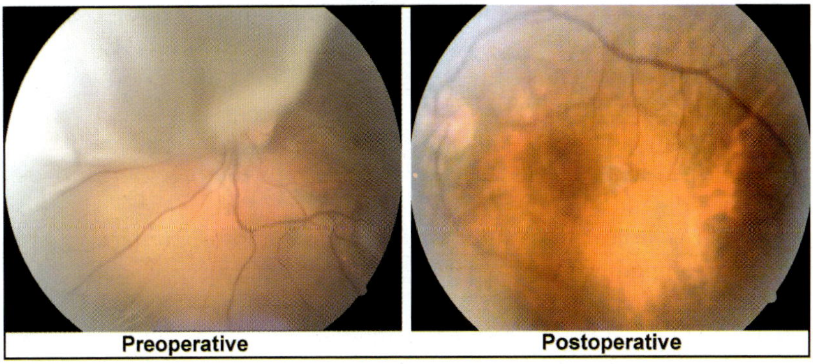

Figure 6: Fundus photograph showing attached retina following scleral buckling

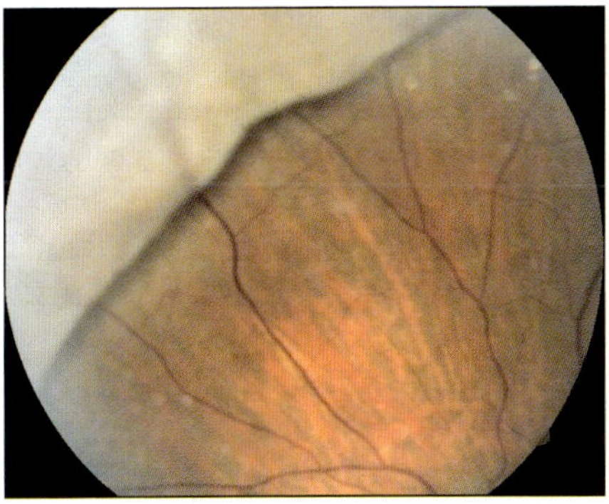

Figure 7: Fundus photograph showing attached retina with buckle indent following scleral buckling

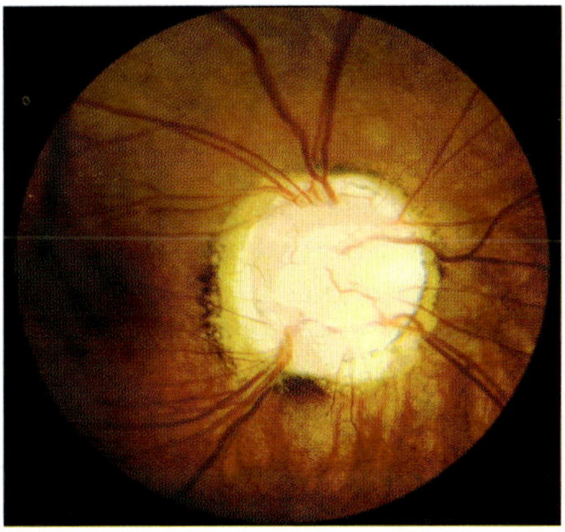

Figure 8: Morning glory disk anomaly

As subretinal exudation increases, exudative RD develops. Eyes with advanced Coat's disease may develop secondary complications such as iridocyclitis, rubeosis, cataract, neovascular, glaucoma and eventually phthsis bulbi in severe cases.

Fluorescein angiography shows peripheral retinal vascular anomalies and is useful for treatment. Fluorescein can be given orally thus avoiding intravenous injection in the child.

Treatment is indicated if exudation is extensive and progressive or if central vision is threatened. The goal of treatment is to preserve visual acuity and eliminate vascular exudation. Less severe cases are treated with laser photocoagulation. A dense scatter is applied to the involved areas. Anterior lesions may be treated with cryoablation. Advanced cases with retinal detachment may be treated with scleral buckling or vitrectomy.

Retinopathy of Prematurity (ROP)

Retinopathy of prematurity was previously called as retrolental fibroplasias. ROP is a proliferative retinopathy of premature and low-birth-weight infants. ROP is an important cause of visual loss in this age group.

Normal retinal vascularization proceeds from the optic disk to the periphery and is complete in the nasal quadrants at approximately 36 weeks of gestation and on the temporal side at 40 weeks. Exposure to excessive concentrations of oxygen during this period can lead to an injury that results in arrest of vascular development, obliteration of newly formed capillaries, and formation of arteriovenous shunt in the eye.

Low birth weight and short gestational age are the principal risk factors for ROP. Other risk factors are exposure to supplemental oxygen, sepsis, blood transfusion, nutritional deficiencies and cardiac defects.

The Joint Statement of the American Academy of Pediatrics; the American Association for Pediatric Ophthalmology and Strabismus; and the American Academy of Ophthalmology recommends at least 2 dilated fundus examination for all infants with a birth weight of less than 1500 g or with a gestational age of 28 weeks or less, as well as for selected infants between 1500 and 2000 g with an unstable clinical course who are believed to be at high risk by their attending pediatrician. The first examination should be performed between 4 and 6 weeks of postnatal age or within the 31st to 33rd week of postconceptional age, whichever is later. Examinations are then generally performed every 1-2 weeks until retina is fully vascularized. One examination is sufficient if retina is vascularized bilaterally.

ROP is classified on four interrelated criteria: stage of the disease, location of the disease, extent and presence or absence of plus disease.

In *Stage 1* ROP, a demarcation line is present between the vacularized and nonvacularized retina, whereas in *Stage 2*, the mesenchymal ridge is elevated. *Stage 3* ROP is distinguished by extraretinal neovascularization. *Stage 4* includes subtotal retinal detachment; 4A is extrafoveal and 4B is retinal detachment involving the fovea. *Stage 5* ROP is total retinal detachment with funnel.

Three zones are described: *Zone 1* encompasses the area included in a circle twice the radius of the optic disk-to-foveola distance. *Zone 2* is the area beyond zone 1 within a circle centered on the optic disk with a radius of the distance from the optic disk to the nasal ora serrata, and *Zone 3* includes the remaining temporal crescent outside zone 1 and 2.

Extent of the disease is measured in number of clock hours of retinal involvement.

Plus disease is determined by the presence of retinal vascular dilation and tortuosity in the posterior pole. Other associated features are vitreous haze, dilated iris vessels and poor dilatation of pupils. It is indicative of an actively progressing phase of the disease. If plus disease is accompanied by vascularization ending in zone 1 or very posterior zone 2, the risk of very rapid progressive disease ("rush" disease) is significant.

Threshold disease is another important term in ROP classification. Threshold ROP as per the cryo-ROP study is the presence of at least 5 contiguous or 8 cumulative clock hours of extraretinal neovascularization in association with plus disease and location of the retinal vessels within zone 1 or 2. Treatment is indicated for threshold ROP.

ROP is a transient disease in the majority of infants, with spontaneous regression occurring in 85% of eyes. Those eyes that demonstrate progression undergo a gradual transition from the active to the cicatricial stage of ROP, which is associated with variable degree of fibrosis, contracture of proliferative tissue, and vitreous and retinal traction, macular distortion and retinal detachment.

Management as defined by Early Treatment for Retinopathy of Prematurity (ET-ROP) supports retinal ablative therapy for eyes with *Type 1 ROP*, which includes zone 1, any stage ROP with plus disease; zone 1, stage 3 ROP without plus disease; or zone 2, stage 2 or 3 ROP with plus disease. A wait-and-watch approach for *Type 2 ROP*, defined as zone 1, stage 1 or 2 without plus disease or zone 2, stage 3 ROP without plus disease.

Most ophthalmologists are now using laser therapy rather retinal cryotherapy as laser therapy is less traumatic and appears to improve the chances for a better visual outcome. The treatment is applied in a full-scatter fashion to the avascular anterior retina with the indirect ophthalmoscope.

Surgery in ROP is reserved for cases that progress to stage 4 and stage 5. Scleral buckling or a lens-sparing vitrectomy is recommended in eyes with stage 4 ROP. For eyes with stage 5 disease, vitrectomy combined with dissection of the fibrovascular membranes and adherent vitreous has been anatomically successful in approximately 30% of eyes .

Juvenile Retinoschisis

Juvenile retinoschisis or congenital hereditary retinoschisis is a rare, X-linked recessive, bilateral condition, which affects only boys. The disease presents early in life with poor vision, strabismus and nystagmus. The retinoschisis gene, XLRS 1 is mapped to X-chromosome (Xp22). The disease is characterized by splitting of the nerve fiber layer resulting in both foveal and peripheral retinal findings. The disease has no systemic associations.

Bilateral inferotemporal retinoschisis is found only in 50% of the cases, while foveal schisis is found in virtually all cases. In the fovea, early signs are slight elevation of the retina with microcystic changes and stellate maculopathy. The retinal folds radiating from the fovea give the typical spoke-wheel appearance. Peripheral schisis does not extend but may undergo the secondary changes. The inner layer, which consists only of the internal limiting membrane and retinal nerve fiber layer, may develop oval defects. In extreme cases, the defects coalesce, leaving only retinal blood vessels floating in the vitreous (vitreous veils). These vessels may give rise to recurrent vitreous hemorrhages. The vitreous is syneretic with vitreoretinal tractional bands.

Retinal detachment occurs in 16 to 20% of the cases by outer retinal breaks. The disease progresses slowly resulting in macular atrophy, diffuse chorioretinal degeneration with pigmentation similar to that seen in retinitis pigmentosa, and optic atrophy.

ERG shows marked reduction of the b-wave amplitude with normal or moderately reduced a-wave. Oscillatory potentials are absent in all cases, confirming the selective involvement of the inner retina. Visual fields show absolute scotomas corresponding to the areas of peripheral schisis.

Treatment is undertaken only when there is retinal detachment or vitreous hemorrhage. Scleral buckling is done cases of retinoschisis with RD. Vitrectomy is undertaken for cases with posterior breaks or vitreous hemorrhage.

Goldmann-Favre Syndrome

Goldmann-Favre syndrome is a rare, autosomal recessive, bilateral condition that affects both sexes equally. It exhibits features similar to juvenile retinoschisis and retinitis pigmentosa. There are no systemic associations.

The patient presents with night blindness in the first decade of life, followed by progressive loss of vision.

The characteristic ocular findings are foveal and peripheral retinoschisis similar to that found in juvenile retinoschisis. Pigmentary chorioretinal degeneration although resembles retinitis pigmentosa, is characterized by pigment spots rather than bone-spicule pattern as seen in retinitis pigmentosa. Vitreous liquefaction gives rise to an optically empty appearance.

ERG is markedly abnormal and is often unrecordable. EOG may also be abnormal. RD in these patients has a poor prognosis. Genetic counseling and family screening are essential.

Retinal Detachment with Systemic Associations

Patau' Syndrome

Trisomy 13 (Patau' syndrome) is a sporadic, bilateral disorder of ocular, cerebral and multisystemic developmental abnormalities. Ocular involvement is frequent and always bilateral.

Ocular signs include microphthalmos, coloboma, cataract, persistence of fetal vasculature and primary vitreous, and retinal detachment. Most affected infants die in the first month of life, usually from cardiovascular abnormalities.

Walker-Warburg Syndrome

Walker-Warburg syndrome is an oculocerebral disorder with ocular manifestations similar to trisomy 13 but distinguished by its autosomal recessive inheritance and distinctive cranial malformations. Ocular involvement is always bilateral, although may be asymmetric.

Ocular findings include microphthalmia, choroidal coloboma, Peter's anomaly, cataract, persistence of fetal vasculature, optic nerve hypoplasia, vitreous hemorrhage, and retinal detachment or fold.

Walker-Warburg syndrome is uniformly lethal. Death occurs in early childhood.

Norrie's Disease

Norrie's disease is a bilateral X-linked recessive syndrome of ocular dysgenesis with progressive auditory and mental impairment. The disease appears to result from fundamental developmental abnormalities of the inner layer of the optic cup.

The disease is always is bilateral and highly symmetric.

Ocular findings include bilateral total RD often present at birth. Surgical interventions have been disappointing.

Meckel's Syndrome

Meckel's syndrome is a bilateral disorder of ocular, cerebral and multisystem developmental abnormalities similar to trisomy 13 but distinguished normal chromosomal karyotype and an autosomal recessive inheritance.

Ocular findings include microphthalmia, aniridia, posterior staphyloma, persistence of the tunica vasculosa lentis, cataract, optic nerve hypoplasia, and sclerocornea.

Affected infants do not survive infancy. No treatment of ocular findings is indicated.

Incontinentia Pigmenti

Incontinentia pigmenti is an X-linked dominant disorder linked to Xp11.21 and Xq28, presenting with the triad of retinal vasculopathy, dermatological features (vesicles, whorl-like pigmentation, alopecia) and central nervous system disease (seizures and mental retardation). Ocular features are retinal neovascularization, tractional RD and vitreous hemorrhage.

Heredofamilial Vitreoretinopathies

Stickler syndrome

Stickler syndrome or hereditary arthro-ophthalmopathy is a disorder of collagen connective tissue with autosomal dominant inheritance. One of the genes implicated in Stickler syndrome, COL2A1, maps to chromosome 12q and encodes for type 2 collagen . The disease has ocular as well as systemic features which include a variable degree of orofacial abnormalities, deafness and arthropathy.

The ocular signs include an optically empty vitreous cavity due to liquefaction and syneresis, myopia, radial lattice-like degeneration, presenile cataracts, glaucoma, strabismus and retinal detachment. Retinal detachment often bilateral, develops in approximately 30% of the cases due to multiple or giant tears.

Systemic manifestations include midfacial hypoplasia and flattened nasal bridge, Pierre-Robin anomaly (micrognathia, glossoptosis, cleft soft palate and high arched palate. Skeletal involvement includes a marfanoid habitus, arthropathy and joint hyperextensibility. Deafness and mitral valve prolapse may also be present.

Retinal detachment is difficult to manage and prognosis is poor. Hence patients should be examined regularly and breaks treated prophylactically. Genetic counseling and family screening also have a major role.

Wagner's Syndrome, Jansen's Syndrome and Erosive Vitreoretinopathy

These disorders have ocular manifestations similar to Stickler's syndrome; however, it is not associated with systemic features. Wagner's syndrome is mapped to chromosome 5q. Erosive vitreoretinopathy also maps to chromosome 5 but at a different locus. The ocular features include myopia, optically empty vitreous, retinal degeneration, progressive chorioretinal atrophy and presenile cataracts. Retinal detachment is very rare in Wagner's syndrome, while rhegmatogenous and tractional RDs occur more frequently in Jansen's syndrome and erosive vitreoretinopathy.

The ERG and dark adaptometry are initially normal in most young patients, but become abnormal as the disease progresses. In late stages, ERG may be markedly reduced.

Management is similar to that of Stickler's syndrome.

Retinal Detachment Associated with Optic Nerve Anomalies

Morning Glory Disk Anomaly

Morning Glory Disk Anomaly (MGDA) is a rare, usually unilateral sporadic condition with a characteristic lesion of the optic nerve often associated with serous retinal detachment.

Ocular features include a funnel-shaped excavation containing an enlarged optic disk. A white, elevated, hyperplastic glial tuft emerges from the center of the disk. Blood vessels emerge from the rim of the excavation in a radial pattern. Serous retinal detachment develop in about 30% of cases.

Systemic associations are present in some patients. Association with basal encephalocele, frontonasal dyplasia and neurofibromatosis type 2 has been reported.

Optic Disk Coloboma

An optic disk coloboma results from incomplete closure of the choroidal fissure. It is a rare, mostly sporadic condition, although AD inheritance may occur. Optic disk coloboma may have profound systemic implications.

Serous retinal detachment at the macula may occur. Rhegmatogenous retinal detachments may occur in eyes with associated chorioretinal colobomas.

Systemic associations are numerous. Important ones include chromosomal anomalies like Patau's syndrome, Edward syndrome and Cat-eye syndrome; CHARGE syndrome comprising coloboma, heart defects, choanal atresia, retarded growth, genital and ear anomalies; Meckel syndrome, Walker-Warburg syndrome and Goldenhar syndrome.

Miscellaneous Syndromes

Infantile Giant Retinal Tear Associated with Lenticular Abnormalities

In 1968, Hovland and Schepens reported eight cases of bilateral giant retinal tear associated with nasal coloboma of the lens. They proposed that the pathogenesis of giant tear formation could be due to abnormal development of the "marginal bundle of drault," or that portion of the secondary vitreous that precedes the development of the vitreous base and lens zonule in the fourth month of gestation.

Aicardi's Syndrome

Aicardi's syndrome is a bilateral, X-linked dominant disorder of cranial, choroidal-pigment epithelium and skeletal development. Ocular features include multiple depigmented chorioretinal lacunae clustered around the disk. Other features are microphthalmous, persistent pupillary membranes, cataract and iridofundal coloboma. Although retinal detachment is rarely seen in this syndrome its occurrence has been reported.

Chapter 45

Juvenile Diabetic Retinopathy

Rajpal Vohra (India)

Epidemiology

The presence of diabetes mellitus is the major risk factor for diabetic retinopathy. Although there have been some claims of "diabetic retinopathy"without diabetes, following publication of the results of the Diabetes Control and Complications Trial (DCCT), this concept is not valid.

The complications of diabetes are direct consequences of long-term hyperglycemia, was decisively confirmed by the results of the DCCT, a randomized, controlled clinical trial involving 27 clinical centers in the USA and Canada. Although the DCCT, and the more recent UK Prospective Diabetes Study (UKPDS), conclusively demonstrated the importance of hyperglycemia in the development of retinopathy and other complications of diabetes, they did not eliminate the possible ancillary role of genetic factors.

Duration of Diabetes and the Development of Diabetic Retinopathy

The duration have been more difficult to determine in type 2 (noninsulin-dependent) diabetes precisely, so that patients with newly diagnosed type 2 diabetes occasionally present with retinopathy as the initial sign of their diabetes, or are found to have retinopathy soon after the diagnosis of their systemic disease.

Study have shown that the prevalence of minimal retinopathy individuals with type 1 diabetes approaches 100% after 20 years. However, the prevalence of proliferative retinopathy is not greater than about 50% in subjects with type 1 is much less in persons with type 2 diabetes of similar duration. There are at lease two possible explanations for this observation. First, proliferative disease may be the result of prolonged, very high average blood glucose levels, which are more likely to occur in persons with type 1 diabetes than in those with type 2. Second, proliferative retinopathy may result from a certain metabolic state of the retina that is more likely to be present in young persons with type 1 diabetes than in (the usually) older people with type 2 disease.

In addition to proliferative retinopathy, the other major vision-threatening form of diabetic retinopathy is macular edema. Macular edema has generally been assumed to be more common in older people with type 2 diabetes than in those with type 1 and, as such, is related to the age of the person affected.

Systemic Factors that may Affect Diabetic Retinopathy

Knowles et al were the first to suggest that the onset of puberty might be important.

The mechanism by which puberty might exert its effect on the development of retinopathy is unknown, but several studies suggest a role for hormonal

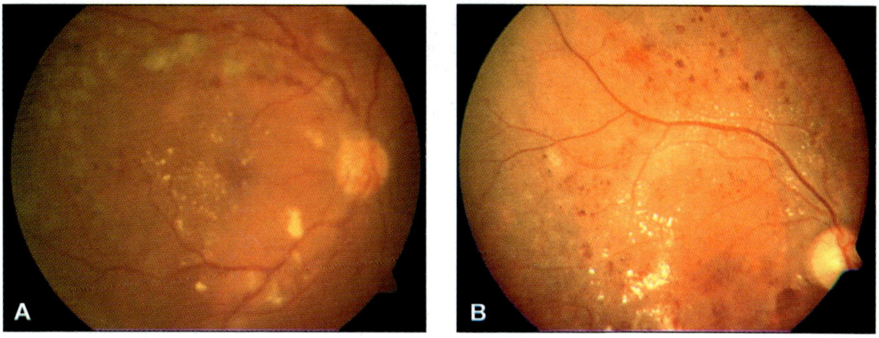

Figures 1A and B: Management of juvenile diabetic macular edema

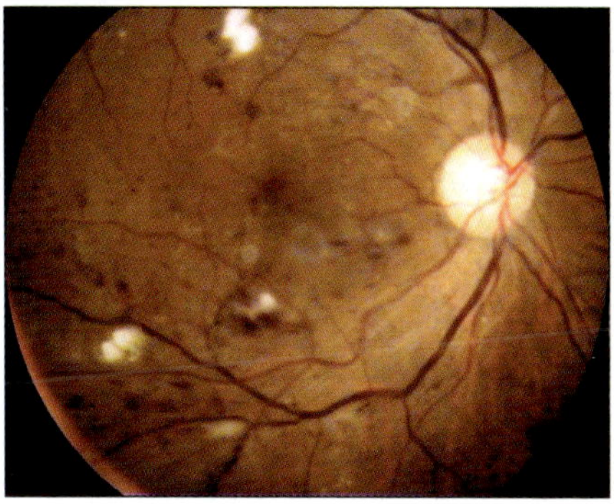

Figure 2A: DDME Pre-IVTA

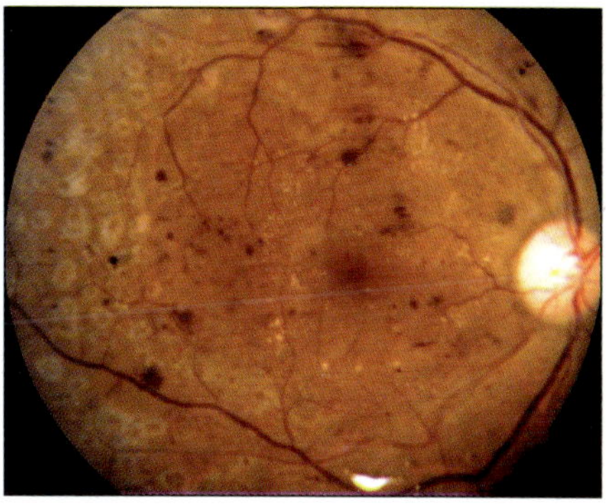

Figure 2B: Post-IVTA (6 months)

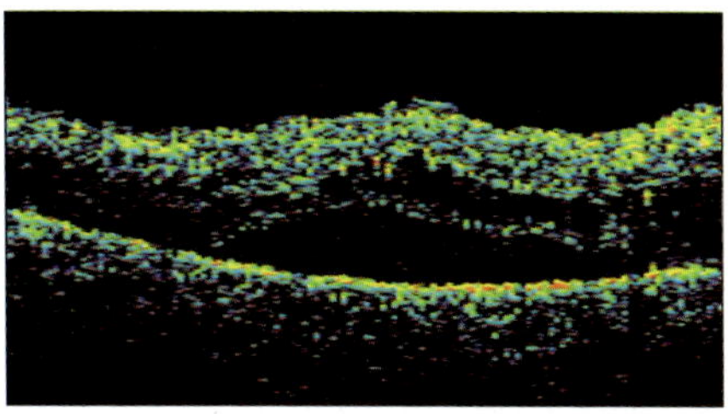

Figure 3A: Pre-IVTA OCT

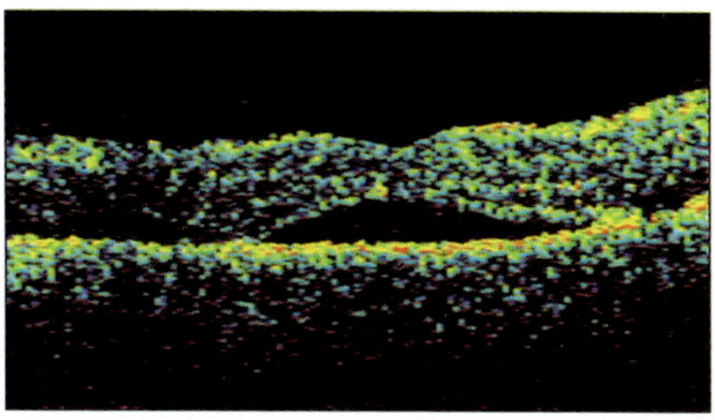

Figure 3B: Post-IVTA OCT

factors related to growth in the pathogenesis of proliferative retinopathy in young people.

Daneman et al described five young patients with Mautic syndrome, a rare form of extremely brittle type 1 diabetes fatty liver, and delayed growth and puberty.

The IGFs have several effects on cells, but one of the most important seems to be to enhance mitogenesis. Thus, elevated levels of IGFs may enhance the development of proliferative diabetic retinopathy, in particular, the rapidly progressive, or florid, retinopathy that is occasionally seen in young people late in adolescence or in young adulthood.

The reduction in IGF levels after destruction of the pituitary gland may also account for the remission of proliferative retinopathy that has been reported after pituitary addition occuring spontaneously, or after intervention by surgery or radiation.

Growth hormone and IGF-1 are important permissive factors for the development of retinal neovascularization but are most likely not directly causal.

Increased blood pressure as well as increased blood sugar levels present an increased risk for the development and progression of diabetic retinopathy.

The effects of pregnancy on diabetic retinopathy have been controversial. Some authors claim that it accelerates the course of the disease, while others believe that it has no effect Klen et al. Have provided the best evidence that pregnancy does promote the progression of diabetic retinopathy.

Ocular Factors

Becker reported in 1967 that glaucoma reduced the prevalence and severity of diabetic retinopathy in affected eyes. It has also been reported that myopia reduces the prevalence and severity of diabetic retinopathy.

Eyes with a great deal of retinochoroidal scarring from trauma, inflammatory disease, etc. had markedly reduced prevalence and severity of diabetic retinopathy. The effect is unexplained, but the most widespread current hypothesis is that it results from decreased retinal metabolism—in particular decreased need for oxygen, with a resultant diminished protection of a vasoproliferative (angiogenic) factor.

Retinopathy in Different forms of Diabetes

Proliferative retinopathy is more prevalent at any given duration of the systemic disease in type 1 than in type 2 diabetes. It is not clear whether this is due to different metabolic factors in the two types of diabetes, to differences in the ages of the patients (type 1 patients are, on average, much younger), or to the higher mean blood glucose levels in type 1 patients. Macular edema probably occurs with equal prevalence as a function of disease duration in both type 1 and type 2 diabetes. Type 2 diabetes is more common after the age of 30 (although "type 2 diabetes of yongh" is becoming increasingly frequently recognized) but, despite

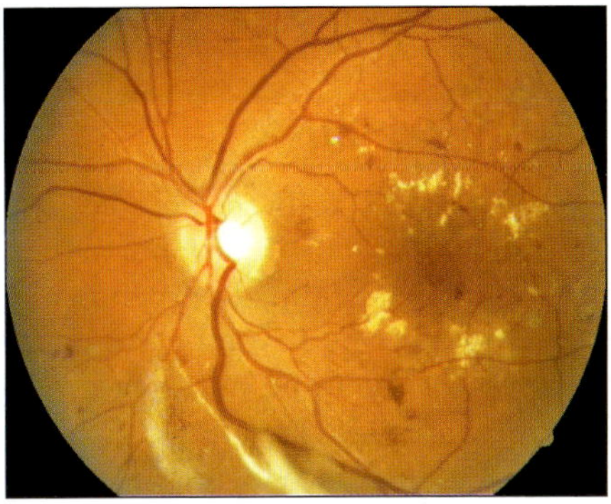

Figure 4A: Pre-IVTA

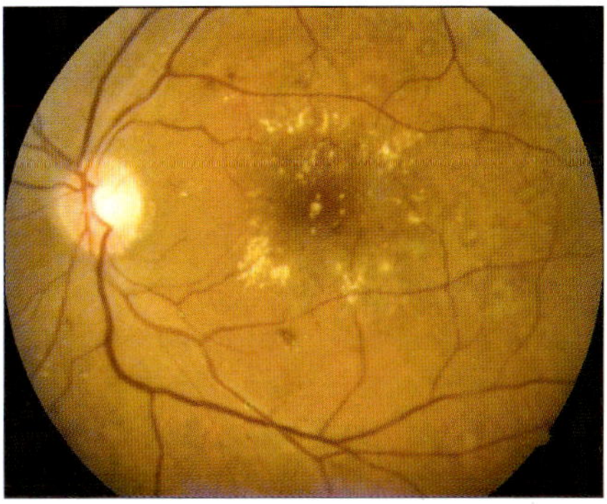

Figure 4B: Post-IVTA

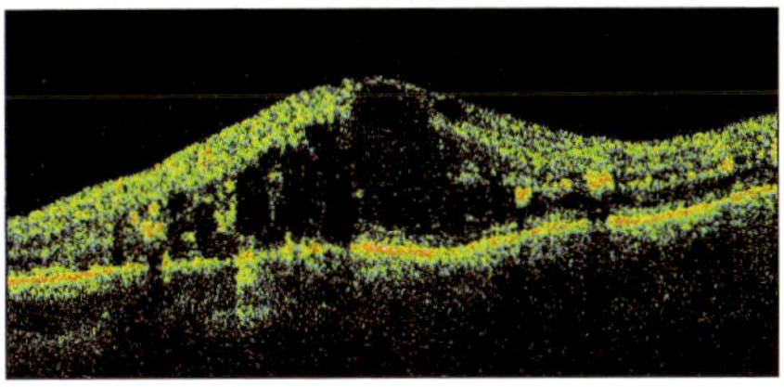

Figure 5A: Pre-IVTA OCT

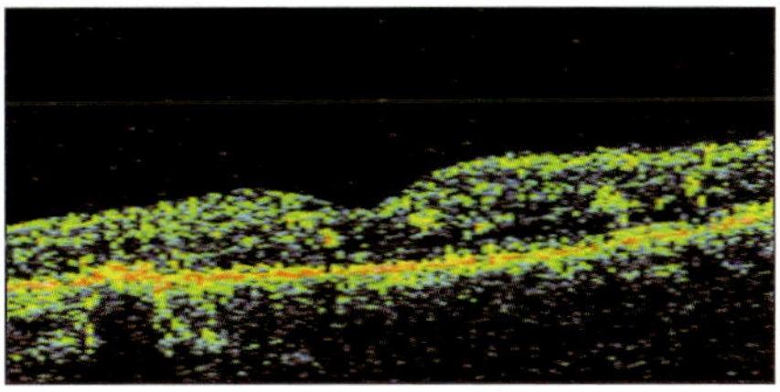

Figure 5B: Post-IVTA OCT

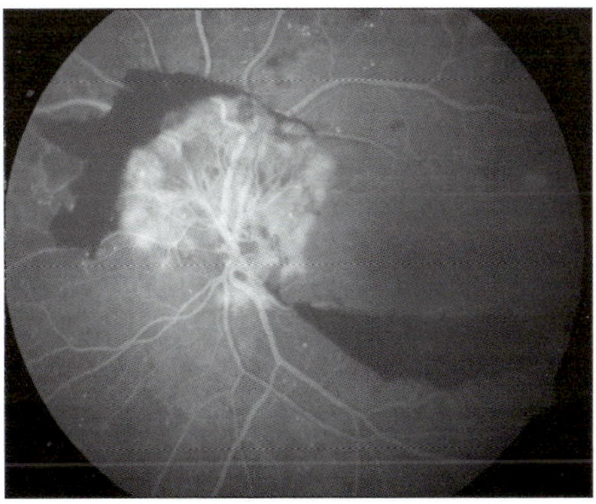

Figure 6: FA of NVD

the apparently mild metabolic defect, proliferative retinopathy can occur as well in this form of the disease Similarly, vision threatening retinopathy can occur in patients with "secondary" diabetes — that which occurs, for example, following pancreatitis, hemochromatosis, or acromegaly.

Techniques to Study Retinal Blood Flow

One of the earliest functional lesions in the eyes of diabetic persons is a breakdown of the blood retinal barrier detected by Vitreous fluorophotometry.

Laser Doppler velocimetry uses an argon laser beam, aimed perpendicular to the direction of blood flow in major retinal vessels (usually the major quadrantic arteries and veins near the margins of the optic nerve head), to measure flow in these vessels by means of the Doppler effect.

The blue-field entoptic phenomenon is a method of studying blood flow in the perifoveal capillary network (The subject looks with one eye at a bright, uniform field of blue light and can then observe a pulsatile pattern of moving particles).

Hyperglycemia per se impairs retinal vascular autoregulation diabetes produces a further impairment of autoregulation. When "tight" blood glucose control is suddenly imposed on a person with chronic diabetes, the impaired retinal vascular autoregulation caused by the prolonged diabetic state may cause a sudden decrease in the retinal oxygen supply, producing areas of retinal infarction. This may result in the "early worsening" of retinopathy that has been observed in some cases clinically.

Anatomic Lesions and the Pathogenesis of Diabetic Retinopathy

Capillary Basement Membrane Thickening

The basement membrane thickening may be a nonspecific, secondary response to a primary biochemical lesion in one of the types of cells that borders the basement membrane. In some cases, as in the retinal microcirculation, this primary lesion may involve the sorbitol pathway. In other cases, as in the renal glomerulus's, it apparently does not.

It has been proposed that an important biochemical lesion of basement membranes in diabetes is a marked decrease in the production of the heparan sulfate proteoglycan, with a resultant secondary over production of basement membrane collagen. Quantitative electron microscopic immunocytochemical studies how that the increased retinal and renal capillary basement membrane thickness in galactosemic rats is accompanied by an surcease in the relative concentrations of types IV collagen and while the relative concentration of HSPG core protein did not change.

One obvious function of basement membranes is to serve as a "skeleton," giving structural rigidity to organs like blood vessel. This is unlikely to be altered by the basement membrane thickening of diabetes. Basement membranes may also serve as filtration barriers for molecules of various size and electrical charges. Perhaps alterations in the amount or degree of sulfation, or in the anatomic distribution of the highly negatively charged heparan sulfate proteoglycan molecules within basement membranes, can affect their permeability properties to various ions. A third function of basement membranes is to regulate cell proliferation and differentiation. A fourth function of basement membranes is their ability to bind various growth factors. In particular, the fibroblast growth factors (FGFs) are potent mitogens that are especially active toward vascular endothelial cells, and are found in many tissues throughout the body.

Since the retina is rich in these growth factors, their sequestration by HSPG residues may serve to restrain neovascularization. If the relative or actual quantity of HSPG is reduced in retinal microvascular basement membranes, then the ability of the basement membranes to prevent neovascularizations may also be decreased.

Loss of Microvascular Intramural Pericytes

Akagi et al have proposed that loss of microvascular intramural pericytes may be related to the action of the sorblted pathway, since they find aldose reductase specifically in mind capillary pericytes but not inendothelial cells in humans

Since PDGF- B has now been described as essential for pericyte development in fetel life, it is possible that much lower concentrations of this molecule are required as a "maintenance factor" for the viability of these cells postnatally.

Microaneurysms

The earliest clinically observable lesion of diabetic retinopathy is the microaneurysm, which appears as tiny, red dot by ophthalmoscopic examinations, and as a hyperfluorescent dot by fluorescein angiography. By light microscopy, in retinal muscular digest preparations, microaneurysms appear as grape like or spindle-shaped dilation of retinal capillaries. Retinal capillary microaneurysms may represent focal regions of endothelial cell proliferation, where the antiproliferative effect of pericytes has been lost. They may arise form weak points in the capillary wall following the loss of pericytes. Pricytes are contractile elements in the capillary wall, much like the smooth-muscle cells of larger vessels, the tonus exerted by the myofibrils in the pericytes may counteract the transmural pressures produced by the flowing blood, and when this tonus is lost, the microvessel wall may dilate focally, producing a microaneurysm.

Capillary Acellularity

A more advanced microvascular lesion of diabetic retinopathy (and one that is not unique to this disease) is the complete loss of all cellular elements from the retinal microvessels.

Breakdown of the Blood-retinal Barrier

Breakdown of the blood-retinal barrier may occur early in the course of diabetes, before retinopathy is observed clinically, and it is certainly present when retinopathy is observed clinically, and it is certainly present when retinopathy is clinically evident.

One possible cause of blood-retinal barrier breakdown is opening of the tight junctions (zonulae occludentes) between adjacent microvascular endothelial cell processes. Several proteins are closely involved with tight junction formation and function.

Clinical Signs of Diabetic Retinopathy

History

In the initial stages, patients are generally asymptomatic; however, in the more advanced stages of the disease, patients may experience symptoms, including blurred vision, distortion, or visual acuity loss.

Signs

Microaneurysms

Earliest clinical sign of diabetic retinopathy detected by direct ophthalmoscope. It is because of capillary wall outpouching due to pericyte loss. Clinically it is seen as small red dots in the superficial retinal layers.

Dot and Blot Hemorrhages

It occurs as microaneurysms rupture in the deeper layers of the retina such as the inner nuclear and outer plexiform layers. It appears similar to microaneurysms if they are small; may need fluorescein angiography to distinguish between the two.

Flame-shaped hemorrhages—splinter hemorrhages that occur in the more superficial nerve fiber layer.

Retinal edema and hard exudates—caused by the breakdown of the blood-retina barrier, allowing leakage of serum proteins, lipids, and protein from the vessels.

Cotton-wool Spots

Nerve fiber layer infarction from occlusion of precapillary arterioles.
Fluorescein angiography—no capillary perfusion.
Frequently bordered by microaneurysms and vascular hyperpermeability.

Venous Loops, Venous Beading

Frequently adjacent to areas of nonperfusion These signs reflects increasing retinal ischemia and significant predictor of progression to PDR.

Intraretinal Microvascular Abnormalities

Remodeled capillary beds without proliferative changes. Usually confused with neovascularization, but can be differentiated on that these do not leak and found intraretinal.

Usually can be found on the borders of the nonperfused retina.

Diabetic Macular Edema

This condition is the leading cause of visual impairment in patients with diabetes. Diabetic macular edema is seen in both type I and II diabetes mellitus and is the most common cause of visual loss in the latter.

Focal macular edema refers to localized areas of retinal thickening caused primarily by focal leakage from microaneurysms, dilated retinal capillaries, and less commonly from intraretinal microvascular abnormalities. Complete or partial rings of hard exudates often demarcate it. Clusters of microaneurysms are seen in the center of circinate exudates and fundus fluorescein angiography demonstrates both their presence and their abnormal permeability. Infrequently a fibrous plaque may develop beneath the macula, resulted from fibrous metaplasia of the retinal pigment epithelium stimulated by the subretinal exudates.

In contrast, in diffuse macular edema there is generalized leakage from dilated capillaries throughout the posterior pole. Occlusion of a considerable portion of the capillary bed leads to widening of the intercapillary spaces and compensatory dilation of the patent capillaries that tend to leak diffusely and cause edema. Diffuse macular edema is usually symmetric in both eyes and without significant exudation.

Classification of Diabetic Retinopathy

The fundus changes that occur in diabetic retinopathy follow a progressive course from non-proliferative to proliferative stage. All fundus changes described as a result of diabetic retinal microangiopathy are characterized in their earlier stages by vascular occlusion and in their later stages by fibrovascular proliferation and scar formation.

Grading of Diabetic Retinopathy on Fundus Photograph/ 90D by Early Treatment of Diabetic Retinopathy Study (ETDRS)

1 Non-proliferative diabetic retinopathy
- Mild
- Moderate
- Severe
- Very severe

2 Proliferative diabetic retinopathy
- With high-risk characteristics
- Without high-risk characteristics

3 Maculopathy
- Clinically significant macular edema (CSME)
- No clinically significant macular edema (CSME)

Definitions

Macular Edema

Thickening of retina within one disc diameter of the center of the macula or hard exudates greater than standard photograph 3 in a standard 30 degree photographic field centered on the macula, with some hard exudates within one disc diameter of the center of the macula.

Clinically Significant Macular Edema

Retinal thickening at or within 500 micrometer of the center of the macula or hard exudates at or within 500 micrometer of the center of the macula if associated with thickening of adjacent retina or a zone of retinal thickening one disc area in size at least part of which was within one disk diameter of the center.

Mild Nonproliferative Retinopathy

At least one microaneurysm.

Moderate Nonproliferative Retinopathy

Hemorrhage or microaneurysm greater than standard photograph 2a or soft exudates, venous beading or intraretinal microvascular abnormality definitely present.

Severe Nonproliferative Retinopathy

Soft exudates, venous beading and intraretinal microvascular abnormality all definitely present in at least two of the fields 4 through 7, or two of the preceding three lesions present in at least two of the fields 4 through 7 and hemorrhage and microaneurysm present in these 4 fields equaling or exceeding standard photo 2a in at least one of them or intraretinal microvascular abnormality present in each of the fields 4 through 7 and equaling or exceeding standard photograph 8a in at least two of them.

Early Proliferative Retinopathy

Proliferative diabetic retinopathy without DRS high-risk characteristics, with neovascularization.

High-risk Proliferative Retinopathy

Proliferative retinopathy with Diabetic Retinopathy Study (DRS) high-risk
 Conditions (HRC). New vessels on or within one disc diameter of the optic disc

(NVD) about one fourth to one third disc area, with or without vitreous or preretinal hemorrhage accompanied by new vessels, or new vessels elsewhere (NVE) that is at least half disc area in extent and associated with preretinal or vitreous hemorrhage.

Risk Factors for Diabetic Retinopathy

Duration of the Diabetes

In patients with type I diabetes, no clinically significant retinopathy can be seen in the first 5 years after the initial diagnosis of diabetes is made. After 10-15 years, 25-50% of patients show some signs of retinopathy. This prevalence increases to 75-95% after 15 years and approaches 100% after 30 years of diabetes.

In patients with type II diabetes, the incidence of diabetic retinopathy increases with the duration of the disease. Of patients with type II diabetes, 23% have NPDR after 11-13 years, 41% have NPDR after 14-16 years, and 60% have NPDR after 16 years.

Glucose Control

The Diabetic Complications Control Trial (DCCT) has demonstrated that intensive glucose control reduced the incidence and the progression of diabetic retinopathy in patients with insulin-dependent diabetes mellitus (IDDM).

Although no similar trials for patients with noninsulin–dependent diabetes mellitus (NIDDM) have been completed, the American Diabetes Association (ADA) has suggested that glycosylated hemoglobin levels of less than 7% (reflecting long-term glucose levels) should be the goal in all patients to prevent or slow down the onset of diabetes-related complications.

Renal disease, as evidenced by proteinuria and elevated BUN/creatinine levels, is an excellent predictor of the presence of retinopathy. This probably is due to the fact that both conditions are caused by DM-related microangiopathies such that the presence and severity of one reflects that of the other. Evidence suggests that aggressive treatment of the nephropathy may have a beneficial effect on the progression of diabetic retinopathy and neovascular glaucoma.

Systemic hypertension, in the setting of diabetic nephropathy, correlates well with the presence of retinopathy. Independently, hypertension also may complicate diabetes in that it may result in hypertensive retinal vascular changes superimposed on the preexisting diabetic retinopathy, further compromising retinal blood flow.

Proper management of hyperlipidemia (elevated serum lipids) may result in less retinal vessel leakage and hard exudate formation. The reason behind this is unclear.

Pregnant women without any diabetic retinopathy run a 10% risk of developing NPDR during their pregnancy. Of those with preexisting NPDR, 4% progress to the proliferative type.

Investigations

Lab Studies

Fasting glucose and hemoglobin A1c (HbA1c) are important laboratory tests that are performed to help diagnose diabetes. The HbA1c level is also important in the long-term follow-up care of patients with diabetes and diabetic retinopathy. Controlling diabetes and maintaining the HbA1c level in the 6-7% range are the goals in the optimal management of diabetes and diabetic retinopathy. If the levels are maintained, then the progression of diabetic retinopathy is reduced substantially, according to the DCCT.

Imaging Studies

Fluorescein angiography is an invaluable adjunct in the diagnosis and management of diabetic retinopathy.

Microaneurysms would appear as pinpoint hyperfluorescence that does not enlarge but rather fades in the later phases of the test.

Blot and dot hemorrhages can be distinguished from microaneurysms because they appear as hypofluorescent rather than hyperfluorescent.

Areas of nonperfusion appear as homogenous dark patches bordered by occluded blood vessels.

IRMA is evidenced by collateral vessels that do not leak, usually found in the borders of the nonperfused retina.

Medical Care

Glucose Control

The DCCT has found that intensive glucose control in patients with IDDM has decreased the incidence and progression of diabetic retinopathy. Although no similar clinical trials for patients with NIDDM exist, it may be logical to assume that the same principles also apply. In fact, the ADA has suggested that all diabetics (NIDDM and IDDM) should strive to maintain glycosylated hemoglobin levels of less than 7% to prevent or at the very least to minimize the long-term complications of DM, including DM retinopathy.

The Early Treatment for Diabetic Retinopathy Study (ETDRS) found that 650 mg of aspirin daily did not offer any benefit in preventing the progression of DM retinopathy. Additionally, aspirin was not observed to influence the incidence of vitreous hemorrhage in patients who required it for cardiovascular disease (CVD) or other conditions.

Further Outpatient Care

The frequency of follow-up care is dictated primarily on the baseline stage of the retinopathy and its rate of progression to PDR.

Only 5% of patients with mild NPDR would progress to PDR in 1 year and, thus, could be monitored every 6-12 months.

As many as 27% of patients with moderated NPDR would progress to PDR in 1 year; therefore, they should be seen every 4-8 months.

More than 50% of patients with severe NPDR (preproliferative stage) would progress to PDR in a year; thus, follow-up care as frequent as 2-4 months is mandated to ensure prompt recognition and treatment.

Management of Diabetic Macular Edema

Photocoagulation treatment for diabetic maculae edema using a variety of wavelengths and treatment techniques has been used foe a number of years with varying reports of success. The Early Treatment Diabetic Retinopathy Study (ETDRS) addressed several issues regarding photocoagulation and provided several guidelines regarding timing and type of laser in patients with diabetic macular edema which are followed today

ETDRS Guidelines for Management of Diabetic Macular Edema (ETDRS Report no.2 1987)

ETDRS, one of the trend setting trials in the field of ophthalmology has stated with respect to diabetic macular edema:

1. After 3 years of follow-up, 12% of eyes that had been assigned to treatment for macular edema had experienced significant visual loss versus 24% of eye that had not received treatment. The differences were even greater with clinically significant macular edema.
2. ETDRS defined clinically significant macular edema (CSME) as (any of the following characteristics) :
   a. Thickening of the retina at or within 500 μ from the center of the macula.
   b. Hard exudates at or within 500 μ from the center of the macula, if associated thickening of adjacent retina
   c. A zone of retinal thickening one disc area or larger, any part of which is within 1 disc diameter of the center of the macula
3. Fluorescein angiography is not absolutely necessary in the treatment of diabetic eyes with localized edema, especially when associated with discrete circinate rings, but is necessary in eyes with diffuse edema.
4. Treatable lesions associated with macular edema are:
   A. Discrete points of retinal hyper fluorescence or focal leakage that were 500 μ or more from the center of the macula and thought to be causing retinal thickening and/ or hard exudates.
   B. Focal leaks 300—500 μ from the center of the macula and thought to be causing retinal thickening and/ or hard exudates
   C. Areas of diffuse leakage within the retina (intraretinal microvascular abnormalities or diffusely leaking retinal capillary bed).
   D. Thickened retinal avascular zones.
5. Direct focal photocoagulation is recommended for fluorescein leaks.
6. Grid treatment for diffuse edema or nonperfused thickened retina

7. Focal photocoagulation reduces the risk of moderate visual loss by 50% or more.
8. Treatment is more effective in preventing visual loss than restoring vision already lost.
9. The risk of visual loss is especially high in eyes with initially decreased visual acuity.
10. The risk of visual loss is greater when the treatment must be placed closer to the center of the macula.

ETDRS Guidelines for Laser Photocoagulation

All eyes with CSME should be considered for photocoagulation.

a. Direct treatment of focal fluorescein leaks – involves focal photocoagulation of individual microaneurysms. Goal is to obtain closure of the leak with preferred end point being whitening or darkening of microaneurysms. Spot size 50–200 µ.
b. Grid treatment of diffuse edema – areas of retinal thickening and associated with areas of less intense leakage being treated with more widely spaced grid. The grid is not placed within 500 µ of the center of the macula or within 500 µ of the disc margin, but it can be placed on the papillomacular bundle. The grid can extend in all directions up to 2 disc diameters from the center of the macula. Spot size 50-200 µ.
c. Modified grid laser treatment for diffuse edema – primarily involves grid treatment to areas of diffuse leakage with occasional treatment of focal leakage located within or outside the areas of diffuse edema. Modified grid is applied using 2/3 rows of 100 µ spots to all areas of perifoveal thickening up to and including the edge of foveal avascular zone, these initial spots places 100 µ apart. Then, 150-200 µ spots are placed approximately 200 µ apart to the remaining areas of retinal thickening and capillary non perfusion. Focal leaks are treated with 100-150 µ spots to achieve mild whitening of micro aneurysms.

The complications of focal and grid laser therapy include the following:

- Decreased central vision
- Paracentral scotomas
- Choroidal neovascularization
- Epiretinal membrane formation
- Further increase in macular edema

Prognosis

Several other authors have also evaluated grid laser photocoagulation in treatment of diabetic macular edema.

Ladas ID et al concluded in their study that modified grid laser photocoagulation is not an effective procedure for the long-term management of diffuse diabetic macular edema compared with the natural course of the disease.

Guyot-Argenton C et al analyzed clinical and tomographic features of diabetic macular edemas (DME) unresponsive to laser photocoagulation. They retrospectively studied 43 eyes presenting with severe DME defined by a macular thickening 450 micron or more, involving the fovea, and associated with either cystoid spaces and/or hard exudates threatening the center of the macula. All 43 eyes underwent sub threshold grid laser therapy (a mean of 2.3 sessions).

Results: Photocoagulation was beneficial in 39% of the eyes (n=17) and failed in 60% (n=26). Comparing these two groups, they found that some tomographic and clinical signs were strikingly more frequent in the unresponsive eyes than in the responsive ones. OCT findings reported foveal thickening greater than 700 μ (38%), subclinical serous foveal detachment (65%), sub clinical vitreomacular interface abnormalities (19%) and as clinical signs, 44% of the unresponsive eyes exhibited rapid progression of retinal ischemia preceding ME constitution.

Conclusion: Long-standing diffuse DME carries an unfavorable prognosis. In cases of unresponsive DME exhibiting these tomographic and clinical signs, alternative therapies such as intravitreal injections of steroids and/or vitrectomy with posterior hyaloid removal should be considered, instead of useless repetitive grid laser treatments.

Shimura M et al evaluated thirty-five eyes of 23 patients with diffuse diabetic macular edema that underwent laser grid photocoagulation excluding the papillomacular bundle area.

Results: Six months after treatment, the visual acuity improved by 2 or more lines in 16 eyes (43%) and the foveal thickness decreased in 32 eyes (91%).

Conclusions: Grid pattern photocoagulation without treatment to the papillomacular bundle area was effective in treating diffuse diabetic macular edema, especially in eyes with an initial mean deviation showing moderate dysfunction.

Degenring R F et al evaluated the clinical outcome of macular grid laser photocoagulation in the treatment of diffuse diabetic macular edema by retrospectively studying 30 consecutive patients (41 eyes) who were treated by macular argon green grid laser photocoagulation for diffuse diabetic macular edema.

Results: Visual acuity decreased from 0.25 +/- 0.18 to 0.20 +/- 0.18 (P = 0.045), 5 (12.2 %) eyes gained in visual acuity, visual acuity remained unchanged for 23 (56.1 %) eyes, and 13 (31.7 %) eyes showed a visual loss of more than one line.

Conclusions: visual acuity decreased in the whole population and especially in the subgroup with a baseline visual acuity of > or = 0.2 after macular grid laser photocoagulation for diffuse diabetic macular edema. Mean visual loss was just below the predefined 2 lines. In view of these results and upcoming new pharmacological and surgical treatment modalities, the significance of grid laser photocoagulation should be re-discussed.

ETDRS report 23 (Early Treatment Diabetic Retinopathy Study Research Group) pointed out the complication of sub retinal fibrosis due to laser photocoagulation in Diabetic macular edema. Presence of hard exudates was found out to be the strongest risk factor for the development of sub retinal fibrosis which consecutively led to extremely poor visual outcome.

Majority of the studies have opined about the poorer prognosis after laser treatment for diffuse edema. The pathogenesis of diffuse edema is more complex than that of other forms of macular edema and includes poorly demarcated leakage from abnormal retinal capillaries and micro aneurysms. Besides the influence of the duration of diabetes mellitus, HbA1c, proteinuria, hypertension the role of the posterior hyaloid has become increasingly recognized.

Nasrallah et al observed in 1988 a lower incidence of posterior vitreous detachment in eyes with diabetic macular edema compared with eyes without edema. They retrospectively assessed clinical records of 76 patients (125 eyes), 60 years of age or older with diabetic retinopathy who had undergone a vitreous examination.

Conclusions: Diabetic cases without macular edema have a significantly higher rate of posterior vitreous detachment than those with macular edema. This study demonstrated that the vitreous may play a role in diabetic macular edema.

Lewis H et al conclude that vitreous surgery can improve the visual prognosis of some eyes with diabetic macular traction and edema associated with a thickened and taut posterior hyaloid. They were the first to report encouraging results after vitrectomy in diabetic eyes in 1992.

Tachi N et al: In eyes with diffuse diabetic macular edema and without posterior vitreous detachment, vitrectomy with posterior vitreous detachment may be effective.

***Pendergast SD et al*:** In eyes with persistent diffuse diabetic macular edema with a taut premacular posterior hyaloid face unresponsive to laser therapy, vitrectomy with removal of the posterior hyaloid appears to be beneficial in some cases.

Ikeda T et al reported the success of vitrectomy in eliminating cystoid macular edema and improving vision in three eyes of two patients with diabetic cystoid macular edema. In all of the eyes there was no ophthalmoscopic evidence of traction from a posterior hyaloid membrane or from proliferative tissue. and conclude that vitrectomy can be effective in some patients with diabetic cystoid macular edema even in patients who lack evidence of traction by ophthalmoscopy.

Sato Y et al conclude that diabetic cystoid macular edema is a good indication for vitrectomy regardless of the posterior vitreous membrane condition.

Vitreous surgery may improve perifoveal microcirculation in the eyes of diabetic patients with cystoid macular edema and resolve the macular edema. Improvement of perifoveal microcirculation may be an important factor affecting visual outcome.

La Heij EC et al concluded that in eyes with diabetic macular edema without evident macular traction from a thickened vitreous membrane, vitrectomy resulted in the resolution of macular edema, with an improvement in visual acuity in the majority of cases. Eyes without preoperative macular photocoagulation had a significantly higher percentage visual improvement than eyes without preoperative macular laser treatment.

Gandorfer A et al were the first to demonstrate encouraging results after vitrectomy with peeling of the inner limiting membrane in patients with diffuse non resolving diabetic macular edema. concluded that vitrectomy including removal of the ILM leads to expedited resolution of diffuse diabetic macular edema and improvement of visual acuity without subsequent epiretinal membrane formation. Complete release of tractional forces and inhibition of reproliferation of fibrous astrocytes seem to be prudent in the eyes of patients with diabetes and advanced vitreoretinal interface disease of the macula.

Recchia FM et al concluded that limiting PPV with ILM removal may provide anatomic and visual benefit in some eyes with chronic diabetic macular edema unresponsive to additional laser photocoagulation.

Yamamoto T et al compared the efficacy of surgically removing or not removing the internal limiting membrane (ILM) during pars plana vitrectomy on the visual acuity and retinal thickness in eyes with diabetic macular edema.

Conclusions: Vitrectomy in eyes with diabetic macular edema without ILM removal was as effective in reducing the retinal thickness and improving the visual acuity as eyes with ILM removal. They concluded that ILM need not be removed to treat eyes with diabetic macular edema.

Yanyali A et al compared the effectiveness of pars plana vitrectomy (PPV) and removal of the internal limiting membrane (ILM) with modified grid laser photocoagulation in diabetic macular edema.

Conclusions: PPV with ILM removal appears to be more effective than a single session of modified grid laser photocoagulation in the treatment of diabetic macular edema.

Kolacny D et al concluded in their study that pars plana vitrectomy with peeling of the ILM stained with If CG leads to good postoperative results in young diabetic patients with recent vision loss due to macular edema and without previous macular laser treatment.

The usefulness of trypan blue in improving the efficiency and safety of membrane identification **(ERM and ILM)** and removal during vitrectomies has been shown by Brendan and others.

Vitrectomy with and without ILM peeling in diffuse diabetic macular edema has also been evaluated by others like ***Avci*** , ***Grigorian*** and ***Mochizuki*** and mostly favorable results have been reported.

Optical coherence tomography has been found to be very useful in evaluating macular edema and assessing improvement in it following laser or surgery.

Several authors like ***Browning DJ*** , ***Panozzo G*** , ***Massin P*** and ***Lattanzio R*** have shown the usefulness of OCT in the diagnosis and management of diabetic macular edema.

Investigations and Current Management of DME

Slit-lamp examination with contact or non-contact lens, makes it possible to detect retinal thickening, localized or extending to the posterior pole. Clinical suspicion of macular edema can be confirmed with the aid of a wide variety of investigations.

Table 1: Current techniques for investigation of macular edema used in clinical practice and research

Technique	*Principle*	*Advantages*	*Disadvantages*	*Others*
Fluorescein angiography	Leakage of dye from capillaries via damaged endothelial cells and/or	Allows visualization of area covered by cystoid formations	Small risk to patient	Qualitative Invasive
		Leakage associated with breakdown of the tight junctions between adjacent retinal pigment epithelium cells	Correlates well with acuity	Improves accuracy of treatment
Vitreous fluoro-photometry	Slit-lamp fluorophotometer	Quantifies fluorescein leakage	Inconsistent results	Quantitative Non-invasive
Laser flare cell photometer	Alteration in Blood-Aqueous barrier	Quantifies blood– aqueous disruption	Non specific	Quantitative Non-invasive
Ocular coherence tomography	Visible light interference	Quantification of retinal thickness	Poorer resolution than ligh microscopy	Quantitative Non-invasive Visualization of undisturbed retinal structure
Retinal thickness analyzer	Laser projected at oblique angle to retina	Retinal thickness $\alpha\alpha$ to acuity	Affected by clarity of media	Quantitative Non-invasive
Scanning laser ophthal-moscope	Scans small focused spot to provide high contrast image	Able to image through small pupils and hazy media	Affected by optics of eye	Quantitative Non-invasive
Contrast sensitivity	Small letter contrast Sensitivity varied	More sensitive than Snellen to mascular edema	Unreliable	Qualitative Non-invasive
Electro diagnostics	Stimulates foveal cones only	Amplitude correlates well with acuity	Qualitative	Qualitative Non-invasive

Management

There are currently four accepted modalities of treatment for DME:

1. Intravitreal Triamcinolone
2. Macular grid potocoagulation
3. Vitrectomy
4. Cytokine (PKCβ, VEF) inhibitors

Intravitreal Triamcinolone

Intravitreal injection of triamcinolone acetate has been used alone or in combination with laser photocoagulation for treatment of diffuse diabetic macular edema. Martidis et al in a prospective, noncomparative, interventional case series reported improvement in visual acuity of 2.4 and 1.3 Snellen lines at the 3-month and 6-month follow-up reviews after intravitreal injections of 4 mg of triamcinolone acetate. More recently Jonas et al administered 25 mg of triamcinolone acetate as opposed to 4 mg that all previous studies had used for the treatment of diabetic macular edema. In a mean follow-up of just over 6 months, they reported significant improvement in visual acuity and reduction of fluorescein leakage when compared with pre-injection levels. However, the investigators pointed out that visual improvement showed a tendency to decline 5 months after the triamcinolone acetate injection. Although 36% of the cases developed intraocular pressure greater than 21 mm Hg following injection of triamcinolone acetate, ocular hypertension was successfully controlled by topical antiglaucoma agents until triamcinolone acetate crystals had disappeared. Other potential complications that intravitreal steroid injection may entail is hastening of cataract formation and deposition of cortisone crystals on the macular region. However, the latter can be avoided should patients be instructed to maintain an upright position for at least 2 hours following the injection.

Macular Grid Photocoagulation

Photocoagulation is a therapeutic technique using a strong light source to coagulate tissue. Several theories attempted to explain the beneficial effect of laser photocoagulation to macular edema. Laser lesions in experimental animals show a temporary breakdown of the BRB and a subsequent repair, as the retinal pigment epithelium cells adjacent to the burns proliferate and slide to replace the necrotic cells. The new retinal pigment epithelium cells produce tight junctions within several weeks, which restores the integrity of the retinal pigment epithelium barrier. An alternative hypothesis states that the grid laser by destroying photoreceptors reduces the oxygen consumption of the outer retina and allows oxygen to diffuse from the choroid to the inner retina, where it raises the oxygen tension and relieves hypoxia. This increased oxygen tension causes retinal arteriolar constriction and increased resistance in the arterioles, leading to reduced hydrostatic pressure in the capillaries and venules. The decreased hydrostatic pressure causes vessel constriction according to Laplace's law, vessel shortening, and less flux of fluid from vessel to tissue as is postulated in Starling's law.

Diabetic macular edema may improve following focal or grid laser photocoagulation. Laser treatment is not indicated for predominantly ischemic maculopathy. Most authors agree that the prognosis is best with localized leakage with or without circinate rings of hard exudates. Should PRP be also needed, this should be carried out after or in conjunction with macular treatment, because post-PRP inflammation and altered retinal blood flow may result in deterioration of macular edema.

The Early Treatment for Diabetic Retinopathy Study (ETDRS) provided the indications for laser treatment of diabetic macular edema.

Side effects such as scotomas, corresponding to the laser burns, have been frequently noticed by the patients following photocoagulation. These scotomas generally fade over a period of several weeks. Symptoms are more likely to occur if laser burns are placed too close to each other.

Vitrectomy

It has been postulated that intractable diabetic macular edema unresponsive to laser treatment may be due to posterior hyaloid traction and not traditional mechanisms.Vitreous surgery may improve perifoveal microcirculation in the eyes of diabetic patients with CME and resolve the macular edema improving the visual acuity. OCT has been proposed to be particularly useful in the detection of shallow, subclinical, macular detachment in eyes with diabetic macular edema associated with posterior hyaloid traction. It has been suggested that vitrectomy should be considered when shallow macular detachments can be demonstrated by OCT. Furthermore, clinical recovery with resolution of macular edema and improvement of visual acuity following PPV has been reported, even when there was no evidence of macular traction on ophthalmoscopy. Based on the available published data, 38–100% of the patients who underwent vitrectomy for diabetic macular edema showed improvement in visual acuity. However, there are significant confounding parameters, including small sample size, short duration of macular edema, retrospective and non-randomized studies, and visual acuity not measured by masked observers using a specific protocol.

Proliferative Diabetic Retinopathy: Surgical Management

Increased level of growth factors (VEGF, b-FGF, IGF-1) result in retinal anginogenesis: the development of neovascular buds, also known as vascular epicenters, from retinal blood vassels. This vascular tissue proliferates in the potential space between the retina and vitreous. Eventually the continued growth of this tissue leads to the invasion of the posterior lamellae of the cortical vitreous, producing a very firm adhesions, vessels continue to proliferate in size and extent, with subsequent development of an increasingly fibrous component. The fibrous element of this fibrovascular complex may contract, causing the vitreous to exert traction on the friable vascular tissue and retina. This could potentially result in a vitreous hemorrhage, which may stimulate further fibrosis and vitreous contraction, and eventually lead to a traction retinal detachment. Significant tracional force is exerted on the neovascularization from adhesions at the vitreoretinal junction, a retinal break may form. Therefore, in a combined traction/rhegmatogenous retinal detachment, the retinal break is often located near fibrovascular proliferative epicenters.

Indication for Surgical Intervention

1. Severe nonclearing vitreous hemorrhage
2. Traction retinal detachment recently involving macula
3. Combined tractional and rhegmatogenous retinal detachment
4. Dense premacular hemorrhage

5. Dense fibrovascular proliferation
6. Diabetic macular edema associated with posterior hyaloid traction
7. Ghost cell and hemolytic glaucoma
8. Anterior segment neovascularization with media opacity.

Severe Nonclearing Vitreous Hemorrhage

The recommended timing for vitrectomy for severe diabetic vitreous hemorrhage is before 3 months for type 1 diabetics and 6 months for type 2 patients. More recently, vitrectomy has been advocated even earlier. Surgical goals include removal of vitreous hemorrhage to provide a clear medium, excision of posterior hyaloid and epiretinal membranes to relieve vitreoretinal traction, and application of endolaser to achieve regression of proliferative tissue.

Traction Retinal Detachment Recently Involving Macula

DRVS defined tractional retinal detachment as retinal elevation at least 4 disc areas in extent, at least a part of which was within 30 degrees of the center of the macula, or retinal elevation less than 4 disc areas if one or more vitreoretinal adhesions causing elevation of the retina were present within 30 degrees of the center and in the presence of active new vessels or fresh vitreous hemorrhage. Traction retinal detachment recently involving macula is currently the most common indication for diabetic vitrectomy Surgery is generally not undertaken in eyes with extra-macular traction detachment and eyes with chronic macular detachment except in special circumstances.. Studies have shown that in some patients with progressive traction detachment that threatens the macula, early vitrectomy is beneficial. Favourable preoperative prognostic factors include short duration of macular detachment, limited extent of detachment, presence of panretinal photocoagulation, and the absence of vitreous hemorrhage and severe neovascularization.

Combined Tractional and Rhegmatogenous Retinal Detachment

Sudden visual loss generally occurs in such cases as the rhegmatogenous component often progresses rapidly. Prompt vitrectomy is required regardless of the macular status. Conventional scleral buckling surgery methods are insufficient because of posterior location of the breaks and persistent vitreoretinal traction.

Dense Fibrovascular Proliferation

In some patients with an attached hyaloid, active neovascular and fibrovascular proliferations may progress rapidly despite extensive panretinal photocoagulation. This typically occurs in patients with poorly controlled type one diabetes. Vitrectomy may be indicated in such patients as neovascularization of the disc and posterior fundus rarely occur after surgical excision of the posterior cortical vitreous.

Dense Premacular Hemorrhage

In cases with nonresolving premacular hemorrhage, surgery is indicated to prevent severe surface wrinkling involving the fovea or traction macular detachment.

An alterenative treatment to surgery may be Nd:YAG laser membranectomy to the posterior hyaloid face: This has been shown to result in drainage of dense premacular hemorrhage into the vitreous cavity.

Diabetic Macular Edema Associated with Posterior Hyaloid Traction

Some patients with macular edema have macular traction associated with a thickened and taut premacular posterior hyaloid. The surgical goals include opening, elevating and removing the posterior hyaloid.

Ghost Cell/Hemolytic Glaucoma

This occurs typically in aphakic eyes with a disrupted anterior hyaloid face. It may also occur after vitrectomy for nonclearing vitreous hemorrhage, as the peripheral residual vitreous skirt acts as a reservoir for degenerated erythrocytes and blood products.

Role of Avastin

Retinal photocoagulation is a destructive therapy with adverse side effect such as loss of peripheral visual fields and night vision as well as exacerbation of macular edema and subsequent reduction in central vision also PRP is not possible in media opacity. Patients with iris neovascularization and neovascular glaucoma often present with hyphema and with cornal edema which prevents any laser treatment. A dramatic and rapid response to intravitreal bevacizumab has shown a complete resolution of vascular leakage in most cases of iris neovascularization and severe PDR.

Surgical Steps in Diabetic Vitrectomy

Vitrectomy is started by removing the central vitreous gel to create space for maneuverability. The central gel should be removed from the central posterior to the peripheral anterior region, making small circular motions with the vitrectomy probe over the entire globe. Next, a button hole is opened in the hyaloid, which is then enlarged across its 360 degree to relieve all anterior-posterior traction on the hyaloid. When we open the hyaloid, we may find blood deposited on the retina. This can be removed if we are going to work on retina. If not, the blood is removed at the end of surgery since it will protect the retina against the phototoxicity of endo-ocular light. At this stage, a peripheral vitrectomy should be performed to remove as much as vitreous possible. Then, with the vitrectomy probe, proliferative tissue can be cut between epicenters and if small, the epicenter can also be removed.

Ocassionally, the hyaliod detaches completely as the vitreous is removed such that surgery is almost complete. Usually, the hyaloid produces traction on retina, which may be raised due to fibrovascular proliferations requiring other techniques such as segmentations. This may be done with vertical blade scissors by resectioning tissue between the traction epicenters with care taken to lift the tissue a little before cutting to avoid damaging the retina. Then, using curved scissors we can delaminate the rest of this tissue. Bimanual surgery can be performed with the two instruments, one for tractioning and other for cutting. The light may be fitted to the infusion cannula or illuminated instruments or a chandelier light may be used.

During dissection, retinal vessel bleeding may occur. To control this bleeding, intraocular pressure may be raised by increasing infusion bottle height. If bleeding persists, the vessel can be coagulated with unimanual bipolar diathermy. In some cases, the tissue manipulator with a source of light, aspiration cannula and diathermy is useful. It should be remembered that when the intraocular instruments are removed under ocular hypertension, the vitreous gel can pull away from the periphery provoking tears in retina and eventually its detatchment.

Another technique exists known as en bloc dissections, whereby anterior-posterior traction of hyaloid is maintained to identify points of traction for their selective removal using scissors. After completing vitrectomy, pan-photocoagulation should be completed. This can be done using curved probe allowing the photocoagulation of anterior sites. We use the laser probes with light that the indentation allow us to reach the ora serrata. In areas of difficult access, retinal ablation can be completed with cryotherapy.

Triamcinolone is sometimes used to facilitate vitrectomy in proliferative diabetic retinopathy. Its use helps visualization of the hyaloid and its posterior removal, stabilizing the blood ocular barrier.

Chapter 46

Hereditary Vitreoretinopathies

Soumen Mondal, Supriya Dabir,
S Natarajan (India)

Stickler's Syndrome

Introduction

First reported in 1965, Stickler's syndrome or hereditary progressive arthro-ophthalmopathy is a progressive, debilitating connective tissue disorder with systemic and ocular manifestations and is of varying severity. It is inherited in an autosomal dominant fashion with variable penetrance.

Clinical Symptoms and Signs

Ocular: Progressive axial myopia with vitreous syneresis is seen. A characteristic finding in the posterior segment is the presence of an optically empty vitreous cavity. Vitreous membranes can be seen which are relatively dense, avascular and freely mobile. In the retina, peripheral radial lattice — like degeneration are seen which are often associated with RPE hyperplasia, vascular sheathing and sclerosis. Single large or multiple retinal breaks can be seen. Retinal detachment occurs in 30% patients in the first decade of life. Other ocular associations are presenile cataract, ectopia lentis and glaucoma.

Systemic: Maxillary hypoplasia, bifid uvula, high-arched palate, Pierre-Robin sequence (micrognathia, cleft palate, glossoptosis) abnormal teeth and malocclusion are some of the orofacial abnormalities seen. Musculoskeletal abnormalities like osteoarthritis, spondyloepiphyseal dysplasia, muscular hypoplasia and hypotony, marfanoid habitus are commonly manifested. Conductive and sensorineural hearing loss are other common systemic findings.

Investigation

ERG: ERG is reduced.

FFA: Areas of paravascular pigmentary degeneration manifests zone of window defect with blockage of choroidal fluorescence at the areas of pigment deposits.

Treatment

Barrage laser or cryopexy should be done irrespective of presence or absence of symptoms. In case of retinal detachment, repair by buckling or vitreous surgery is done (as appropriate) though results are not very encouraging (inadequate drainage of subretinal fluid due to liquefied vitreous).

Inference

A hereditary arthro-ophthalmopathy, Stickler's syndrome manifests with liquefied, optically empty vitreous cavity, peripheral radial or paravascular lattice — like retinal degenerations and retinal breaks. They frequently lead to rhegmatogenous retinal detachment. All peripheral degeneration seen in Stickler's syndrome is to be aggressively treated.

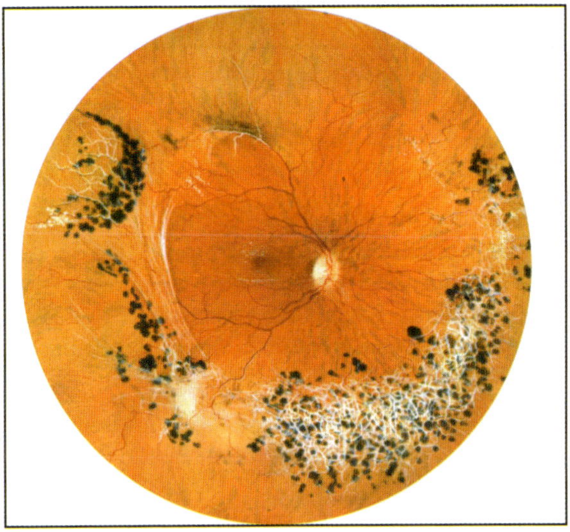

Figure 1: Peripheral retinal degeneration in Wagner's disease

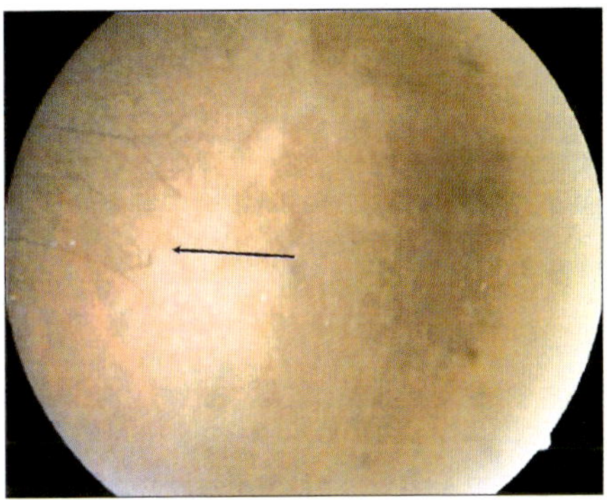

Figure 2: FEVR — typical abrupt cessation of vessels at midperiphery with fimbriated edge of vessels

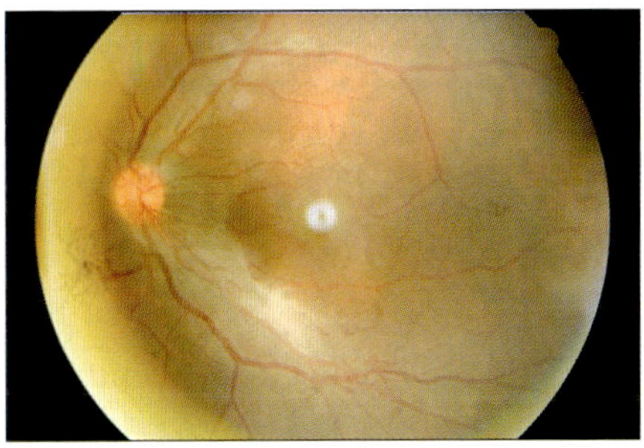

Figure 3: FEVR — thick preretinal vitreous causing minimal TRD

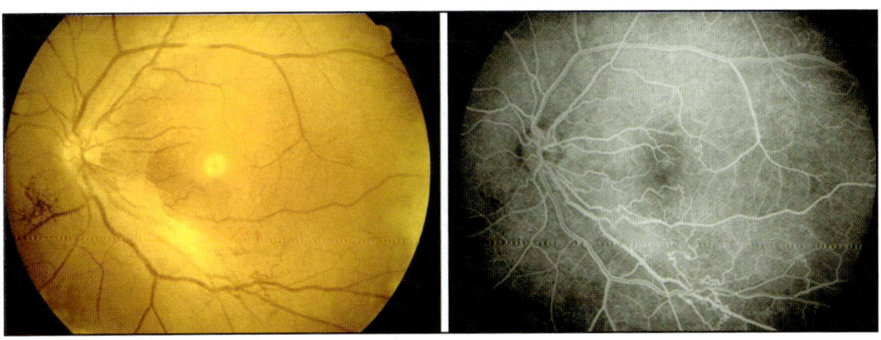

Figure 4: FEVR — thick preretinal vitreous causing minimal TRD, vascular distortion also seen

Wagner's Disease

Wagner's hyaloideoretinal dystrophy or Wagner's disease is a rare vitreoretinopathy with autosomal dominance inheritance pattern.

Clinical Signs and Symptoms

Liquefaction of vitreous with absence of scaffolding is seen most commonly, which presents as an optically empty vitreous. Also seen are equatorial, preretinal grayish white membranes. With time, progressive chorioretinal atrophy is seen. Patients with Wagner's disease have an increased risk of having rhegmatogenous retinal detachment. Other associated ocular findings are low myopia and cortical cataract. Unlike Stickler's syndrome, there is no systemic association.

Treatment

Prophylactic treatment to all breaks should be done. Contrary to Stickler's syndrome, rhegmatogenous retinal detachment in Wagner's disease has a better outcome following scleral buckling surgery.

Familial Exudative Vitreoretinopathy

Inherited in an autosomal dominant pattern, familial exudative vitreoretinopathy is characterized by failure of the temporal retinal periphery to vascularize.

Clinical Signs and Symptoms

Presenting in late childhood, initially, areas of white without pressure are seen which are associated with peripheral attachments and vitreous degeneration. Later on, telangiectasis is seen in retinal periphery which may further progress to fibrovascular proliferation and ridge formation due to vitreous traction. These in turn, may lead to tractional retinal detachment and subretinal exudation.

Investigation

FFA: Peripheral nonperfusion with vascular straightening and abrupt termination.

Treatment

Prognosis of this condition is generally poor. Vitrectomy for tractional retinal detachment has been successful in selected cases.

Fabre-Goldmann's Disease

Fabre-Goldmann's tapetoretinal dystrophy or Fabre-Goldmann's disease is a bilateral, progressive disease inherited in an autosomal recessive pattern.

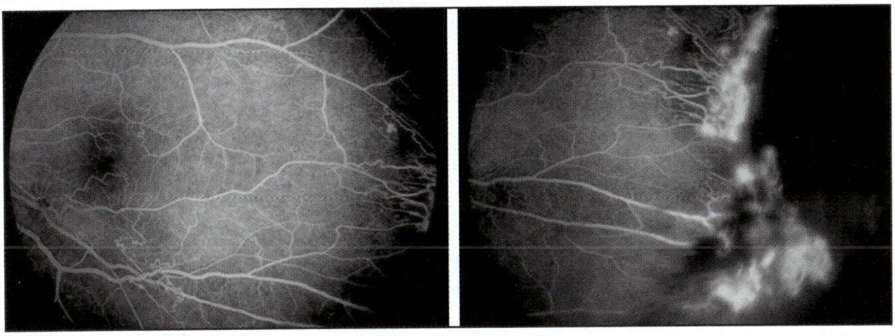

Figure 5: FFA of the same patient showing avascular retina at midperiphery with diffuse leakage from abnormal vessels

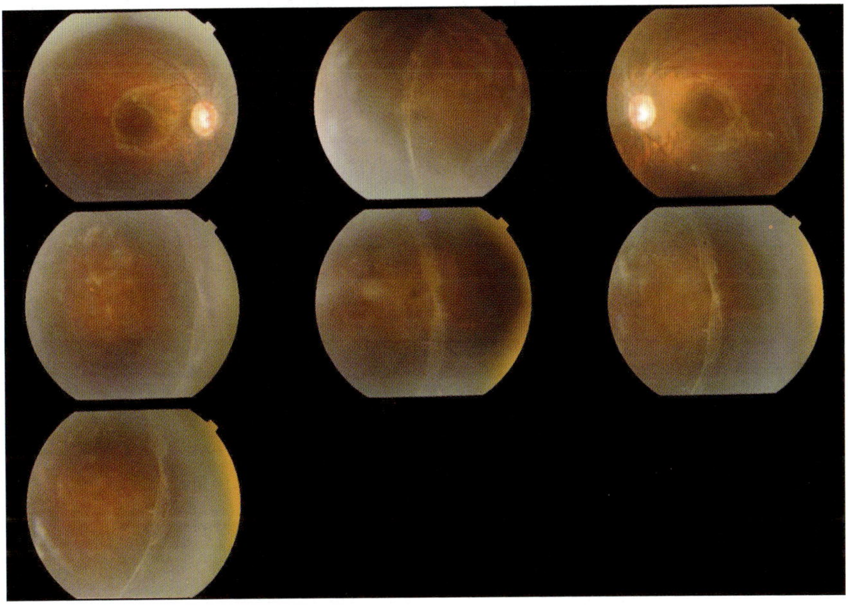

Figure 6: Fabre-Goldmann's disease

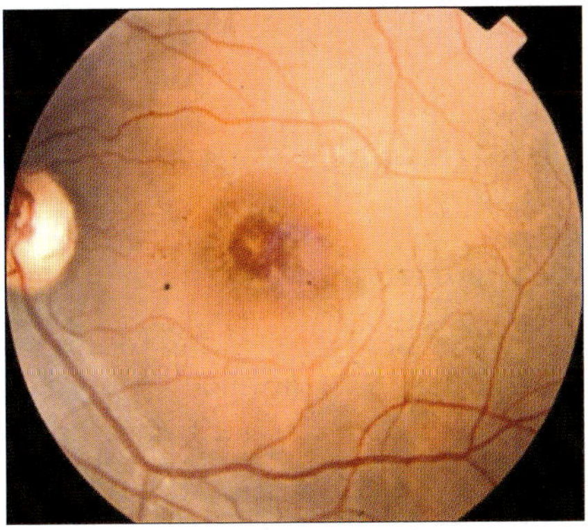

Figure 7: X-linked retinoschisis – cystoid changes at Macula

Clinical Signs and Symptoms

Usually the child presents with defective vision and nyctalopia. Clinical examination reveals features of peripheral congenital retinoschisis as well as pigmentary retinopathy.

Peripheral retinal degenerative changes like chorioretinal atrophy and pigment clumping are seen in areas of schisis, along with arteriolar attenuation and occasionally waxy disc pallor. There may be associated vitreous syneresis. Retinal detachment may occur at any time.

Investigation

ERG: Markedly reduced or absent α-wave and β-wave amplitudes.

Treatment

Early diagnosis, genetic counseling and vigilance for retinal detachment is warranted.

Hereditary Retinoschisis

A rare vitreoretinal dystrophy with an X-linked transmission pattern, hereditary retinoschisis presents in the first or early second decade.

Foveal retinoschisis is seen in almost 100% cases. Initially the foveal lesion may have a stellate appearance formed by intraretinal microcystoid spaces which enlarges overtime to coalsce and rupture. Peripheral schisis predominantly involves the inferotemporal quadrant. The inner layer contains the internal limiting membrane and the nerve fibre layer whereas the outer layer contains the rest of the outer retina. Avascular or vascular vitreous viels may appear in extreme cases which probably represents various combinations of retinoschisis and inner layer holes. There may also be peripheral perivascular sheathing, dendritiform lesions and neovascularizatin of the retina.

Complications of the dystrophy include vitreous and intra-schisis hemorrhage and retinal detachment.

Investigation

ERG: In eyes with peripheral schisis, there is decrease in β-wave amplitude in photopic and scotopic testing.

OCT: Cystoid changes characterizing the foveal retinoschisis can be documented by OCT.

Management: Prophylactic laser to peripheral retinoschisis has been found to be of no benefit. Scleral buckling surgery for retinal detachment has a variable success rate. Vitreous hemorrhage and posterior break might require a vitrectomy procedure. Genetic counseling is a must for patients and family members.

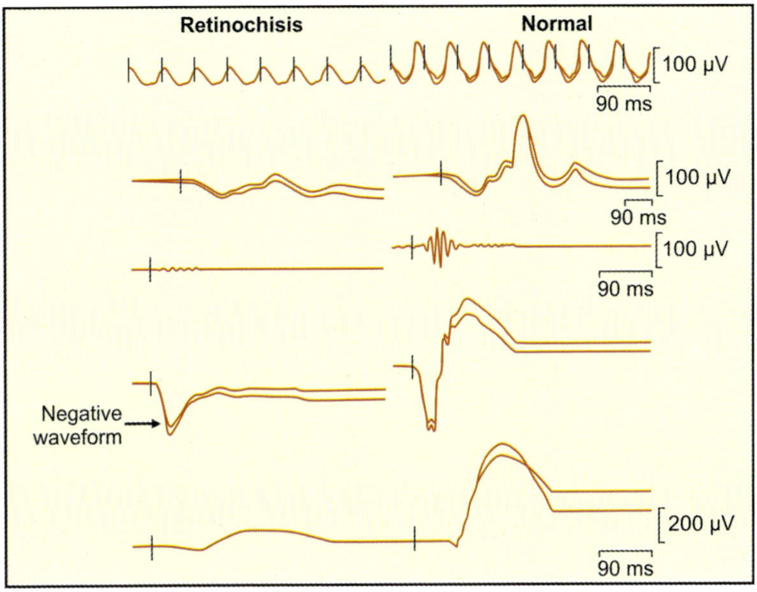

Figure 8: ERG — β wave amplitude reduced

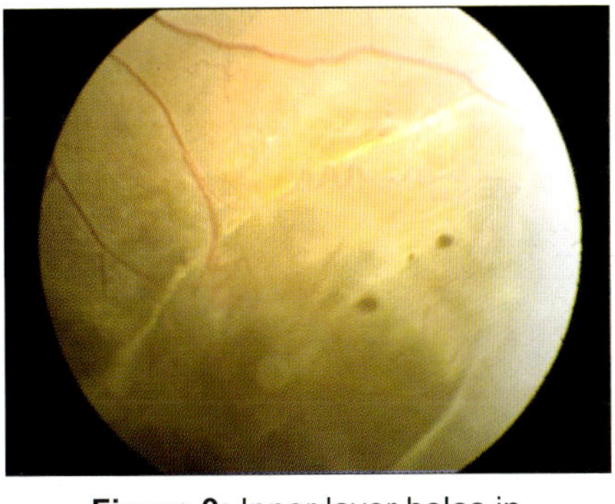

Figure 9: Inner layer holes in retinoschisis

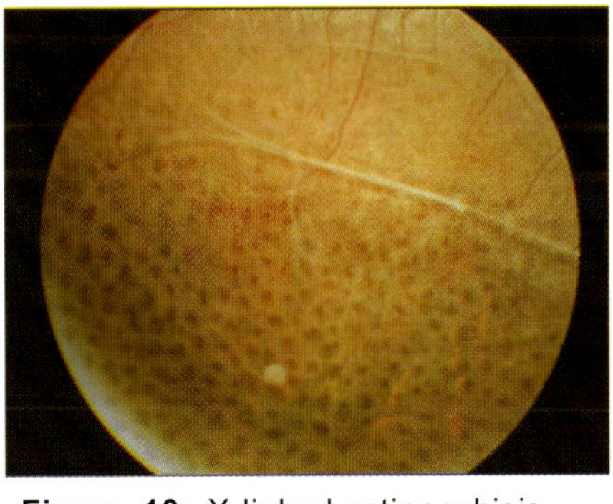

Figure 10: X-linked retinoschisis — mottled appearance of retinal pigment epithelium

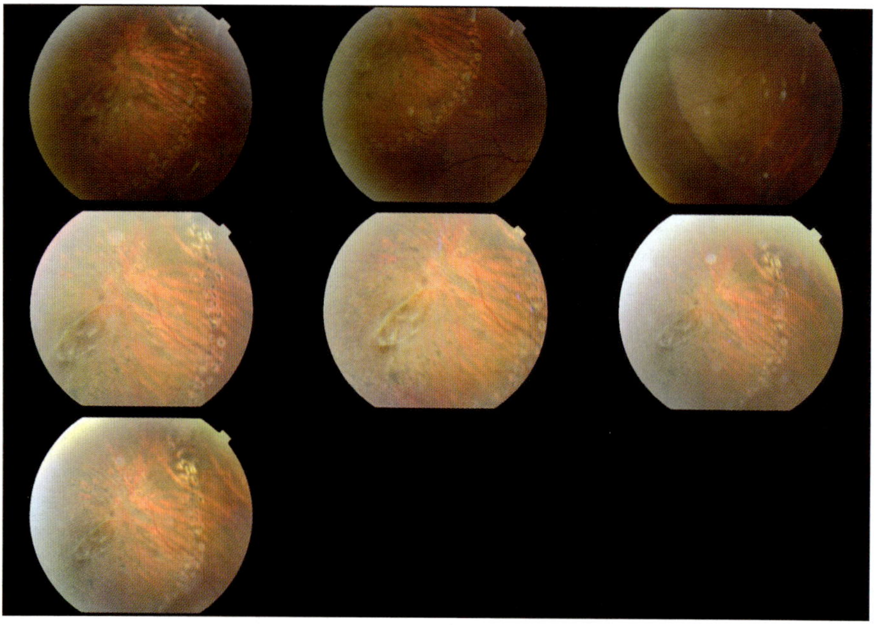

Figure 11: Peripheral retinoschisis

Chapter 47

Retinitis Pigmentosa and Allied Disorders

Ajay Aurora, Neeraj Sanduja (India)

Introduction

Retinitis pigmentosa (RP) is a generic term used for a group of disorders that are characterized by progressive destruction of the photoreceptors and the retinal pigment epithelium which in turn damage the inner retinal layers. These patients initially present with night blindness and varying degrees of loss of field. The visual loss gradually advances. The patient may have a profound peripheral visual defect (amounting to tunnel vision) and in late stages in most cases, central vision also gets affected. The age of onset of disturbance in vision ranges from infancy to late adulthood. *Retinitis pigmentosa* is not an inflammatory disorder as the name may suggest, but is a dystrophy/degeneration that is genetically determined. It has been given other names like: *tapeto retinal degenerations (Leber 1916), rod cone dystrophy and pigmentary retinopathy.*

The incidence of RP world wide is 1:5000; There is no sex predilection, however of the X-linked RP, males may be slightly more affected than the females. RP that occurs alone with no systemic association is called *Typical Retinitis pigmentosa* while the RP that occurs in association with systemic disease is known as *Complicated Retinitis pigmentosa.* At present RP is classified clinically based on the findings of complete ophthalmologic evaluations and special function tests.

It certainly would be attractive to classify RP based on the gene defect as a large number of forms of RP are becoming understood at the molecular level. However at present our knowledge of these disorders at the molecular level is, not sufficient to enable a complete classification of various forms of RP.

Patients with various forms of typical RP may have many clinical features in common, but the genetic inheritance is one of three types. Typical or classic RP can be inherited as an autosomal recessive, autosomal dominant or X-linked recessive trait. The percentage of each inheritance type has been found to vary from author to author and with country of origin of the study.

Although all cases of true RP are believed to be genetic, there is no family history of affected relatives in from 15 to 63% of cases (the average across studies is 35% in the United States, 42% in England, and 48% in China). The estimates of percentage of all RP attributed to autosomal recessive inheritance(arRP) has ranged from 13 to 69% (average: 41% in the United States, 15% in England, and 33% in China). Autosomal dominant RP (adRP) is believed to account for from 10 to 24% (16% in the United States, 24% in England, and 11% in China). X-linked RP (XLRP) accounts for from 5 to 21% (9% in the United States, 18% in England, and 8% in China).

Clinical Features

Nyctalopia

Night blindness is one of the hallmark symptoms of RP. Usually, patients with typical RP experience night vision difficulties beginning in their first or second decade of life. In arRP the symptoms (Tanino and Ohba) of nyctalopia, occurred

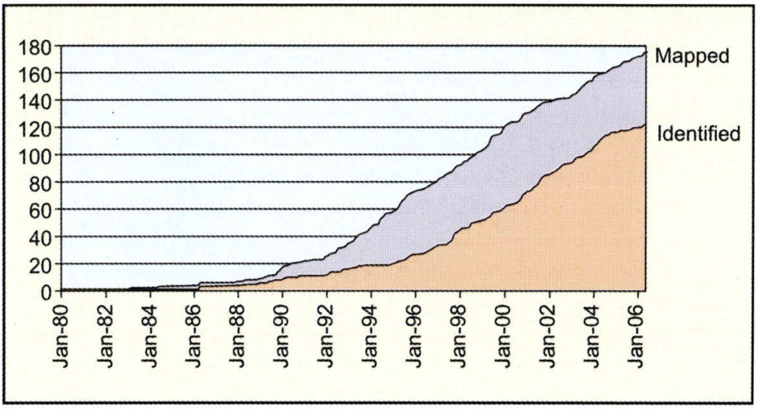

Mapped and identified retinal diseases genes 1980-2006 (*Courtesy:* Dr Stephen P. Daiger accessed from: http://www.sph.uth.tmc.edu/Retnet)

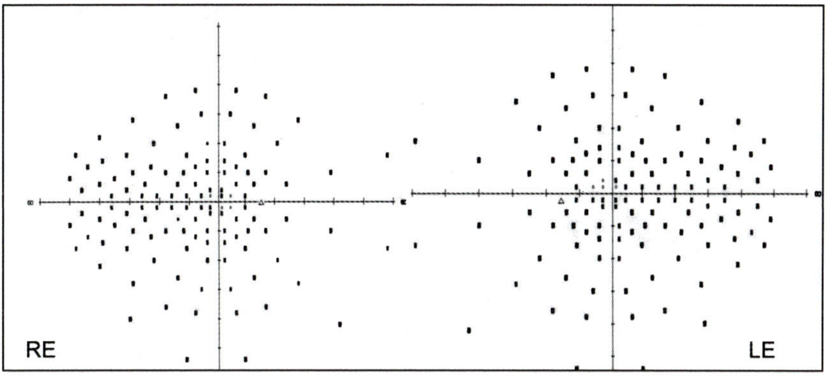

Figure 1: Humphreys visual fields 60-4 in a case of advanced RP with tunnel vision. VA in both eyes 6/9

at a median age of 10.7 years and in adRP at 23.4 years. The symptom of nyctalopia should not be confused with the symptom of blurred vision with uncorrected refractive error.

Patients with RP, when tested with dark adaptometry, may show elevation the cone segment, the rod segment, or both, to varying degrees. Also, in some patients there may be delay in reaching what eventually for them is a relatively good final dark adaptation rod threshold.

Kinetic analysis of dark adaptometry has been performed in patients with ADRP and prolonged dark adaptation associated with certain of the recently described mutations of rhodopsin (Thr17Met, Pro23His, Thr58Arg). These studies suggest that each of these mutations produces specific abnormalities in the rate of reactions within the rods that limit the recovery of scotopic sensitivity. In patients with delimited or regional forms of RP, zones of more normally functioning retina may allow reasonably good final rod thresholds. Abnormal cone threshold or cone segments of the curve, even if they are mild, are more likely to result in the complaint of poor dark adaptation than mild to moderate elevation of rod thresholds. Recent studies indicate that abnormalities in the normal interactions between rods and cones may underlie the symptoms of poor night vision in some patients.

Visual Field Loss

The second characteristic feature of RP is the slowly, progressive loss of visual field. This may happen over years or decades. Cases with a high index of suspicion, even before the appearance of pigmentary changes, the midperipheral depressions of retinal sensitivity is most readily documented as decreased retinal thresholds in the midperiphery (30 to 50 degrees from fixation) on static perimetry. In the initial stages it may be diagnosed as islands of defects in the midperiphery that enlarge, deepen and coalesce over time into a ring scotoma. The ring scotomata gradually enlarge, and break out to the periphery, leaving peripheral islands of vision, usually temporal but occasionally inferior or nasal. Often the superior visual field is more abnormal, reflecting the earlier involvement of the inferior retina. Occasionally the visual field loss is greater temporally, nasally, or inferiorly. Typically, in advanced state of RP patient may have 6/6 vision but a field contracted to the 20-degree horizontal central diameter (Considered legally blind in the US with III-4e test target on a Goldmann perimeter). Rarely some patients of may develop visual field defects in the pericentral region between 5 and 30 degrees from fixation. These are cases of Central Pericentral or Inverse RP. These patients may not be legally blind based on the definition of Vision or Visual field, yet are severely handicapped. *Krauss and Heckenlively* found this type of visual field loss more frequently in those patients with RP who have a predominance of cone loss as compared with rod loss on the electroretinogram (ERG).

Massof et al. found that, in most forms of generalized RP, the visual field seeing area shrank approximately 50% over 4.5 years. *Massof and Finkelstein* argue that the time course for all major genetic and functional classes of RP is nearly identical if one corrects for the critical age, which they define as the age

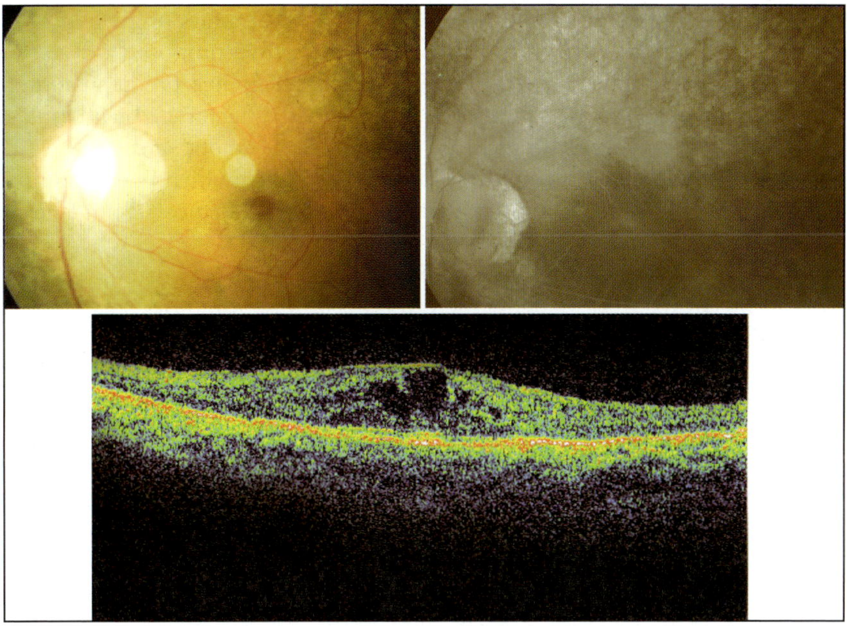

Figure 2: A case of RP with cystoid macular edema as seen in late phase of FFA and on optical coherence tomography that is showing fluid filled cysts (*Courtesy:* Grewal Eye Institute)

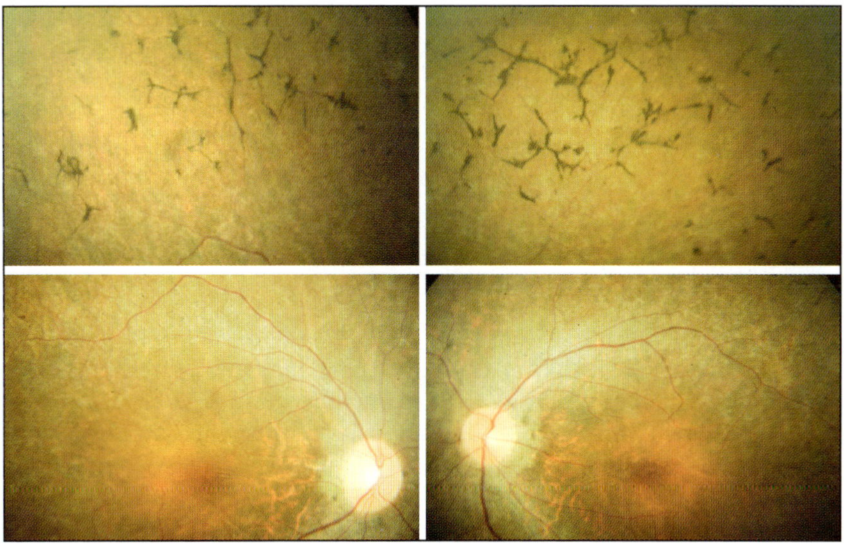

Figure 3: Shows characteristic bony spicule with narrowed arterioles in a patient of typical retinitis pigmentosa

when visual field loss would be first detected by a test target of given size and brightness. In conjunction with this concept, they have proposed a two-stage hypothesis for the natural course of RP. The first stage is a predisposition for retinal degeneration, such as genetic or environmental factors, which would be different for the separate types of RP and possibly among individuals. The second stage involves the actual retinal degeneration, which proceeds on its own internal time course, and which would be common to most, if not all forms of RP.

RP patients usually have a symmetric visual field loss between the two eyes. However in X-linked RP patients there can be striking differences between the two eyes. This may be because of:

a. Lyonization (X-chromosome inactivation) is a random event and occurs close to the time of lateralization in the developing embryo. Hence two eyes may be differently affected.
b. Random nature of the Lyonization (X-chromosomal inactivation) of cells in the retina, may lead to patchy distribution of retinal cells expressing the abnormal gene-containing X-chromosome resulting in unusual patterns in visual field loss. However, even in these cases the visual fields usually correspond quite closely to the fundus appearance, with the greater visual field loss in the eye with greater pigmentary abnormalities.

Central vision

It is a widely held that RP patients retain **Central vision** till late even if most of the peripheral field is lost. This is dependent on the type of RP. Patients with sector RP may retain good visual acuity all their life. Patients with adRP are more likely than patients with arRP or X-linked RP to retain good acuity beyond 60 years of age. Central vision can be seriously affected early in otherwise typical RP in following situations:

1. Cystoid macular edema (CME)
2. Diffuse retinal vascular leakage
3. Wrinkling of the internal limiting membrane
4. Macular preretinal fibrosis
5. Certain subtypes of RP
   i. XLRP
   ii. Inverse RP
   iii. Certain arRP

Sandberg and Berson using testing for cone increment thresholds, found that reduced cone spatial density (reduced numbers of cones per unit area) is a major determinant of reduced visual acuity in patients with RP. However, the reduction in number of functioning cones does not appear to be even across the posterior pole. Relatively early involvement of the macula with visual acuity loss is especially seen in certain subtypes of RP, such as XLRP, one of the forms of early-onset recessive RP, and inverse RP which is an entity that some investigators consider may represent a cone-rod dystrophy rather than RP.

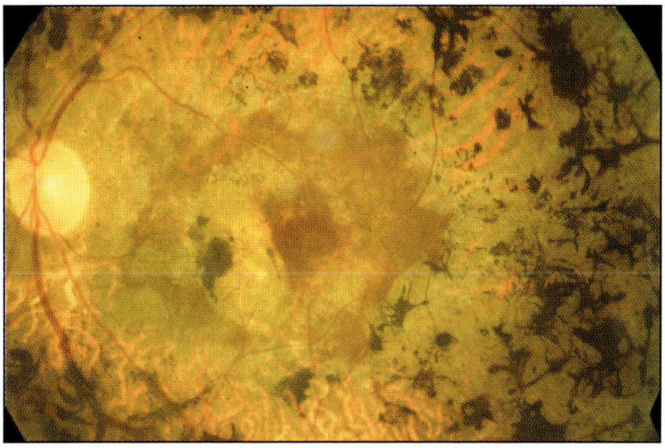

Figure 4: Left eye of a 65 years female with BCVA of 6/18 showing advanced retinitis pigmentosa with macular involvement

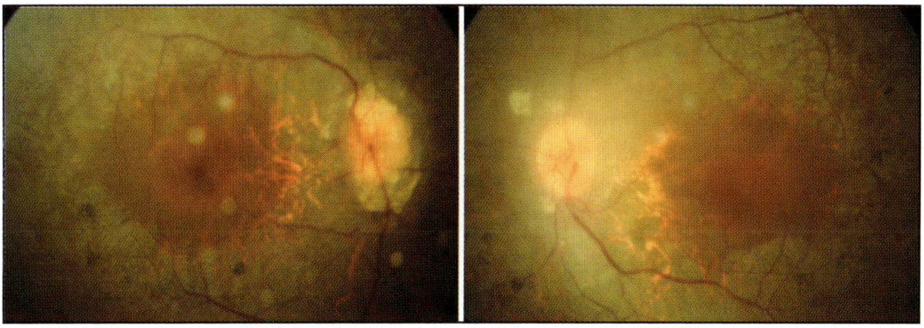

Figure 5: Shows characteristic bony spicule with narrowed arterioles in a patient of typical retinitis pigmentosa with Drusens of the optic disks in both eyes

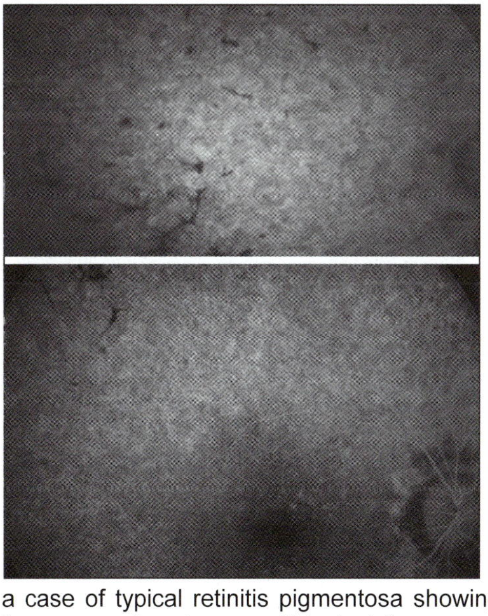

Figure 6: FFA in a case of typical retinitis pigmentosa showing window defects (transmitted hyperfluorescence) and areas of blocked fluorescence corresponding to bony spicules

Color Vision

Color vision in typical RP remains good until the vision has fallen to a level of 20/40 or worse. However, the color vision may fail early in juvenile Batten disease and Bardet-Biedl syndrome, in which central cones appear to be abnormal from the beginning. In some patients of atypical RP, the pericentral scotomata encroach very close to fixation early in the disease. These patients, even though they show a rod-cone loss on ERG, may show more significant color vision defects even when the vision is relatively good.

Photopsia

About 35 % of all RP patients experience flashes of light that usually occur in the midperipheral field adjacent to the areas of scotomas (both relative and absolute), are continuous in nature (those that are associated with migraine are episodic) and usually disappear with advancing disease and enlarging scotomas. Patients describe these photopsias as tiny blinking lights or as coarse sparkling graininess in vision. In the series presented by Heckenlively 170 of 500 (35%) patients developed photopsias and of these eight patients developed retinal detachment. Hence a good fundus exam should be a routine in all these cases. The cellular cause for photopsias is not clear but could be due to photoreceptor dysfunction, neurite sprouting, aberrant synapse formation and secondary remodeling of the retina.

Fundus Findings

In early stages the retina may appear near normal , even when the visual field shows relative scotomata or areas of decreased retinal thresholds on static perimetry. Patients who have very early RP without fundus pigmentary abnormalities are often diagnosed as having retinitis pigmentosa sine pigmento, which is not a specific subtype of RP but a stage through which most, patients of RP pass. In most, if not all, pigmentary deposits in the retina will develop eventually. The sine pigmento stage may exist for decades. In those patients with high myopia along with RP, often the presence of the typical findings of high myopia delays the appreciation of other abnormalities. The earliest findings of RP on fundus examination are attenuation of retinal vessels and the appearance of fine mottling or granularity of the RPE in the midperiphery and far periphery. The macular may exhibit increased luster due to the reflection of light off the internal limiting membrane of the retina, or wrinkling, suggesting the presence of edema of the retina in the posterior pole or early preretinal fibrosis. This edematous or wrinkled appearance to the retina may change over a few years to a drier or smoother appearance, perhaps because of either a change in the vascular permeability or atrophy of retinal elements.

Classically a moderately advanced RP would show attenuated retinal vessels, mottling and granularity of the retinal pigment epithelium (RPE), migration of pigment into the inner retina and its accumulation in the interstitial spaces surrounding retinal vessels, especially at vessel branching, producing

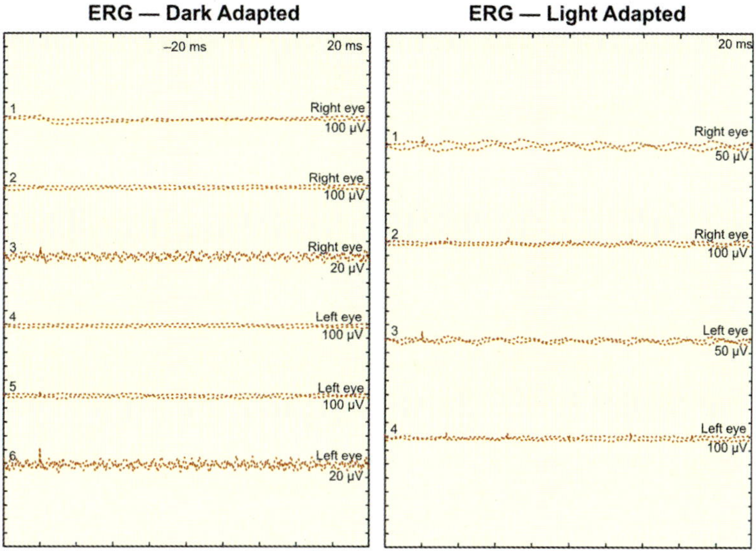

Figure 7: Three years male,fixing and following light; ERG showing extinguished responses in both eyes for both dark adapted and light adapted conditions. Suggestive of retinitis pigmentosa in both eyes.(*Courtesy:* Shroff Eye Centre, New Delhi)

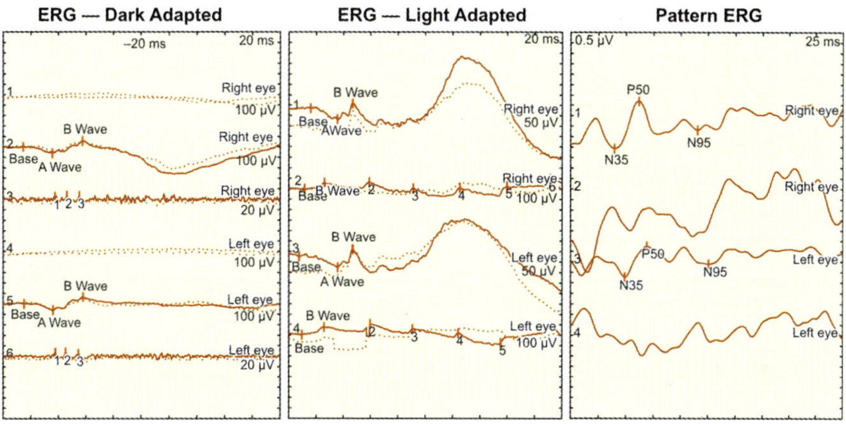

Figure 8: Symptomatic 12 years female with VA both eyes of 6/9. Flash ERG shows grossly reduced amplitudes for both dark adapted and light adapted conditions in both eyes. Pattern ERG shows normal amplitudes in both eyes.These are suggestive of early retinitis pigmentosa in both eyes. (*Courtesy:* Shroff Eye Centre, New Delhi)

perivascular pigmentary cuffing and bone-spicule formation. The RPE and choriocapillaris gradually atrophy leading to larger choroidal vessels becoming prominent and overall fundus appearing greyer. At this stage, usually, the fundus in two eyes appears symmetrical. In the late stages the peripheral and far peripheral fundus is replaced by dense bone-spicule pigmentary formations; vessel attenuation that may have been mild in earlier stages becomes severe, so that the retinal vessels appear threadlike.

Women who are carriers of X-linked form of RP may have a yellowish-white metallic tapetal reflex or sheen in the midperiphery or far periphery or even in the posterior pole.This may sometimes be seen in young males with early RP as well. Women who are carriers for XLRP may show patchy bone-spicule pigmentation with associated visual field defects. In carriers for XLRP, the fundus appearance may be quite asymmetric between the two eyes, consistent with expected normal variation in X-chromosomal inactivation or lyonization. With time, in males who show the tapetal reflex as well as in carrier women, regional or diffuse mottling and atrophy of the RPE eventually replace the tapetal sheen.

The optic disk may be normal in early RP. As the disease progresses the optic disk tends to become pale and this pallor is described as waxy pallor. Histologic studies have shown that the peculiar appearance of the disk patients with RP is associated with gliosis (astrocytic proliferation) overlying the disks. The optic nerve head cup-to-disk ratio has been reported to be significantly smaller in RP patients of all types (0.19 compared to 0.35 in normals).

Drusenlike globular excrescences may develop on the optic nerve or adjacent retina. These globular excrescences were believed to represent astrocytic hamartomas but histologic studies support the concept that these are typical drusen that occur presumably as a manifestation of aberrant axoplasmic transport.

Fundus Fluorescein Angiography

Fluorescein angiography will often reveal transmission defects of the RPE with later diffuse leakage. Some patients may show extravasation of dye from perifoveal capillaries. Angiographically evident CME occurs not infrequently in RP, even in younger patients at an early stage of their disease and even with visual acuity of 20/25 or better. Uncommonly, peripheral retinal vasculopathy with lipid exudations can be seen in RP, leading to the diagnosis of Coats' disease

Anterior Segment Abnormalities

Cataracts are the most frequent of anterior-segment complications that can be seen with RP. The prevalence of cataracts in RP patients aged 20 to 39 years varied with the inheritance type, being roughly 52% for autosomal dominant, 39% for autosomal recessive, and 72% for X-linked cases. The incidence of cataracts in RP is highly age-dependent. The most frequent type of cataract is the posterior subcapsular opacity, which was found in 49% of one group of patients with ADRP. Keratoconus is generally accepted as occurring more frequently with Leber's congenital amaurosis. Some claim that keratoconus is more frequent among patients with RP glaucoma is also allegedly more frequent in RP, with roughly only half the cases representing chronic open-angle glaucoma. One form of sector RP appears to be associated with hyperopia and angle-closure glaucoma. Because of the other abnormalities of the disk and fundus, and because of the already abnormal visual fields, the diagnosis and management of glaucoma are more difficult in association with RP.

Bietti's crystalline dystrophy of the cornea and retina is an autosomal recessive, presumably metabolic disorder. Patients develop RP, which can be either regional, with a predilection for the posterior pole, or diffuse, involving the entire retina. The peripheral corneal stroma characteristically shows myriads of yellow-white crystals of unknown composition; these crystals are also present in various layers of the retina.

Vitreous Abnormalities

On careful examination of the vitreous with a contact lens/90D exam, fine dust like pigmented opacities that represent pigment released from the degenerating RPE cells may be found. In some patients one may find "cottonball" opacities, interwoven filaments in the retrocortical space and spindle-shaped vitreous condensation are seen more frequently than in normal population.There is only a single report of a patient with opacity so dense that vitrectomy was required.

Refractive Status

High myopia and astigmatism are more frequent in many forms of RP, especially XLRP, one form of Leber's congenital amaurosis, and at least one form of autosomal recessive RP. High hyperopia occurs with what may be a specific form of uncomplicated Leber's congenital amaurosis and preserved para-arteriolar RPE-RP.

Other Associated Features

Approximately 30% of all patients with RP will experience mild to severe hearing loss as adults. This does not include those with Usher's syndrome, which is congenital hearing loss plus RP. Patients with RP appear at a greater than normal risk for thyroid disease. Several studies have reported immunologic abnormalities in patients with RP, but it is not known whether these are important in the pathogenesis or merely epiphenomena.

Psychophysical Findings

Perimetry

Visual field assessment is an important aspect of the management of RP. Visual field is able to quantify the affected patient's visual deficit.

Most studies in the past have used Goldman Kinetic primetry to quantify the visual deficit, and lately Humphrey's visual field analyzer or Octopus perimeter is being used.Now two color static perimetry is being increasingly used to assess the dark adapted visual field in an RP patient.This technique allows evaluation of rod and cone retinal sensitivities in different regions of the retina. Based on this technique *Massof and Finkelstein* have classified the RP patients into two categories 1) Type 1 RP: is characterized by early diffuse loss of rod sensitivity relative to cone sensitivity and childhood onset nyctalopia 2) Type 2 RP characterized by regional and combined loss of both rods and cone sensitivity and adult onset nyctalopia. No patients have been reported to changeover from one type to another and the sibs within a family maintain the type. Two color scotopic static perimetry is useful in monitoring disease progress, response to therapy and to understand the pathophysiology in a case.

Dark Adaptometry

Normal subjects when placed in dark after exposure to a strong adapting light, rapidly reduce their psychophysical threshold using their cone system, reaching a plateau in about 5 minutes. Thereafter rod adaptation slowly increases, and rods determine retinal threshold for another 3 log units of sensitivity before a second plateau occurs at about 30 minutes of dark adaptation.When RP patients are tested on dark adaptometry, there may be an elevation of cone segment, rod segment or both in varying degrees.In some patients there may be a delay in reaching their final drak adapted rod threshold. Various studies have documented rhodopsin mutation that produce specific abnormalities in he rate of reaction within the rods that limit the recovery of scotopic sensitivity.

Retinal Densitometry

This technique aims to assess photoreceptor photopigment density by measuring the difference between the light shone into the eye and the light reflected from the eye. These measurements can be made and compared at different loci, at different times so as to evaluate the process of progressive depigmentation and may be compared to a definitive retinal standard.

Electrophysiology

The standing(resting) potential of the eye was first described by DuBois-Reymond in 1849. In 1945 Karpe reported that the ERG was "extinguished" in RP. Riggs in 1954 reported that the resting potential was decreased in pigmentary degeneration of the eye.

In 1962 Arden et al developed the currently used technique of measurement of light- induced rise of the resting potential of the eye (EOG), which is considered a function of the RPE.Gouras in 1970 based clinical ERG on the use of Ganzfield stimulation.Standardized conditions and assessment protocols have now been established for electrodiagnostic investigations.

The ERG responses in RP patients can range from normal to extinguished. Younger patients and those in the early stages of their disease have more sizeable responses. Marmor has suggested that RP patients with scotopic ERG amplitudes of 100 mV or greater have a "delimited" form of the disease with a better prognosis. Most patients with advanced RP will have undetectable responses (typically less than 10 mV) to single-flash, nonaveraged techniques. Computer averaging, however, can usually detect small ERGs in even moderately advanced stages. Berson et al while studying the natural course of RP, found that patients lost an average of 16% to 18.5% of their remaining ERG amplitude to bright white light flashes (a mixed rod-cone response) per year. Massof and Finkelstein found that the scotopic rod-dominated ERG was affected to a much more severe degree than the photopic cone-mediated ERG in type I RP, whereas the scotopic and photopic ERGs were more equally abnormal in type II RP. Arden et al also concluded that the presence or absence of rod ERG may supplement psychophysical testing in the categorization of patients with ADRP. It has been found that the ERG was more likely to be recordable in older patients with ADRP than autosomal recessive RP. Also ADRP was significantly less likely to show progressive ERG loss of amplitude over time.

It has been reported that the rod-mediated b-wave implicit time is significantly prolonged in all inheritance types of typical RP. However the validity of this is questioned by others. *Birch and Fish* found that for a given stimulus intensity, the rod-mediated b-wave implicit times are prolonged in those RP patients with a greater rod than cone loss on the ERG, but not RP patients with greater cone than rod loss on the ERG. Most patients with RP have losses of retinal ERG sensitivity that are related to loss of rhodopsin. If adjusted for the loss of retinal sensitivity as detected by the Naka-Rushton half-saturation coefficient, log k, rod implicit times are for the most part, normal in RP. Birch and Fish also found that the criterion (87 ms) rod b-wave implicit time correlated well with the half-saturation coefficient, log k. There is reasonable agreement that the cone-mediated implicit times are significantly prolonged in various forms of RP.It is believed that when normal rod andcone b-wave implicit times are recorded in an RP patient, the disease is most likely to have limited progression or may be stationery.

Newer models of analysis of ERG that attempt to isolate from the ERG the photoreceptor and bipolar contributions are being used. These models of analysis are being used to quantify the visual deficit attributable to outer and inner retinal disease. Arden, Barrada, and Kelsey in 1963 developed the currently widely used technique for measurement of the light-induced rise of the resting potential of the eye. Fast oscillations of the resting potential can be recorded and these offer another measure of RPE function In general, the electrooculogram (EOG) is abnormal in diffuse hereditary rod-cone degenerations of the retina.In typical RP, the slow and fast light-induced oscillations of the resting potential are usually decreased simultaneously early in the disease. The EOG, in most cases of RP, is abnormal when the ERG is abnormal. In most cases, the EOG serves as an adjunct test for the ERG.

Classification

Historically, retiitis pigmentosa patients have been classified by the findings on clinical examination and by the results of specific functional studies. The RP disorders can be classified by predominant photoreceptor involvement on the ERG (rod-cone or cone-rod), by inheritance type (autosomal recessive, autosomal dominant, or X-linked), by distribution of retinal involvement (central, pericentral, sector, or peripheral), and by age of onset (Leber's congenital amaurosis, childhood onset, juvenile onset, adult onset, or late onset).

There has been an explosion of information of molecular genetics in the patients of RP. It would be ideal to subdivide RP based on their biochemical characteristics and correlate these observations with characteristic clinical features. However present day knowledge does not allow us to have a unified classification system that may be used by the clinicians, molecular geneticists and researchers with ease.

Subdivision by Mode of Inheritance

This is the most useful way of classifying RP.Typical RP may be inherited as adRP (autosomal dominanat RP), arRP (autosomal recessive RP) and X-linked recessive trait(XLRP). Though mitochondrial inheritance is associated with pigmentary retinal degeneration, typical non-syndromic RP is yet to be associated with this type of inheritance. The percentage of inheritance of each RP varies amongst authors as well as countries. Despite the fact that typical RP is always genetic, family history may be lacking in 15-63% cases. Such cases are labeled as "simplex RP". On an average about 40% of all RP patients are of simplex variety and it seems that most of these patients are of autosomal recessive variety.

Subdivision by Age of Onset

This may be classified as:

1. Early onset RP
   a. Congenital RP: These patients present with nystagmus.
   b. Childhood onset form
2. Juvenile or early adult onset: Usually present in the first three decades.
3. Adult Onset or Late onset form: May have a non-genetic basis. If inherited this form is usually autosomal recessive.

Subdivision by Molecular Defect

In the past decade there has been a rapid advancement in the understanding of the genetic basis of various retinal diseases particularly of the molecular genetic basis of Retinitis pigmentosa and allied disorders.

This has become possible due to the advances in the methods that have become available for understanding the human genome. Particularly useful is the development of genetic markers which are based on DNA polymorphism identified throughout the genome and their application through polymerase chain reaction methodology in linkage analysis. In linkage analysis the unknown human disease—gene locus is compared with a marker locus. Earlier restriction fragment length polymorphism (RFLP) was used. Now, newer techniques like polymorphic minisatellites or polymorphic microsatellites, or single nucleotide polymorphism are being employed. We now understand that a mutant allele for a gene can behave in different ways, depending on where the sequence change resides within the gene and the status of the other allele. Gene mutations that produce no gene product (*null alleles*) may exhibit autosomal recessive inheritance, if one good copy of the gene is sufficient to produce enough product to maintain normal function. Some of the genetic localizations for RP patients are listed below. Detailed latest information of gene assignments and localizations, list of cloned and mapped genes causing retinal degenerations or allied disorders that has been compiled by Dr Stephen P Daiger and may be accessed at: http://www.sph.uth.tmc.edu/Retnet

Disease category	*Mapped Loci (not Identified)*	*Mapped and Identified Genes*
Retinitis pigmentosa, autosomal dominant	RP31, RP33	CA4, CRX, FSCN2, GUCA1B, IMPDH1, NRL, PRPF3, PRPF8, PRPF31, RDS, RHO, ROM1, RP1, RP9, SEMA4A
Retinitis pigmentosa, autosomal recessive	RP22, RP25, RP28, RP29, RP32	ABCA4, CERKL, CNGA1, CNGB1, CRB1, LRAT, MERTK, NR2E3, NRL, PDE6A, PDE6B, PRCD, RGR, RHO, RLBP1, RP1, RPE65, SAG, TULP1, USH2A
Retinitis pigmentosa, X-linked	RP6, RP23, RP24, RP34	RP2, RPGR
Usher syndrome, autosomal recessive	USH1E, USH2B	CDH23, MASS1, MYO7A, PCDH15, USH1C, USH1G, USH2A, USH3A
Bardet-Biedl syndrome, autosomal recessive	None	ARL6, BBS1, BBS2, BBS4, BBS5, BBS7, BBS10, MKKS, PTHB1, TRIM32, TTC8

(*Coutesy:* Dr Stephen P. Daiger accessed from: http://www.sph.uth.tmc.edu/Retnet)

It most unlikely even today and more so in the Indian circumstance that a patient will present with information on the specific gene mutation for their disease. Hence it is most unlikely that a classification based on molecular genetic defect will at present replace the popular subdivision of RP based on clinical grounds. However, molecular information will certainly be immensely helpful in defining the true spectrum and natural history of a specific form of RP.This will help in prognostic counseling and the patient may be able toplan his or her life based on the natural history of the disease predicted by the genetic basis of the disease.The ability to detect the presence of gene defect by examining the DNA taken from the blood samples will allow earlier and more accurate diagnosis, facilitate genetic counseling, open ways of prenatal diagnosis and eventually guide the patient to specific gene defect-relted therapies.

Subdivision Based on Distribution of Retinal Involvement and Fundus Appearance

Retinitis Pigmentosa Sine Pigmento

This is RP without signs of intraretinal pigmentation.Usually this represents an early form of RP.

Retinitis Punctate Albescens

Fine white punctate lesions are seen in the mid and far periphery at the level of RP. This usually happens in the early stages of RP and may be seen in the younger members of the family while the older members show typical features of RP.White dots on the fundus associated with stationery night blindness are characteristic of *Fundus albipunctatus*. Patients with vitamin A deficiency may also demonstrate white dot lesions on the fundus.

Sector and Sectorial Retinitis Pigmentosa

Sector RP was first described by Bietti in 1937. It is characterized by RP changes that are limited to one or two quadrants. The visual field defect corresponds to the retinal quadrant that is involved and there is no extension of retina linvolvement with time. The ERG responses are good. However it has been shown that the absolute retinal thresholds are elevated throughout retina.Rods and cones appear to be equally affected. With time the viual field defect may worsen. The overall visual prognosis is good and the affected patients can lead a healthy normal life.

Retinitis Pigmentosa Inversus (Pericentral and Central Retinitis Pigmentosa)

Classically this entity is RP involving only the posterior pole. However since cases of cone-rod dystrophy , RP with macular lesions have been also labeled as RP inversus the true incidence of this disease is unknown.

The proper classification of cone-rod dystrophies is debated. Since most if not all cone retinal dystrophies with time will develop rod abnormalities, some authors have stated that this distinction has limited value and would classify cone-rod dystrophies as a subset of cone retinal dystrophy Others would classify cone-rod dystrophies as a subset of RP because rods are eventually severely affected as well and the end visual burden is often as severe as any cases of RP Moreover, the precise separation of cone-rod vs. rod-cone involvement depends upon the criteria that one accepts, since often persons affected with cone-rod dystrophies will have some features in common with rod-cone dystrophies. Few histopathologic studies exist for cone-rod dystrophy, but Rabb et al reported a case with loss of photoreceptors in the periphery and macula with preservation of both rods and cones in the equatorial regions. This distribution of photoreceptor loss differs from typical RP, in which the usual zone of greatest loss in the midperiphery or equatorial retina.

Complicated Retinitis Pigmentosa

Most RP patients are not associated with manifestations outside the eye. About one third of RP patients experience hearing loss of varying degrees as adults.It is not known how many of these are cases of Ushers syndrome as in many cases it is a coincidental association.Patients of RP have a greater than normal risk of Thyroid disease.

Usher's Syndrome

Usher's syndrome is an autosomal recessive congenital deafness with typical RP von Graefe in 1858 descibed this condition but it was the British ophthalmologist Charles who described it as a distinct familial entity. Usher's syndrome accounts for 18% of all cases of RP and 50% of those persons who are both deaf and blind in the US have Usher's syndrome.

Usher's syndrome can be divided clinically into three major groups:

Type 1: Profound congenital sensorineural deafness (prelingual deafness), vestibular symptoms, and prepubertal onset of RP.

Type 2: Partial congenital non-progressive deafness, absence of vestibular symptoms, and the RP is slightly milder and of late onset.

Type 3: Progressive deafness starting in the second to fourth decade, adult onset retinopathy and hypermetropic astigmatism.

These types have not been reported to be mixed in the same sibship and in most, if not all, cases, probably represent nonallelic, different genotypes.

The two most common settings where the diagnosis is missed are early disease, where bone-spicule fundus pigmentation is lacking, and disease with fine to medium pigment clumping, where the diagnosis is mistaken for rubella retinopathy. ERG must be done to confirm the diagnosis of Usher's syndrome.Other syndromes that can be associated with deafness and RP must be considered when the diagnosis is entertained. These include infantile Refsum's disease (also called infantile phytanic acid storage disease), adult Refsum's disease, Cockayne's syndrome, Bardet-Biedl syndrome, Alström's disease, Flynn-Aird syndrome, Friedreich's ataxia, and Kearns-Sayre syndrome.

The photoreceptors of the retina and the hair cells of the inner ear are both ciliated epithelial cells. Sperm, photoreceptors, and inner ear hair cells all contain axonemes. *Hunter et al* in 1986 found abnormal axonemes in sperm from subjects with Usher's syndrome and abnormal axonemes on histologic examination of retinal sections from a patient with Usher's syndrome. Abnormal connecting cilia have been found on electron microscopy of retinal sections from a male with type 2 Usher's syndrome. These findings suggest that both the cilium of the inner ear and the cilium of the photoreceptors may share axonemal components that are necessary for formation of ciliated structures and whose genes would be candidates for the defective gene in Usher's syndrome.

Leber's Congenital Amaurosis

Leber's congenital amaurosis (LCA) is a group of disorders characterized by severe visual impairment or blindness from infancy with no discernible other cause. Theodor Leber in 1869 described children with severe visual impairment before age 1 year, nystagmus, poor pupillary reflexes, either normal fundi or a tapetoretinal degeneration, and an autosomal recessive inheritance pattern The ERG is profoundly abnormal or absent and is a requirement for the diagnosis. Eye rubbing, the oculodigital sign is commomly associated.

LCA could be divided into two subtypes:

Uncomplicated LCA: is characterized by congenital blindness, nystagmus, high hyperopia and extinguished ERG responses.

Complicated LCA: is LCA with other ocular or systemic features.

The fundus in LCA could be entirely normal, show RPE granularity and mild vessel attenuation. Various retinal abnormalities that have been described in LCA include, macular coloboma, "salt and pepper" retinopathy, retinitis punctata albescens and nummular pigmentation.LCA often (about 30% cases) has associated keratoconus.Systemic association of LCA include deafness, renal abnormalities, infantile cardiomyopathy (Alström's syndrome), hepatic dysfunction, skeletal abnormalities and neurological abnormalities. Recent studies suggest that 20% of the

Bardet-Biedl Syndrome

Bardet in 1920 described a patient with RP, polydactyly, and congenital obesity. Biedl in 1922 added the fourth and fifth cardinal features of the syndrome: mental retardation and hypogenitalism. Most authors today regard Bardet-Biedl syndrome as distinct from the syndrome described by Laurence and Moon in 1866, which, as later reported by Hutchinson, had paraplegia as a prominent feature and which did not have polydactyly or obesity.

Forty to fifty percent of all cases have incomplete manifestation of the five cardinal features. It has been suggested that at least four of the five cardinal features, of which RP must be one, must be present to conclusively establish the diagnosis. Following are the incidence of various features:

1. Pigmentary retinopathy is reported in from 90% to 100% of cases.
2. Abnormal ERG in all patients.
3. Tendency for obesity is nearly universal but patients have been able to control their weight by dieting and exercise.
4. Polydactyly (postaxial) in 75% of cases. and may involve any or all extremities. Syndactyly or brachydactyly was present in 14.4% of patients.
5. Hypogenitalism in 50% of patients over the age of 15.

Deafness occurs in approximately 5% of patients. The retinal dystrophy in Bardet-Biedl syndrome differs in most patients from typical RP in that the visual acuity fails early in the course of the disease and usually the fundus shows little pigmentary dispersion until later stages. Color vision may also be defective early. Macular lesions and atrophy of the RPE or choriocapillaris often develop as the disease progresses. Macular abnormalities may include macular wrinkling, preretinal membrane formation, and leakage on fluorescein angiogram from paramacular capillaries. When detectable, the ERG may show a rod-cone loss or in some cases a cone-rod loss pattern, which has led authors to call the retinal dystrophy in Bardet-Biedl syndrome a cone-rod retinal degeneration. The absence of pigmentary deposits early has led to the retinal dystrophy being called RP sine pigmento or, if patchy whitish RPE lesions are evident, retinitis punctata albescens. Approximately 73% of patients reach legal blindness status by age 20 years and 86% by the age of 30 years.

Neuronal Ceroid Lipofuscinosis (Batten disease, Amaurotic Idiocy)

Neuronal ceroid lipofuscinosis are a group of progressive neurodegenerative disorders characterized by accumulation of complex storage material within the lysosomes. These are the commonest neurodegenerative disorders to affect the children with a worldwide incidence of 1:1, 25000.These patients characteristically have severe psychomotor deterioration that eventually leads to a vegetative state , seizures, visual failure from retinal degeneration and premature death.Four classic forms exist: three childhood-onset forms which are all autosomal recessive, and one adult onset form which may be autosomal recessive or dominant.

1. *Infantile onset neuronal ceroid lipofuscinosis* (INCL) also called Haltia-Santavuori disease, Hagberg-Santavaouri disease or Finnish form of NCL. Manifests at 8-24 months with severe psychomotor retardation, blindness and microcephaly.
2. *Late Infantile onset Neuronal ceroid lipofuscinosis* (LINCL) also called Jansky-Bielchowsky disease. Manifests at 2 to 4 years of age with ataxia, loss of speech, regression of development milestones, seizures and later loss of vision.
3. *Juvenile onset neuronal ceroid lipofuscinosis* (JNCL) also called Batten-Mayou syndrome, Spielmeyer-Vogt disease or Spielmeyer-Sjogren syndrome; manifests at 4-8 years of age with progressive loss of vision to virtually no vision after one to two years.
4. *Adult onset neuronal ceroid lipofuscinosis (ANCL)* also called Kuf's disease, usually manifests as a motor disturbance without visual symptoms.

Bassen-Kornzweig Syndrome (Abetalipoproteinemia)

First described in 1950 includes malformed erythrocytes (acanthocytosis), neuromuscular disturbance with ataxia, fat intolerance and retinitis pigmentosa. Strabismus and nystagmus are seen in several patients and may be related to the central nervous system defect.All psychological and electrophysiologic findings are quite similar to typical RP. It is an autosomal recessive disorder in which apolipoprotein B is not synthesized, leading to fat malabsorption, fat-soluble vitamin deficiencies, spinocerebellar degeneration, and retinal degeneration. In abetalipoproteinemia, the mutated protein is microsomal triglyceride transfer protein (MTP). This protein catalyzes the transport of triglyceride and cholesteryl ester from phospholipid surfaces. It is present in the lumen of the microsomal fraction of liver and intestine. The role of this protein in the RPE is unknown.High-dose therapy with the fat-soluble vitamins A and E can prevent or ameliorate the retinal degeneration. In order to establish that vitamin A deficiency alone is responsible for the retinal degeneration in this disorder, it is impotant to maintain normal serum vitamin A levels in these patients from earliest possible age and do ERG periodically.

Refsum's Disease

Refsum's disease is a peroxisomal disorder associated with progressive neurologic deficit, deafness, skeletal abnormalities and pigmentary retinopathy. Peroxisomes are cytoplasmic single membrane organelles present in almost all eukaryotic cells. They contain a number of enzymes such as catalases, hydroxylases and oxidases involved in many oxidative reactions. Serum phytanic acid levels are elevated either moderately (Infantile form) or dramatically (adult form).The biochemical hallmarks are defective oxidation and accumulation of very long chain fatty acids.

Infantile Refsum's Disease (IRD)

IRD presents with severe visual impairment in infancy, craniofacial malformations, severe hypotonia, psychomotor retardation, bleeding episodes and liver dysfunctionare usually evident by 6 months of age. Severe deafness is also evident in the first year of life. The disease is fatal by second or third decades of life. Ocular manifestations include nystagmus, retinal disease, optic atrophy and cataract. Early in the disease, white flecks are evident in the midperipheral retina (leopard spots). These abnormalities are replaced by coarse posterior-pole pigment clumping

Zwellweger syndrome (similar to IRD), the prototype of these disorders, is characterized by infantile retinal degeneration that is associated with hypotonia, psychomotor retardation, seizures, characteristic facies, renal cortical cysts, and hepatic interstitial fibrosis. In 1994, Masuno et al mapped Zellweger syndrome to chromosome band 8q21.2. The human gene is known as PAF-1 (peroxisome assembly factor-1), and at least 9 different genes are involved in the assembly of peroxisomes. No obvious relationship was noted between genotype and phenotype. A second form of Zellweger syndrome was identified in peroxisomal membrane protein-70, which mapped to chromosome 1. Another form was mapped to chromosome 7 by demonstration of chromosomal rearrangement in 2 cases. A third disorder known as pseudo-Zellweger syndrome has been mapped to the peroxisomal thiolase gene in chromosome 3. The role of these proteins in the RPE remains elusive.

Neonatal adrenal leukodystrophy (resemble IRD) may present in infancy, but they generally survive until age 7-10 years.

Adult Onset Refsum's Disease

It is an autosomal recessive disease also called *heredopathia atactica polyneuritiformis* was first described in 1946. It is characterized by cerebellar ataxia, polyneuropathy, anosmia, deafness, ichthyosis, and cardiac myopathy with arrhythmias. Night blindness may be an early symptom.Ocular features include cataract, miosis with por pupillary dilatation and retinopathy. Nyctalopia in thesecond dcade of life is followed by peripheral field defects. Pigmentary retinpathy is evident in the third decade. ERG corresponds to classic RP.

Phytanic acid levels in blood and urine are always elevated due to deficiency of phytanic acid α oxidation. Protein levels in the CSF are characteristically elevated. Restriction of dietary phytanic acid (which is present in dairy products and ruminant fat) can limit progression of disease and often improve icthyosis, neurologic deficits, and cardiac disease.

Mitochondrial Myopathy (Chronic Progressive External Ophthalmoplegia, (Kearns-Sayre Syndrome)

Barnard and Scholz first reported the association of external ophthalmoplegia and retinal dystrophy in 1944 and Kearns and Sayre subsequently added cardiomyopathy as a feature is condition is part of a group of diseases collectively termed mitochondrial myopathies in which the mitochondria are increased in number and distorted; "ragged-red" fibers may be evident in muscle. The metabolic defect(s) is (are) in the mitochondrial DNA (mtDNA).

Affected children may have a progressive external ophthalmoplegia, an atypical retinitis pigmentosa, and, in the Kearns-Sayre syndrome, cardiomyopathy. Onset is usually prior to age 10 years, and most children are symptomatic by the second decade of life (usually 14 years).

The pigmentary retinopathy may be typical of retinitis pigmentosa or atypical with development of a maculopathy early in the course of the disease Korner and Probst reported cases of chronic progressive external ophthalmoplegia and found an atypical pigmentary retinopathy in 36% of patients and bone spicule-like formation in 7%. In another study, the retinal dystrophy occurred in approximately one-third of patients with mitochondrial myopathy and, in some cases, occurred without the progressive external ophthalmoplegia. Most patients with retinal changes had a salt-and-pepper appearance with abnormalities of retinal pigment epithelium a consistent feature. The ocular course is variable and some patients have normal visual acuity. The electroretinogram is frequently subnormal and may become extinct.

Autopsy studies of the eyes have shown loss of retinal pigment epithelium and the photoreceptor cell layers which has been more severe in the posterior pole.

Pseudoretinitis Pigmentosa

1. Retinal inflammatory diseases
   a. Rubella retinopathy
   b. Syphillis
   c. Infectious retinitis

2. Autoimune paraneoplastic retinopathy
3. Drug toxicity
   a. Thioridazine
   b. Chlorpromazine
   c. Chloroquine
   d. Hydroxychloroquine
   e. Quinine
4. Pigmented parvenous retinochoroidal atrophy
5. Traumatic retinopathy
6. Diffuse unilateral subacute neuroretinitis.

Retinal Inflammatory Diseases

Rubella Retinopathy

Rubella retinopathy, the most common ocular manifestation of congenital rubella, is often mistaken for a panretinal degeneration such as RP. Conversely, true RP may be mistakenly called rubella retinopathy. This latter situation is especially likely to occur in the case of Usher's syndrome (RP with partial or complete congenital deafness); often the child is erroneously thought to have rubella retinopathy and deafness rather than RP and deafness. Rubella retinopathy may take any of several forms. In some, the macula will be the only site of abnormality, with a speckling of fine pigment granules. In others, the involvement may involve the posterior pole to a much greater extent, or may involve the periphery. The correct diagnosis can be established by a combination of clinical features and the ERG, which is either normal or only mildly abnormal in rubella retinopathy but which is usually severely abnormal in RP as part of Usher's syndrome. Rubella retinopathy is believed to be a disease capable of progression with increase in pigmentary changes or subretinal neovascularization. Juvenile-onset glaucoma is a significant risk for patients with rubella syndrome.

Syphillis

Congenital or acquired syphilis can present as a pigmentary retinopathy that may appear similar in some respects to advanced RP, but careful examination usually establishes the correct diagnosis. Congenital syphilis usually includes interstitial keratitis, and the pigmentary changes in the fundus appear more patchy and postinflammatory in nature. Usually the pigment deposits are clumps or large patches of black pigment associated with chorioretinal scars; typical bone-spicule pigment formations are uncommon. The posterior pole may be as equally involved as the periphery. There may be evidence of past or present overlying vitreous reaction. Acquired syphilis can present with a diffuse retinal involvement that simulates an advanced retinal degeneration

Infectious Retinitis (Cytomegalovirus Infections, Toxoplasmosis, Herpes Infections)

These entities usually produce extensive full-thickness chorioretinal scars, but may, in certain areas, produce only mottling and pigment granularity of the RPE.

Usually, the random patchy distribution of the lesions and the appearance will allow the correct diagnosis. The ERG is usually normal or only minimally affected in postinfectious retinopathies—unless extensive retina is severely damaged, in which case the ERG will be accordingly decreased in amplitude.

Autoimmune Paraneoplastic Retinopathy

Several reports have documented the existence of severe panretinal degeneration as a remote effect of cancer, either small-cell (Oat cell) carcinoma of the lung or small-cell undifferentiated cervical carcinoma. In at least two cases the vision loss preceded the diagnosis of the cancer. The cancer-associated retinopathy (CAR) can be extremely rapid or slow, resulting in loss of vision over a period of several months or years. The ERG is markedly to severely abnormal and vision may be totally lost. The fundus appearance may be normal even when the ERG is extinguished and the vision severely decreased. Evidence is strong that the retinal degeneration is immunologically mediated from cross-reactive antigenicity between the retina and certain carcinomas. The autoantigen in the human retina identified with a CAR appears to be recover in and retinal enolase.

A paraneoplastic form of night blindness with a characteristic ERG has been reported with malignant melanoma.This association has been called melanoma-associated retinopathy (MAR). The scotopic ERG to maximum-intensity flash has a "negative" configuration, identical to that seen with congenital stationary night blindness.

Drug Toxicity

Thioridazine

Thioridazine is the only phenothiazine that has been definitely linked to severe, blinding retinal toxicity. Phenothiazines, in general, bind to melanin and concentrate in the uveal tract and presumably the RPE. The retinal toxicity of thioridazine is believed to result from the presence of a piperidyl group at position 10 of the molecule, similar to the drug NP-207, which was withdrawn from the market because of severe toxicity to the retina. Thioridazine can cause a pigmentary retinopathy that early in the course can be confused with RP, or, perhaps even more so in advanced stages, choroideremia. In most patients with thioridazine retinopathy the drug has been taken at high doses (1000 mg/day or greater) for many months to years. However, one article documents the occurrence of toxicity at 800 mg/day.

The earliest symptoms include blurring of central vision, poor night vision, and a brownish discoloration to the vision. Early toxicity produces fine, deep retinal pigment posterior to the equator, which becomes more coarse as the condition progresses, often producing large "signal" plaques of pigment deposition. The characteristic appearance of advanced thioridazine retinopathy is diffuse, patchy atrophy of choriocapillaris, RPE, and overlying retina, simulating the fundus appearance of early choroideremia. The ERG may show decreased amplitudes of both cone- and rod-mediated responses; responses of both a-waves and b-waves are subnormal. One report of the histopathologic changes in advanced thioridazine toxicity showed patchy loss of choriocapillaris, RPE, and photoreceptor outer segments.

Chloropromazine has been reported to produce a pigmentary retinopathy when taken at high doses for prolonged times. The pigmentary retinopathy does not significantly affect retinal function, and the retinopathy appears to regress when the drug is stopped.

Chloroquine

Chloroquine, similar to the phenothiazines, binds to melanin and can cause a toxic retinal degeneration if taken over a prolonged period of time. Very few cases have been reported with patients taking a total dose of less than 300 g. The risk for chloroquine retinal toxicity appears minimal if the dose is kept at or below 250 mg/day. Early in the course of toxicity the ERG, EOG, and visual fields can be normal, although in late, severe toxicity they can become markedly abnormal. Unlike RP, in advanced chloroquine retinopathy the dark adaptometry may be either normal or only minimally abnormal. The typical picture of advanced chloroquine toxicity is that of a bull's eye maculopathy, although pigmentary changes with bone-spicule formations can occur in the midperiphery and far periphery.

Quinine

Quinine toxicity of the retina can lead to a fundus appearance than can enter into the differential diagnosis of RP. Usually such a dramatic retinopathy results from large doses of quinine ingested during either a suicide attempt or an attempt to abort a pregnancy. Often, the diagnosis is aided by the history of acute loss of vision and the finding of characteristic pallor and edema of the retina early, with later development of attenuation of retinal vessels and optic nerve head pallor. At this stage, quinine toxicity may be misdiagnosed as RP sine pigmento. The ERG in quinine toxicity usually is of a "negative" configuration, with far greater depression of the scotopic β wave than α wave. With time, the β wave may recover somewhat, but usually remains mildly to moderately subnormal.

Pigmented Paravenous Retinochoroidal Atrophy

Pigmented paravenous retinochoroidal atrophy (PPRCA) was first described in 1937 as retinochoroiditis radiata. PPRCA is a pigmentary retinopathy that is presently poorly understood, but may represent an acquired response pattern to an infectious or inflammatory disease rather than a genetic retinal dystrophy. A number of infectious agents or inflammatory disease processes may trigger this pattern of retinochoroidal atrophy. PPRCA has been reported in association with meningoencephalitis, tuberculosis or a family history of tuberculosis, syphilis, and rubeola.

As the name implies the pigmentary changes are closely associated in distribution of the retinal veins. Most cases are stable over time although progression has been reported in one case. this may have been the natural evolution of originally involved retina. Most cases are relatively stable with time. The ERG in PPRCA is usually only mildly to moderately abnormal, if at all, but the EOG is usually abnormal and can be severely affected.

Unilateral Pigmentary Retinopathy (Unilateral RP)

Traumatic Retinopathy

The RPE and retina have only a limited range of responses to a traumatic insult. One of these is regional or generalized loss of the RPE with migration of melanin into the retinal layers where it accumulates along vessels, especially at branching points, creating a bone-spicule pattern. Thus patients with post-traumatic injury to the eye can present with a fundus appearance in the traumatized eye that mimics RP.

Diffuse Unilateral Subacute Neuroretinitis

Diffuse unilateral subacute neuroretinitis (DUSN) is the term used for the disorder that previously was called "unilateral wipe-out syndrome" and that probably is identical to what others have called unilateral RP. True unilateral genetic RP probably does not exist, except possibly as an example of extreme lyonization of retinal involvement in a carrier of XLRP. DUSN is believed to result from the panretinal degeneration that takes place in eyes that have been infected by any of several possible worms. The raccoon Nematode (*Baylisascaris procyonis*) has been incriminated but other worms such as *Toxocara canis* have been suspected as well. The cases are all sporadic; none have had other, similarly affected family members.

The patients classically have normal vision until a certain age, at which time a visual disturbance (loss of central acuity, reduction of visual field, or poor night vision) is noted. At this time the examination of the retina may be either normal or show early evidence of retinal degeneration (mottling of retina, edematous-appearing retina, or narrowing of retinal vessels). Sometimes one may see an elevated gliotic mass in the mid or far periphery that may represent the encased worm. The visual field will often show abnormalities early in the course of the disease, but these are usually patchy, involve central defects, or demonstrate a configuration atypical for RP. The ERG, if performed at this time, may show moderate to profound abnormalities limited to the involved eye. With time the visual function may continue to deteriorate in the affected eye but remains normal in the fellow eye. Eventually, the retina develops pigmentary clumping and scarring reminiscent of advanced RP. The entire course of the disease conforms to that expected for an acquired parasitic infection.

Treatment and Management

The fact that only three of the numerous forms of RP and allied disorders (abetalipoproteinemia, Refsum's disease, and possibly gyrate atrophy of the choroid and retina) are treatable has led many ophthalmologists to dismiss their patients with RP with the statement, "I can't do anything for you."

Sometimes, the patient obtains the opinion that, since his disease is untreatable, the physician does not wish to see him again. This is unfortunate, because, as physicians, we can provide these patients with a better understanding of their disease, information about their present level of visual function, what future visual limitations they can expect, and what they can do to minimize the disabilities and manage the possible complications.

Substantial refractive errors or a need for a change in correction may go unattended in patients with RP. Corrections that normally would be too small to recommend may offer significant subjective improvement of vision. Presentation of the manifest refraction in a trial frame is the best way for patients to evaluate the possible benefit of a new pair of eyeglasses. Often adults at younger ages than usual, or even occasionally children, will appreciate the added help of a bifocal add for their glasses when reduction of visual field or central acuity reduces accommodative and fusional reserves. Low-vision aids may allow patients to continue to read or work longer than otherwise possible.

Berson in 1971 proposed that protection of the eyes of patients with RP from ordinary daylight might slow the rate of progression of retinal degeneration. He tested this theory by occluding with an opaque scleral shell for 6 to 8 hours per day for 5 years one eye in each of two patients with RP, one patient being autosomal dominant and the other autosomal recessive. Every 6 months both eyes in each patient underwent tests for visual acuity and visual fields, fundus examination and photography, and ERG. In each patient, each eye showed comparable progression over the 5 years of observation. Thus, there is no evidence at present to substantiate the view that light deprivation with any type of sun glasses or an occlusive opaque lens will alter the course of progression for any type of RP. Conversely, there is no conclusive evidence, for human forms of RP, that ambient light exposure is harmful.

Tinted lenses may provide comfort outdoors, and, for some patients with RP, may provide better contrast enhancement. These reasons alone are sufficient to recommend tinted lenses for many patients with RP.

The Night Vision Aid is a monocular, handheld device that amplifies low-level illumination to help patients with defective night vision see under dimly illumination situations. Patients must have at least 20/200 visual acuity and 20 degrees of central field to receive benefit from using this device. The device can only be properly fitted at certain centers and one group found that a wide-angle powerful flashlight was more effective and far less expensive than the Night Vision Aid.

Periodic visual field examinations with compassionate explanation of visual field defects can help patients appreciate the rate of progression and hence plan for future disability. Explanation of statutory visual requirements for driving will help patients who are still driving to plan for the eventuality of quitting driving. Reassurance that the changes seen are typical or usual for patients with RP will often allay fears that they are losing visual function at a rate faster than expected.

Counseling

To manage RP patients it is important to precisely determine the specific subtype of RP in a given family and to assess the visual status of the affected individual in detail. This helps in the management and future lifestyle planning for the patient. Te affected individual needs to have complete retinal evaluation. The retinal function of the affected individual must be determined.

Genetic counseling: All genetic counseling for patients with RP should be nondirective and supportive. The aim of the counseling are: (i) diagnosis (ii) genetic counseling (iii) management of therapeutic options. The clinical diagnosis and molecular genetic defect is established by the techniques and information outlined above and this is followed by the process of counseling.The patient whose diagnosis brought the family to the attention of physicians is called the proband or propositus. The member of the family who is asking the questions is the consultant. Before genetic counseling can be given, the type of RP affecting the proband and other affected family members must be defined as precisely as possible. A complete detailed pedigree is an essential part of the workup before genetic counseling can begin. Examination of other family members may not only be essential for the establishment of the correct diagnosis but will allow better appreciation of the range and extent of the manifestation shown by other family members and the expected rate of progression. For some of the forms of RP and allied disorders, such as Usher's syndrome and Bardet-Biedl syndrome, the inheritance, autosomal recessive in these examples, will be known once the proper diagnosis is made. For others—classic RP, for example—the family work-up may be the only way an inheritance subtype may be uncovered.

Certain patients will benefit greatly by appropriate referral to state, regional, or local agencies that provide services to the blind or visually impaired, such as the programs for the visually impaired child in the school system, state schools for the blind, vocational rehabilitation divisions at these blind schools and others that may be run by non governmental organizations. It will be important to establish a well functioning support groups, such as the National Retinitis Pigmentosa Foundation as this would help him or her to appreciate that others are similarly affected and have coped successfully with the disorder.

Cataract Surgery

Patients with RP often develop cataracts that may become visually significant. They would benefit from phacoemulsification with implantation of intraocular lens. However, before this decision is taken it is important to clinically assess macula with fundus fluorescein angiography and OCT and to assess the chances of visual acuity improvement with laser interferometry and the potential acuity meter (PAM). Occasionally, lens opacities, especially posterior subcapsular cataracts, can become so dense that significant potential improvement in visual acuity cannot be detected by either laser interferometry or the PAM. Before surgery, the patient must be made to realize that any improvement in central acuity will not be associated with improvement in visual field and that the cataract surgery will in no way slow the expected rate of progression of the disease.

Macular Edema and Serous Retinal Detachment

Cystoid macular edema occurring in RP patients can significantly reduce vision. Numerous treatment methods like peribulbar steroids, oral steroids and carbonic anhydrase inhibitors have been assessed. Most satisfactory results have been obtained using oral acetazolamide at a dose of 500 mg/day.

Numerous authors have found an improvement in objective (Snellen's acuity) and subjective vision after treatment of CME in RP patients despite persistence of angiographic changes of the CME. This may be because the angiographic changes correspond to changes in the permeability of retinal capillaries while carbonic anhydrase inhibitors increase fluid passage through the RPE.An induction dose of 500 mg/dat followed by maintainence dose of 250 mg/day is recommended.The major limitation of this treatment is the side-effects produced by acetazolamide.

There have been some reports of laser grid treatment to the macula of RP patients with CME, and this too has been claimed to be beneficial. However, the wisdom of treating, in a destructive manner, any retina within the central field in patients with RP has been challenged. Recently 12 RP patients of refractory CME underwent vitrectomy, posterior hyaloid dissection, removal of posterior ILM after staining with ICG and gas tamponade. They showed three line improvement of vision. It must be remembered that patients with CME may even improve spontaneously with no intervention.

Vitamin A Supplements

Vitamin A supplements are effective in treating retinopathies that are associated with Vitamin A deficiency resulting from intestinal malabsorption or defective transport as occurs in Bassen-Kornzweig syndrome (abetalipoproteinemia). In a randomized prospective trial by Berson et al has found that the groups receiving 15,000 IU/day of Vitamin A showed a slower rate in decline of cone ERG. Interestingly the groups receiving 400 IL/day of vitamin E were found to have a decline in amplitude of 50% or more from the baseline.

Lutein Supplements

Lutein and zeaxanthin are macular pigments that cannot be synthesized in the body and must be derived from dietary sources. Oral supplementation of 20 mg/day of lutein for 6 months demonstrated increased macular pigment in 50% of the subjects with RP or Usher syndrome but no change in central vision.Long term affects of supplementation are unknown.

Medications with Potential Adverse Reaction with RP

Isoretinoin (13-cis-retinoic acid)

Isoretinoin (13-cis-retinoic acid, Acutane) is a synthetic retinoid used to treat acne. It has been shown to produce night blindness. The mechanism of this is by inhibition of visual cycle resulting in decresed rhodopsin chromophore.

Sildenafil (Viagra)

The function of sildenafil (Viagra) as a potent inhibitor of PDE5 is used to treat erectile dysfunction. Sildenafil is a weak inhibitor of PDE6, which is used to hydrolyze cGMP in the photoreceptor outer segments. Its short term effects on vision and ERG are reversible but longterm effect is unknown. Theoretically the newer more selective PDE5 inhibitor such as tadalifil (Cialis) should have safer profile for the RP patients.

Advances in Therapeutics

The aim of this section is to mention the newer modes of therapies that are on the horizon or are being worked at. Knowledge about these will help the ophthalmologist to discuss the future with the patients who has pianstaikingly collected information on the internet.

Much of the newer work is being done on various animal models that are now availaible.It seems one of the greatest handicap in human RP is caused by secondary loss of cone dysfunction. The identification of rod derived cone viability factor offers hope for the preservation of central cones that will preserve central vision.

Gene Therapy

Retina as a target for genetic manipulations has some advantages:

1. Target cells (photoreceptors) are directly accessible
2. Effects of manipulation can be observed
3. Cell population is non-dividing and static, hence once a change has been introduced it will be permanent.

The aim of genetic manipulation is based on consequences of genetic mutation and this could be

1. Those abnormalities that lead to loss of function e.g arRP, XLRP, some adRP. The aim here would be to replace the mutant gene to cure the " loss of function".
2. Those that lead to extrafunction. The aim here would be to block or switch off the diseased gene

The main problem associated with retinal gene therapy is the delivery of genetic material within the target cells and the appropriate expression of this material without any advrse effects.Various options that are being considered are : Ligand-DNA conjugates, DNA- loaded vesicle (liposome) fusion with mutant cells, physical transfer (electroporation) and use of viral vectors. Adenovirus or lentiviruses are under investigation and seem to be promising.

Growth factors like the *basic fibroblast growth factor* (bFGF) have been injected intravitreally and subretinally in animals.Their potential benefits to human disease are promising but poorly understood at present. Side effects of such injections need also to be considered.

Retinal Transplantation

Work done in the last decade has suggested that transplantation may have a functional benefit. The aim of the therapy has been directed either at replacing abnormal RPE cells or by using immature neural cells to replace the defective neuroretina. Some of the useful observations/work in this regard is as follows:

1. **Li and Turner** in 1988 showed that transplanting normal RPE cells into the subretinal space of the RCS rat, an animal model of autosomal recessive retinal dystrophy rescued photoreceptors in the immediate vicinity of the transplant.
2. **Stem cells:** It has been shown that new neurons are continuously being generated from stem cells in the adult mammalian brain. Two approaches are being considered:
   i. Identify the cells in retina that have the potential to redifferentiate to make new photoreceptors. It has been shown by **Fischer and Reh** that Muller glial cells can dedifferentiate, proliferate, express transcription factors normally expressed by embryonic retinal progenitors and produce reinal neurons and glia.
   ii. Transplant stem cells from other sources to replace the missing cells (e.g. embryonic retina precursors, bone marrow derived stem cells).
3. Twelve patients underwent subretinal injection of a suspension of human fetal neural retina in the paramacular space. Patients were followed for 2-20 months and VA improved from to light perception or finger counting only. Some improvement in VA (20/200 at best) was reported from 4 months after surgery. An unexplained result was an improvement in VA in the untreated eye of some of these patients.

Electronic Prosthesis (Artificial Retina)

A retinal prosthesis or phototransducing chip placed on the retinal surface has been investigated for several years. The healthy ganglion cell layer of the retina can be stimulated, and implants in animal models have long-term stability. **Humayun et al** have presented a single human subject implanted with a chronic, epiretinal device (Second Sight, Valencia, CA, USA) with 16 electrodes. Preoperatively the subject had no light perception from RP. Postoperatively, the authors demonstrated that the subject could perceive light in response to electrode stimulation.The subject perceived individual spots in response to stimulation of each of the 16 electrodes.The major issues regarding the development of these devices are inner retinal viability, stimulus threshold, signal encoding, ower requirements, biocompatibility, encapsulation and he best way of testing these implants.Currently, no retinal prosthesis is available for clinical use, and this technology remains investigational.

Chapter 48

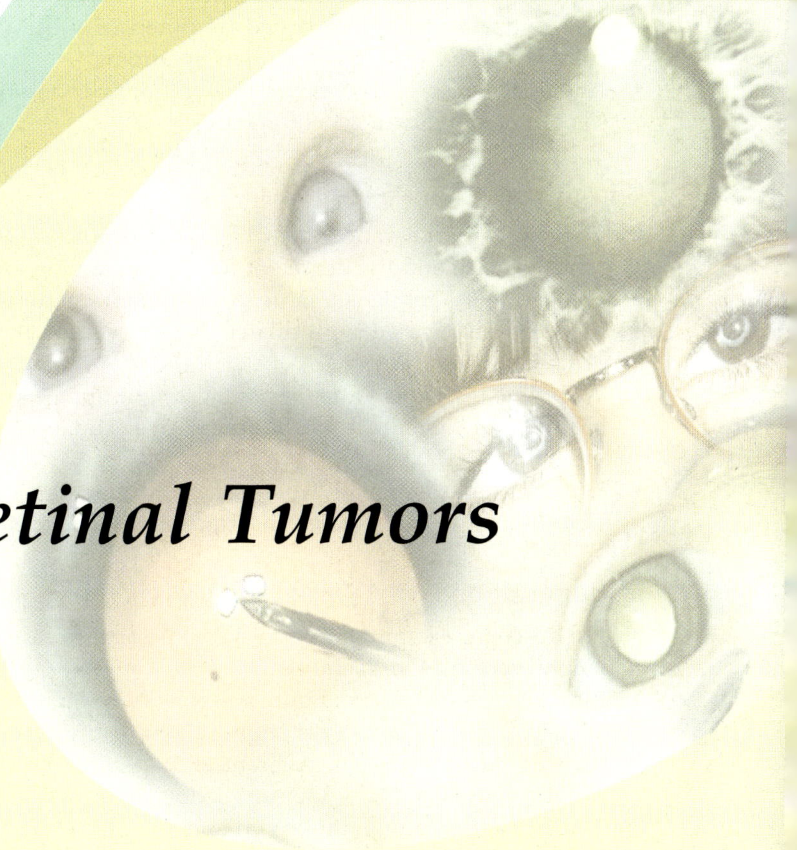

Retinal Tumors

Debraj Shome, Ashok Garg (India)

Retinal Capillary Hemangioma

Introduction

- Retinal Capillary Hemangioma (RCH) are benign angiomatous hamartomas of the retina composed of expansive capillary networks with in the matrices of interstitial cells.
- They may be located in the peripheral retina or associated with the optic Disc and may be accompanied by potentially life threatening systemic condition like Von Hippel–Lindau Syndrome.
- About 50% of occurrences are bilateral or with multiple angiomas in the same eye, implying a genetic etiology.

Clinical Signs and Symptoms

- The clinical appearance of RCHs varies according to its location in the retina, its size and the degree of the accompanying exudative changes.
- The peripheral retina is a more common location for RCHs.
- RCHs are associated with dilated feeder arteries and enlarged, tortuous draining veins.
- With time, RCHs enlarge, becoming bright orange red masses sometimes greater than 8 mm in size with progressive exudation of fluid and lipid into the retina.
- Loss of vision is usually due to cystoid macular edema, Serous retinal Detachment, hard exudates and tractional retinal detachment.

Investigations

- Fundoscopic examination and workup for decreased visual acuity shall help in making the diagnosis.
- Initial ophthalmoscopic appearance of Peripheral capillary Hemangiona (The Von-Hippel tumor) is subtle; a red or grayish dot no larger than a diabetic microaneurysm. Afferent and efferent vessels may be normal to slightly dilated but later they show fine tortuosity or focal telangiectasia.
- The Appearance of Endophytic and Exophytic Juxtapapillary capillary Hemangioma is quite different.
- Endophytic hemangiomas are well circumscribed, bright red sessile tumor that lie on the surface of and partially obscure the optic disc. These tumors may give rise to surface neovascularization, traction and exudation.
- Exophytic Juxtapapillary lesions appear as a diffuse, graying thickening that obscures the border of the optic disc often without prominent vascular channels. Intraretinal exudates are often present.
- Steroscopic Fluorescein angiography. Show early filling of a vascular intraretinal mass with a variable degree of leakage and late edema.
- Ultrasonography optical coherence tomography. Color Fundus Photography, MRI, Blood Tests, Genetic testing are other investigations which can be performed.

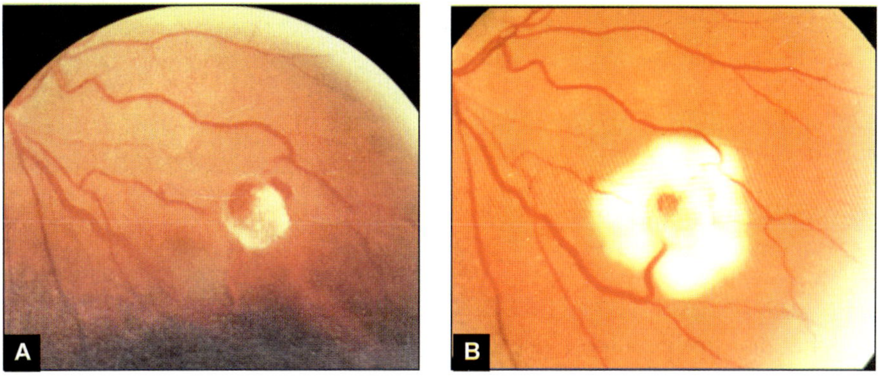

Figures 1A and B: Retinal capillary hemangioma

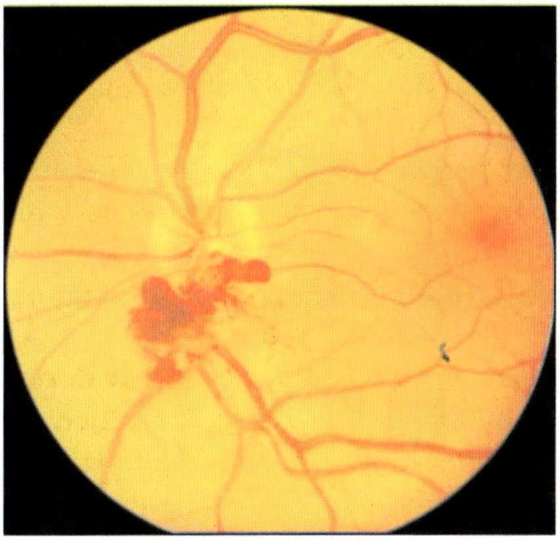

Figure 2: Retinal cavernous hemangioma

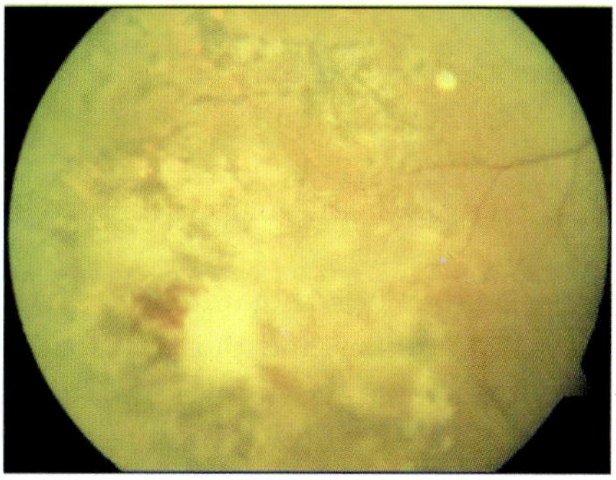

Figure 3: Vasoproliferative tumor of the retina

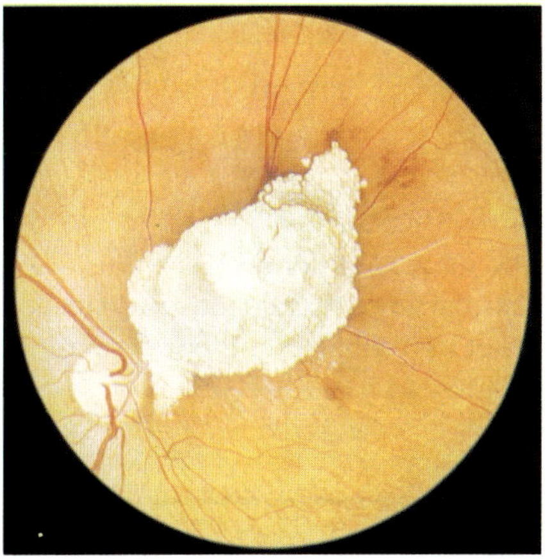

Figure 4: Retinal astrocytoma of larger size

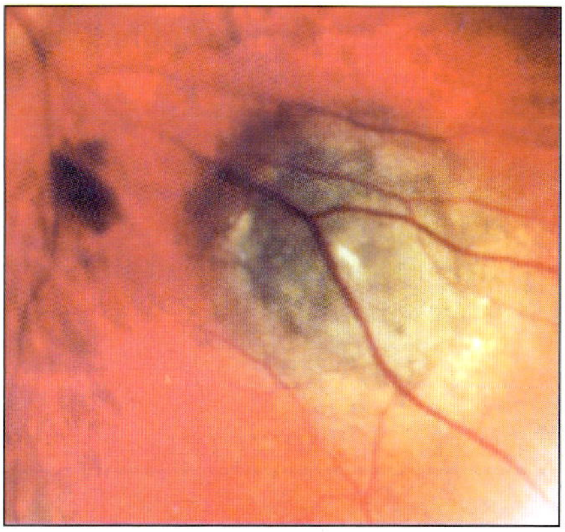

Figure 5: Choroidal melanoma

Differential Diagnosis

These lesions may be confused with:

- Papilledema
- Papillitis
- Choroiditis
- Choroidal neovascularization
- Choroidal hemangioma
- Malignant melanoma
- Vitreous hemorrhage
- Exudate
- Fibroglial proliferation
- Coat's disease
- Neurofibromatosis
- Retinitis pigmentosa
- Inflammatory conditions.

Treatment

- Periperal RCHs may be treated with laser photocoagulation or cryotherapy. Laser Photocoagulation tends to be more effective on smaller tumors with less exudation (that are 1.5 mm or smaller) photocoagulation can be applied directly to the tumor or to the feeder artery or a combination of both techniques can be used.
- Recently Photodynamic therapy has been reported to induce occlusion of Juxtapapillary and peripheral retinal capillary Hemangimas. Cryotherapy is preferable to photocoagulation when the retinal capillary Hemangioma is located anterior with subretinal fluid that might reduce laser energy uptake and is more than 3.0 mm in diameter. In general cryotherapy is effective for RCH up to 4.5 mm in size.
- RCHs that are larger than 4mm show a poor response to cryotherapy and laser photocoagulation. Such tumors are treated successfully with plaque radiotherapy.
- Low dose external beam radiotherapy may be option in cases refractory to other modes of treatment.

Prognosis

- RCHs tumors may remain asymptomatic for a long period.
- Visual loss results from intraretinal exudation, macular edema, surface neovascularization and its consequences or epiretinal membrane formation.

Retinal Cavernous Hemangioma

Introduction

- Cavernous Hemangioma of the retina is a rare vascular Hamartoma.

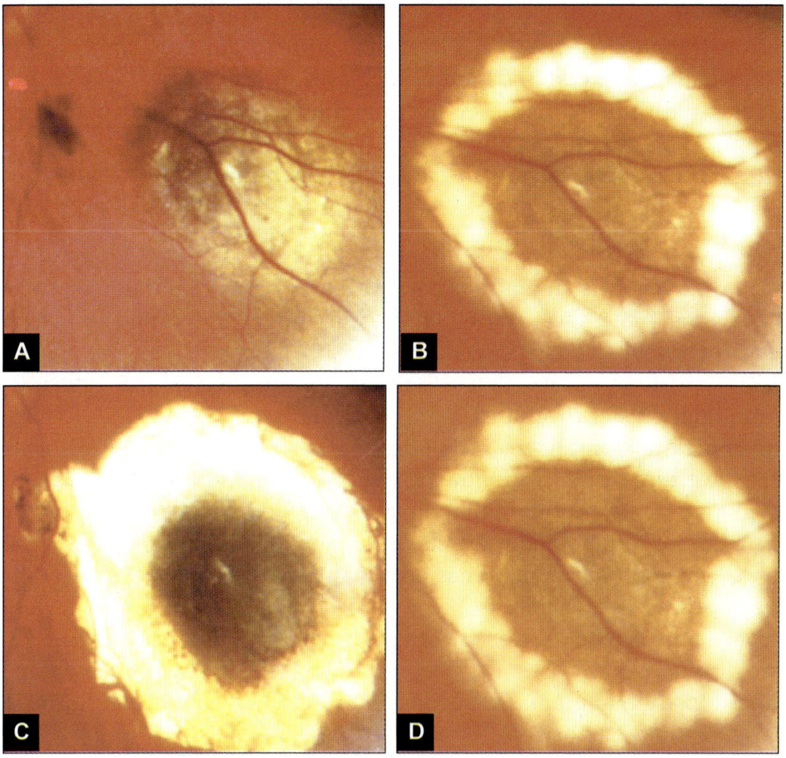

Figures 6A to D: Photocoagulation with argon and krypton laser in choroidal melanoma

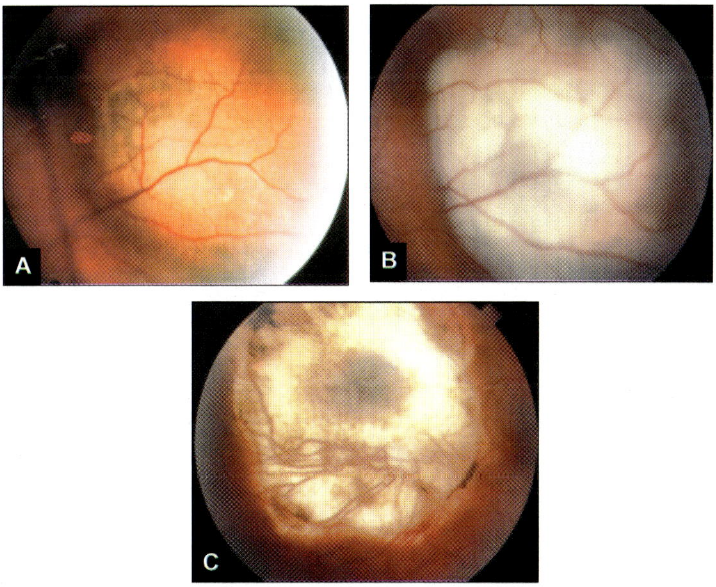

Figures 7A to C: Transpupillary thermotherapy in choroidal melanoma

- The tumor is composed of clumps of dark intraretinal aneurysms that demonstrate a characteristic "Cluster of grapes" appearance.
- It is usually unilateral and rarerly increases in size.
- Patients with this hamartoma also may have hemangiomas involving the skin and nervous system.
- It has an autosomal dominant pattern of inheritance.

Clinical Signs and Symptoms

- Retinal cavernous hemangiomas are composed of cluster of saccular aneurysms filled with dark blood. The aneurysms range in size from microaneruysm to a half disc diameter.
- The typical tumor is isolated, 1-2 disc diameters in size and resembles an intraretinal cluster of grapes.
- The clinical appearance can be quite variable with the wide distribution over the entire fundus or following the course of a major vein.
- Often a white or gray fibroglial membrane covers the surface of the tumor. The adjacent retinal blood vessels appear unaffected by the tumor.
- Retinal cavernous hemangiomas are symptomatic when they are located in or adjacent to the macula.
- Visual acuity can be decreased both on the basis of tumor location as well as amblyopia.
- Cavernous hemangiomas can cause simultaneous subretinal, intraretinal and preretinal hemorrhage.

Investigations

- Fluorescein angiography may show autofluorescence of the gray white epiretinal membrane overlying the tumor. The aneurysms will slowly fill and often incompletely upto 30 minutes after dye injection.
- The plasma-erythrocytic separation often seen on clinical examination is dramatically demonstrated in the later phases of the angiogram.
- In certain cases when diagnosis is made difficult by vitreous hemorrhage ultrasonography is required.
- A scan shows a high initial spike and high internal reflectivity while B-scan shows an irregular surface, large internal acoustic density and absence of choroidal excavation.

Differential Diagnosis

- Retinal telangiectasis.
- Coat's disease
- Lebers miliary aneurysms
- Von Hippel's disease.
- Racemose hemangioma.

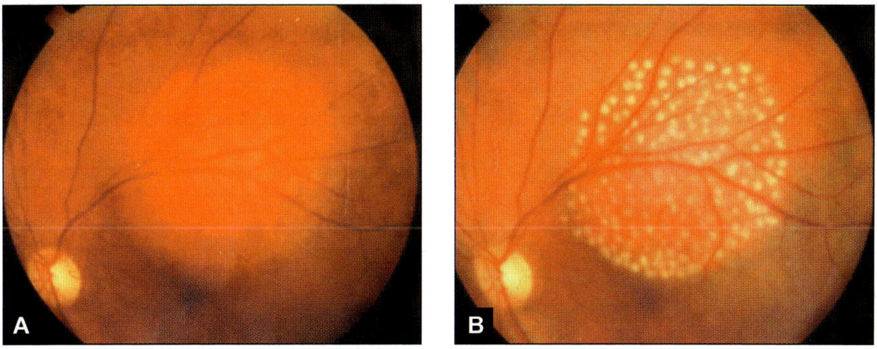

Figures 8A and B: Choroidal hemangioma

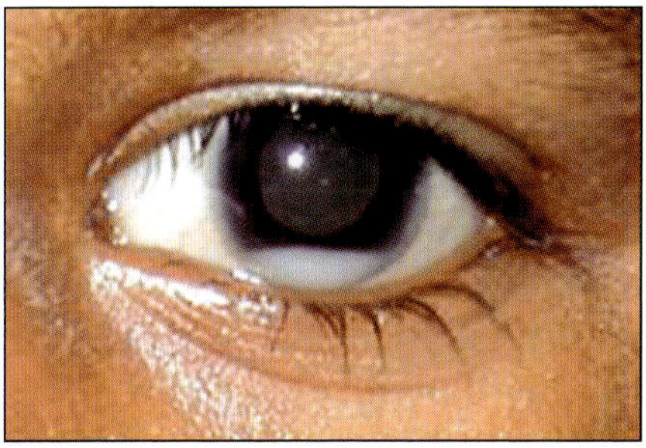

Figure 9: Pseudo Hypopyon due to retinoblastoma cells

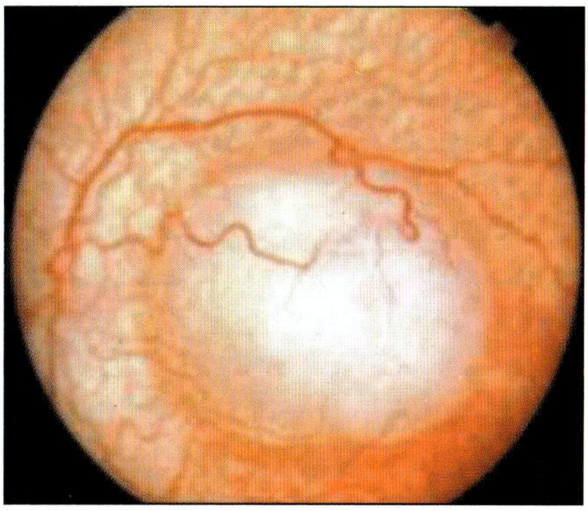

Figure 10: Color fundus photograph of the left eye showing early macular retinoblastoma

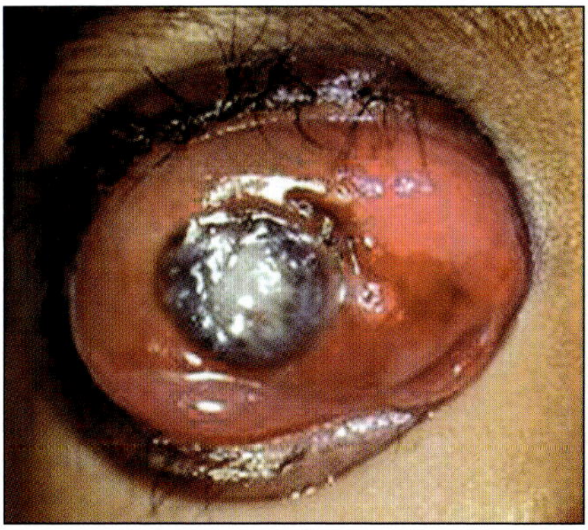

Figure 11: Orbital retinoblastoma

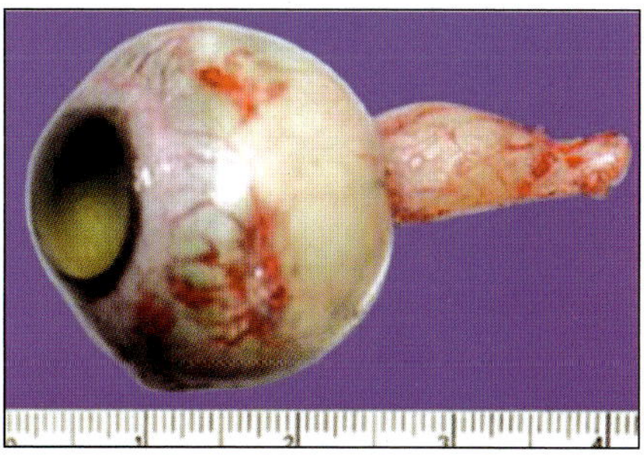

Figure 12: Enucleated eyeball with enlarged optic nerve suggestive of nerve involvement with tumor

Treatment

- As cavernous hemangiomas rarely increase in size or cause Lipid exudation or severe vitreous hemorrhage, these tumors generally do not require treatment.
- Photocoagulation or cryotherapy have been advocated if vitreous hemorrhage occurs.

Prognosis

As cavernous hemangiomas rarely increases in size and are generally asymptomatic the prognosis is good.

Vasoproliferative Tumor of the Retina

Introduction

These are solitary tumors commonly involves the inferotemporal of inferior quadrants of the retina.

- These may occur without any antecedent cause and may be associated with prior Retinitis pigmentosa, Coat's disease, familial exudative vitreoretinopathy and toxoplasma scars.
- These tumors may be multiple or diffuse tumors.
- The pathogenesis of these lesions is unclear.

Clinical Signs and Symptoms

- These tumors appear as solitary mass lesions with minimally dilated feeder vessels associated with intraretinal and subretinal exudation and hemorrhage, secondary retinal detachment, RPE hyperplasia, Macular edema and vitreous hemorrhage.

Investigations

- Fluorescein angiography shows early filling and later leakge and dilated feeder vessels.

Differential Diagnosis

- Racemose hemangioma
- Retinal telangiectasia
- Capillary hemangioma
- Neurofibromatosis.

Treatment

- If progressive exudation causes loss of vision, cryotherapy, photocoagulation, plaque brachytherapy may be required.
- Epiretinal proliferation may need vitreous surgery.

Prognosis

- Good

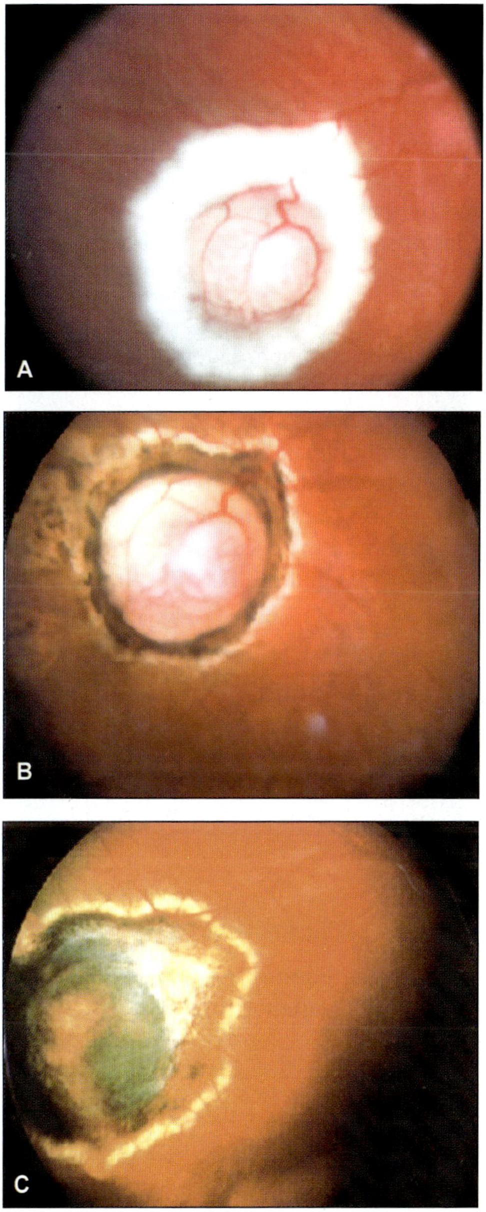

Figures 13A to C: TTT in retinoblastoma (Tumor is heated till it turns subtle gray).

Retinal Astrocytoma

Introduction

- Retinal astrocytoma of the retina rarely occurs.
- It may appear as isolated lesions and are commonly seen in patients with tuberous sclerosis which is one of the phacomatosis.
- Retinal astrocytoma is of autosomal dominant inheritance with new mutations in about 50% of cases.
- It is characterized by the triad of mental retardation, epilepsy and adenoma sebaceum skin lesions.

Clinical Signs and Symptoms

- Retinal lesions arise from the inner layers and can be single or multiple.
- These are usually present at or near the optic nerve head although they may be present in periphery also.
- The tumor may be small and flat or modular and well circumscribed with the size ranging from 0.5 to 1 mm in diameter.
- Early tumors may appear semitranslucent but in later stage they become more dense white color and the occurrence of multiple areas of calcification with in the tumor may give it a mulberry like appearance.

Investigations

- Fluorescein angiography and color fundus photography alognwith ophthalmoscopy are recommended for the diagnosis of the disease.

Differential Diagnosis

- Retinoblastoma
- Hyaline bodies

Treatment

- Generally treatment is not required as the lesions are usually asymptomatic and show only a minimal tendency to grow.

Prognosis

- Good

Choroidal Melanoma

Introduction

- Choroidal (uveal) melanoma is the leading primary eye malignant tumor.
- It arises either from a uveal nevus or may arise de novo without a pre-existing lesions.

- It often strikes without symptoms and carries a risk of spread via metastasis to the liver, lung and skin.
- The average age of patient with choroidal melanoma is about 50 years.
- Patients with ocular or oculodermal melanosis are at increased risk of choroidal melanoma.

Clinical Signs and Symptoms

- The tumor is usually unilateral and clinical features are variable.
- A typical melanoma is characterized by pigmented, elevated, oval shaped mass. The color of tumor is usually brown although it may appear as dark brown or black or may be amelanotic.
- When tumor grows it break through the Bruch's membrane and appear as mushroom shaped mass giving rise to exudative detachment of the retina.
- Other associated features of choroidal melanoma can be choroidal folds, subretinal or intraretinal hemorrhage, hard yellow exudation, vitreous hemorrhage, secondary glaucoma, cataract and posterior uveitis.

Investigations

- The diagnosis of uveal melanoma is best made using Indirect ophthalmoscopy by Expert clinician familiar with ocular tumors.
- Non invasive ancillary testing include transillumination, ocular ultrasonography. Fluorescein angiography, Indocyanine Green angiography, ultrasound biomicroscopy, color Doppler imaging and P_{32} testing. Fine needle biopsy may be employed for difficult cases that pose a diagnostic dilemma.
- Visual field examination, computed tomography and Magnetic resonance imaging are other investigations which are of value in clinching diagnosis.

Differential Diagnosis

- Retinal Detachment
- Metastatic tumor of choroid
- Exudative ARMD
- Choroidal detachment
- Choroidal Hemangioma
- Large choroidal nevus.

Treatment

Tumor growth pattern is a factor in the therapeutic decision if there is diffuse melanoma or if there is extraocular extension, enucleation is of choice but radiation therapy can be employed for less extensive disease. Based on COMS classification the therapeutic opinions for medium sized choroidal melanomas are –

- Plaque radiation therapy.
- External beam, charged particle radiation therapy.
- Local eye wall resection.
- Combined therapy with ablative laser Coagulation or transpupillary thermotherapy (TTT) to supplement plaque treatment.
- Photocoagulation.
- Transpupillary Thermotherapy (TTT)
- Encucleation
- Chemotherapy and immune therapy regimens (using melanoma vaccine).
- Laser photocoagulation has a limited role to play in the treatment of choroidal melanomas.
- Therapeutic options for large choroidal melanomas.
- Radiation therapy plus enucleation
- Enucleation.

Prognosis

- It depends upon on cell type. Spindle A cell tumors have the best prognosis and those composed of epithelioid cells have the worst prognosis.
- Tumor size – large tumors have a worse prognosis than small tumors.
- Diffuse tumors have worst prognosis.
- If Bruch's membrane is ruptured than prognosis is not favorable.
- Patient over the age of 65 years have worst prognosis.
- Extrascleral extension carries a poor prognosis.

Solitary Choroidal Hemangioma

Introduction

- Choroidal hemangiomas are benign and may be circumscribed or diffused.
- Circumscribed Choroidal Hemangiomas are usually unifocal and unilateral while diffuse hemangiomas are commonly associated with Sturge Weber syndrome and may be bilateral.

Clinical Signs and Symptoms

- Choroidal Hemangiomas typically appears as a dome shaped or placoid red orange lesion most commonly situated at the posterior pole.
- Frequent secondary changes include non-rhegmatogenous retinal Detachment, cystoid degeneration and pigment epithelium mottling of the overlying retina.
- A useful clinical sign is blanching of the lesion with pressure on the globe.
- Choroidal hemangiomas can cause decrease in vision and photoreceptor loss.

Investigations

- Ultrasonography

- A scan shows a high initial spike with high internal reflectivity. B scan shows an oval or placoid lesion with a sharp. Anterior border and acoustic solidity.
- Fluorescein angiography usually shows up the large choroidal vessels during the prearterial or arterial phase with late staining of the tumor and cystoid spaces in the retina.

Differential Diagnosis

- Amelanotic choroidal melanoma.
- Metastatic tumour

Treatment

- Laser photocoagulation has been advocated in the management of choroidal hemangioma associated with exudative retinal detachment.
- Both Argon Laser and Dye Yellow Laser can be used in the treatment.
- If there is no secondary retinal detachment than there is no indication for treatment.
- Low dose external beam radiotherapy has also been used in the management of refractory tumors.

Prognosis

Prognosis in choroidal hemangioma without exudative retinal detachment is good. However prognosis in hemangiomas with ERD is gaurded.

Retinoblastoma

Introduction

- Retinoblastoma is the most common primary intraocular malignancy of infancy and childhood.
- Retinoblastoma represents the phenotype expression of an abnormal or absent tumor suppressor gene known as the Retinoblastoma gene (RBI).
- It is second only to malignant Melanoma of the uvea as the most common malignancy of the eye.
- There is no predisposition for Retinoblastoma by race or gender. Both eyes are affected equally.
- The incidence of Retinoblastoma worldwide ranges from 1 in 14000 Live birth to 1 in 34000.
- A substantial proportions of cases of Retinoblastoma are hereditary arising through germ-line mutations in tumor suppressor genes.
- The incidence peaks in the first year of life and declines gradually with age thereafter.

Clinical Signs and Symptoms

- Initially there may be little or no signs or symptoms hence public awareness and regular eye check-ups are essential to catch the disease at an early stage of presentation.
- The tumor first starts in the retina (Neural layer of the eye) and in later stages, involves the entire eye and spreads to the orbital structures and brain and finally spreading to different organs of the body.
- Most infants and children with retinoblastoma are referred for ocular examination at a later stage when physician detects an abnormal while papillary reflex (Leukocoria), crossed eyes (strabismus) or decreased vision.
- Advanced tumor present with spontaneous hyphema, pseudo-hypopyon, secondary glaucoma or chronic inflammation.
- The accuracy of clinical diagnosis is made with indirect ophthalmoscopy when the ocular media is clear.
- Early lesions appear as flat, transparent or slightly white placoid tumor in the neurosensory retina.
- As tumor enlarges, they have a white color with chalky, fleck like deposits of calcium.
- Growth is either Endophytic (into the vitreous) or exophytic (under the neurosensory retina) or combined.
- If vitreous Hemorrhage obscures the fundus view, ultrasonography and computed tomography are indispensable in the workup. Calcium within the tumor is highly characteristic of retinoblastoma and usually is easily demonstrable by both methods.

Differential Diagnosis

Diagnosis of retinoblastoma requires differentiation from other causes of leukocoria. These are as follows :

- Congenital cataract may be hereditary or may result from other conditions like congenital rubella, galactosemia and intraocular infections.
- Anomalous optic disc.
- Coat's disease
- Congenital corneal opacity.
- Coloboma of choroid and optic disc.
- Persistant Hyperplastic primary vitreous
- Developmental retinal cyst
- Retinal glaucoma
- Hematoma under retinal pigment epithelium.
- High myopia with advanced chorioretinal degeneration.
- Juvenile retinoschisis.
- Toxocara canis.
- Medullation of nerve fibers layer.
- Metastatic Endophthalmitis.
- Norrie's Disease
- Retinal Detachment due to choroidal or vitreous hemorrhage.

- Vitreous hemorrhage.
- Oligodendroglioma of the retina
- Retinal Dysplasia
- Retinopathy of prematurity (ROP)
- Secondary glaucoma
- Rhegmatogenous retinal detachment.
- Tapetiretinal degeneration
- Microphthalmia
- Ocular toxoplasmosis
- Traumatic chorioretinitis
- White with pressure sign
- Trisomy 13.

Investigations

The diagnosis of retinoblastoma is best made using indirect ophthalmoscopy. Other investigations to be performed are:

- Ocular ultrasonography.
- Fluorescein angiography.
- Computerized photographic imaging
- Computed tomography
- Magnetic resonance imaging.
- Calcium within the tumor is highly characteristic of retinoblastoma and is easily demonstrable by ultrasonography and computed tomography.
- Computed tomography is also helpful in excluding orbital extension and in demonstrating pineal tumor.

Treatment

- Early diagnosis and recent advances in management have improved the prognosis of this potentially fatal tumor significantly.
- Survival rate has improved to nearly 95% in last decade.
- It is very important to recognize the other causes of white papillary reflex (leukocoria) before starting definitive treatment of RB.
- The most important factor that must be considered in the treatment are the tumor size, number, location and laterality, condition of other eye, threat of metastasis, risk for second malignant neoplasms and systemic status of the patient. The latest international classification is given at the end of this clinical condition.

Treatment modality currently available as classified as:

a. Focal therapy like cryotheraphy, tanspupillary therapy and laser photocoagulation.
b. Local therapy like External beam radio therapy and Enucleation.
c. Systemic therapy like chemotherapy.

Cryotherapy

It involves freezing the tumor leading to ischemic necrosis of tumor. It is performed for small equatorial or peripheral retinoblastoma measuring upto 4 mm in basal diameter and 2 mm in thickness.

Complications include:
- Transient serous retinal detachment.
- Retinal tear
- Pre-retinal fibrosis
- Rhegmatogenous retinal detachment

Laser Photocoagulation

This modality of managing RB has been sidelined with the advent of Thermotherapy as laser involves destruction of retina and retinal pigment epithelium.
- This is usually done for small posterior tumors 4 mm in basal diameter and 2 mm or less in thickness.

Complications includes:
- Vascular occlusion.
- Retinal traction.
- Transient serous retinal detachment
- Retinal hole

Transpupillary Thermotherapy (TTT)

TTT is the delivery of heat using infrared radiation. The goal is to reach a subcoagulative temperature range of 40-60 Celsius thus sparing retinal vessels of photocoagulation.
1. TTT using infrared radiation from a semiconductor diode laser has become a standard practice. It is specially useful in treating lesions at the macula.
2. The large spot adapted indirect ophthalmoscope, operating microscope with a laser delivery system or trans-scleral route using a diopexy probe can be used to deliver it.
3. TTT alone can be used for small tumors measuring upto 4mm in basal diameter and 2mm in thickness. However its major application is an adjunct to chemoreduction.
4. TTT alone is highly effective for relatively small retinoblastomas without associated vitreous or subretinal seeds.

The Chief complications of TTT are:
1. Focal iris atrophy.
2. Peripheral focal lens opacity.
3. Retinal traction.
4. Retinal vascular occlusion.
5. Transient serous retinal detachment.

Brachytherapy Plaque

Retinoblastoma is a radiosensitive tumor. In Brachytherapy, a radioactive implant is placed on the sclera over the base of the tumor to irradiate the tumor transclerally. The goal is to deliver a radiation dose of 4000-5000 cGy to the apex of the tumor selectively without irradiating the remaining ocular structures.

- The radioactive materials used commonly are 125 Iodine and 106 Ruthenium.
- Plaque brachytherapy can be performed as primary or as secondary treatment. It is generally reserved for the tumors less than 16 mm in diameter and 8 mm in thickness ideally situated > 3 mm from the optic nerve and fovea.

1. The Radiation associated problems of papillopathy and retinopathy usually become clinically manifest at above 18 months after irradiation.
2. Custom design of plaques have reduced the incidence of radiation induced complications.

External Beam Radiotherapy (EBRT)

1. EBRT was conventionally indicated for moderately advanced unilateral or bilateral retinoblastoma.
2. Currently EBRT is indicated in eyes where chemoreduction and/or local therapy have failed and in rare conditions where chemotherapy is contraindicated due to poor systemic status.
3. EBRT is also used as a standard adjunct following enucleation in patients with retinoblastoma with gross or histopathological involvement beyond the optic nerve transaction, sclera infiltration and orbital extension.

Enucleation

1. About a decade ago primary enucleation was standard procedure in majority of unilateral retinoblastoma. However the advent of chemotherapy has changed this radical Management of Retinoblastoma. Enucleation is thus the second or third line of management and is reserved for patients who fail focal therapy, chemotherapy and EBRT. However tumors where there characteristics are not visualized are primarily managed by by enucleation.

- Minimum manipulation surgical technique should be necessarily practiced. Optic nerve head should be examined carefully post enucleation for thickening, suggestive of tumor involvement.
- Non integrated orbital implants like PMMA or silicon or biointegrated implants like hydroxypatite or porous polyethylene promotes orbital growth, provides better cosmeses and enhances prosthetic motility.

Orbital Exenteration

- It is usually done for orbital recurrence after the child has received the maximum dose of radiation and chemotherapy.

Chemotherapy

- With the advent of Chemotherapy, radical methods of management like enucleation have been shifted to second and third place. The introduction of newer chemotherapy protocols has dramatically improved the prognosis for life, eye salvage and residual vision.
- Chemotherapy can be local or systemic. Local Chemotherapy is under Phase III clinical trials. The role of systemic Chemotherapy in the management of retinoblastoma includes Chemoreduction, adjuvant Chemotherapy and treatment of metastasis.

Systemic Chemotherapy Drugs and Disc Schedules

a. Standard chemotherapy :
Vincristine 0.05 mg/kg on day 1 of Chemotherapy
Etoposide, 5 mg/kg on days 1 and 2 of Chemotherapy
Carboplatin, 18.6 mg/kg on day 1 of Chemotherapy

b. High Dose Chemotherapy :
Vincristine 0.025 mg/kg on day 1 of Chemotherapy
Etoposide, 12 mg/kg on day 1 and 2 of Chemotherapy
Carboplatin, 28mg/kg on day 1 of Chemotherapy

c. Periocular Chemotherapy
One of the main concern in systemic chemotherapy is that chemotherapeutic agents may not be able to penetrate the blood retinal barrier. The other route suggested to the deliver Chemotherapy locally thereby allowing transscleral penetration of drugs and high intraocular concentrations.

- Carboplatin administered subconjunctivally has been shown to be efficacious in the management of retinoblastoma specially in the presence of vitreous seeds as it can penetrate the sclera and achieve effective concentrations in the vitreous cavity. However response may be short lived with tumor recurrences.

Follow-up Schedule

- The usual protocol is to schedule the first examination. 3-6 weeks after the initial therapy. In cases where chemoreduction therapy has been administered, the examination should be done every 3 weeks with each cycle of Chemotherapy.
- Patients under focal therapy are evaluated and treated after every 4-8 weeks until complete tumor regression.
- Following tumor regression, follow up examination should be done 3 monthly for the first year, 6 monthly for three years or until the child attains 6 years of age and yearly thereafter.

Prognosis

- Early detection and recent advances in the management of retinoblastoma along with customized multispeciality management for individual patient have yielded gratifying outcomes in terms of preservation of life, salvage of the eye and optimal residual vision.

International Classification (New)

Group	Quick reference	Specific features
A.	Small Tumor	RB < 3 mm
B.	Larger tumor Macula Juxtapapillary Sub-retinal fluid	RB > 3 mm • Macular RB location (<3mm to Foveola) • Juxtapapillary RB location [< 1.5 mm to the disc] Additional sub-retinal fluid <3 mm from margin.
C.	Focal seeds	RB with : • Sub-retinal seeds < 3 mm from RB • Vitreous seeds < 3 mm from RB • Both sub-retinal and Vitreous seeds <3 mm from RB
D.	Diffuse seeds	RB with : • Sub-retinal fluid > 3 mm from RB • Sub-retinal seeds > 3 mm from RB • Vitreous seeds > 3 mm from RB • Both sub-retinal and Vitreous seeds > 3 mm from RB.
E.	Extensive RB	Extensive RB occupying > 50% of the globe or • Neovascular glaucoma • Opaque media from hemorrhage in anterior chamber, vitreous or sub-retinal space. • Invasion of post-laminar optic nerve, choroid (>2 mm), sclera, orbit and anterior chamber. • Pthisis bulbi post RB • Orbital cellulitis due to aseptic tumor necrosis.

Chapter 49

Ocular Trauma

Rupal H Trivedi, M Edward Wilson (USA)

Introduction

Ocular trauma is an important cause of monocular blindness in children. It is more frequent in children as compared with adults and boys are more frequently affected compared to girls. Children are often not able to cooperate for the kind of detailed clinical examination done on adults after trauma. In addition the tendency to develop amblyopia makes it harder to manage children after ocular trauma. Clinical signs and symptoms, investigations, differential diagnosis, management and prognosis vary greatly in patients with ocular trauma—mainly attributed to the extent of the initial injury.

Clinical Symptoms and Signs

The patient may complain of dimness of vision, diplopia, or pain (due to glaucoma, retrobulbar hemorrhage or iritis) etc. The parent may report leucokoria or an abnormal shaped pupil. Mechanism of injury, time and place of injury, visual status prior to trauma, child's general medical status and tetanus immunization status should be documented. The goal is to quickly determine the extent of the injury, without risking further damage to the eye. Noncontact portion of the examination should be performed first. If open globe is suspected, aim would be to prevent any more injury to the eye. External pressure should not be applied on the globe at any time during the examination. Anesthesia is occasionally needed for detailed evaluation.

Commonly observed signs are corneal tear, corneal foreign body, hyphema, iritis, hypopyon, secondary glaucoma, vitreous hemorrhage, or retinal detachment. Signs suggestive of scleral rupture include: Intraocular or subconjunctival hemorrhage, hypotony, light perception or worse vision, an abnormally deep or shallow anterior chamber.

Examination should include documentation of visual acuity (if the child is verbal and conscious), IOP and details on pupil (size, shape and reaction to light). The detailed examination should be customized based on the type of ocular injury. These examinations may include an evaluation of the eyelids and lacrimal system; orbital rim palpation (for any irregularities); ocular motility (especially in orbital fractures and traumatic nerve palsy); conjunctivae and sclera (to identify lacerations, perforations or foreign bodies); corneal staining (to identify abrasions); anterior chamber (for hyphema, hypopyon or any other abnormalities); lens (for subluxation, dislocation, anterior and posterior capsular integrity, extent and type of cataract or phacodonesis); fundus (for retinal detachment, choroidal rupture, commotio retinae, preretinal hemorrhage, intraretinal hemorrhage, subretinal hemorrhage, optic nerve pallor, optic nerve avulsion).

Investigations

Appropriate radiologic studies should be obtained if orbital fracture, intraocular or intraorbital foreign body, or other intracranial injury is suspected.

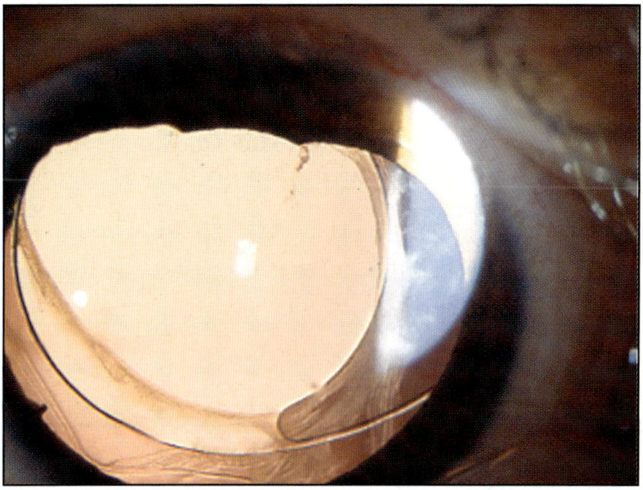

Figure 1: IOL implantation in an eye with traumatic cataract

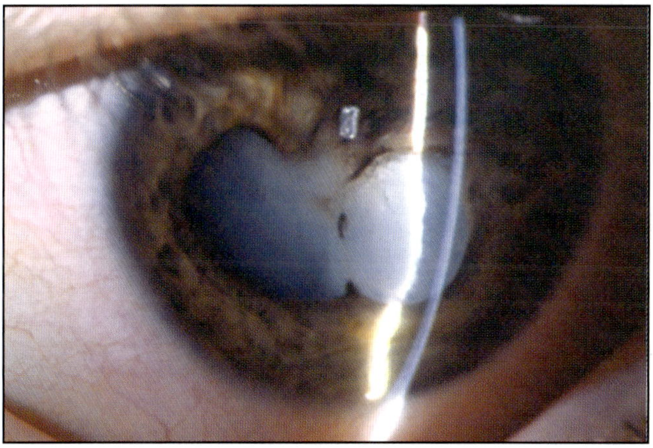

Figure 2: Traumatic cataract

B-scan ultrasound should be done if the posterior pole cannot be visualized. It can also be helpful in identifying IOFB. A-scan ultrasound axial length measurements would be needed prior to cataract extraction. Orbital imaging studies are done if necessary to rule-out fractures and foreign bodies. Patients with corneoscleral lacerations should have cultures performed in the operating room if the wound appears infected. Cultures from the wound should be obtained before the patient is prepared for surgery with Betadine. Cultures can also be obtained from any IOFBs or tissue resected during surgery. UBM is often useful to rule out a foreign body embedded in the anterior sclera. These foreign bodies may not be visible because of their nature (e.g. glass) or the presence of an overlying opacity (e.g. conjunctival hemorrhage).

Differential Diagnosis

Hyphema without a history of significant trauma should raise the suspicion of bleeding diatheses, leukemia, juvenile xanthogranuloma, iris neovascularization, or retinoblastoma. For a patient with a history of ocular trauma, associated injuries should also be looked for. For example, a patient with a traumatic cataract should be evaluated for globe rupture, orbital fractures, retinal detachment, secondary glaucoma, or traumatic optic neuropathy. Other presenting ocular disorders may be first noticed after minor trauma (preexisting leukocoria, strabismus or proptosis). One should search for nontraumatic preexisting conditions when performing evaluation of an injured child.

Treatment

- Superficial corneal foreign bodies can be removed with a moistened cotton-tipped applicator or with the help of 26G needle.
- Most traumatic corneal abrasions should not be patched. Topical NSAID are helpful in reducing the associated pain. Because of the increased risk of developing bacterial keratitis, the use of antibiotic ointment is recommended until the corneal epithelium has fully healed.
- While treating hyphema the goal is to prevent increase in IOP, secondary hemorrhage, and corneal blood-staining. The management of traumatic hyphema is controversial in that a universally agree-upon protocol does not exist. A moderate restriction of physical activities is often recommended. Topical steroids and cycloplegics are usually started to decrease anterior chamber inflammation. Aminocaproic acid is reported to reduce the incidence of rebleeding, however, its role is somewhat controversial. Surgical intervention may be required in children with a hyphema if the IOP cannot be lowered with medical therapy or if the hyphema persist long enough to put the eye at risk of developing corneal blood staining or amblyopia. In some cases, a wash-out of the anterior chamber is sufficient. If a clot is present, it may need to be surgically excised using a vitreous cutting instrument. IOP should be monitored on a regular basis.

- For open globe injury — the defect in the eyewall should be closed surgically as soon as possible to restore the structural integrity of the globe. A delay in closing the wound may increase the risk of endophthalmitis or result in prolapsed uveal tissue becoming epithelized. In case where no light perception is present postoperatively, secondary enucleation may be indicated to prevent sympathetic ophthalmia. This is less commonly done now that sympathetic ophthalmia has shown to be a more treatable condition.
- If IOFB is present, the eye is usually closed primarily, but a reoperation is scheduled soon afterward to remove the IOFB. The administration of intravitreous or oral antibiotics may decrease the risk of traumatic endophthalmitis.
- Traumatic cataract surgery is usually not performed concurrently with the primary repair of an open globe. If cataract surgery is delayed for several weeks, the procedure can be combined with the removal of the sutures used to close the corneal laceration. An IOL should be implanted whenever possible in children with traumatic cataracts. The IOL will ensure that at least a partial optical correction is present at all times. A rigid gas permeable contact lens is occasionally needed postoperatively to neutralize irregular corneal astigmatism after a laceration repair.
- Mild vitreous hemorrhage (VH) can often be treated with topical corticosteroids and safely observed. However, dense VH involving the posterior segment may leads to a poor visual outcomes. Early vitrectomy is used to clear the visual axis in children who are at risk for form deprivation amblyopia. Vitrectomy is also useful in identifying and treating underlying pathology such as retinal tears, choroidal rupture, and macular holes.
- When a retinal tear or dialysis is identified, prophylactic photocoagulation or cryopexy is recommended. Traumatic retinal detachments are treated with conventional scleral buckling and with vitrectomy. Treatment can be difficult in children and poor outcomes are frequently associated with postoperative proliferative vitreoretinopathy.
- Spontaneous closure of traumatic macular holes is not uncommon, especially in children, and therefore the timing of treatment is somewhat controversial. If the hole is small, observation is extended for several months. Vitrectomy with fluid-gas exchange is the current surgical approach.

Prognosis

Poor prognostic indicators include poor visual acuity on presentation, vitreous hemorrhage, retinal detachment, and endophthalmitis. The presence of IOFB, a delay in wound closure, an injury to the crystalline lens, and the occurrence of the injury in a rural setting have been shown to increase the risk of endophthalmitis. Open globes secondary to blunt trauma are associated with particularly poor visual outcomes. Posterior segment injuries are more visually devastating than anterior segment globe injury.

Chapter 50

Hereditary Retinal Dystrophies

Supriya Dabir, Soumen Mondal
Priyanka Doctor, Nikoloz Labauri
S Natarajan (India)

Retinitis Pigmentosa

Introduction

Retinitis pigmentosa (RP) is a term used for a group of disorders characterized by inherited, progressive dysfunction, cell loss and eventual atrophy of retinal tissue.

Genetic heterogenicity is known to exist within a given hereditary pattern.

Genetic types in a state in the United States were found to be 19% autosomal dominant, 19% autosomal recessive, 8% X-chromosome linked, 8% undetermined and 46% isolates with only one affected member in the family.

Clinical Signs and Symptoms

The initial symptom is usually defective dark adaptation or "night blindness". Central visual acuity is usually preserved until the end stages of retinitis pigmentosa. This can however be affected, if there is cystoid macular edema (CME) diffuse retinal leakage and retinal pigment defects in the macula. Color vision in typical RP remains good until visual acuity is 20/40 or worse. Color vision may fail early in cases where central cones appear to be abnormal from the beginning.

Myopia was found to be more common in the X-linked group. Posterior subcapsular cataracts characterized by yellowish crystalline changes within the peripheral lens cortex in the visual axis are common. All the patients have changes in the vitreous, as reported by Pruett-like fine colorless dust-like particles, posterior vitreous detachment; vitreous condensations and collapse of the vitreous with greatly reduced volume.

The earliest observed changes in the fundus are arteriolar narrowing, fine dust-like intraretinal pigmentation and loss of pigment from the pigment epithelium. In the past the term retinitis pigmentosa *sine pigmento* was applied when the retina appeared normal despite documented abnormalities of photoreceptor function; however, this term is now regarded as confusing because it implies a separate disorder rather than the early stages of RP. As photoreceptor deterioration progresses, there is increasing loss of pigment from the pigment epithelium with intraretinal clumping of melanin, appearing most often as coarse clumps in a "bone spicule" configuration. A golden ring or yellowish halo can be seen surrounding the disc in early RP, which is replaced by peripapillary mottling, hyperpigmentation and atrophy of the RPE as the disease progresses. Retinal vessel attenuation and waxy pallor of the optic nerve become apparent in patients with advanced RP. The cause of the retinal vessel attenuation is unknown, but it appears to be a secondary change and not the primary disease process. Other retinal changes include white dots deep in the retina at the level of the pigment epithelium. These deposits are believed to be a nonspecific manifestation of pigment epithelial degeneration and may account for the retinal appearance termed *"retinitis punctata albescens,"* which is considered a manifestation of RP.

Fishman, et al reported three types of macular lesions in RP patients: Atrophy of the macular area with thinning of the retinal pigment epithelium, cystic

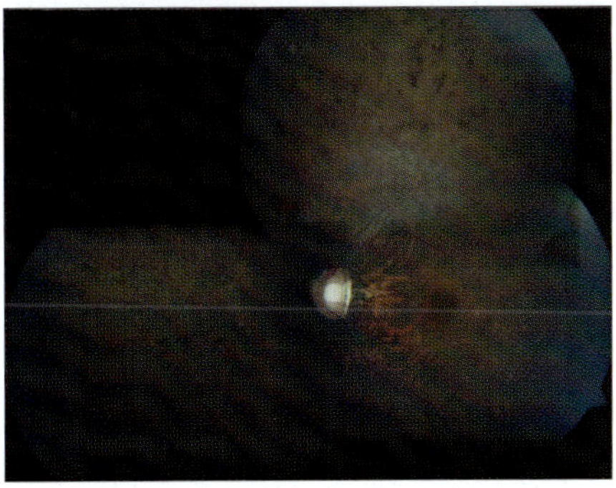

Figure 1: Fundus photograph with arteriolar attenuation, coarse clumps in a "bone spicule" configuration and waxy pallor of the disc

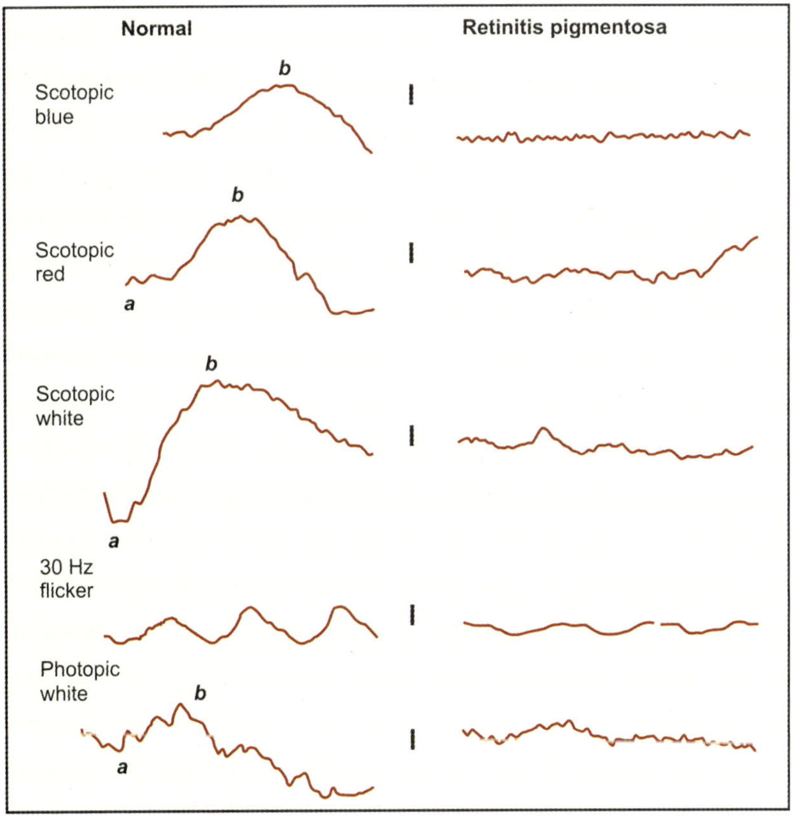

Figure 2: ERG recordings of retinitis pigmentosa

lesions or partial thickness holes within the macula with radial, inner retinal traction lines and/or various degrees of preretinal membranes causing a "surface wrinkling phenomenon and cystoid macular edema.

Choroidal changes in advanced RP generally include loss of the choriocapillaris and eventually all but the largest choroidal vessels.

Classification of RP

I. Subdivision based on inheritance type
- Autosomal dominant RP
- Autosomal recessive RP
- X-linked recessive trait RP

II. Subdivision by age of onset
- Congenital RP
- Childhood onset RP
- Adult onset RP

III. Subdivision by molecular defect
- Genes expressed predominantly in photoreceptors or in RPE (e.g. rhodopsin)
- Genes associated with RPE and disease in other tissue (e.g. Usher's syndrome)
- Genes widely expressed but for which mutations cause a retinal phenotype

IV. Subdivision by fundus appearance
- RP sine pigmento
- Retinitis punctata albescens
- RP inversus (pericentral and central RP)
- Sector RP

V. Systemic associations like Usher's syndrome

 I. **Nonprogressive**
 1. Usher's syndrome Type I
 2. Usher's syndrome Type II
 3. Congenital adrenoleukodystrophy
 4. Infantile phytanic acid storage disease

 II. **Progressive**
 1. Usher's syndrome Type III
 2. Cockayne's syndrome
 3. Alstrom's syndrome
 4. Mitochondrial myopathy (Kearns-Sayre's syndrome)
 5. Refsum's syndrome
 6. Mucopolysaccharidoses I-H, I-H/S, I-S, II, II
 7. Edwards' syndrome

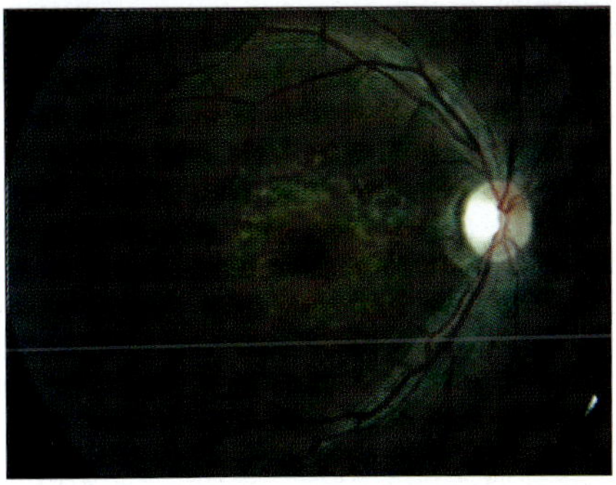

Figure 3: Beaten bronze appearance seen in Stage 1

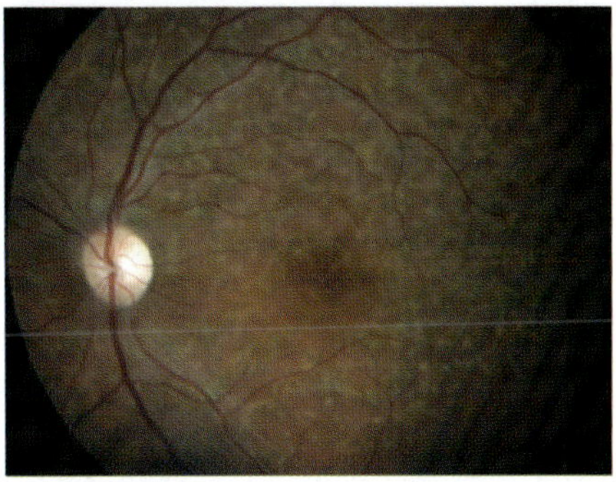

Figure 4: Pisciform flecks seen

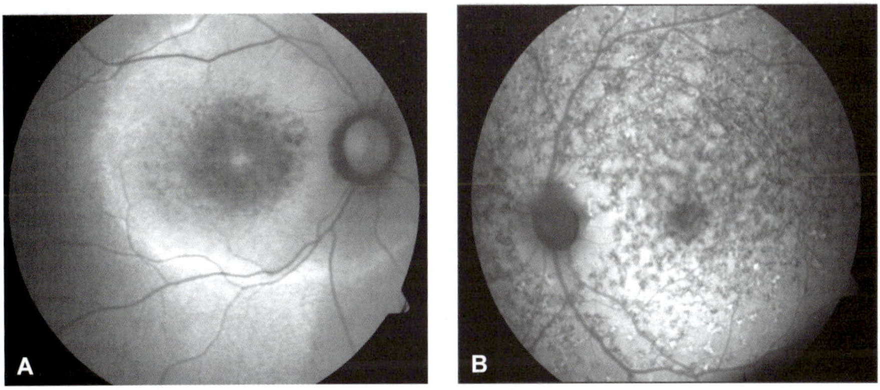

Figures 5A and B: Hypoautofluorescence at the macula and periphery respectively

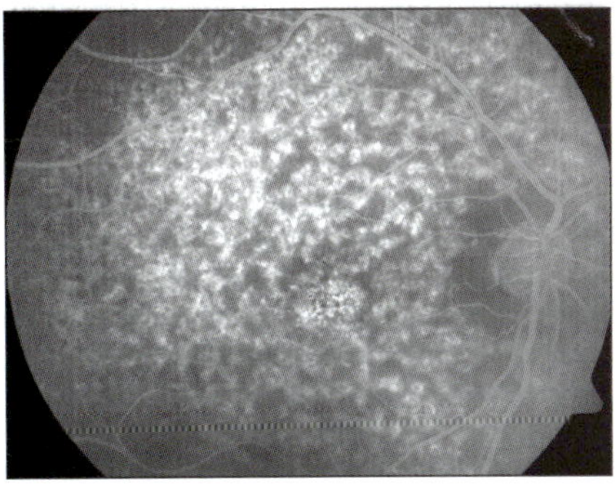

Figure 6: Choroidal silence with hyperfluorescent flecks

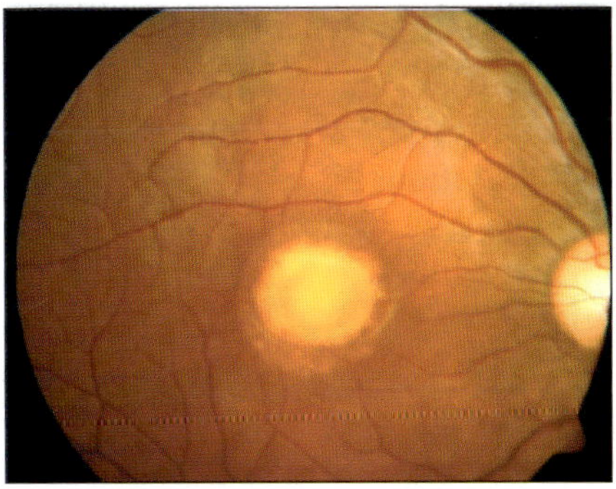

Figure 7: Classic Vitelliform stage with the egg yolk appearance at the macula

Tests of Visual Function

Electroretinography

In patients with early disease the α- and β-waves generated by the photoreceptors in response to white light under dark-adapted conditions are reduced in amplitude. Figure shows that patients with advanced RP have nondetectable rod and cone responses.

The scotopic rod-dominated ERG was affected more than the photopic cone-mediated ERG in type I RP, whereas the scotopic and photopic ERGs' were more equally abnormal in type II RP.

In general, the EOG is abnormal in diffuse hereditary rod-cone degenerations of the retina.

Dark Adaptometry

Patients with RP, when tested with dark adaptometry, may show elevation of the cone segment, rod segment, or both, to a varying degree. There may be a delay in reaching a relatively good final dark adaptation rod threshold.

Visual Fields

Characteristic ring scotomas are seen in the midperiphery of the visual field. It usually starts as a group of isolated scotomas in the area 20 to 25 degrees from fixation. These gradually coalesce to form a partial and then a complete ring. The outer edge of the ring expands fairly rapidly to the periphery, while the inner margin contracts slowly toward fixation. Long after the entire peripheral field is gone, there remains a small oval of intact central field.

Differential Diagnosis

I. Genetic disorders that cause retinal degeneration
   1. Gyrate atrophy of choroid and retina
   2. Choroideremia
   3. Cone dystrophy
   4. Lebers congenital amaurosis
   5. Congenital stationary night blindness

II. Drug exposure—thoridazine chorioretinopathy

III. Infections
   - Syphilis
   - Rubella

Treatment

1. *Cataract extraction*
2. *Macular edema:* Peribulbar, oral and intraocular steroids have produced temporary reduction in CME. Grover, et al found oral acetazolamide was found to be more effective than topical dorzolamide. Vitrectomy with inner limiting membrane peeling with gas tamponade may lead to resolution of refractory CME.

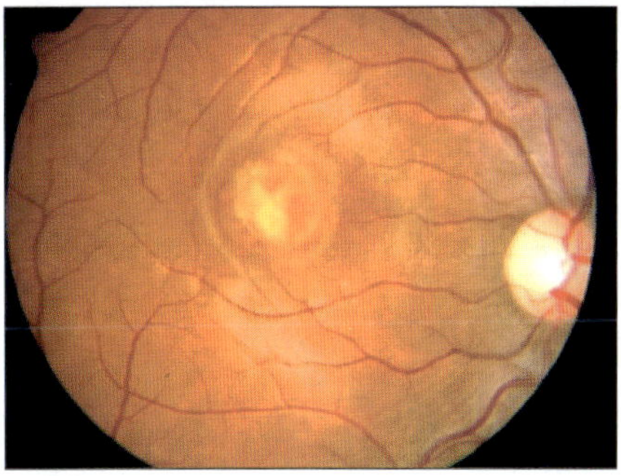

Figure 8: Scrambled-egg stage where the yellowish material in the disc has disintegrated

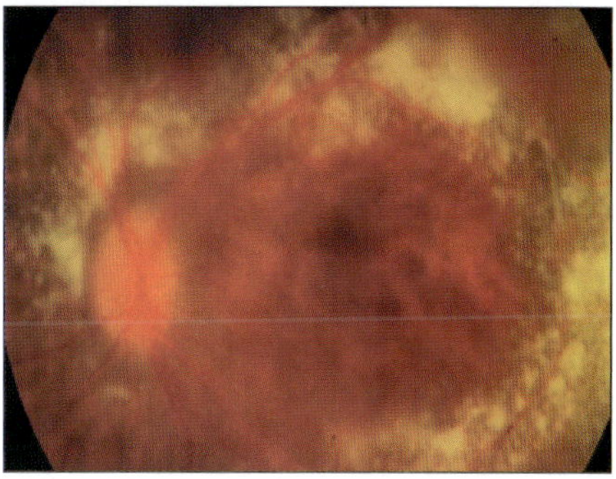

Figure 9: Showing multiple hard exudates all over the posterior pole as a fundus variant in LCA

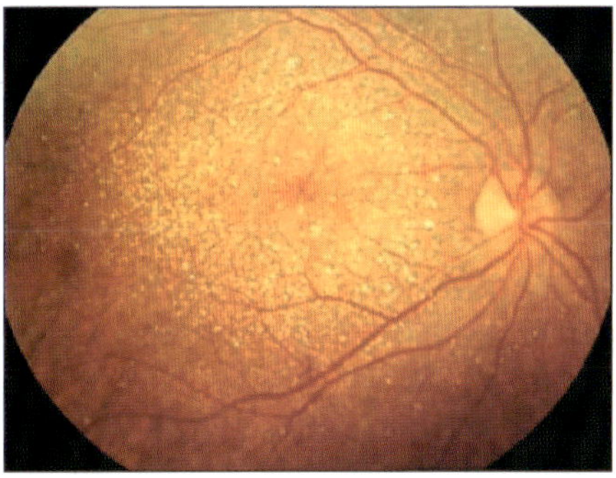

Figure 10: Bietti crystalline dystrophy

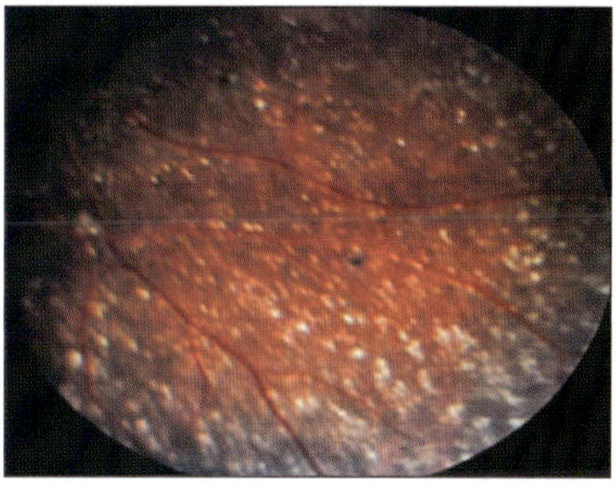

Figure 11: Grade 1 of North Carolina macular dystrophy

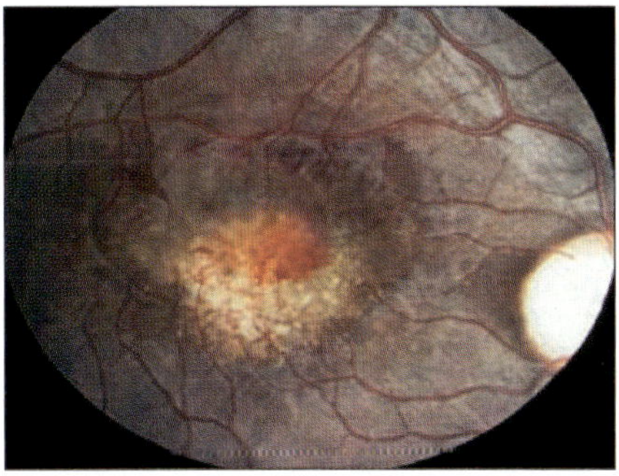

Figure 12: Exudative maculopathy in Grade 2 North Carolina macular dystrophy

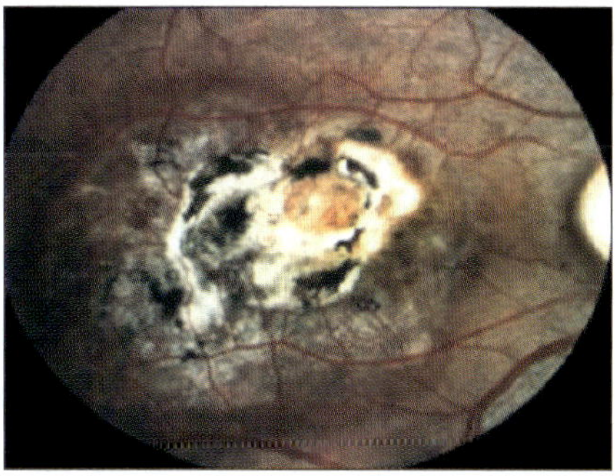

Figure 13: Subretinal scarring in North Carolina macular dystrophy

3. **Vitamin A Supplements** treat retinopathies associated with Vitamin A deficiency resulting from intestinal malabsorption or defective transport.
4. **Lutein supplements** may covey protection from oxidative damage and light induced photoreceptor cell death. Long-term effects of such supplementation is unknown.
5. **Docosahexaenoicacid (DHA) supplements.** DHA is an abundant lipid in photoreceptors accounting for 30-40% lipids in rod outer segments. Its synthesis is impaired in few of the X-linked recessive patients and its supplementation in these patients may be beneficial.

Advances in Therapeutics

1. *Gene therapy:* It involves replacing the mutant in "loss of function"-type disease and switching off of the disese gene in the "gain-of-function" disease. Adenoviruses have been extensively studied gene transfer vector for the eye. Intravitreal and subretinal injections of the vector have been attempted. Ribozymes, RNA enzymes, are being-designed for destroying mutant mRNA in dominant disease.
2. *Growth factors:* Injections of intravitreal and subretinal basic fibroblast growth factor have been promising.
3. *Retinal transplantation:* This is directed at replacing abnormal RPE cells or by using immature neural cells to replace defective neuroretina. Mueller glial cells can dedifferentiate and produce new retinal neurons. Bone marrow derived stem cells can also be injected to integrate into host retina and differentiate.
4. *Artificial retina:* Perception of light and cortical responses can be elicited in patients with advanced RP. Thus, electronic prosthesis may help. Subretinal, epiretinal, optic nerve and cortical implants have been studied. Patients have reported improvement in vision, color vision and fields.

Stargardt's Disease and Fundus Flavimaculatus

Introduction

Karl Stargardt, in Graefes Archives of Clinical and Experimental Ophthalmology in 1909 described a familial degeneration which was associated with an atrophic macular dystrophy surrounded by yellowish, ill-defined subretinal lesions. Later on, in 1962, A Franceschetti introduced the term fundus flavimaculatus to characterize a fundus with yellow irregular subretinal "flecks" scattered diffusely throughout the posterior pole, and only half of the patients in his series had macular atrophy. Examination of multiplex families uncovering intrafamilial presence of both Stargardt's disease (SD) and Fundus flavimaculatus (FFM), and seemingly caused by the same gene (ABCR4 gene) on the short arm of chromosome1, it is now assumed, (not without controversy) that the two disease entities are temporally variant expressions of each other.

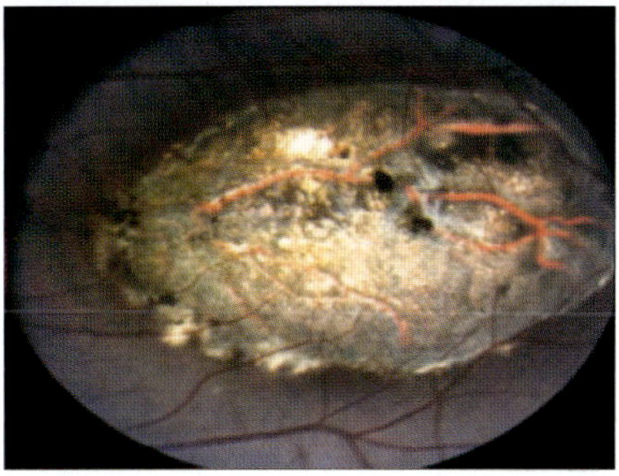

Figure 14: Grade 3 of North Carolina macular dystrophy

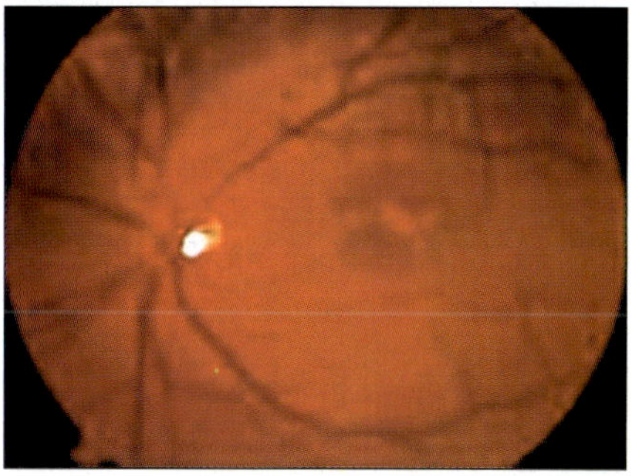

Figure 15: Butterfly dystrophy

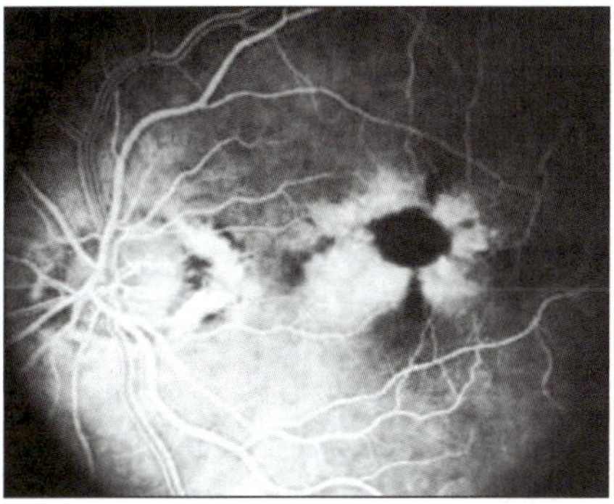

Figure 16: Fluorescein angiography shows reticular hypofluorescent pattern corresponding to the yellow and yellow-grey deposition material with pigment epithelial transmission leading to a hyperfluorescence pattern

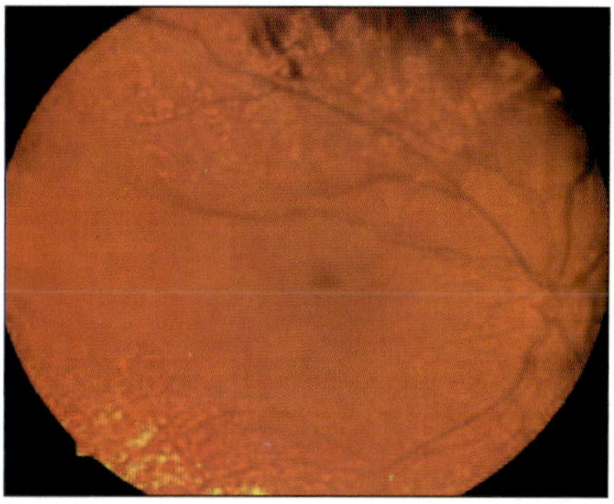

Figure 17: Early Sorsby pseudo-inflammatory macular dystrophy showing confluent spots along the arcades

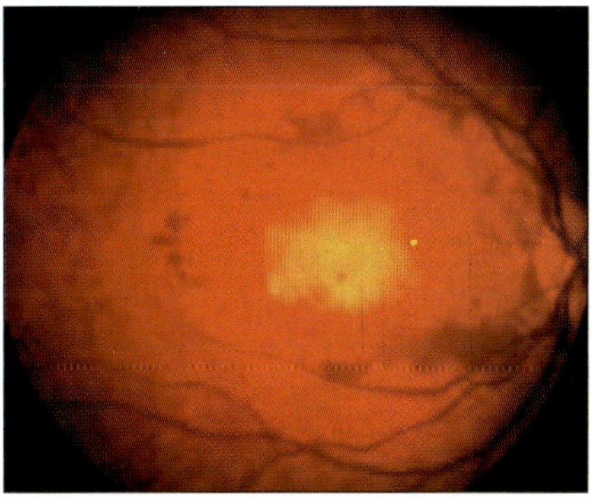

Figure 18: Exudative maculopathy in Sorsby pseudo-inflammatory macular dystrophy

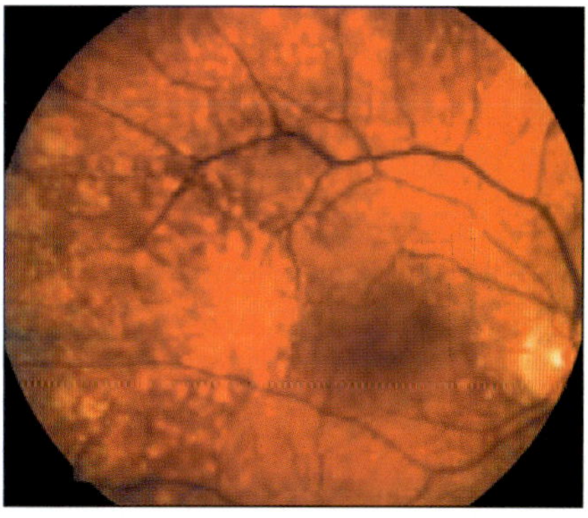

Figure 19: Sharply delineated drusens are distributed in the macula and around the optic nerve head

Clinical Symptoms and Signs

As visual loss due to macular atrophy forces the patient to go for check-up, SD is detected in childhood. On the contrary, FFM is detected in adulthood, as macular atrophy is a late manifestation in FFM. So, onset of symptoms occurs in the first or second decade of life in SD and in FFM it is generally after the third decade. Bilateral symmetric gradual dimness of vision is the most common presenting symptom. Some patients with advanced disease may complain of a central scotoma.

In the initial stage, the clinical appearance of fundus can be deceptively normal. There can be loss of foveal reflex and symmetric atrophic retinal pigment epithelial changes. A tapetal reflex (beaten bronze), granularity or RPE destruction all manifests atrophy of the macula. This is accompanied by adjacent flecks. They are irregularly shaped yellow subretinal lesions varying in shape (described as round, linear, crescentic or pisciform) and size (100 to 200 µm) extending as far as midperiphery. As the disease progresses the flecks disappear leaving behind RPE atrophy, and new flecks appear at a different location. In long-standing cases flecks become less yellow and pigmentations may occur. The central annular focus of atrophy may extend to the deeper layers of posterior pole resulting in extensive atrophy of the choriocapillaries.

Classification (Fishman)

Stage 1: Central macular atrophy of RPE and choriocapillaris often associated with ring of flecks.

Stage 2: Central macular atrophy and flecks of different stages of development often extending to equator.

Stage 3: Extensive fleck resorption in the posterior pole with early chorio-capillaris atrophy.

Stage 4: End stage; flecks completely replaced by diffuse RPE and choriocapillaris atrophy throughout the fundus.

Investigations

Autofluorescence: Hypofluorescence suggesting RPE atrophy in the area noted to have beaten metal appearance clinically and it ascertains the extent of the condition.

FFA: In early cases, central oval zone of hyperflourescence which may be surrounded by some hyperfluorescent flecks. "Choroidal silence" is often seen which is because of increased filtering action of the RPE secondary to the absorption by lipofuscin of the excitatory blue wavelength emitted by the camera during FFA. As the disease progresses, there are more flecks until the entire posterior pole shows a blotchy pattern of hyperfluorescence, which may later on show confluence suggestive of widespread RPE atrophy. In late stages, central choroidal atrophy is seen.

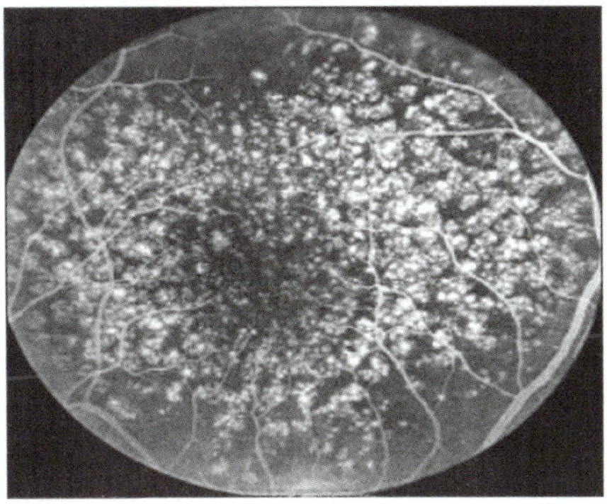

Figure 20: FFA of familial drusen

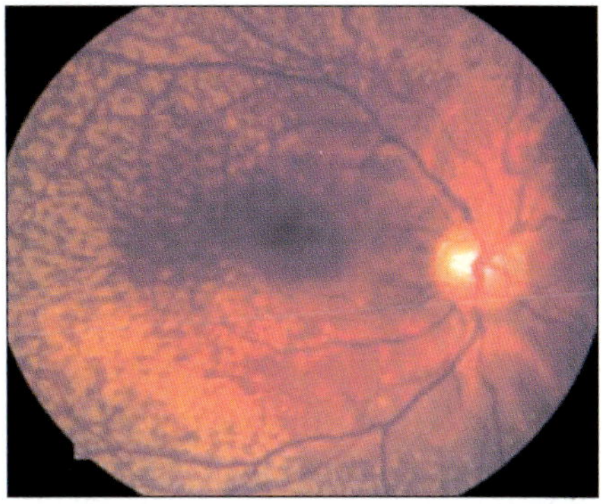

Figure 21: Central lesions, which spare the fovea in benign familial fleck retina

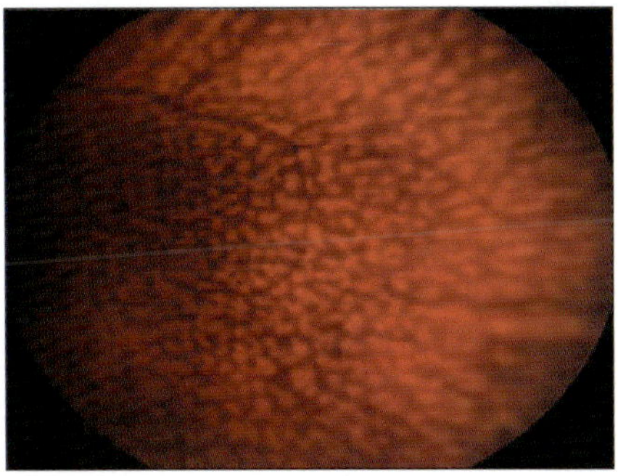

Figure 22: Peripheral lesions in benign familial fleck retina

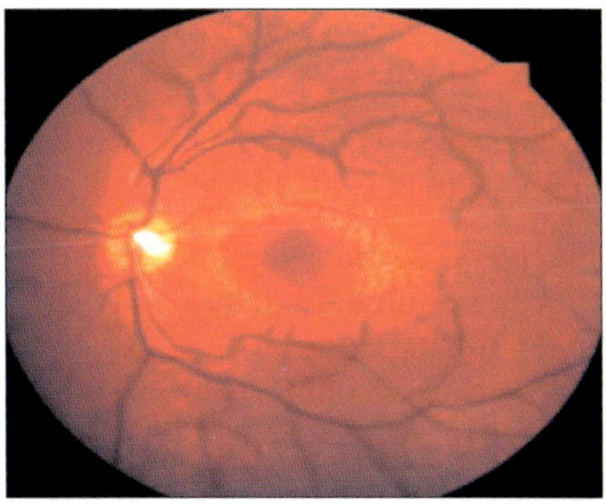

Figure 23: Macular flecks in Alport's syndrome

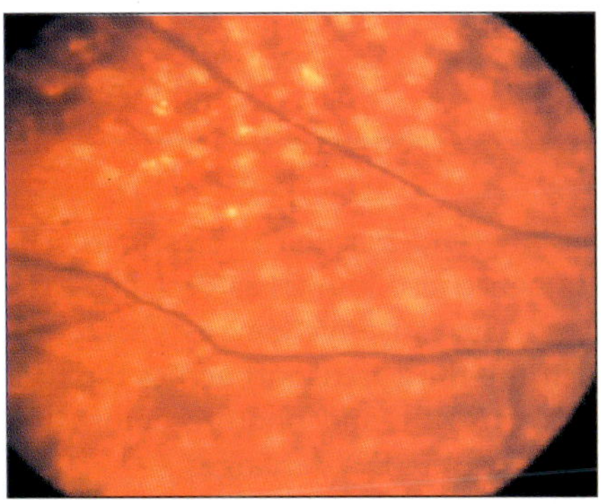

Figure 24: Larger peripheral flecks in Alport's syndrome

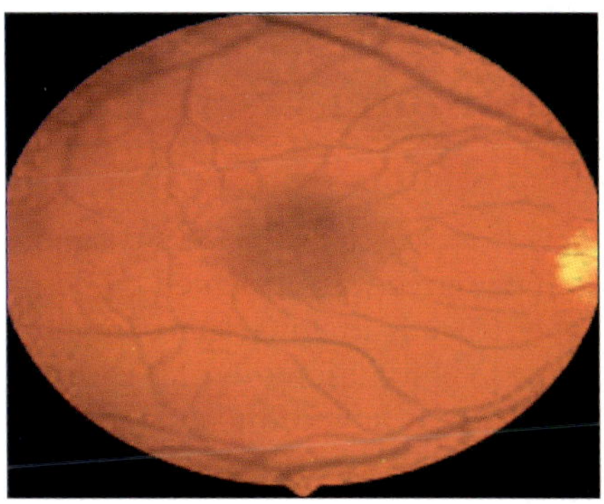

Figure 25: Dominant cystoid macular edema

Retinal Function Tests

Visual Acuity: The majority of patients with stage 1 and stage 2 Stargardt's disease maintains 20/200 or better VA at their initial and most recent visits. When fundus flecks show a notable degree of resorption, VA will decreases below 20/200.

Visual fields: Initially relative central scotoma followed by absolute central scotoma.

Color vision: Mild red-green dyschromatopsia.

ERG: Early in the disease process normal photopic and scotopic response. Later on ERG amplitudes may decrease, and the degree of abnormality correlates with the clinical severity of the disease.

EOG: Subnormal in most cases suggesting a diffuse disturbance in RPE function.

Differential Diagnosis

Variants of retinitis pigmentosa: Abnormal or extinguished ERG response as opposed to SD

Progressive cone dystrophy: Abnormal single/flicker photopic response as opposed to SD

Vitteliform Macular Dystrophy:
- Chloroquine Toxicity
- Familial Drusen
- Bietti Crystalline Dystrophy

Treatment

No known treatment. In case of considerable visual loss, low visual aids can be tried. It is mandatory to undergo genetic counseling if the patient is contemplating marriage or having children.

Vitelliform Dystrophy

Introduction

This is a clearly distinct entity among the inherited macular dystrophies. The first pedigree was presented by Best and is hence also known as Best's disease. Inheritance is irregular autosomal dominant. The causative gene is VMD2 and maps to chromosome 11q13. Disturbance in the fluid transport across the RPE could result in accumulation of debris between RPE and photoreceptors and between RPE and Bruch's membrane, leading to the EOG changes.

Clinical Features

Visual acuity is often minimally affected and the typical vitelliform structures may be noted during routine ophthalmoscopy. Severely diminished visual acuity may occur particularly in older age groups. Occasionally, light flashes and retinal detachment may be associated. Refraction is often hyperopic with astigmatism.

The vitelliform changes are usually noted bilaterally. The evolution of vitelliform dystrophy is schematically as follows:

1. Normal fovea, EOG pathologic
2. *Previtelliform stage:* Small, round yellowish dot at the site of the foveola or a tiny honeycomb structure centrally
3. *Vitelliform stage:* The classic vitelliform structure is an egg-yellow, sometimes orange, round, slightly elevated structure surrounded by a darker border. This macular disc may measure 0.5 to 3.0 disc diameters, with a resemblance to the intact yolk of a fried egg. The disk may disappear completely, leaving a normal-appearing macula.
4. *Scrambled-egg stage:* The yellowish material in the disc may disintegrate, leaving a scrambled-egg appearance. The disc may appear to rupture at a certain spot, with a decrease in visual acuity as viewed in Figure 8.
5. *Cyst stage:* The disc may in some cases give the appearance of a cyst
6. *Pseudohypopyon stage:* The disc may disintegrate or demonstrate syneresis, giving rise to a cyst with a fluid level, thus resembling a hypopyon.
7. *Round chorioretinal atrophy stage:* Subretinal neovascularization may occur accompanied with visual decline. Ultimately either round areas of chorioretinal atrophy or marked pigmentation may occur.

Multifocal vitelliform dystrophy: Lesions typically are manifested as sharply demarcated yellowish cysts in the macula, near the retinal vascular arcades and surrounding the optic disc. A variation in size and number (as many as 20) can be observed. Lesions may grow and merge with neighboring lesions. The evolution of the peripheral lesions may parallel the evolution of the central lesion but may also have a different time course.

Adult-onset foveomacular vitelliform dystrophy (AOFVD) is a rare macular condition that usually results in slow progressive bilateral vision loss. First described by Gass in 1974, these bilateral macular lesions are usually symmetrical, one third to one half disc diameter in size, round or oval, slightly elevated grayish-yellow subfoveal lesions that occur with or without a central pigmented spot in the fovea of each eye. AOFVD typically occurs in adults between the ages of 30 and 50 years old and has an autosomal dominance inheritance pattern with variable expression and incomplete penetrance. In the early stages of the disease, patients with AOFVD are usually visually asymptomatic or have mild complaints of visual blur or metamorphopsia in one or both eyes. As the disease progress, vision loss may become more drastic when the vitelliform lesion disrupts and leads to geographical atrophy similar to that seen in ARMD, or infrequently if the patient has choroidal neovascularization (CNV).

Investigations

Fluorescein angiography: Hypofluorescence corresponding to the macular disc in the intact disc stage is seen as the yellowish material does not transmit choroidal fluorescence. As the disc disintegrates, areas of hyperfluorescence indicating atrophic retinal pigment epithelium become visible.

At autofluorescence imaging, areas of highly increased autofluorescence within lesions correspond with the yellow-white material as seen at ophthalmoscopy. More advanced lesions show loss of autofluorescence centrally with an increased amount of autofluorescence at the outer border of the ovoid lesion.

Color vision: As in most macular diseases, colour vision is affected with a mild red-green dyschromatopsia.

ERG — is completely normal.

EOG — is subnormal even in carriers and is an important diagnostic tool. The light-dark ratio is rarely higher than 1.5.

Differential Diagnosis

Central serous chorioretinopathy, in individuals aged 20-60. It is usually unilateral, seen as a dome-shaped elevation at the macula. Hyperfluorescence with a smock-stack or inkblot pattern is noted. OCT reveals elevated neurosensory retina separated from the intact RPE by optically empty subretinal fluid and is associated with a normal EOG.

- Pigment epithelial detachment in individuals over 40 years. It is seen as a round elevated lesion, hyperfluorescent on angiography. OCT reveals elevated RPE layer without separation from photoreceptor.
- Fundus flavimaculatus in which pisciform flecks and beaten-metal appearance of the macula may be noted. Angiography is characterized by early stage: Dark silent choroid and late stage: Central hyperfluorescence
- Basilar laminar drusen in which numerous, small, uniform sized, round, slightly raised, yellow subretinal lesions may be visualized with early discrete hyperfluorescence corresponding to these lesions on angiography.
- Geographic AMD is usually seen in older individuals (>60 years) bilaterally with hyperfluorescence on angiography and absence of reflective band of photoreceptor layer with enhanced reflectivity of the choroid on OCT.
- Central areolar atrophy is visualized as atrophic macula 1-3 DD in size with visible choroidal vasculature

Treatment

No therapy exists for halting the progression of the disease with the possible exception of treatment of complications such as choroidal neovascularization, macular hole and retinal detachment. However, an accurate diagnosis and pedigree analysis is important for allowing the physician to perform adequate family and genetic counseling to affected patients.

Leber's Congenital Amaurosis

Introduction

Leber's congenital amaurosis (LCA) is a clinically and genetically heterogeneous disorder characterized by severe loss of vision at birth. It was first described by Theodor von Leber in 1869 and is the earliest and most severe form of all the inherited retinal dystrophies responsible for congenital blindness Its incidence is 2–3 per 100 000 births

Clinical Features

The currently recognized (although still debated) criteria for a diagnosis of LCA are the ones proposed by De Laey in 1991

- Onset of blindness or poor vision (appearing early in the first year of life, before 6 months of age);
- Sluggish pupillary reactions;
- Roving eye movements/nystagmus;
- Oculo-digital signs (eye poking, eye rubbing, eye pressing, etc.);
- Extinguished or severely reduced scotopic and photopic electroretinogram (ERG);
- Absent or abnormal VEPs;
- Variable fundus (for example, normal, marbled, albinotic with pigmentation).

In addition to these ocular symptoms a series of symptoms has been variably described that includes: Neurodevelopmental delay, mental retardation, associated systemic anomalies.

Investigations

The specific hallmark of LCA is seen in the ERG, which, in this disease, is extinguished or severely reduced in both the scotopic and photopic components.

Autosomal recessive inheritance is commonly found and six genes with disparate functions have been implicated in LCA.

Neuroradiological studies: The only consistent finding is hypoplasia of the cerebellar vermis, which can be seen in 10% of infants affected by LCA. Electroencephalography reveals epileptiform abnormalities on EEG.

Differential Diagnosis

A. Differential diagnosis of the ocular phenotype of LCA without a syndrome

	Features	Tests	Inheritance
LCA		ERG-not detectable	AR, rare AD
Complete achromatopsia	Striking photoaversion and blepharospasm	ERG-nondetectable or absent cone response, D15, FM 100-absent color vision	AR

Blue cone monochromatism	Less severe photoaversion and blepharospasm	ERG-nondetectable or absent cone response, D15, FM 100-tritanopia	XR
Complete CSNB	High myopia, good central day vision	ERG-absent rod responses, normal cone ERG, electronegative ERG	XR,AR,AD
Incomplete CSNB	High myopia, good central day vision	ERG-absent rod responses, abnormal cone ERG, electronegative ERG	XR,AR,AD
Oculocutaneous Albinism	Iris transillumination, blond fundus, foveal hypoplasia, hyperopia with oblique astigmatism		AR

B. Differential diagnosis of the ocular phenotype of LCA associated with a syndrome

Syndrome	*Features*
Bardet-Biedl's syndrome	Polydactyly, mental retardation, obesity, retinitis pigmentosa, kidneys often abnormal
Alstrom's syndrome	Cone-rod dystrophy, hearing loss, obesity, diabetes mellitus, cardiomyopathy
Abetalipoproteinemia	Rod-cone degeneration, celiac syndrome, ataxia, demyelination, steatorrhea, RBC acanthocytosis
Peroxisomal disorders	Malformation syndrome, hypotonia, liver failure, kidney failure, brain malformations, leopard spot retinopathy, Urine testing for very long chain fatty acids
Batten disease	Neurodegeneration, Bull's eye maculopathy. Rectal, conjunctival biopsy
Senior-Loken's syndrome	Nephrophthisis
Saldino-Mainzer's syndrome	Phalangeal cone-shaped epiphyses of hand, ataxia
Joubert's syndrome tachypnea	Agenesis of cerebellar vermis, hypoplasia of corpus callosum, neonatal
Lhermitte-Duclos' syndrome	Macrocephaly, seizures

Treatment

Various lines of investigation are currently open. These include retinal and stem-cell transplantation, drug therapies (for patients with normal but inactive retina) and gene therapy.

Inference

LCA is a highly heterogeneous disorder in which much remains to be clarified. In particular, an adequate classification is yet to be developed and the differences between the various clinical forms need to be established, as does the relationship between these and the genetic subtypes, in order to devise therapies for this disorder.

Bietti Crystalline Dystrophy

Introduction

Bietti crystalline dystrophy is a very rare condition, which predominantly affects males. Inheritance may be either X-linked or autosomal recessive.

Clinical Signs and Symptoms

It is characterized by the deposition of crystals in the peripheral cornea and retina. Presentation is in the third decade of life with progressive visual loss.

Signs in Chronological Order

- Yellow-white crystals scattered throughout the posterior fundus.
- Localized atrophy of the RPE and choriocapillaris at the posterior pole.
- Diffuse atrophy of the choriocapillaris.
- Gradual confluence and expansion of the atrophic areas into the retinal periphery.

Investigation

ERG and EOG are subnormal.

Treatment

No known treatment is available.

Inference

Prognosis is variable, because the rate of disease progression differs in individual cases.

North Carolina Macular Dystrophy

Synonym: Lefler-Wadsworth-Sidbury dystrophy

Introduction

In 1971, Lefler and colleagues described an autosomal dominant foveal dystrophy found in 25 of 70 members of a family spanning four generations.

By 1974, this pedigree had been expanded to include 545 individuals spanning seven generations; 130 were studied ophthalmoscopically, and 50 were found to be affected by the dystrophy. As this pedigree has been traced back to a family originating in North Carolina, it is now referred to as North Carolina macular dystrophy.

Clinical Signs and Symptoms

The dystrophy develops during the first year of life, and the foveal lesions were thought to progress throughout childhood to reach their final stage by late puberty. The final visual acuity is also reached by late puberty. Marked variations are noted in the final stage achieved by different siblings. Some individuals have foveal lesions arresting at an early or intermediate stage, whereas the lesions of others progress to a final atrophic stage.

Ophthalmoscopically, the macular changes can be divided into three stages:

Stage 1: Scattered drusen and pigment dispersion within the fovea Visual acuity is usually 20/20, and central or paracentral scotomas are not present. Fluorescein angiography reveals transmission defects within the fovea corresponding to the drusen.

Stage 2: Confluent drusen with or without pigment clumping within the central macula. RPE atrophy and partial choroidal atrophy may be seen. The visual acuity is usually in the 20/50 range, and small central or paracentral scotomas may be present. Fluorescein angiography shows a more confluent pattern of transmission defects with no evidence of dye leakage or pooling.

Stage 3: Choroidal atrophy. Total RPE and choriocapillary atrophy of the fovea, parafovea, or entire macula may develop.

Visual acuity is usually in between 20/50 to 20/200. Large central or paracentral scotomas are present. The foveal lesion is always moderately severe before any decrease in visual acuity occurs. Thereafter, the decrease in visual acuity closely parallels the severity of the foveal lesion. Likewise, the size and development of central scotomas correspond closely to the stage and size of the foveal lesions.

Investigation

The ERG and EOG are normal, as are dark adaptometry and color vision testing.

Differential Diagnosis

The differential diagnosis includes dominant progressive foveal dystrophy (dominant Stargardt's), familial drusen, central areolar choroidal dystrophy, and congenital macular colobomas.

Treatment

There is no known therapy for this dystrophy.

Inference

Small in 1989 reexamined 22 members of the original family and reported that only 1 patient demonstrated progression of macular disease. Gass, who examined two families with this entity who originated from North Carolina, also emphasized the generally stationary nature of this dystrophy.

Butterfly-shaped Pigment Dystrophy of the Fovea

Introduction

Deutman and associates in The Netherlands in 1970 first described this autosomal dominant dystrophy with a peculiar pigmentary pattern in the central macula.

Clinical Signs and Symptoms

This disorder manifests itself in the second to fifth decades and is accompanied by normal or only slightly decreased vision between 20/20 to 20/25. The predominant feature of this dystrophy is the presence of a bilaterally symmetric reticular pattern of pigmentation (the so-called butterfly-shape) within the central macula, which is best seen with fluorescein angiography. Pigment stippling in various configurations and drusen-like changes may also be noted in the peripheral retina.

Investigations

Fluorescein angiography demonstrates a reticular hypofluorescent pattern corresponding to the areas of hyperpigmentation with no obvious hyperfluorescence or dye leakage. In cases in which the pigmented structures are barely visible on fundus examination, the lesions can be seen clearly on fluorescein angiography, a characteristic shared by all the pattern dystrophies of the retinal pigment epithelium.

The ERG is normal, while the EOG may demonstrate abnormal values, suggesting a more widespread disturbance of the retinal pigment epithelium than is appreciable ophthalmoscopically. Dark adaptometry and color testing are normal, while visual field studies may reveal a relative central scotoma with normal peripheral fields.

Differential Diagnosis

The clinical findings, however, suggest a primary dystrophy of the retinal pigment epithelium. Butterfly-shaped pigment dystrophy of the fovea, as well as pattern dystrophy of the pigment epithelium of Marmor and Byers, foveomacular vitelliform dystrophy: Adult type, dominant slowly progressive macular dystrophy of Singerman-Berkow-Patz, macroreticular dystrophy, fundus *pulverulentus*, the reticular dystrophies of Benedikt-Wernerand of Kingham-Fenzl-Willerson-Aaberg, and autosomal dominant dystrophy of the retinal pigment epithelium of O'Donnell-Schatz-Reid-Green demonstrate remarkably similar characteristics, both clinically and pathophysiologically.

Treatment

No known treatment is available.

Inference

Prognosis is generally good, although a minority of patients may develop visual impairment.

Sorsby Pseudo-inflammatory Macular Dystrophy

Introduction

Sorsby pseudo-inflammatory macular dystrophy, which is also referred to as hereditary hemorrhagic macular dystrophy, is a very rare but serious condition. Inheritance is autosomal dominant.

Clinical Signs and Symptoms

Presentation is during the second and fourth decades with initially unilateral impairment of central vision and metamorphopsia.

Signs are yellow-white, confluent spots located along the arcades and nasal to the optic disk.

Investigation

ERG is normal.

Differential Diagnosis

Age-related macular degeneration

Treatment

No known treatment is available.

Inference

Prognosis is poor due to the development, during the fifth decade of life, of exudative maculopathy and subsequent subretinal scarring similar to that seen in age-related macular degeneration.

Dominant Drusen

A spectrum of disease characterized by dominantly inherited drusen, it is variously named as Doyne's honeycomb dystrophy, Mallatia Levantinese,

Hutchinson-Tay choroiditis, Holthouse-Batten superficial chorioretinitis or familial drusen.

Symptoms and Signs

Initially, no symptoms. Later, decrease in visual acuity and metamorphopsia

Affected persons present in the second and third decade with drusens in the fundus and have a history of conditions affecting several generations. These sharply delineated drusens are distributed in the macula and around the optic nerve head with a nasal predominance (pathognomonic of familial drusens). There is a halo of drusen surrounding the foveola. Later these spots coalesce and retina shows atrophic RPE. In late stages, oval white plaques surrounding the discs are characteristic findings in this dystrophy.

Investigation

Fluorescein Angiography

In the arterial phase sharply defined fluorescent spots are seen corresponding to lesions observed during ophthalmoscopy. Also RPE atrophy is revealed by window defects. Occasionally, large drusens (hyaline bodies consisting a large mass) may not show hyperfluorescence. No leakage is seen in the late phases.

Retinal Function Tests

Diminution of visual acuity is rarely seen before 40 years. In advanced cases there may be central scotoma. Mild red-green dyschromatopsia in HRR test is seen. Dark adaptation and ERG are usually normal. EOG is normal at initial stages but may be subnormal later on, depending upon the extent of involvement.

Benign Familial Fleck Retina

Introduction

Benign familial fleck retina is a rare autosomal recessive disorder which is asymptomatic and therefore, usually discovered by chance.

Clinical Signs and Symptoms

Widespread, discrete, yellow-white, flecks at the level of the RPE, which spare the fovea.

The flecks have variable shapes and extend to the far periphery.

Investigation

ERG is normal.

Differential Diagnosis

Differential diagnosis of fundus flecks:

1. *Benign familial fleck retina:*
   Differences — shape of flecks is highly variable: Many are larger and spare the macula.
2. *Alport's syndrome:*
   Differences — macular flecks are pale and punctate; periphery flecks are confluent.
3. *Early North Carolina macular dystrophy:*
   Differences — flecks at the macula are smaller and tightly packed together.
4. *Fundus albipunctatus:*
   Differences — flecks are punctate and spare the macula.
5. *Basal lamina drusen:*
   Differences — flecks are more numerous, smaller and more subtle.

Treatment

No known treatment is available.

Inference

Prognosis is excellent.

Alport's Syndrome

Introduction

Alport's syndrome is a rare abnormality of glomerular basement membrane which is characterized by chronic renal failure and sensorineural deafness. Inheritance is X-linked dominant.

Clinical Signs and Symptoms

Scattered, pale, yellow, punctate flecks at the macula with normal visual acuity.

Larger flecks, some of which may be confuent, are seen at the periphery.

Investigation

ERG is usually normal.

Treatment

No medical treatment is available.

Inference

Prognosis is excellent because the retinal changes are innocuous.

Dominant Cystoid Macular Dystrophy

Introduction

Reports from The Netherlands indicate that cystoid macular edema can be inherited as an autosomal dominant trait. An additional report describes an affected Greek family.

Clinical Signs and Symptoms

Dominantly inherited cystoid macular edema is characterized by an early onset in the first and second decades with a prolonged course of macular cystoid change and progressive loss of central vision. Hyperopia from +2.00 to + 10.00D is frequently seen along with hypopigmentation within the central macula. Macular atrophy is a fairly prominent finding late in the disease. Occasionally, a bull's-eye pattern of atrophic change may be seen. Vitreous cells, strands, and veils, and peripheral retinal pigmentary disturbances ranging from a slight hyperpigmentation and depigmentation to the formation of bone spicule changes have also been reported. Late in the disease, vision may be reduced to the 20/200 to finger counting range and a relative-to-absolute central scotoma may be present.

Investigation

Fluorescein angiography reveals leakage from perifoveal capillaries with dye pooling in a cystoid pattern. Later in the disease, transmission defects are seen in areas of RPE atrophy. In some cases, fluorescein leakage from optic disc capillaries has also been noted.

The ERG has been normal in all patients studied to date. The EOG and results of dark adaptometry, however, are subnormal in most, but not all, patients. The subnormal EOG would indicate widespread dysfunction of the retinal pigment epithelium. Color testing usually shows mild-to-moderate deuteran-tritan defects.

Differential Diagnosis

The pathogenesis and prevalence of this dystrophy are as yet undetermined. The condition should be differentiated from other hereditary retinal disorders that are associated with cystoid macular edema, especially retinitis pigmentosa (rod-cone dystrophy), and dystrophies characterized by the presence of foveal retinoschisis (which may be mistaken for cystoid macular edema) such as X-linked juvenile retinoschisis and familial foveal retinoschisis.

Treatment

No known treatment is available.

Inference

Prognosis is poor because the disease is progressive with the eventual development of pericentric pigmentary changes and a decline of visual acuity to counting fingers.

Chapter 51

Uveitis

Rupal H Trivedi, M Edward Wilson (USA)

Introduction

The incidence of uveitis in children has been reported to be less than that of adults and up to 10% of the total number of uveitis patients belong to the pediatric age group. For childhood uveitis, anterior uveitis accounted for 30-40%, posterior uveitis for 40-50%, intermediate uveitis for 10-20%, and panuveitis for 5-10%. Common causes of childhood uveitis are juvenile idiopathic arthritis, toxoplasmosis, toxocariasis, sarcoidosis, Vogt-Koyanagi-Harada's syndrome, acute retinal necrosis, Reiter's syndrome, lupus, and Fuchs' heterochromic iridocyclitis.

Clinical Signs and Symptoms

Children with uveitis may not present until late stage. Patients may present complaining of dimness of vision (secondary to cataract, vitreous haze, etc.), sensitivity to light or glare, redness, pain, photophobia, floaters, etc. Obtaining proper history can help the clinician narrow the differential diagnosis and to locate the etiology.

The cornea should be examined for keratic precipitates (KP) (stellate vs mutton fat), endothelial pigment dispersion, or stromal changes. Anterior chamber cell or flare should be noted and graded. The iris should be examined for synechia, iris nodules (Busacca/Koeppe), areas of atrophy or discoloration. Iris atrophy may be sectorial, diffuse, superficial or very subtle with minimal shallowing of the crypts. Filiform synechiae with a 'festooned pupil' are common in long-standing anterior uveitis cases. In chronic cases of anterior uveitis, complicated cataract, band-haped keratopathy (often seen in JIA-associated uveitis), and secondary glaucoma are common. Vitreous cell and haze can be present. The existence of snow banks, large white opacities (snowballs) or pars planitis should also be noted. The retina should be examined for findings such as the presence of masses, serous retinal detachments, areas of acute inflammation, necrosis, vessel sheathing or macular cysts, macular pigment, or macular edema. The optic disc may also show diffuse atrophy or pallor, sectorial atrophy, thinning, neovascularization, hyperemia or edema.

Other systemic associations should be looked for to help identify the etiology of the uveitis.

Investigations

Investigations should be customized to the suspected etiology. If JIA is suspected, obtain an antinuclear antibody test to classify the condition and to determine the risk of recurrent and severe disease. Sarcoid uveitis is investigated with determination of the angiotensin-converting enzyme (ACE) level, with or without serum lysozyme testing, chest roentgenograms, and gallium scanning. Definitive diagnosis requires histopathologic demonstration of noncaseating granulomatous inflammation, in the absence of another possible cause.

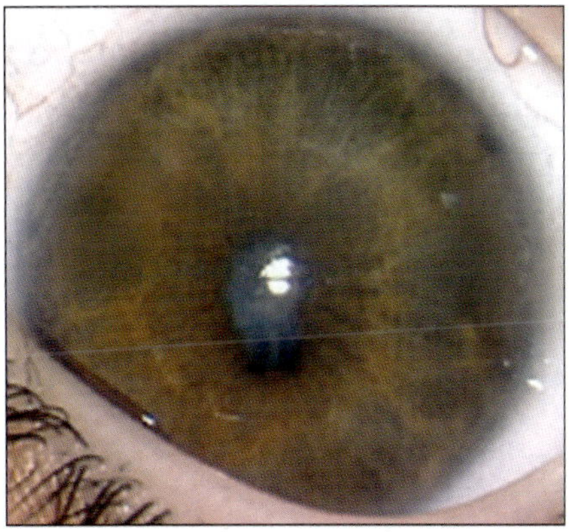

Figure 1: Cataract secondary to uveitis

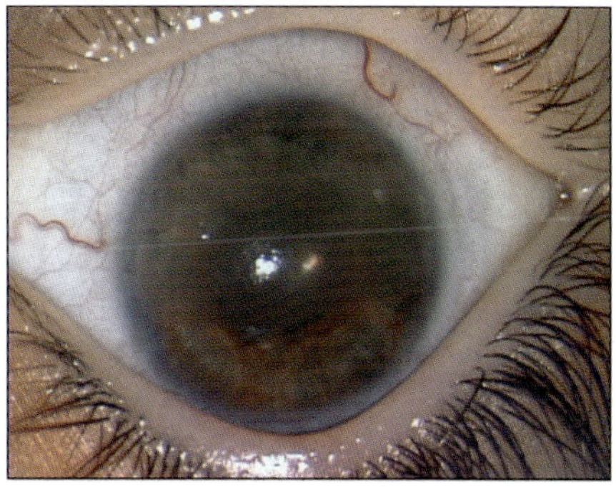

Figure 2: Postoperative view of cataract

Differential Diagnosis

Differential diagnosis varies greatly based on the etiology of the uveitis. A detailed evaluation can help identify the etiology. For example, the diagnostic triad of Fuchs' uveitis syndrome consist of stellate KP, cataract and iris atrophy leading to heterochromia. Lacrimal gland may be enlarged in sarcoidosis and other infiltrative conditions. Mutton-fat KP may be present in granulomatous conditions, but smaller KP occur in JIA-associated uveitis.

Treatment

The goal of treatment is to reduce the intraocular inflammation, relieve pain, prevent vision loss and treat the cause of uveitis if known. For anterior uveitis, a topical steroid is typically the first step. The strength and frequency of topical medications depend on the level of intraocular inflammation. If the uveitis does not respond to topical treatment, injectable steroids should be prescribed. These include sub-tenons or intraocular administration. Rarely, oral steroids will be needed as well. Mydriatic drops may be prescribed, which dilate the eyes to keep the pupils open and help prevent synechaie. IOP lowering drops would be needed if anterior uveitis causes increased IOP.

For intermediate uveitis and posterior uveitis—it is very important to determine the underlying cause of the inflammation. Infectious causes require the use of an anti-infective agent. For non-infectious causes, the goal of therapy is to get the inflammation under control. This can be done by the use of corticosteroids. Oral, injectable, or IV steroids may need to be prescribed.

Side effects of long-term steroid use may cause special problems for children being treated for chronic uveitis. For some patients with chronic uveitis, nonsteroid anti-inflammatory drugs need to be prescribed. Other agents which affect the immune system but which are not steroid based include oral or injectable methotrexate. It is now often used to treat significant eye inflammation (in cooperation with a rheumatologist), so the long-term side effects of steroids can be avoided. Safety profile and success of methotrexate in the pediatric population is well-documented.

In addition to treat ocular inflammation, it is also important to treat the cause of uveitis. For example, standard treatment for toxoplasmosis consists of systemic pyrimethamine and sulfadiazine with folinic acid supplementation. However, these drugs can have significant side effects including bone marrow suppression and Stevens-Johnson's syndrome.

Surgery is required to treat the complications of severe or chronic inflammation. For example, in JIA-associated uveitis, cataract often develops and needs to be removed. Severe band keratopathy, as seen in JIA, may require treatment with Ca EDTA chelation. Development of glaucoma may require trabeculectomy or placement of a drainage implant. In toxocariasis with retinal traction or severe vitreous opacity, vitrectomy may become necessary. In most cases, laser photocoagulation or cryoretinopexy of the larvae is not suggested since destruction of the nematode may cause a severe inflammatory process. The use of antihelminthes medications are common in treating systemic disease, but remain controversial with ocular disease. As with laser photocoagulation, it is believed that the destroyed larvae are responsible for a severe inflammatory reaction.

Prognosis

Uveitis is mostly asymptomatic in the early stages in children and they may be presenting to the ophthalmologist at a very late stage. Complications of uveitis are more common in children because of the chronic and relentless course of the disease in many cases coupled with delayed presentation. Early detection and treatment of uveitis is essential for preservation of normal vision and ocular anatomy. Long-term studies on JIA patients have shown that a majority of the patients had a favorable outcome. However, when untreated due to delayed diagnosis can devastate an eye with permanent cicatricial or inflammatory damage. Prognosis in sarcoid uveitis may vary widely; intractable cases leading to blindness do occur. In general, late onset and delayed treatment are associated with poor prognosis in uveitis cases.

Chapter 52

Ocular Toxoplasmosis

Masoud Soheilian, Rezaei Kanavi
MM Sadoughi, Azimzadeh A (Iran)

Definition

Toxoplasma gondii is an intracellular parasite and may manifest as a systemic infection especially in newborns and immunocompromised patients. It is an important cause of ocular disease in both immunocompetent and immunocompromised individuals. Toxoplasmosis has been considered the most common cause of posterior uveitis in the world.

Ocular toxoplasmosis is usually a self-limited cause of posterior uveitis. If optic nerve and macula are involved, vision may be severely decreased.

Most cases of ocular involvements are due to the recurrence of a congenital infection, although acquired toxoplasmosis is more common than what previously suspected. Ocular infection, in immunocompetent patients, produces acute retinochoroiditis together with vitreous inflammation and focal retinal necrosis. Recurrence of ocular toxoplasmosis is frequent and usually occurs at the borders of old retinochoroidal scars.

History and Classification

Toxoplasma gondii was first observed by Nicole and Manceaux in 1908 in North African rodent. Subsequent study on ocular tissue of a child who died from congenital infection revealed *Toxoplasma gondii* in the retinal tissue.

The name of toxoplasma has been derived from the Greek word of toxon-means arc shaped and gondii is the name of the animal in which the parasite was found.

Traditionally, it was thought that ocular toxoplasmosis was a reactivation of congenital toxoplasmosis that was transmitted from placenta. Recently, it has been shown that the acquired forms occur more frequently than what previously suspected. Toxoplasma infection is asymptomatic in most immunocompetent patients and if it occurs, the clinical course usually will be benign and self-limited. The infection may manifest as a devastating disease in fetus and immunocompromised patients.

Toxoplasmosis is one of the most frequently identifiable causes of uveitis and is also the most common pathogen of posterior infectious uveitis.

Fetus may be infected during pregnancy and the disease is benign and self-limited as in other immunocompetent patients; however, it may cause variable manifestations in children such as retinochoroiditis, strabismus, blindness, cerebral involvement, thrombocytopenia, and anemia.

Clinical Characteristics

Systemic Manifestation

Clinical features of systemic toxoplasmosis in the immunocompetent patients may be different from those seen in immunocompromised patients.

The presentation of acquired disease in an immunocompetent patient may be varied from a symptom-free condition to a form of flu-like syndrome with

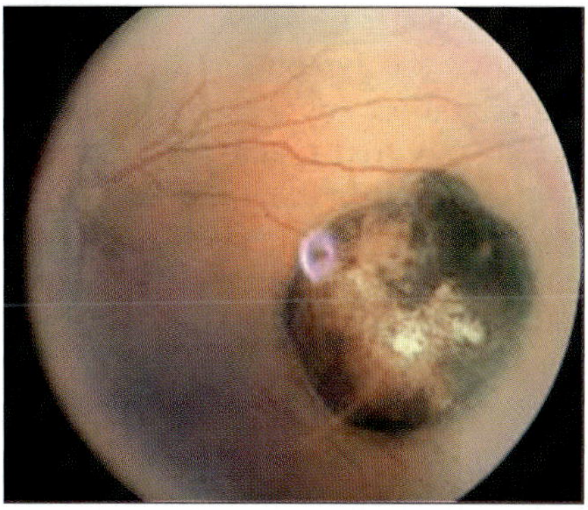

Figure 1: A typical quiescent congenital toxoplasmosis retinochoroiditis scar in a young adult in the left eye, the other eye was normal

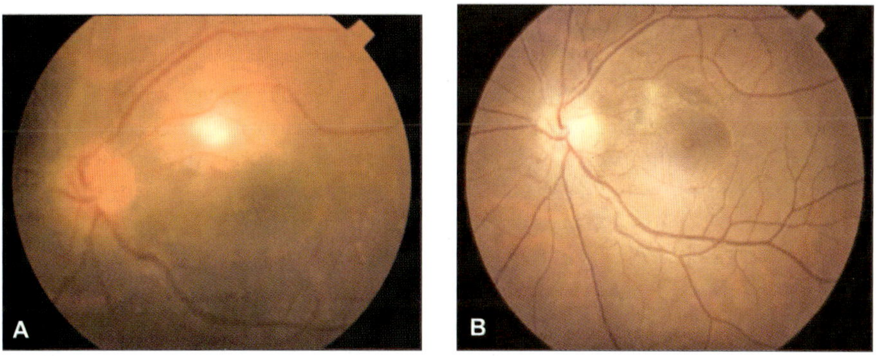

Figures 2A and B: Typical acquired toxoplasma focal retinitis adjacent to macula. (A) Before and (B) After classic treatment with pyrimethamine, sulfadiazine and prednisolone

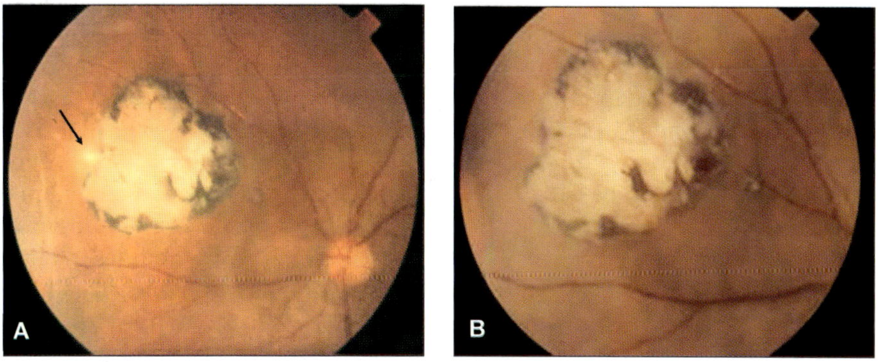

Figures 3A and B: A new active lesion (arrow) adjacent to a large pigmented retinal scar in a 39-year-old man before and after treatment. This picture somehow demonstrate intraretinal migration of trophozoites

fever, malaise and sore throat; up to 90% of the patients may develop lymphadenopathy. The involved lymph nodes are usually bilateral and non-tender. Severe disease may affect any organ such as meninges, muscle, skin, brain, heart and kidney. Acquired toxoplasmosis in an immunocompetent person is usually benign and self limiting; lasting 2 to 4 weeks. Death due to toxoplasmosis in immunocompetent patients is very rare and may be the result of encephalitis, pneumonitis, myocarditis or hepatitis. Since acquired toxoplasmosis in most of the cases is asymptomatic, its true incidence is unclear. The interval between the systemic disease and ocular manifestations is variable, and ranges from days to years.

Toxoplasmosis in immunocompromised patients including HIV-positive patients, transplant recipients and those on chemotherapy, may induce a severe, fulminant course and may be fatal if untreated. It may be caused by reactivation of a chronic infection or may be newly acquired. Since the parasite has an affinity for central nervous system, the common manifestation in the immunocompromised patients is intracranial involvement with diffuse neurologic dysfunction, seizures and meningoencephalitis. Immunocompromised patients may develop multi-organ involvement, especially pneumonitis and myocarditis. In one study, 40% of the Acquired Immunodeficiency Syndrome (AIDS) patients had intracranial toxoplasmic abscess at autopsy. When toxoplasmic retinochoroiditis occurs in AIDS patients it is frequently associated with encephalitis, therefore, all the AIDS patients who have ocular toxoplasmosis should undergo a neurologic work up, including computed tomography (CT) or magnetic resonance imaging (MRI) with contrast and lumbar puncture. Serologic tests in the diagnosis of toxoplasmosis may not be helpful because the IgG or IgM titers may not be elevated in the AIDS patients.

Ocular Manifestations

Ocular presentation usually depends on age, severity, size and location of toxoplasmic retinochoroiditis. It may present with decreased visual acuity, strabismus, nystagmus or leukocoria in children. Ocular manifestations in adults include floaters and blurred visual acuity. Decreased visual acuity may occur due to macular involvement or severe vitreous opacification. Patients with bilateral disease often have active lesion only in one eye at the time of presentation unless an immunocompromised condition influences the clinical course. In immunocompromised population, the clinical presentation may be rather atypical, particularly with fewer vitreous cells and less vitreous opacification than otherwise would be expected. Mild to moderate inflammation of anterior segment may be another presenting feature. In proportion to the posterior segment disease, some patients may present with Koeppe nodules, stellate keratic precipitates, and posterior synechiae formation. A syndrome very similar to Fuchs' Heterochromic iridocyclitis may be seen in patients with toxoplasmosis. More severe inflammation may be accompanied by granulomatous mutton fat keratic precipitates. Elevated intraocular pressure is commonly seen in patients with acute toxoplasmosis. Glaucoma may be caused by obstruction of trabecular meshwork by cellular debris and inflammatory

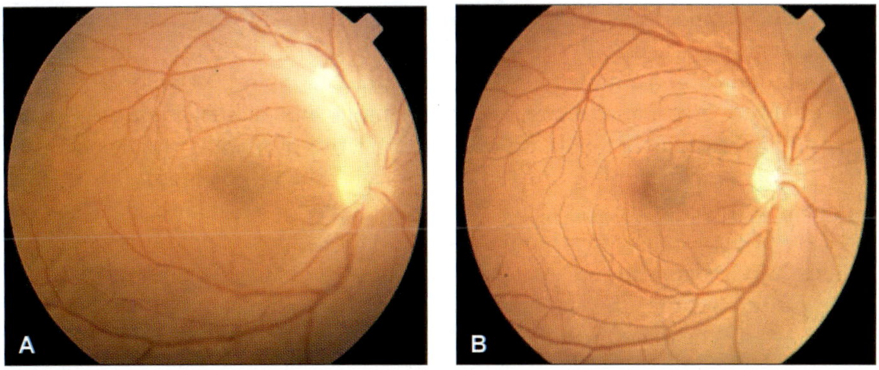

Figures 4A and B: Toxoplasma neuroretinitis and papillitis in the right eye of a 25-year-old woman before and after treatment with trimethoprim/sulfamethoxazol

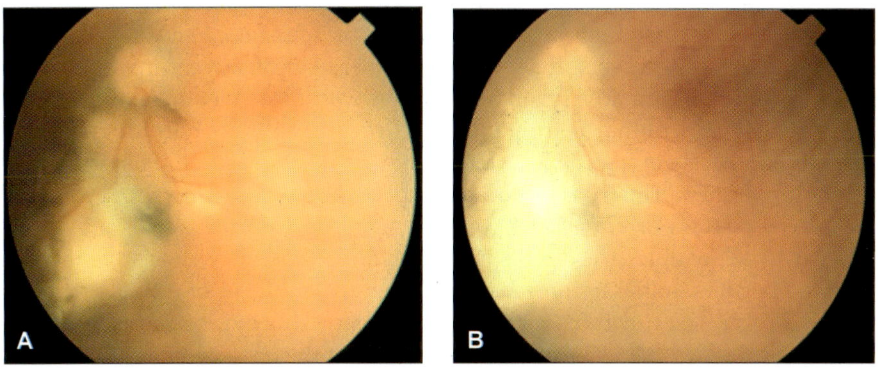

Figures 5A and B: A recurrent, large peripapillary toxoplasma retinochoroiditis in a 29-year-old immunocompromised patient with vitreous hemorrhage and persistent vitreous bands before and after long-term treatment with trimethoprim/sulfamethoxazol

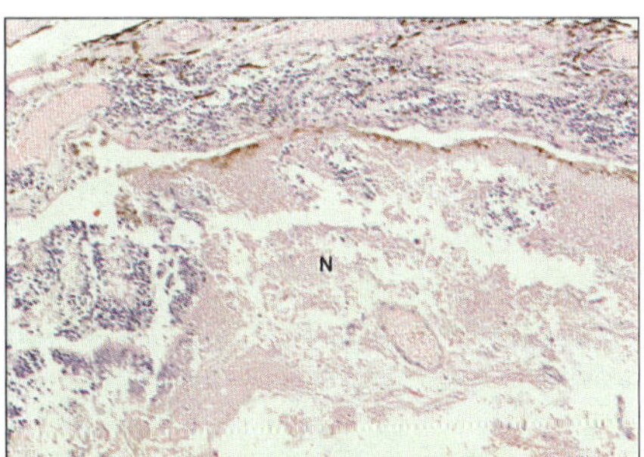

Figure 6: Note the partial retinal necrosis (N) with loss of its lamellar architecture in toxoplasmic retinochoroiditis (H and E staining, magnification × 25)

cells, acute trabeculitis, or chronic peripheral anterior synchiae formation. Secondary cataract, usually of posterior sub-capsular type, may also develop. The anterior vitreous almost always is inflamed, although in mild cases, focal vitritis may overly the small areas of focal retinitis with a quiet anterior vitreous.

The classic lesion of toxoplasmosis is a focal area of retinitis and it is believed that it occurs as a consequence of reactivation of the congenital infection. Congenital infections may account for about 80-90% of ocular toxoplasmosis.

Toxoplasma gondii has a strong predilection for the posterior pole and macular lesions have been reported in 76% of patients. The reason is unclear but some have postulated that the parasites first invade the eye through the posterior ciliary arteries or the optic nerve. Invasion by the way of optic nerve may give rise the juxta-papillary retinochoroiditis. It is thought that the macular predilection for toxoplasmosis may be related to earlier vascularization of the posterior pole than periphery during fetal development and the fact that fetal vasculature contains end arterioles.

Toxoplasma retinitis is a recurrent disease, occurring in two thirds of the patients. The relapse may be due to release of *Toxoplasma gondii* from cysts. After rupture of the cysts, live organisms release and actively invade normal adjacent retina. Alternatively, an autoimmune response may develop to retinal antigens such as retinal S-antigen, which result in retinochoroiditis. On the basis of another theory, some recurrences may be the result of re-infection because immunity from a primary infection may not be sufficient to prevent re-infection with a new strain of *Toxoplasma gondii*.

An active toxoplasma retinitis is whitish and moderately exudative with ill-defined borders. Initial lesion starts in the nerve fiber layer of retina and as the lesion progresses full thickness retina, adjacent choroid, vitreous and even sclera may be involved. Gradually the borders of the lesion, either as the result of treatment or natural course of the disease, become more defined. Then inflammation diminishes and, after a while, pigmentation develops at the borders of the lesion. The healing time varies and depends on the size of the lesion, treatment delivered, the host immunity, and the *Toxoplasma gondii* strain. During healing process retinochoroidal shunt and even choroidal neovascularization (CNV), gliosis and tractional bands may develop.

Retinal vasculitis in the vicinity of an active lesion or in the distant retina may be seen and is produced by antigen — antibody complex deposition in the vessel wall. The vasculitis primarily involves the veins but the arteries may also be involved less commonly than the veins.

Atypical clinical forms of toxoplasmosis such as punctuate outer retinal toxoplasmosis, neuroretinitis, and papillitis have been described. Optic neuritis demands prompt therapy. Pseudoretinitis is characterized by the retinal edema which is non-contiguous with the active lesion, may be seen in some cases and usually disappears after healing of the true lesion.

Toxoplasma retinal lesions in AIDS patients, unlike the situation in immunocompetent persons, do not develop adjacent to an old retinochoroidal scar. Instead, the lesions occur in perivascular distribution which may be the result of dissemination of parasites from other non-ocular sites in the body.

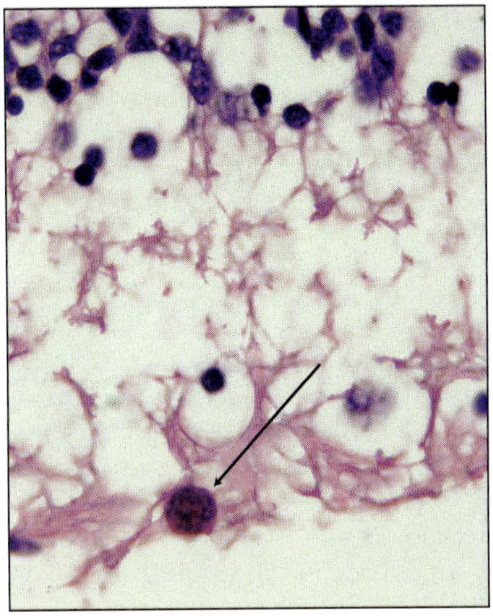

Figure 7: Note a toxoplasmic cyst (arrow) in the inner retinal layer (H and E staining, magnification × 250)

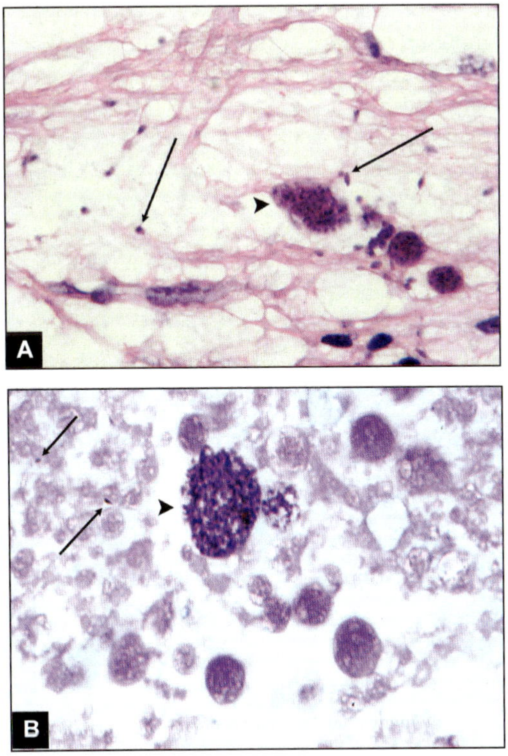

Figures 8A and B: Note the spherical cysts containing toxoplasma organisms (arrowheads) and the free forms of the trophozoites (arrows) on H and E (A) and PAS (B) stainings

Retinochoroiditis in AIDS may take atypical features such as very large areas of severe confluent retinal necrosis and bilateral lesions may also be seen. Ocular inflammation is variable and depends on the patient's lymphocyte count. Toxoplasma retinochoroiditis in AIDS patients may extend into the orbit and cause panophthalmitis and orbital achyzoite. Toxoplasma retinochoroiditis in AIDS patients may resemble acute retinal necrosis, CMV retinitis and even progressive outer retinal necrosis (PORN).

Pathogenesis

Toxoplasma gondii is an obligate intracellular protozoan parasite occurring worldwide in humans and animals. It belongs to the subphylum Sporozoa and is a coccidian parasite. The definitive host of the intracellular protozoan is household cat and other members of the family Felidae, but many intermediate hosts (e.g. humans, rodents, and fowl) are known.

It exists in two forms in nature: An asexual form and a sexual form. Sexual and asexual reproduction occur in the intestine of the cat; only asexual reproduction occurs in human beings and the other intermediate hosts. The result of sexual reproduction is the oocyst, which is passed in cat feces. The oocyst requires 2 to 5 days in the environment to mature and become infective. There are two life cycle stages in human beings: The achyzoites and the bradyzoite. Actively motile and reproducing forms are referred to as tachyzoites. They are crescent-shaped, about 7 microns in length and 2.5 microns in width, and have a prominent nucleus. The infected tissues contain free tachyzoites as well as intracellular forms. Bradyzoites are the slowly growing and reproducing forms found within a cyst-like structure during the dormant phase of the infection.

There are basically three ways in which human beings can acquire infection with *Toxoplasma gondii*, as shown in scheme A.

1. Ingestion or inhalation of the oocyst, which is shed in cat feces
2. Ingestion of undercooked meat containing the cyst with bradyzoites
3. Congenital transmission.

Scheme A: The ways of acquiring toxoplasma infection in human beings

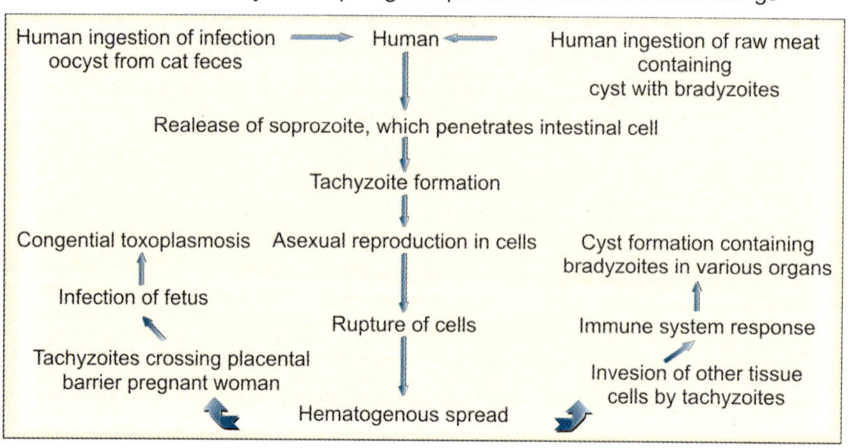

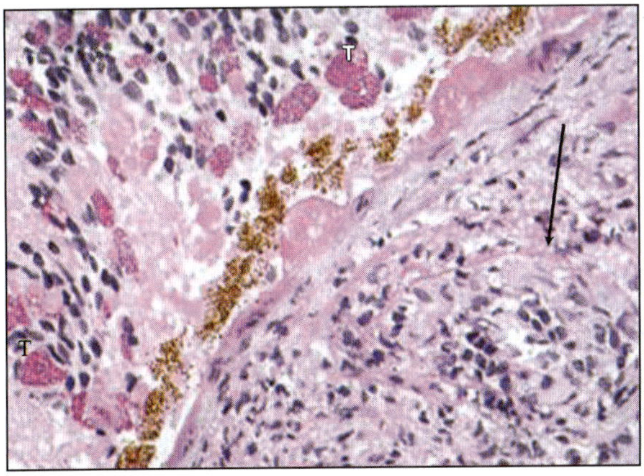

Figure 9: Note the moderate numbers of PAS-positive toxoplasmic cysts (T) within the neural retina and the presence of chronic granulomatous inflammatory cell infiltrate (arrow) within the adjacent choroid (PAS staining, magnification × 100)

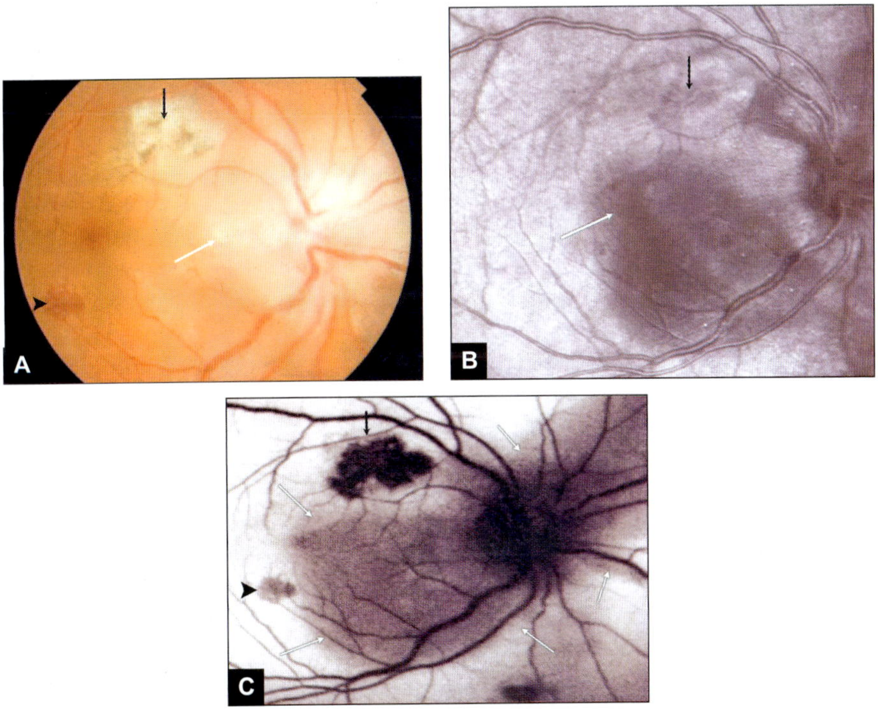

Figures 10A to C: Demonstrate an acute diffuse neuroretinitis in a 27-year-old man (white arrows). A pereretinal hemorrhage (arrow head) and an old toxoplasma retinochoroiditis scar superior to macula (black arrow) are visible. The corresponding infrared, (B) and autofluorescence, (C) photographs are shown. Extent of hypo-autofluorescence (Figure 10 C white arrows) clearly demonstrates the real lesion border that may not be detectable clinically, can be used for monitoring the effect of treatment and resolution of retinal edema

When human being ingests the infective oocyst, sporozoites present in the oocyst are released in the intestine and may multiply rapidly in the intestinal epithelium for several generations before penetrating the intestinal wall. These rapidly multiplying forms, named tachyzoites, invade regional lymph nodes and gain access to the circulation. Some of them, encased in the protective milieu of leukocytes, migrate to the other organs such as skeletal muscle, heart, brain and eye. These tachyzoites invade cells, multiply, and eventually lead to cell membrane rupture and the liberation of tachyzoites to invade other cells. The immune system response and conditions of cell nutrition, such as availability of the oxidative metabolism, result in formation of a large cyst-like structure that contains the slowly growing and reproducing bradyzoites. At this point, the infection remains in a dormant state, unless the immune system is compromised. In the immunocompromised patient, the bradyzoites are released from the cyst and become active tachyzoites that invade multiple organs, resulting in disseminated infection. The wall of the tissue cyst is composed of complex proteins and polysaccharides arranged to permit the passage of water, gases, electrolytes, and amino acids across the tissue-cyst-wall barrier but substances of higher molecular weight, such as proteins, are probably prohibited.

In the second method of infection, a human being ingests raw or undercooked meat containing the cyst with bradyzoites. The cyst wall is broken up, and bradyzoites are released. The organisms appear to be resistant to digestive tract enzymes for about 6 hours, during which time they convert to tachyzoites and invade the intestinal wall. They then gain access to the circulation and subsequently invade various organs. It appears that *Toxoplasma gondii* tissue cysts, tachyzoites, and oocysts are all capable of initiating systemic disease in humans. Ingestion of tissue cysts contained in undercooked meat is likely the most frequent cause of disease whereas tachyzoites and oocysts have only a relatively minor role.

The parasite, encased in the protective milieu of leukocytes, is brought to the retina by the bloodstream, deposited in the retinal capillaries and invades retinal cells directly. All types of leukocytes may be infected. These leukocytes may be arrested temporarily in the terminal capillary loops of areas such as the macula, only to release their burden of parasites. The parasites then proliferate locally at the site of their release. Reproduction of the parasite is a primary factor in the pathogenesis of the retinal lesion. It has been reported that the destructive activities of the parasite are more significant in retinal cells than in cells of the intestinal villi or liver because the latter cells tend to be substituted quickly, whereas retinal cells are never replaced. The eye is an immune-privilege site, and the pathogenesis of ocular toxoplasmosis is complex and poorly understood. Ocular toxoplasmosis may also be considered an immune-mediated process. Host resistance to *Toxoplasma gondii* infection is complicated and may involve a number of different cellular and humoral immune responses. Cell-mediated immunity is the major defense against *Toxoplasma gondii* infection. Several studies have demonstrated the importance of cell-mediated immune response and specific cytokines in the pathogenesis of ocular toxoplasmosis. T-lymphocytes liberate cytokines on stimulation by toxoplasmic antigens and accelerate the killing of parasites within macrophages. Tachyzoites have four major antigenic proteins (designated P43, P35, P30, and P22) on their membrane surfaces that seem to have a role in stimulating the host's immune response. The major surface antigen, P30, appears to induce cytotoxic reactions against infected macrophages and antibody-dependent complement-mediated lysis of tachyzoites. Antibodies against P30 reduce the ability of tachyzoites to invade mammalian cells. $CD4^+$ T cells are essential to the pathogenesis of ocular toxoplasmosis and are the major source of production of interferon-γ (IFN-γ) and tumor necrosis factor-α (TNF-α) and subsequent tissue inflammation. Resistance depends on both $CD4^+$ and $CD8^+$ T-lymphocytes. A variety of cytokines is involved; particularly important are Interleukins 2, 10, and 6. IL-10 is important in the regulation of inflammation during acute ocular toxoplasmosis. TNF-γ and IFN-γ work together to activate macrophages, which are necessary for killing the parasite. By slowing tachyzoite divisions, IFN-γ may also have a role in tissue-cyst formation. $CD4^+$ and $CD8^+$ T-lymphocytes, IFN-α, and TNF-α have all been shown to have a role in protection against ocular disease in animal models.

Inflammation, as a response to the proliferation of trophozoites, occurs at the region of infection. Within several hours after infection in the retina, macrophages can be identified in the tissue. The macrophages engulf the parasites and release lytic enzymes (principally acid hydrolases and proteinases). The function of these enzymes is to clear the lesion from cellular debris. In individuals with no previous immunity to *Toxoplasma gondii*, these macrophages are somewhat ineffective in controlling the infection. The macrophages activity is enhanced by stimulated T-lymphocytes. Natural killer (NK) cells, monocytes, polymorphonuclear leukocytes, eosinophils and other lymphocytes are soon attracted to the site of lesion. Natural killer cells may attack and kill the parasite, and then shift to another parasite. The numbers of natural killer cells may diminish early. Polymorphonuclear leukocytes may predominate when severe necrosis occurs. It is not known why *Toxoplasma gondii* prefers the retina over the choroid as a site for multiplication. It has been speculated that the retina, like the brain, is isolated from the free flow of serum antibodies into the tissue spaces. Normally, little IgG and no IgM can be identified in the retina. Low reproduction rate of brain and retinal cells and the presence of certain metabolic factors within the cells favor the tissue cyst formation *in situ* after initial establishment of infection in these tissues. Various types of antibodies are generated in response to *T. gondii* infection. Organisms that become coated with antibody and complement are soon lysed but this action appears to offer little protection against intracellular organisms. Extracellular organisms in tissues such as the retina and brain do not seem to be affected by intravascular circulating antibody.

Although no association was found between any HLA types and ocular toxoplasmosis, there is an association between HLA Bw62 and manifestations of severe ocular disease (bilaterality and macular involvement) in patients with congenital toxoplasmosis.

Congenital transmission occurs when tachyzoites in the maternal circulation cross the placenta and enter the fetal circulation and tissues. Antibody-negative women of child-bearing age are at risk for acquiring the infection and transmitting the parasite to their fetuses. The rate of transmission to the fetus actually is higher during the later months of pregnancy than the first trimester, possibly due to the presence of a more vascularized placenta in the later months. Fortunately, the incidence of acquired toxoplasmosis during pregnancy is low (0.2 to 1%), although there is a 40% chance of transplacental infection in pregnant women who contract toxoplasmosis. The fetus is significantly more damaged when infection occurs in the first trimester, presumably due to immature fetal immune response and higher vulnerability of fetal organs such as brain and eye during the first trimester. Infants born of women who acquire toxoplasmosis during pregnancy may appear to be perfectly normal at birth and develop retinochoroiditis later in childhood, adolescence, or early adulthood. In general, a woman who has given birth to one child with congenital toxoplasmosis will never give birth to another congenitally infected child. If the women have previously been infected with *Toxoplasma gondii*, they will be at little or no risk for transmitting the infection to their fetus because of the protective effects of maternal antibodies. It appears, however, that maternal infections acquired within the last several weeks before conception can be transmitted to the fetus, even in immunocompetent women.

Pathology

Ocular toxoplasmosis begins as unifocal or multifocal retinitis together with marked coagulative necrosis and severe inflammatory changes in the retina and exudation into the vitreous. The lesions are mostly located in the posterior pole of retina. On histopathologic evaluation, toxoplasma organisms are almost always found in three forms: Free, in pseudocysts, or in true cysts. The free parasites, called trophozoites, may rarely be found in the free form within the neural retina at the region of acute lesions. The protozoa are most commonly found in the inner retinal layers; in the area of coagulative necrosis of the neural retina. They also may be seen in the optic nerve but not in the uveal tract, except in patients with AIDS.

When a protozoan enters a retinal cell (neural retina or retinal pigment epithelium), it multiplies within the cell. Therefore, histologically, there is a pseudocyst composed of a group of protozoa surrounded by the retinal cell membrane. If the environment becomes unfavorable for the organism, the intracellular protozoan (trophozoite) may transform itself into a bradyzoite, surround itself with a self-made membrane, multiply, and then form a true cyst that extrudes from the cell and lies free in the tissue. The cysts may contain 50 to 3000 viable, resting bradyzoites, surrounded by a zone that is argyrophilic and is often positive on PAS staining. The cysts have a diameter of up to 250 μ. The organisms increase in number within the cyst in the retina, and once the cyst wall breaks down; the free organisms invade adjacent cells.

A secondary diffuse granulomatous inflammation is almost always present in the adjacent choroid, and occasionally, the sclera is thickened and inflamed.

Obliterative arteritis has also been reported. After the inflammatory process subsides, severe retinal destruction together with chorioretinal adhesion occurs and a pale atrophic scar with pigmented borders will remain. The chorioretinal scars are characterized by gliosis, obliteration of blood vessels, and hyperpigmentation of the borders. Adjacent to the retinochoroidal scar, the cysts may be found in the relatively normal tissue. Rupture of these cysts may lead to reactivation of the ocular disease.

Retinal dysplasia together with rosette formation has been reported in histopathologic examination of fetus and infants with ocular toxoplasmosis. Toxoplasma retinochoroiditis is more destructive in the immunocompromised patients than what seen in the immunocompetent hosts. As with the immunocompetent patients, the predominant site of infection appears to be the inner retina. The lesions may be unifocal or multifocal in one or both eyes, and they may be associated with diffuse areas of retinal necrosis.

Remarkable miliary toxoplasma retinitis was noted in a patient with AIDS. Most lesions do not arise from the borders of old healed lesions. Organisms can occasionally be seen in the uveal tissue and there is scant inflammatory cell infiltrate within retinal tissue. The density of parasites is frequently greatest near blood vessels, suggesting newly disseminated disease rather than recurrence from tissue cysts within the retina in contrast to the features observed in immunocompetent patients.

Diagnosis

The diagnosis of ocular toxoplasmosis is made by clinical observation of the focal necrotizing retinochoroiditis.The lesion is white to yellowish-colored with or without adjacent scar.

In atypical cases of ocular toxoplasmosis, serologic tests such as serum anti-toxoplasma titers of IgM and IgG may be helpful to support the diagnosis although the antigen load of a small active lesion in one eye may not be sufficient to motivate increased systemic antibody titers. In ocular toxoplasmosis, the serum titers of anti-toxoplasma antibodies are poorly related to the active lesion. Finding low or negative antibody levels is not unusual in patients with acute symptomatic or recurrent ocular toxoplasmosis. Therefore, it should be remembered that undiluted serum should be used for serologic tests in these patients. In atypical cases, positive serology results only suggest a presumptive ocular toxoplasmosis because of the high prevalence of antitoxoplasma antibodies in general population. Negative results are of importance to exclude atypical ocular toxoplasmosis. In cases with uncertain diagnosis, demonstration of anti-toxoplasma antibody titers in the aqueous humor or vitreous can be helpful. The ratio of serum levels of the anti-toxoplasma antibodies to the aqueous or vitreous levels, when corrected for total protein concentration, is known as the coefficient of Witmer-Desmonts. No active ocular toxoplasmosis is present when the coefficient is less than 2 in an immunocompetent patient. The ratio between 2 and 4 is suggestive of an active ocular infection. The ratio of 4 or more is diagnostic for active ocular toxoplasmosis.

An immunoassay for *Toxoplasma gondii* IgG should be performed routinely in AIDS patients. The positive results suggest the risk of reactivation of the infection; however, patients with a negative result should be instructed on how they can prevent upcoming infection. The IgG titer in AIDS patients may be relatively low and serologic test for IgM, IgA, and IgE may be negative.

When the serologic results are ambiguous, Polymerase Chain Reaction (PCR) is a powerful tool with high sensitivity and specificity in demonstrating the toxoplasma DNA sequences within the aqueous and vitreous samples. PCR of the amniotic fluid is also necessary to confirm the diagnosis and initiation of the treatment of infected fetuses with congenital toxoplasmosis.

Fluorescein angiography (FA) and indocyanine green angiography (ICG) findings in toxoplasma retinochoroiditis are nonspecific with hypo- and hyper-fluorescence depending on the stage of the lesion. Retinochoroiditis scars in early phase of FA may be seen as a hypofluorescent lesion due to blockage by RPE hypertrophy or as a window defect due to RPE atrophy. ICG of an old lesion is also hypofluorescent. FA in acute stages of the disease may disclose disc and vascular leakage because of papillitis and retinal vasculitis. Both FA and ICG are very essential for diagnosis and decision making for treatment of choroidal neovascularization (CNV). In addition ICG has been reported to be useful for early diagnosis of recurrent toxoplasma retinochoroiditis because it may be able to identify an area of reactivation not detectable by fundus examination and FA. Two recent non-invasive photography techniques, i.e. infrared and autofluorescence also may further enhance our ability to diagnose the extent of retinitis not detectable by clinical examination and FA. Toxoplasma retinochoroiditis scar in an autofluorescence photography demonstrates a dark area (hypo-autofluorescence) due to lack of functional RPE. Acute retinitis lesion also may show hypo-autofluorescence due to overlying retinal edema that is more extended than what is clinically observed. This autofluorescence photography is helpful for monitoring the effect of medical therapy, because it may better demonstrate the resolution of retinitis and resultant adjacent retinal edema.

Differential Diagnosis

Differential diagnoses of congenital ocular toxoplasmosis include: Macular coloboma, persistent hyperplastic primary vitreous and retinoblastoma. Recurrent toxoplasma retinochoroiditis adjacent to a scar area may be confused with serpiginous choroiditis. In the latter, there is no considerable inflammatory reaction in the anterior segment or vitreous and a single helicoid chorioretinal scar is usually present. Necrotizing retinitis due to cytomegalovirus, herpes simplex and herpes zoster virus, fungal retinitis (candidiasis, blastomycosis), septic retinitis, ocular toxocariasis, sarcoidosis, syphilis and tuberculosis are other differential diagnoses of ocular toxoplasmosis. Punctuate outer retinal toxoplasmosis is an atypical form of ocular toxoplasmosis and may be confused with acute posterior multifocal placoid pigment epitheliopathy (APMPPE), punctuate inner choroidopathy (PIC), multifocal choroiditis and diffuse unilateral subacute neuroretinitis (DUSN).

Treatment

Ocular toxoplasmosis is a self-limited disease. The following criteria are generally accepted for medical treatment of ocular toxoplasmosis:

- Optic nerve involvement or threatened by an adjacent lesion within 2 disc diameter
- A lesion within the temporal arcade
- A lesion threatening a large retinal vessel
- Concomitant subretinal hemorrhage and toxoplasma lesion
- Severe inflammatory reaction in a lesion
- Excessive chronic exudative lesions regardless of location
- Severe vitreous haze
- Loss of more than 2 lines in visual acuity
- Persistent inflammation for more than one month
- Congenital toxoplasma retinochoroiditis in the first year of life
- A newborn diagnosed with congenital toxoplasmosis regardless of the presence of ocular lesions
- Any lesion in an immunocompromised host.

However, some authorities believe that all the active lesions should be treated. One of their reasons is that active lesions even far from macula may be associated with loss of visual acuity due to macular edema, intense vitritis, macular tractions or retinal detachment. Furthermore, the tachyzoites in the active lesions may spread to the other sites of retina and encyst. Some believe that treatment of any active lesion theoretically may be associated with decreased number of tachyzoites and decrease the risk of reactivated disease. A recent evidence-based literature review concludes there is inadequate evidence to support the routine use of antibiotics in the treatment of acute toxoplasmic retinochoroiditis. Even though the active lesion may be self-limited; treatment with antibiotic agents and steroids has been well established in clinical practice. Considering the long-term consequences of irreversible visual loss and suggestive evidence that treatment can reduce the size of retinal scars, it would seem reasonable to treat active ocular toxoplasmosis when side effects of treatment are limited.

The goal of treatment is to arrest the multiplication of the parasite during the period of active retinochoroiditis to prevent irreversible damage to the retina and optic nerve. Response to treatment was identified as sharpening of the lesion border with or without hyperpigmentation and resolution of vitreous inflammation. There are many treatment options to arrest the parasite but none of them do eliminate the parasite. The most common treatment is classic therapy consisted of pyrimethamine and sulfadiazine plus corticosteroids. Classic treatment consisted of an initial dose of 75 to 100 mg of pyrimethamine daily for two days followed by 25 to 50 mg dose daily, 2 to 4 g of sulfadiazine daily for two days followed by 500 mg to 1 g dose every six hours and 5 mg of folinic acid daily, for 4 to 6 weeks and oral prednisolone 1 mg/kg daily starting from the third day and tapered over 2 to 6 weeks. The other alternative treatment is trimethoprim (80 mg)/sulfamethoxazole (400 mg) every 12 hours plus steroid (1mg/kg started after 3 days) that works like classic therapy and has shown similar efficacy in a randomized clinical trial. Other available treatments include quadruple drug therapy (classic treatment plus clindamycin), clindamycin, spiramycin, minocyline, azythromycin, atovaquone (hyroxynaphthoquinone), clarithromycin and intravitreal injection of clindamycin and dexamethsone. Laser photocoagulation and pars plana vitrectomy may also be considered as other treatment options.

In immunocompromised patients, the treatment regimen is partially modified. It should be emphasized that any active retinal lesion in these patients demands treatment because the risk of dissemination of the infection and related complications is high. Since there is no remarkable inflammation in the immunocompromised patients, corticosteroids are not included in the treatment regimen. Pyrimathamine has an antagonistic activity against ziduvudine that is an antiretroviral agent used in the treatment of AIDS. For this reason and because of the risk of drug-induced bone marrow suppression, it sometimes may be avoided or used in lower dosage in the treatment regimen of the AIDS patients who receive highly active antiretroviral therapy (HAART). Lifetime maintenance therapy including either lower dosage of pyrimethamine combined with sulfadiazine/clindamycin, or trimethoprim/sulfamethoxazole is crucial to prevent relapse and dissemination of the infection.

In pregnant patients, spiramycin is the drug of choice with no reported teratogenic effects. It achieves a high concentration in the placenta and may reduce the incidence of congenital transmission. Combined intravitreal injection of clindamycin and dexamethasone with systemic sulfadiazine has been reported as a successful management of ocular toxoplasmosis in pregnancy.

In newborns and infants with congenital ocular toxoplasmosis confirmed by PCR of amniotic fluid, there has been a concept that these patients should have been received treatment during fetal life as well as during the first year of life. The recommended regimen includes a combination of pyrimethamine, sulfadiazine and folinic acid.

Prevention

Prevention of the initial infection is the most effective way for reducing toxoplasma-related morbidity. The strategy of prevention is based on the understanding the *Toxoplasma gondii* life cycle and involves avoiding ingestion of live tissue cysts or oocysts. Therefore, raw meat, raw eggs and unpasteurized milk should not be consumed. Cooking meat at the temperature over 66°C and washing fruits and vegetables before ingestion is important for prevention of parasite. Freezing meet below –20°C for 24 hours will destroy tissue cysts of the parasite. Hand washing should be performed after touching uncooked meat and after contact with cats or soil that could be contaminated with cat feces. Contaminated water may be a source of infection in some patients. Daily cleaning of cat litter box should be performed by non-pregnant person. Blood transfusions and organ transplants from sero-positive donors should be avoided if the recipient is sero-negative. Prevention of disease transmission is also crucial for immunocompromised individuals and sero-negative pregnant women.

The goal of prevention is to achieve an effective vaccine against the parasite. Vaccines derived from the major surface antigen (p30) of *Toxoplasma gondii* result in partial protection in laboratory animals. Cats' vaccination may interrupt the parasite life cycle.

Complication

The course of the ocular toxoplasmosis may be complicated by development of glaucoma. On review of literature, glaucoma has been reported as the most common complication of ocular toxoplasmosis. Most of the cases are of open angle type due to obstruction of trabecular meshwork by inflammatory cells; angle closure glaucoma may rarely occurs due to peripheral anterior synechiae formation.

Decreased vision and visual field defects secondary to retinal necrosis and involvement of optic nerve and macula, cataract and other rare vitreoretinal problems may also occur.

Sub-retinal neovascularization, vascular occlusion and neovascularization, vitreous hemorrhage, tractional and rhegmatogenous retinal detachment have been reported as rare complications of ocular toxoplasmosis. Phthisis bulbi may eventually occur in ocular toxoplasmosis.

Prognosis

Prognosis of ocular toxoplasmosis usually depends on location and size of retinochoroiditis lesion. In the lesions far from optic nerve and macula, the prognosis is usually favorable. However, large lesions close to macula with frequent relapse have the worst prognosis. Sometimes peripheral lesions also may produce epiretinal membrane formation, vitreous haze, macular edema and even retinal detachment. Early diagnosis and therapy may diminish such unfavorable complications.

Conclusion

Toxoplasmosis is the most common cause of infectious posterior uveitis in many countries. The responsible organism *T. gondii* is a neurotrophic organism and has a tendency for the retinal and CNS tissues. This disorder is a recurrent and destructive ocular and systemic disease that may have fatal consequences particularly in immunocompromised patients. Classic ocular disease usually is unilateral with focal retinitis with or without associated uveitis. The diagnosis of ocular toxoplasmosis is clinical and is based on observation of typical foci of retinitis.

A positive toxoplasmosis titer at any dilution is further additional supportive for the diagnosis. In immunocompromised patients the diagnosis of toxoplasmosis may be confused with CMV retinitis. Preventive strategies are important especially for sero-negative pregnant women and immunocompromised patients. If chronic infection has been established tissue cysts usually lay in a dormant state, however, these cysts may become reactivated by various mechanisms such as physiologic stress, pregnancy, life threatening illness, major surgery and even emotional strain.

There is no effective treatment to eradicate the organism, although active lesion may be self limited. The decision to treat toxoplasma retinitis depends on the location and activity of lesion. Several therapeutic regimens are available and most are suited to the majority of patients. A most recent published study has shown trimethoprim/sulfamethoxazol as an alternative to classic treatment with pyrimethamine and sulfadiazine in treatment of ocular toxoplasmosis with fewer side effects. Trimethoprim/ sulfamethoxazol have been used for prophylaxis of toxoplasmosis encephalitis in AIDS patients and has shown efficacy in preventing recurrence of ocular toxoplasmosis retinochoroiditis.

Acknowledgments: The authors thank L Azadvari for her assistance with preparation of this text.

Chapter 53

Pediatric and Adolescent Refractive Surgery

Belquiz A Nassaralla
João J Nassaralla Jr (Brazil)

Introduction

Although many ophthalmologists viewed the field of refractive surgery with skepticism only a few decades ago, refractive surgery is now highly accepted and much practiced. Excimer laser refractive surgery has been successfully used for treatment of myopia, hyperopia, and astigmatism in adults. As advances in excimer laser surgery occur, new indications for refractive surgery are expected, including its use in children. One indication currently investigated is its use in treating children and adolescents with anisometropia.

Clinical Signs and Symptoms

Anisometropia occurs because of uncorrected unequal refractive error between fellow eyes. Uncorrected anisometropia produces image blur in one eye (form vision deprivation) and/or abnormal binocular interaction by producing dissimilar images on the fovea of each eye. High degrees of anisometropia cause disparity in image size between the two eyes (aneisokonia). The brain cannot be able to reconcile the difference in images coming from the two eyes. It develops a preference for the image coming from one eye and suppresses the image from the other eye and, in time, the brain loses the ability to "see" the image from that eye (amblyopia).

Anisometropic amblyopia is often detected later than other forms of amblyopia because vision is generally good in the fellow eye, the eyes are typically orthotropic, and the child functions well with the use of the sound eye. The level of anisometropia required to cause amblyopia has been well-studied. In general, anisomyopia of more than 2 diopters, anisohyperopia of more than 1 diopter, and anisoastigmatism of more than 1.5 diopters may result in amblyopia.

Conventional Treatment for Anisometropia

Refractive correction of anisometropia often leads to aniseikonia, with each diopter of spectacle refractive correction changing the image size by approximately 2%. The actual difference between the image sizes in the 2 eyes depends upon whether the refractive error is axial or refractive, however, and the amount of aniseikonia is difficult to determine without special subjective tests. Aniseikonia may be symptomatic simply from the difference in retinal image sizes —or, more commonly, the anisometropic spectacle correction causes anisophoria or anisotropia in different directions of gaze because of the different prismatic effect induced by the 2 lenses. Thus, glasses for moderate-to-severe anisometropia are commonly not well-tolerated.

Contact lens is an alternative treatment for anisometropia. It essentially eliminates the issue of aniseikonia for most patients, provide better quality of vision and larger visual field with improved contrast sensitivity. Unfortunately,

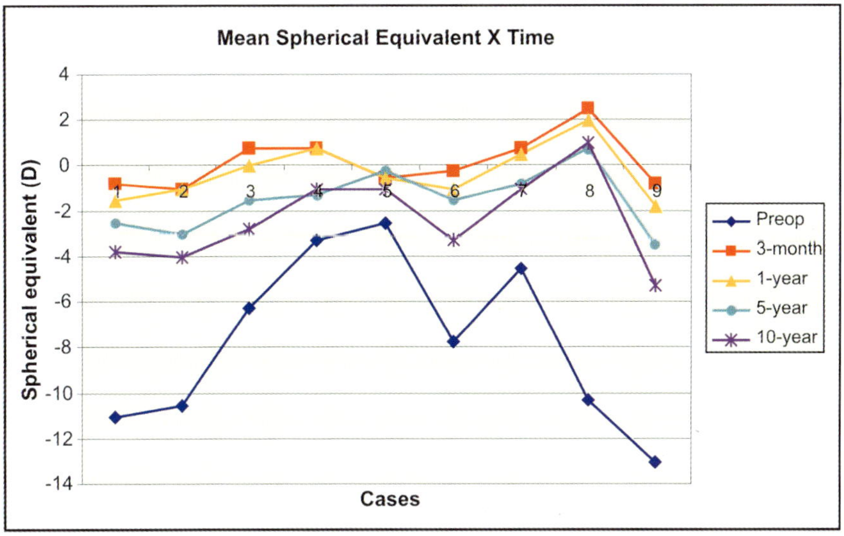

Figure 1: Mean spherical equivalent refraction overtime

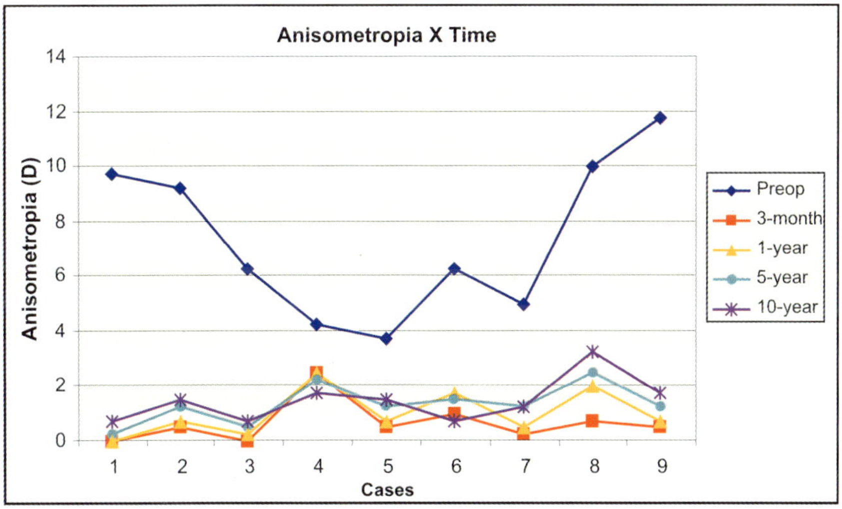

Figure 2: Mean anisometropia overtime

because of the young age and co-existing ocular or medical problems, compliance with contact lens use during all waking hours is not always optimal or possible. Besides, contact lenses are often difficult for parents to insert and remove, loss is frequent, the costs are relatively high and there is a higher risk of microbial keratitis.

However, there has been no effective alternative to treat high anisometropia in children and adolescents who refuse conventional therapies or in whom these methods have failed. In these cases, refractive surgery may provide a better option that should not be discarded.

Investigations

Excimer Laser Refractive Surgery

The 193-nm argon-fluoride excimer laser decreses refractive error by ablating the anterior corneal stroma to create a new radius of curvature. Three major refractive surgical techniques use excimer laser ablation. In photorefractive keratectomy (PRK), the epithelium is debrided with a variety of techniques, including metal blades, brushes, and laser. In laser subepithelial keratomileusis (LASEK) and epi-LASIK, the epithelium may be preserved as an epithelial flap or excised with an epithelial microkeratome. All these forms are considered surface ablation. In laser *in situ* keratomileusis (LASIK), the excimer laser ablation is performed under a lamellar flap formed with a microkeratome or scanning pulsed laser.

PRK, underwent extensive preclinical investigation before it was applied to sighted human eyes. Results of early animal studies provided evidence for relatively normal wound healing in laser-ablated corneas. The popularity of PRK faded rapidly when LASIK began to be performed in the late 1990s because of LASIK's faster visual recovery, decreased postoperative discomfort, better stability and lack of corneal haze. In the case of reoperation, when there is enough residual stromal bed, it is easy to lift the LASIK flap and perform another ablation.

Although more LASIK than surface ablation procedures continue to be performed, surface ablation is an attractive alternative in specific indications, such as irregular corneas, epithelial basement membrane disease, and thin corneas, and for treatment of some LASIK flap complications, such as incomplete or buttonhole flaps. Surface ablation eliminates the potential for stromal flap-related complications. With the advent of new epithelial removal techniques and wavefront-guided laser ablations, the popularity of surface ablation has been increasing. However, haze continues to be the most challenging complication after PRK. Persistent severe haze is usually associated with greater amounts of correction or smaller ablation diameters. Specially in children and adolescents, there is an increased risk of haze related to the more vigorous wound-healing response that occurs in this age group.

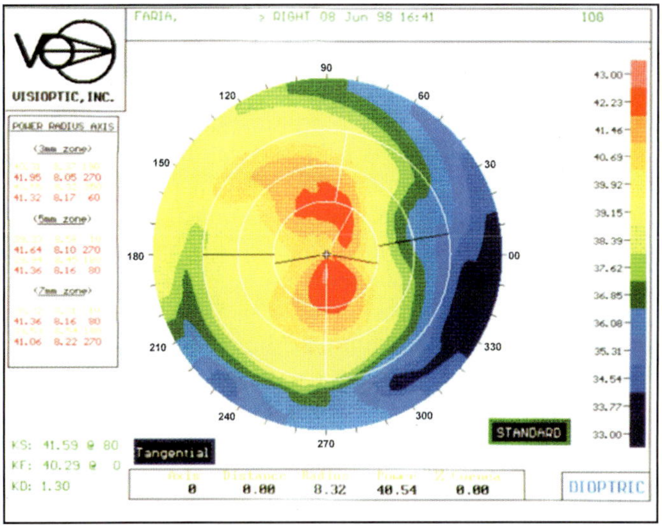

Figure 3: Preoperative topography of the right eye of patient 6. Before surgery, spherical equivalent refraction was –7.75 D

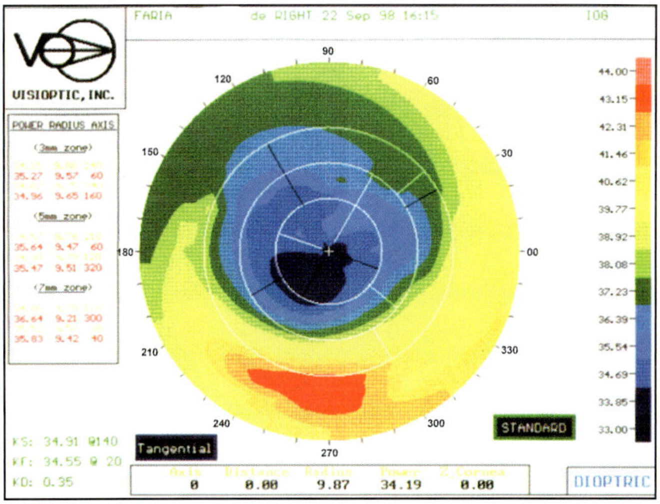

Figure 4: Corneal topography of the right eye of patient 6, 3 months after LASIK. Spherical equivalent refraction was –0.25 D

Refractive Surgery in Children

While the surgical treatment of adult ametropias has gained increasing acceptance in the ophthalmic community, experience with the surgical correction of pediatric and adolescent ametropias is limited.

Refractive surgery in children is controversial; the major areas of concern are unstable refraction due to ongoing growth of the eye, poor cooperation and long-term implications. Besides, there are technical difficulties involved in performing these procedures because of smaller palpebral apertures and the need for general anesthesia in younger children.

Although, recent reports suggest that PRK is relatively safe and effective in reducing high refractive error in children, the main concern with PRK in the pediatric population is the risk of haze, due to the reactive nature of children's corneas.

Our Personal Experience

We have reported our experience with LASIK to correct high myopia or high myopic astigmatism in eyes with high anisometropia in whom conventional treatments have failed. The report is based on the study of a series of LASIK procedures performed at the Goiania Eye Institute, Goiania, GO, Brazil, between, 1996 and 1997 by a single surgeon (BAN).

This study was composed of nine eyes of nine patients, three boys and six girls, with a mean age of 11.5 years (range, 8 to 15 year). In each patient, the eye with the higher refractive error was treated with LASIK using the Technolas 217 excimer laser (Bausch and Lomb Surgical, Claremont, CA). Minimum follow-up was 10 years.

To be eligible for the study, patients should be able to cooperate for surgery under topical anesthesia and have had high anisometropia (>3.5 diopters [D]) secondary to high myopia or myopic astigmatism. The fellow untreated eye in all patients had uncorrected visual acuity (UCVA) of 20/40 or better and best spectacle-corrected visual acuity (BSCVA) of 20/20. Poor compliance to spectacles and unstable contact lens fitting were, in all cases, the conditions that made surgery the only possible option. Preoperative diagnoses for anisometropia were: congenital myopia or myopic astigmatism (66.6%), cataract surgery after trauma (22.2%) and corneal transplantation for corneal scar (11.1%). Time of LASIK after PKP was 24 months and after cataract surgery was 16 months in one eye and 13 months in the other. Table 1 shows the preoperative data.

Mean preoperative spherical equivalent refraction with cycloplegia was –7.63D (range –2.50 to –13.00D). All patients had a preoperative UCVA lower than 20/300 and a BSCVA of at least 20/150 (range 20/150 to 20/30). Target refraction was emetropia in all patients.

The automated corneal shaper (ACS, Bausch and Lomb Surgical, Claremont, USA) was used to create a corneal flap of approximately 8.5 mm diameter and 160 μm thickness. The LASIK procedure was performed using our standard technique for all cases.

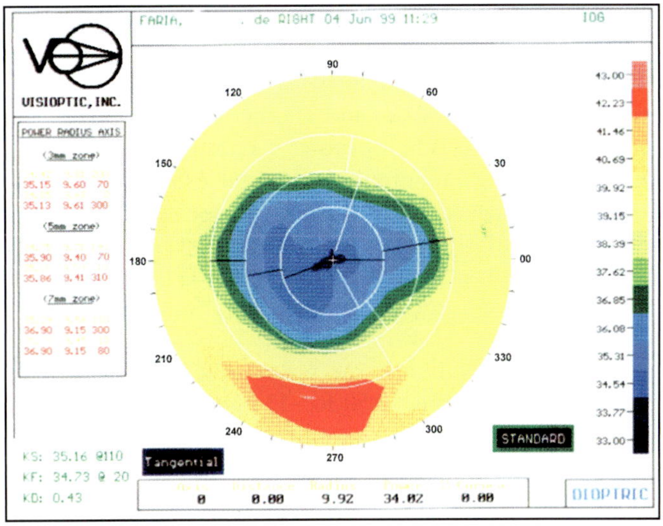

Figure 5: Corneal topography of the right eye of patient 6, 1 year after LASIK. Spherical equivalent refraction was –1.00 D

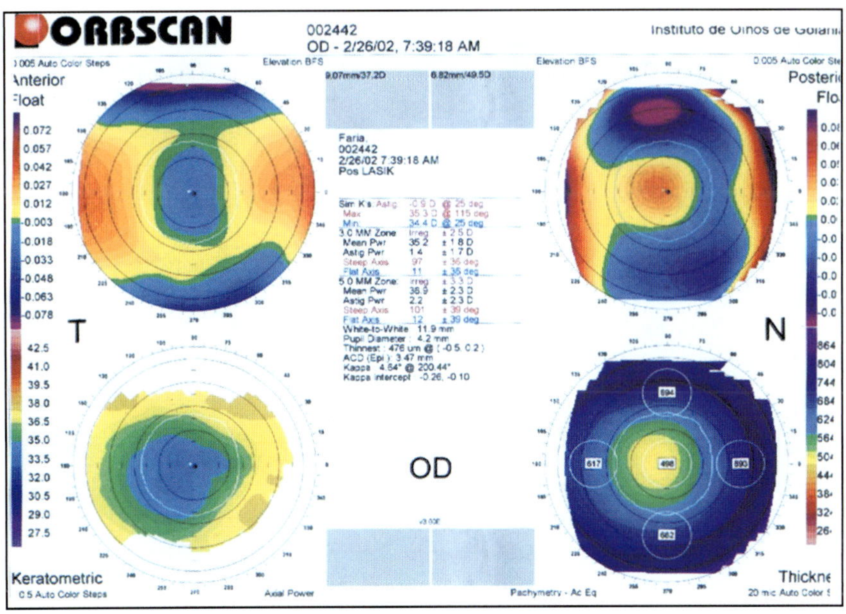

Figure 6: ORBSCAN of the right eye of patient 6, 5 years after LASIK. Spherical equivalent refraction was –1.50 D

Postoperatively, the patients were examined everyday until the corneal epithelium healed. They were then examined 1 month after the procedure and every 3 months for 12 months, and again once a year for at least 10 years. Two patients were followed for 12 years and another for 11 years.

No eyes experienced intraoperative complications. Postoperative complications were epithelial ingrowth in patient 7 (11.1%), which was limited to within 1.0 mm of flap edge and did not require treatment, and Bowman's layer wrinkles in patient 9 (11.1%), that disappeared completely by 1 month after surgery. Ten years after LASIK, all corneas remained clear with no displacement of the flap and the cut on the cornea was barely detectable on slit lamp microscopy.

Three months postoperatively, the mean spherical equivalent refraction decreased from –7.66 D (range, –2.50 to –13.00 D) to 0.16 D (range, +2.50 to –1.00 D), and the mean preoperative astigmatism decreased from –3.11 D (range, 0 to –6.00 D) to –0.69 D (range, 0 to –1.50 D). Three eyes (33.3%) were within ± 0.50 D of the desired outcome and eight eyes (88.8%) were within ± 1.00 D. Table 2 shows the 3-month and 1-year postoperative data.

Ten years after surgery, mean spherical equivalent refraction was –2.33 D (range, +1.00 to –5.25 D). Figure 1 shows the mean spherical equivalent refraction overtime.

The mean preoperative anisometropia decreased from 7.36 D (range, 3.75 to 11.75 D) to 1.47 D (range, 0.75 to 3.25 D). Figure 2 shows the mean anisometropia overtime.

Comparing the 3-month with the 10-year results, a slight-to-moderate regression of effect in spherical equivalent refraction was noted in all patients. Mean regression of effect was –2.1 D (range, –0.50 to –3.50D).

Corneal topography revealed no decentered ablation. In all eyes, there was a decrease in central corneal power that correlated closely with the change in manifest refraction. Figures 3 to 7 show the corneal topographic change overtime in patient 6.

Ten years after surgery, best spectacle-corrected visual acuity (BSCVA) did not change in four eyes (44.4%) and improved in five eyes (55.5%) by at least one Snellen line. Four eyes (44.4%) were 20/40 or better with spectacles. No patient had decreased best spectacle-corrected visual acuity. This increase in vision was attributed to an increase in magnification and a decrease in optical aberrations, since all patients were beyond the sensitive period of visual development. Table 3 shows the 5-year and 10-year postoperative data.

In this study we included an evaluation of endothelial cell count overtime. The percentage of cell loss after surgery was 3.6% at 1 year, and 3.8% at 10 years, both in respect to the preoperative count.

Discussion

It has become increasingly evident that children with severe visual impairments that cannot be treated otherwise, such as high anisometropia, both amblyopic

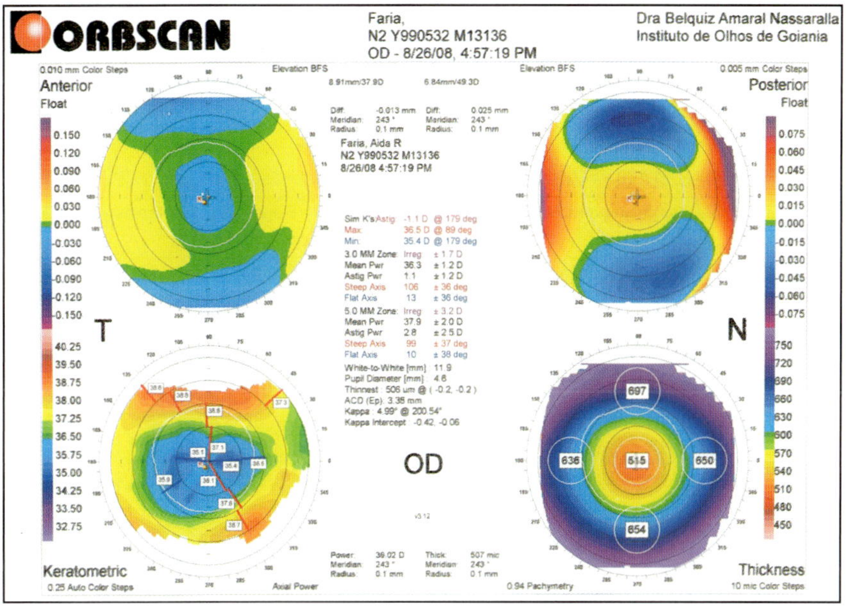

Figure 7: ORBSCAN topography of the right eye of patient 6, 10 years after LASIK. Spherical equivalent refraction was –3.25 D

Table 1: Preoperative data

Case/ Sex/Age	Remarks	Manifest refraction (D)	Spherical equivalent (D)	Uncorrected visual acuity	Best spectacle corrected visual acuity	Fellow eye spherical equivalent refraction (D)
1/F/8	Ambl/Anis	–10.00 –2.00 x 100	–11.00	20/800	20/80	–1.25
2/F/9	Ambl/Anis	–8.00 –5.00 × 15	–10.50	20/800	20/150	–1.25
3/F/9	Ambl/Anis	–6.00 –0.50 × 110	–6.25	20/400	20/60	plano
4/M/10	Post IOL	–0.50 –5.50 × 160	–3.25	20/400	20/40	+1.00
5/M/12	Post IOL	pl – 5.00 × 175	–2.50	20/400	20/30	+1.25
6/F/12	Ambl/Anis	–6.75 –2.00 × 180	–7.75	20/800	20/40	–1.50
7/M/14	Post PKP	–1.50 –6.00 × 150	–4.50	20/300	20/50	+0.50
8/F/15	Ambl/Anis	–10.25	–10.25	20/800	20/60	–0.25
9/F/15	Ambl/Anis	–12.00 –2.00 × 180	–13.00	20/1200	20/150	–1.25

Ambl//Anis = amblyopia/anisometropia; IOL = Intraocular lens; PKP = Penetrating keratoplasty; D = diopter.

Table 2: Postoperative data

	3-month follow-up			1-year follow-up		
Case	UCVA	BSCVA	SE (D)	UCVA	BSCVA	SE(D)
1	20/80	20/60	–0.75	20/100	20/60	–1.50
2	20/150	20/150	–1.00	20/150	20/150	–1.00
3	20/40	20/40	+0.75	20/40	20/40	plano
4	20/30	20/30	+0.75	20/30	20/30	+0,75
5	20/30	20/25	–0.50	20/30	20/25	–0.50
6	20/50	20/40	–0.25	20/60	20/40	–1.00
7	20/50	20/50	+0.75	20/50	20/50	+0.50
8	20/70	20/50	+2.50	20/70	20/50	+2.00
9	20/150	20/150	–0.75	20/150	20/150	–1.75

SE= spherical equivalent; UCVA= uncorrected visual acuity; BSCVA= best spectacle corrected visual acuity; Ambl//Anis= amblyopia/anisometropia; D = diopter.

Table 3: Postoperative data

	5-year follow-up				10-year follow-up			
Case	UCVA	BSCVA	SE (D)	Fellow eye SE (D)	UCVA	BSCVA	SE (D)	Fellow eye SE (D)
1	20/200	20/60	–2.50	–2.25	20/400	20/60	–3.75	–3.00
2	20/200	20/150	–3.00	–1.75	20/300	20/150	–4.00	–2.50
3	20/150	20/40	–1.50	–1.00	20/200	20/40	–2.75	–2.00
4	20/100	20/30	–1.25	+1.00	20/100	20/30	–1.00	+0.75
5	20/30	20/25	–0.25	+1.00	20/150	20/25	–1.00	+0.50
6	20/100	20/40	–1.50	–3.00	20/200	20/40	–3.25	–4.00
7	20/80	20/50	–0.75	+0.50	20/80	20/50	–1.00	+0.25
8	20/60	20/50	+0.75	–1.75	20/60	20/50	+1.00	–2.25
9	20/300	20/150	–3.50	–2.25	20/800	20/150	–5.25	–3.50

SE = Spherical equivalent; UCVA= Uncorrected visual acuity;
BSCVA = Best spectacle corrected visual acuity; Ambl//Anis = amblyopia/anisometropia; D = diopter

or not, have the potential for useful vision. We should initially consider clinical visual rehabilitation. If the patient is unable to wear spectacles or contact lenses, surgical treatment should be considered.

The cornea reaches adult size by about 2 years of age. Myopia often develops between 6 to 9 years of age and increases throughout adolescence, with the greatest change at the time of puberty. Because myopia is not stable in children, refractive surgery is usually deferred until refraction is reasonably stable, which is assumed to occur in early adulthood. However, in older children, especially in those that are unilaterally highly myopic, LASIK can be an acceptable alternative to reduce high anisometropia.

The primary goal of LASIK in older children and adolescent is resolution of sufficient myopia and astigmatism to allow spectacle correction of the residual refractive error and return to binocularity. In our series, all nine patients were able to function binocularly with spectacles.

An accurate assessment of the patient's true refraction is important. Especially in children, it is not an easy job, particularly if the patient has had a corneal transplant. In such cases, true refraction depends on the donor cornea returning to its normal shape after suture removal. In patient 7, LASIK was performed 2 years after penetrating keratoplasty for corneal scar and 6 months after suture removal. According to our data from another study of LASIK after penetrating keratoplasty, we agree with other authors in recommending this prolonged period to allow the corneal wound to stabilize. Other authors have suggested that after corneal transplantation, the LASIK flap be cut first and then laid back down to allow the eye to settle and the residual refractive error and astigmatism to adjust. Once the eye is stable, after several days to a week, the refractive error is reassessed and then the corrective LASIK ablation is performed. Although this technique may improve results, it also requires two procedures, each with potential complications, including graft rejection and wound dehiscence. If the correction is performed with the first keratectomy, the patient has the chance of needing only one procedure—important for young patients.

Although we were able to perform this series of procedures with oral sedation and topical anesthesia, surgeons should consider using general anesthesia in a patient who is not expected to cooperate.

Endothelial alterations after LASIK have been studied. Pallikaris and Siganos believe that endothelial loss of up to 4.11%, related to the quantity of the desired correction, was probably caused by the shock waves produced by the excimer laser photoablation and corneal manipulation during keratomileusis. Other studies, however, have demonstrated no significant endothelial alterations following LASIK after penetrating keratoplasty. The 10-year postoperative endothelial cell loss of 3.8% should probably be regarded with caution as an acceptable percentage.

Another major concern in performing LASIK in eyes with prior corneal surgery is the risk of damage to the wound. Wound dehiscence after penetrating keratoplasty or cataract extraction is a well-described phenomenon and can occur years after surgery. In LASIK, intraocular pressure (IOP) is elevated to more than 65 mmHg and there is a risk of wound dehiscence with the possibility of extrusion of the intraocular contents. During surgery, we tried to minimize the suction time. In our series, elevation of IOP during LASIK did not affect the wound either in cases of corneal transplantation or cataract extraction.

No complication was noted during follow-up. It may seem likely that traumatic displacement of the flap would be more common, simply because of less careful behavior of children and adolescents, but we did not see any trend toward postoperative flap displacement for any reason. Haze was not observed in any patient.

Successful reduction of myopia and myopic astigmatism was independent of preoperative refractive error. A slight-to-moderate regression of effect in spherical equivalent refraction was noticed in all patients and was probably related to the natural change in refraction with maturation.

It was our goal to equalize the refractive errors, decrease the anisometropia and improve binocularity. The small amount of regression did not affect our goal, since all patients were able to wear spectacles.

It is difficult to compare this heterogeneous young population to other populations reported in the literature. The ten-year data resulted from this series of young patients are encouraging and support previous reports.

More studies on the growing eye and the effect of excimer laser on the pediatric corneal endothelium are needed before the effect of refractive surgery in the pediatric age group can be fully understood. We are enlarging this study to include more patients and a longer clinical follow-up.

Chapter 54

Refractive Surgery in Children: When and How?

Antonio Marinho (Portugal)

Introduction

Refractive Surgery is defined as a permanent change in the refractive status of the eye by means of surgical intervention. The normal human eye has two main refractive structures: The cornea and the lens. The cornea is responsible for 2/3 of the refractive power of the eye and the lens for 1/3. Changing the refractive power of the cornea by mechanical or incisional means has been the goal of the pioneers of refractive surgery (keratomileusis, radial and arcuate keratotomies, etc.). Today we still change the refractive power of the cornea, but using the excimer laser as in PRK, LASEK or LASIK. Changing the power of the natural lens is not possible, but it is today very safe to extract the lens and to replace it by an IOL of desired power. This is the basis of our routine refractive lens exchange or refractive cataract surgery. But there is still another option to modify surgically the refractive status of the eye: To introduce a new refractive structure in the eye, not disturbing the cornea or the lens. This is the concept of a phakic IOL (PIOL).

According to the above mentioned definition of refractive surgery and regardless the used technique, the modification of the refractive status of the eye must be permanent. As we know refraction is not strictly stable, although in most cases a high degree of stability is maintained between the second and the fourth decades of life. This is why most textbooks point to a minimum age of 18 and a stable refraction for at least 18 months, as conditions required to perform refractive surgery.

The immediate conclusion of this introduction is that refractive surgery is not a routine practice for people younger than 18. However, as we will see in this chapter there are particular situations in young age, where refractive surgery is indicated.

Refractive Surgery in Children: When?

Anisometropia

Anisometropia is a situation, where there is a difference in refraction between the 2 eyes. Slight anisometropia is common and is only considered significant if the difference is at least 3 diopters. Important anisometropia causes a difference in the size of the retinal images called aniseikonia. This aniseikonia turns fusion impossible leading to suppression of the poorer image, ultimately leading to amblyopia.

As it is well-known amblyopia is difficult to reverse, and when possible it is only during childhood. So, to avoid the development of amblyopia, or at least minimize its extent, we must be very careful with anisometropia in children.

Slight anisometropia can be easily controlled with glasses, but the aiseikonia induced by important anisometropias precludes the use of glasses. Contact lenses are often a solution, but many young children refuse them. These cases are the indications of refractive surgery in anisometric children.

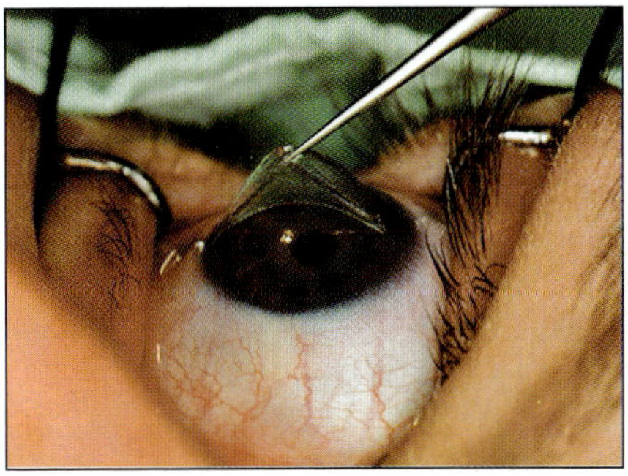

Figure 1: Lasik (the most common refractive surgery in children)

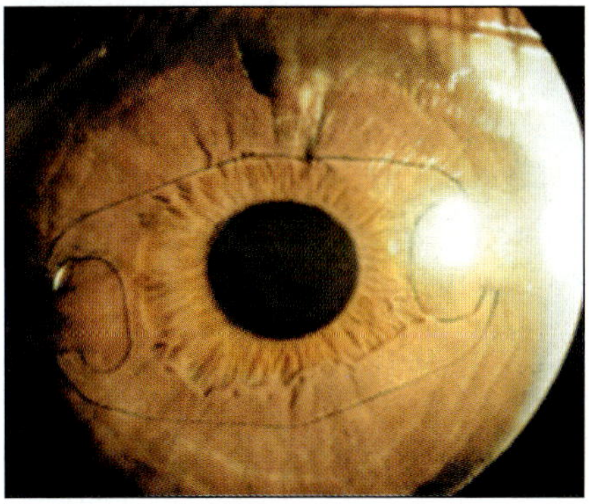

Figure 2: Artisan (mod 206)

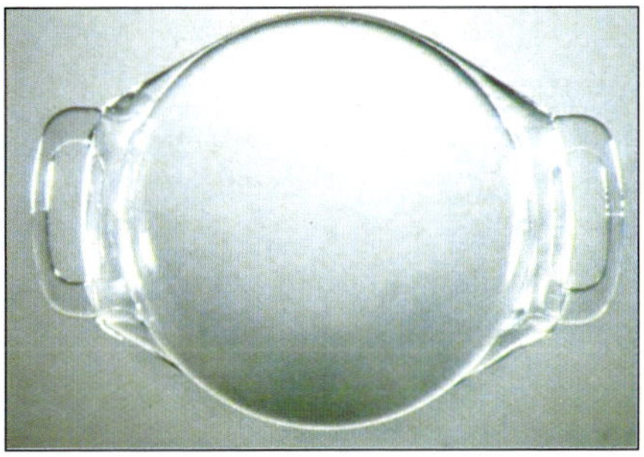

Figure 3: Artiflex (the new iris supported foldable IOL, particularly fitted for children)

In summary, refractive surgery is indicated in anisometric children, if:

1. Anisometropia is greater than 5 diopters (myopia or astigmatism) or 3 diopters (hyperopia)
2. Contact lens is not perfectly tolerated

Of course in these eyes the goal is not a "permanent" correction of the refractive error, but to reduce or eliminate the aniseikonia, enabling the child to use both eyes simultaneously. Future developments of the refractive error will be dealt in adulthood.

Accommodative Esotropia

In this situation, we have a hyperopic child that develops esotropia between 3 and 4 years of age. The correction of the hyperopia (often greater than 3 diopters) achieves ortophoria. These children do not generally present amblyopia, but are only ortophoric with glasses, the esotropia reappearing immediately once they take off their glasses. It has been suggested that in these cases, surgical correction of the hyperopia during the adolescence will solve the problem.

As we conclude from the previous paragraphs, the 2 indications for refractive surgery in children are:

- Anisometropia
- Accommodative esotropia

Refractive Surgery in Children: How?

Corneal Refractive Surgery

Literature Review

There are several published papers dealing with PRK, LASEK and LASIK to correct myopic or hyperopic anisometropia in children. Most of these papers present very good refractive results in children despite the myopia being in some cases very high. (mean > –7.00). The corneal refractive surgery have been done with topical anesthesia in most cases, and after amblyopia treatment (occlusion) has been performed. The follow-up period is generally short, usually between 12 and 24 months. Although the refractive results reported are very good, the improvement in BSCVA is mild, specially in important amblyopias. Only 1 paper shows some kind of regression (mild) during the follow-up period.

When general anesthesia is used, there are reports of a decreased effect of the laser. This may be due to poor centration of the laser beam (no fixation available) or to changes in corneal hydration leading to poorer impact of the laser energy in the cornea. Another possible explanation for this fact, is that the anesthetic drugs (gases) interfere with the laser energy. Two papers report better results with general anesthesia, either by using only sedation instead of full anesthesia or inducing the anesthesia in a different room.

Concerning the use of LASIK for accommodative esotropia, the literature shows good refractive results and achievement of ortophoria in a great percentage of patients. There are no reports of regression with time even at a 7 year follow-up.

Comments and Personal Experience

Reviewing the literature on corneal refractive surgery in anisometropic children, we may assume that it is a very good solution to solve the problem. My personal experience is on the contrary, quite disappointing. Let us go on detail through that experience and then we will try to give some explanations, why in my opinion corneal refractive is seldom of use in these cases.

As it was stated before, the candidates for refractive surgery are children with myopic aisometropia of at least 5 diopters or hyperopic anisometropia of 3 diopters. As we also know the limits of LASIK in adults are –7.00 and +3.50, so the vast majority of the children needing surgery will fall out of the range. The minor anisometropias of 2 to 3 diopters are easily corrected with glasses and do not need surgery.

Another important issue (disregarded in most papers) is the anesthesia. To perform a LASIK under topic anesthesia in a young child seems difficult. I did my cases under general anesthesia leading to important undercorrections (laser energy ? centration ?). If we want to prevent amblyopia, we need to do the surgery as young as possible, so general anesthesia must be used. Topical can be used during adolescence, but in that age if amblyopia is present, the possibility of reversion is scarce.

Most of the papers show a short follow-up. Everyone who has operated adults with myopia above –7.00 has seen cases with important regression. Is regression not present in high myopic children ? Certainly it is.

My personal experience with LASIK in children was done from 1996 to 1999 in myopic anisometropic children (–7.00 to –16.00). No surgical complications were observed, but important undercorrection and regression overtime were present.

Since 1999, I have not performed LASIK in these cases, and I do not think it is the best option.

Concerning accommodative esotropia, I do not have personal experience, but as we all know hyperopic treatments tend to regress, mostly in young people, so it seems odd that in high hyperopes, no regression is observed with the consequent reappearance of some esotropia.

Phakic IOLs

Literature Review

There few reports of implantation of phakic IOLs in anisomtropic children. The IOL used was the ICL (collamer posterior chamber IOL, STAAR Switzerland) in 3 papers and the ARTISAN (iris-fixated anterior chamber IOL, OPHTEC. The Netherlands) in 2 papers. The refractive results reported are very good and stable. Despite the relatively short follow-up (6 to 48 months), here we are not concerned with regression, as no tissue healing process is important to the refractive result.

No complications are reported, except an important endothelial cell loss in 1 eye.

Comments and Personal Experience

My personal experience with phakic IOLs in children is small (6 eyes) but highly rewarding. I used the Artisan (model 206) in all cases. The Artisan is an iris fixated anterior chamber phakic Iol made of PMMA with an optic of 5.0 mm and an overall diameter of 8.5 mm. There are available powers from –23.00 to +12.00. To implant this IOL we need a large incision (5.2 mm). This incision turns the surgery difficult in young children, where because of high vitreous pressure, we are often confronted with shallow anterior chamber and difficulties in manipulating the IOL. This probably the cause for the case of important endothelial loss reported in the literature. In my experience, I was able to achieve the desired refractive result without complications and with improvement of BSCVA in all cases.

The ICL is a foldable posterior chamber phakic IOL, that has 2 advantages over Artisan. First, it only needs a small incision, permitting an easier surgery and second as it sits on the posterior chamber it is further away from the endothelium. However, its proximity to the natural lens may lead to cataracts. We must remember that the natural lens will grow with age eventually reducing its distance to the ICL and cause cataract. The safest Phakic IOL for this case is now the Artiflex. This IOl is similar to the Artisan, but made of polisyloxane (silicone) enabling it to need only a 3 mm incision, turning the surgery easier and safer.

Although, I do not have personal experience of correcting accommodative esotropia with phakic IOLs, it seems to me, that phakic Iols may be ideal for the purpose, because they ensure the full correction of the hyperopia without regression. The only problem in some cases may be the shallow anterior chamber (<2.8 mm) common to hyperopes, that does not allow the implantation of phakic IOLs. In these cases is better not to do surgery.

Conclusion

Refractive surgery is not a routine practice for people younger than 18 years of age. It should be reserved for important anisometropia, that cannot be solved by classical optical means (glasses or contact lenses).

Corneal refractive surgery (mostly LASIK) and implantation of phakic IOLs (ICL and Artisan) have been used in quite small numbers. According to the fact that we are usually dealing with high ametropias and also data from our personal experience, it seems to us that phakic IOLs are more promising, because of higher predictability and stability than corneal refractive surgery.

Phakic IOLs (Artisan and mostly Artiflex) are for us the procedure of choice for treating myopic and hyperopic anisometropia in children, as well for correction of accommodative esotropia in adolescents and young adults.

However, we must not forget that implantation of phakic IOLs follows some important rules such as:

1. Healthy eye
2. Endothelial cell count > 2500 cells/mm
3. Anterior chamber depth > 2.8 mm (endothelium/natural lens)
4. Nonconvex iris (most important in Artisan/Artiflex)

These rules, that are very important in adults, are even more in children, as the time the implant will be inside the eye is longer.

In summary, refractive surgery in children must still go a long way before it becomes clinical routine, but the present possibilities done carefully and in selected patients can help many children in visual rehabilitation of eyes otherwise condemned to irreversible amblyopia.

Chapter 55

Implantation of Phakic Refractive Lenses (PRL) in Pediatric Myopic Eyes Associated with Scleral Reinforcement Surgery

Dimitrii Dementiev (Italy)

Introduction

High myopia in early childhood can impede development of normal binocular vision and cause irreversible amblyopia. Myopic anisometropia, a condition in which there is more than 2-2.50 diopters (D) of difference between the refractive power of two eyes induces anisoconia resulting in difference of retinal image size. Left untreated, the perfect fusion of the two images is impossible, causing loss of binocular vision and deep amblyopia. The amount of amblyopia is usually correlated with the amount of anisometropia. Several times strabismus easy occurs in these patients. It is well known that amblyopia cannot be treated in adult age. That is why the correct treatment of anisometropia in childhood is important for the prevention of amblyopia and strabismus. Current modalities to treat high ametropia in pediatrics are limited. At present, the refractive amblyopia in children is treated with spectacles or contact lenses associated with occlusive patching of the dominant eye. Various surgical treatments used successfully in adults as RK, LASIK or PRK have limited use in pediatric cases due to irreversibility of these refractive procedures, as well as the need for further refractive correction of progressive ametropia. However, significant impairment of life quality exists in this group of patients, as early intervention to prevent development of amblyopia is critical, especially in cases of unilateral myopia.

Phakic refractive lenses to treat ametropia have been in evolution since 1986. Current designs include anterior chamber lenses: iris-fixated, angle-supported and posterior chamber lenses. The benefit of phakic refractive lenses in pediatrics is reversibility of the procedure. The potential concerns include lack of long-term information on complications, especially on cataractogenesis, iridocyclitis, glaucoma and retinal detachment.

Refractive procedures used in pediatric patients have included RK, PRK, LASIK and ICL posterior chamber lens implantation.

The posterior chamber Phakic Refractive Lens (PRL™) has been used extensively in our practice in over 800 adult patients to treat high myopia and hyperopia. Results have included accuracy and stability of refraction, good vision quality and a low incidence of complications in these cases. The objective of this series was to evaluate the use of the PRL, following scleral reinforcement surgery to retard/prevent progression of axial myopia and to prevent/reversal of amblyopia in a small series of pediatric cases.

Patients and Methods

Patients

Implantation of the PRL was performed in 11 eyes of 11 pediatric patients. The mean age of the 7 females and 4 males was 9.5 years (range 7 to 12 years). The preoperative mean spherical equivalent was -10.6 diopters (D) ranging from –7.0 D to –17.5 D. The refractive goal was emmetropia. The mean follow-up was 22.2 months.

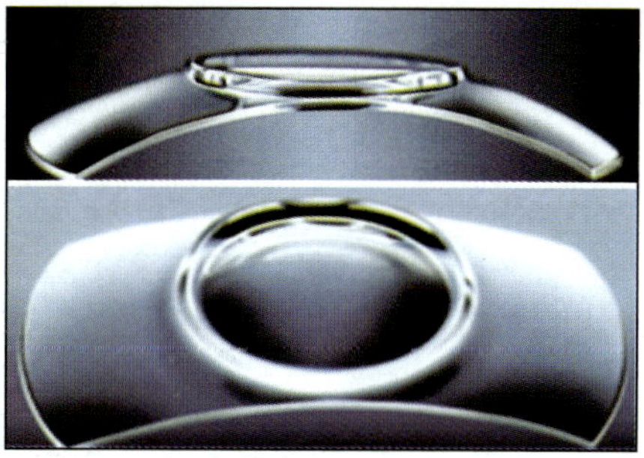

Figure 1: Myopic PRL IOLtech/Carl Zeiss meditec

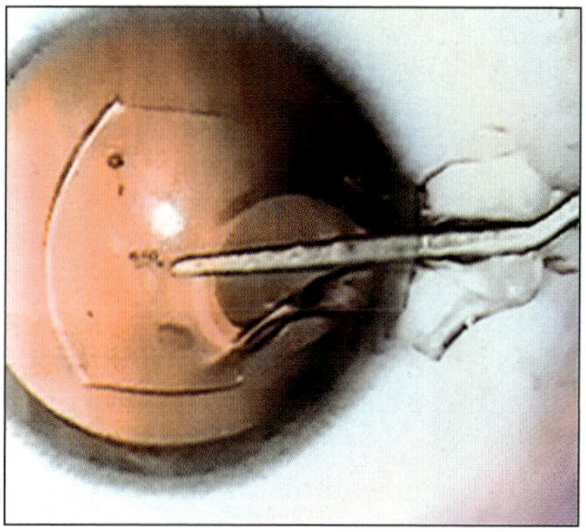

Figure 2: PRL insertion with the forceps

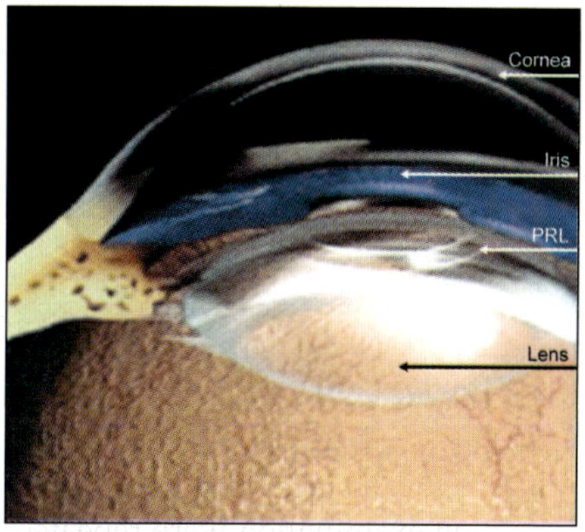

Figure 3: Implant is floating in the posterior chamber, no sulcus fixation

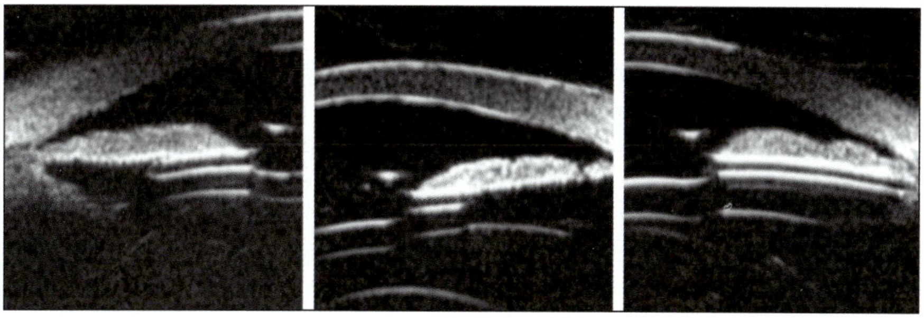

Figures 4 to 6: UBM picture, evidence of the free space between PRL and anterior capsula, Aqueous easy passes, no voulting is seen,-floating in the posterior chamber

Inclusion criteria were: All the patients had unilateral (anisometropic) axial myopia, amblyopia with the BCVA not less than 20/60 and not more than 20/40, strabismus was observed in 5 cases, progressive axial myopia were observed in all cases. Only the eyes with the clear media and no macular changes were chosen for this study. In all patients, all methods of amblyopia therapy had failed.

Unsuccessful occlusion therapy was observed partially due to high anisometropia and partially due to the psychological factors, 6 of the patients refused the occlusion and it was impossible to be sure that the eyes were patched in a right way. No prior procedures were performed to correct strabismus before the implantation of phakic implant.

Anterior chamber depth was 3.85 mm (+/- 0.42); in all the eyes the anterior chamber angle was seen open during the gonioscopy examination.

The exclusion criteria were: Shallow anterior chamber (less than 3.0 mm), chronic inflammation, significant amblyopia with low BCVA and no potential for visual improvement, maculopathy, and persistent eye hypertension-glaucoma.

Preoperative Evaluation

Preoperative evaluation included:
The best spectacle-corrected visual acuity (BSCVA) using Snellen chart, cycloplegic refraction, keratometry, tonometry (Tonopen), slit lamp examination, axial length and anterior chamber depth with A-scan method, gonioscopy, specular microscopy and fundus examination.

Six months after the first visit the AXL measurements and cycloplegic refraction examination were repeated to verify the progress of myopia.

The surgical procedure and its possible complications were explained to the parents, who signed the informed consent.

Surgical Procedure

The PRL *(IOLTECH /CARL ZEISS MEDITECH, FRANCE)* is a posterior chamber silicone lens for treatment of high myopia and hyperopia. The high refractive index (1.46) enables a slim optic profile and flexible design. The PRL diopteric power required for each case was determined using formulas developed that incorporate the patient's refraction and vertex distance. The length of the implant was 11.3 mm, the width was 6.0 mm, and the optic center diameters were different: from 4.5 mm to 5.0 mm according to the optic power of the implant. The lens is not fixed in the sulcus straightly, but "floats" in the posterior chamber touching the zonule with the distal and proximal edge. Being manufactured from the hydrophobic material the aqueous humor can move it easy towards the iris avoiding the contact with the anterior capsule of the crystalline lens. Space between PRL and lens is well seen during slit lamp examination and Ultrasonic Biomicroscopy (UBM). I believe that free aqueous circulation in the posterior chamber even in presence of the PRL permits to maintain the normal lens metabolism and not to create its opacification.

Prior to implantation of the PRL, all the patients underwent unilateral scleral reinforcing surgery (scleroplasty) in highly myopic eye to prevent or at least strongly retard progression of axial myopia.

All surgeries were performed under general anesthesia. No complications were noticed. In the period of 1-3 months after the scleroplasty all the patients underwent the next step of the treatment- PRL implantation for the correction of myopia.

Every patient started to install the antibiotics drops (Tobramicin) 3 days before the surgery; the pupil was dilated (min. 8.0 mm) with midriacyl and fenelefrin 20 minutes before the procedure.

The PRL implantation was also performed under general anesthesia.

The clear cornea 3.0 mm incision was performed with *PRL Dementiev trapezoid blade (Rumex International, USA)* temporally, Following injection of viscoelastic (Ophtaline® Ciba Vision), the paracentesis 1.0 mm large was done at 12.00 in order to have the second access in AC for implant manipulation and peripheral iridectomy performance. The PRL was inserted through a temporal 3.0 mm. clear corneal incision using *Dementiev PRL forceps (Janach, Italy)* specially designed to insert the implant. Haptics were positioned posteriorly to the iris with a *Dementiev PRL manipulator (Janach, Italy)* and the PRL was centered. After viscoelastic removal with irrigation only and pupil constriction *(Miochol®)*, a surgical iridectomy was performed through the previously created paracentesis at 12.00. No stitches were applied to the incision.

Tobradex **and** Pilocarpin **drops with the eye patching were the final steps of the surgery.**

The postoperative regimen included:

1. Eye patched for one night.
2. Diamox **250 mg two times a day for 2 days**
3. Tobradex **drops 5-6 times a day for 10-12 days**
4. Midriacyl **0.5 % drops 2 times a day for 3 days**
5. Voltaren **ofta drops 3 times a day for 7 days starting from the 10th day after procedure.**
6. Patch occlusion of the fellow eye for the amblyopia treatment was starting from the 3rd day after the surgery.

Follow-up examinations were scheduled at 1, 3, 7 and 14 days, and at 1, 2, 3, 6 and 12 months, and thereafter as needed. Postoperative evaluations included slit lamp biomicroscopy, ocular symptomatology, BCVA, cycloplegic refraction at 14 days, 6 month and 1 year visits, IOP, anterior chamber depth all the visits, specular microscopy 6 months and 1 year visits, keratometry and gonioscopy 1 month and 1 year visits. AXL measurement at 1-year visit. Binocular vision testing 3 months, 6 months and 1 year visits.

Postoperative outcomes at the most recent visit are provided in Table 2.

Results

No surgical complications of PRL surgery were experienced. Three eyes developed increased IOP at 3 days postoperatively. Antiglaucoma medications

Table 1: Preoperative parameters

Patient/ Sex (F/M)	Age (years)	Cycloplegic Spherical Equivalent (D)	BCVA [or BSCVA]	Endothelial Cell Count	IOP (mmHg)	A.C. depth (mm)
1/F	8	-11.0	20/50	3475	14	3.87
2/F	11	-10.0	20/50	3340	16	3.68
3/F	9	-7.0	20/40	3105	14	3.69
4/F	10	-14.50	20/60	2980	18	3.90
5/F	8	-9.0	20/40	3578	14	3.84
6/F	7	-17.50	20/60	3160	16	3.95
7/F	11	-10.0	20/50	3014	16	4.01
8/M	12	-9.0	20/40	3246	17	3.81
9/M	10	-8.75	20/50	3437	16	3.90
10/M	9	-13.00	20/50	3349	14	3.85
11/M	9	-7.50	20/40	3298	15	3.90

Table 2: Postoperative parameters

Patient/ Sex (F/M)	Age (years)	Cycloplegic Spherical Equivalent (D)	BCVA [or BSCVA]	Endothelial Cell Count	IOP (mmHg)	A.C. depth (mm)
1/F	8	-0.50	20/40	3365	14	3.67
2/F	11	-0.25	20/40	3150	17	3.57
3/F	9	0	20/20	2978	14	3.48
4/F	10	-1.0	20/40	2847	16	3.70
5/F	8	-0.50	20/20	3429	14	3.61
6/F	7	-1.0	20/50	3051	17	3.73
7/F	11	0	20/40	2989	16	3.89
8/M	12	+0.25	20/20	3104	15	3.65
9/M	10	0	20/20	3321	16	3.80
10/M	9	-1.0	20/40	3189	14	3.69
11/M	9	+0.50	20/40	3127	15	3.64

including Diamox, Trusopt, Timoptol 0.5% were administered, and IOP returned to preoperative status by the 2-4 day after the treatment began. The implants remained centered throughout the follow-up examination period, and anterior chamber depth was maintained.

All patients improved their best corrected visual acuity and uncorrected visual acuity. Eight patients experienced an improvement of at least 4 lines by 3 months postoperatively. Additionally, 6 patients with the preoperative BCVA more than 20/50 developed binocular vision three months postoperatively and after 3 months of occlusion therapy of fellow eye.

Two patients improved 2 lines after 3 month of occlusion therapy.

One patient improved only one line the first day after the surgery and it remained stable BCVA even after 3 month of occlusion therapy without further improvement.

Endothelial cell loss was not more than 4.0% in all the eyes, and no progress was noticed in the period from the 3rd month till the 6 month and 1.5 year visits.

Improvement of UCVA was in all the eyes from the first day after the surgery and was improving with the occlusion therapy till 6 months. At 1 year and 2 years control visit the same UCVA like 6 month control visit was noticed, except one eye of the youngest patient (age 9 YO during last visit) in which the UCVA is improving every visit. This patient is still under occlusion therapy daily 2 hours a day. Strabismus was improved in all 5 eyes of previously strabic patients. No any additional strabismus surgery was necessary. The progress of myopia was not noticed in all the period of follow-up, the measurement of AXL remained the same like after the scleroplasty procedure. Postoperatively, mean refraction was –0.5 D, and ranged from +0.5 to –1.0 D. Gonioscopy revealed open angles. No cataractogenesis was observed, and the status of the crystalline lens remained unchanged throughout the postoperative follow-up period.

Discussion

To date refractive surgery in children remains controversial. The treatment of high anisometropic myopia and the resulting amblyopia however often fails. Current methods used are correction with contact lenses or glasses associated with eye patching. Often the wearing of contact lenses is not well tolerated or the compliance is poor especially if the need for contact lens is for one eye only. Children who have myopic anisometropia and who refuse the conventional therapy are at risk of developing greater amblyopia when left without treatment. In these cases refractive surgery has been proposed. The procedures considered an option for refractive correction in adults in children might be the only way to treat amblyopia in children.

Radial keratotomy has been performed in some cases with poor results and many limits treating not more than 4-5 diopters.

The use of excimer laser has been reported in children. Singh reported PRK results in 10 children, 5 of whom were myopic. The results were good but 2 patients developed corneal haze. Nano evaluated the results of PRK in 5 children with myopic anisometropia with 40% of haze incidence.

Aliò reported results of 5 PRK treatments in myopic anisometropia having one case of severe corneal haze.

The destruction of Bowman's layer during PRK initiates a heavy healing response that is stronger in children than in adults. This process is responsible for the instability of refraction, regression of refractive effect and development of corneal haze. The need of using corticosteroids drops for several months after the procedure can cause a secondary rise of intraocular pressure.

Also the Lasik procedure has been proposed in pediatric patients.

Khaled reported results of Lasik treatment of 14 eyes with myopic anisometropia and amblyopia (mean SE –7.87 D) with BSCVA improved in all eyes. The follow-up was of one year with spherical equivalent manifest refraction from 0 to –1.50 D at that time.

Niteen described the results of three months of follow-up in 3 pediatric eyes of 3 anisometropic amblyopes treated with Lasik with satisfactory outcomes and relative stability.

Performing Lasik in children the progression of myopia after the surgery must be taken into account and the long term safety and predictability need further evaluation.

Our experience with highly myopic adults treated with implantation of Phakic Refractive Lens convinced use of the superiority of phakic IOLs in these cases. After the treatment of 11 pediatric eyes we feel completely satisfied with the results obtained with the PRL even in children. We had several reasons for preferring PRL to treat anisometropic myopia. The procedure is completely reversible; the phakic lens can be exchanged to another one of different power in case of axial myopia progression or wrong power calculation. The quality of vision is often better and there is no fear of corneal haze or ectasia. The surgery is simple and fast. The only transitory post-op adverse effect was transient IOP increase. There is no risk of corneal endothelial cell loss or pigment dispersion as it may happen with anterior chamber phakic lenses using the children rub their eyes. No anatomic complications were observed and BSCVA improved in all eyes implanted with PRL. 6 patients developed binocular vision. During the follow-up no cases of lens opacification, glaucoma or uveitis were noticed. The endothelial cell loss was about 4%, what is considered in the physiological range.

Scleral reinforcement surgery to prevent or limit the progression of axial myopia associated with subsequent PRL implantation to treat anisometropic amblyopia is an effective way to limit the handicap of highly myopic children. The functional outcomes are very satisfying and a marked progress in the child's quality of live was reported us by the parents. Encouraged by the results we are convinced that the procedure is safe and predictable to correct progressive myopia and amblyopia resulting from myopic anisometropia. Additional cases and longer follow-up observation are needed to evaluate the full extent of benefits of this technique in children.

Chapter 56

Multifocal IOLs in Children: A Long-term Analysis

Keiki R Mehta, Cyres K Mehta (India)

Pediatric Cataract Surgery

Most challenging surgery, not only in Ophthalmic speciality but in any branch of surgery. It needs follow up for the rest of life. It has changed considerably in last 20 years, because of early intervention and immediate optical correction.

Though intraocular implants in children are a well established entity, it required the efforts of McClatchey and Hofmesiter (1997, 1998, 2000, 2005) who demonstrated that after the age of 6 months, the intraocular power calculation follows a virtual linear logarithmic pattern thus proving that the refractive status of the eye can be predicted with a high level of accuracy.

Coupled with the ability to achieve this level of accuracy are the advent of the newer more sophisticated computer controlled machines and the availability of alternative modalities to ultrasound like neosonx and aqualase

Until the availability of mutifocal IOLs one had to be content with monofocal IOL for children the most popular being the Alcon single piece and multipiece AcrySof IOL. The material, thanks to its bioadhesive ability and the restriction of capsular growth due to the square edged design made it a very [popular IOL in infants and children.

All was good except that the child had, for practical purposes very limited near vision and since, for children, their proximal horizon accounts for more than 80% of their daily activities, it became extremely problematical. There is nothing sadder than to see a little child with reading glasses or wearing bifocal trying to move his head to focus. It placed a great deal of restrictions on the daily activities and in many ways was psychological reminder to both the children and the parents that the child was a visually deficient.

Stein 2004, critically analyzed and brought out three salient factors which need consideration a) Critical period of visual maturation completes in 3 to 4 months period. b) Upto the age of 8 months the visual apparatus goes on developing at a very rapid rate, and perhaps the most important c) The ability to see near and distance important for the child to be able to develop depth perception and enhance visual development.

Jacobi PC; Dietlein TS2001 from the University of Cologne, Cologne, Germany. evaluated implantation of a zonal-progressive multifocal intraocular lens (IOL) in children. Thirty-five eyes of 26 pediatric patients aged 2 to 14 years with multifocal IOL implantation at one institution with more than 1 year of follow-up using a multifocal IOL (Array SA40-N; Allergan, Irvine, CA) implantation in all eyes. Their results were very encouraging. Twenty-six patients (35 eyes) had an average follow-up of 27.4 +/- 12.7 months (range, 12-58 months). At last follow-up, best-corrected distance visual acuity improved significantly (P = 0.001), 71% of eyes with a visual acuity of 20/40 or better and 31% of eyes with a visual acuity of 20/25 or better. In the 9 bilateral cases, spectacle dependency was moderate, with only 2 children (22%) reporting the permanent use of an additional near correction. The remaining children were either using distance-correction only (4 patients; 44%) or no glasses at all (3 patients; 33%). Stereopsis also improved significantly after multifocal IOL implantation (P = 0.01. concluded: Multifocal IOL implantation is a viable alternative to monofocal pseudophakia in this age group.

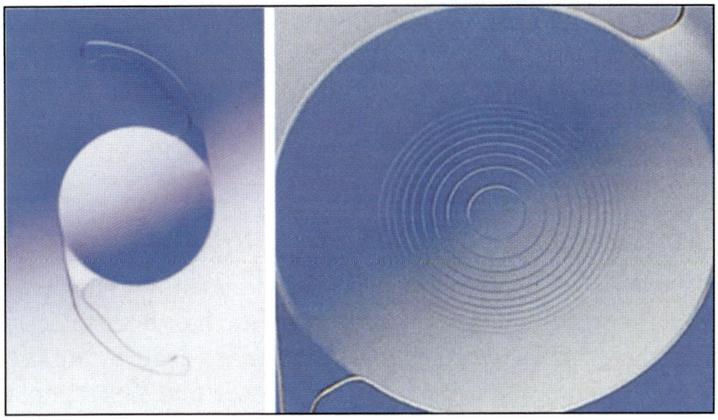

Figure 1: ReStor IOL

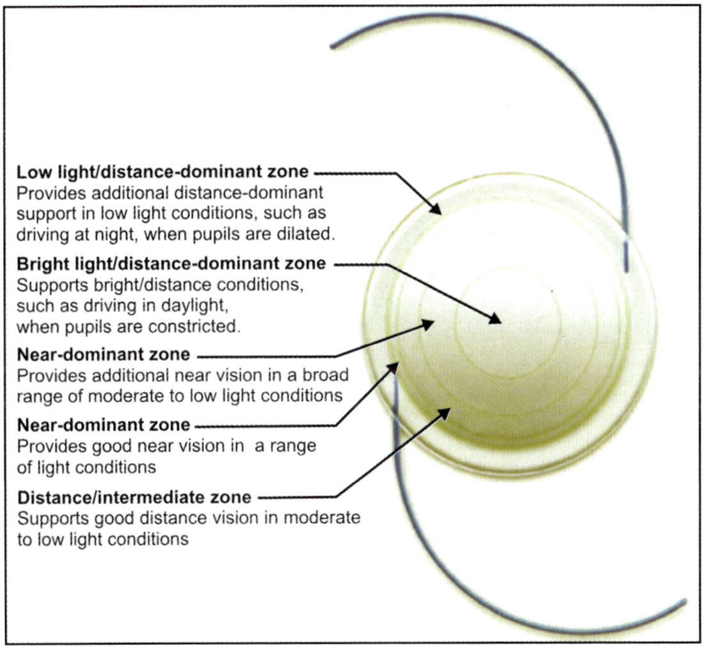

Figure 2: Five focusing zones for a full range of vision

With all the above factors described started a thought towards the use of multifocal implants in infants and children. In the earlier days, the Array (AMO) had the problems of decentrage, typical to silicone based IOLs. The newer hydrophobic acrylic material, the allergen ReZoom ReStor, do not suffer from that problem.

Can Children and Infants Manage Multifocality?

The Institute runs a well established contact lens clinic. However for many years, fitting contact lenses in small children has been a labor of love. Unfortunately the success rates with contact lenses even in the best of hands has been poor. Implants were the obvious answer and were implanted in all cases unless contraindicated with nystagmus, microphthalmos, uncontrolled glaucoma. It has been a practice that following implantation that the children were always fitted with varifocal glasses. Children adapt to varifocality very easily. There is never the problems of adaptation. Even a 4-year-old once he perceives the obvious benefits will wear his glasses. Not having separate reading glasses or having glasses with a bifocal segment obvious, makes wearing of the glasses easier with no social stigma attached to them.

Considering how easily children accept varifocality, and with the encouraging results in the ophthalmic literature we had decided on the concept of multifocal IOL for all children over the age of 2 years. An additional small power could be worn over as single vision glasses, in those whom we had calculated as an excess, which would over time, with the myopic shift achieve Emmetropia in adulthood. Naturally as the reading addition in the implants sufficed for all.

Multifocal IOLs in Children

We commenced multifocal IOLs in 2002 February. The one good IOL available was the Allergan Array IOL. A year later came the Preziol, which was a three zone refractive IOL, made by the CareGroup.

The results were immediate. The children were very contented and there was no immediate problem. The long-term problem of the Array was the tendency to shift out from the center (decenter) due to eccentric bag contraction typical of silicone IOLs.

In 2005 came the newer ReZoom, 5 zone multifocal and in early 2006 came the ReStor IOL made by Alcon, the first 2 infants were implanted with the ReStor in India in March and June of 2006. Implantation of a zonal-progressive multifocal IOLs in pediatric cataract patients provides a high level of distance-corrected far, intermediate and near vision, reduced spectacle dependence and improved binocular vision

Again the acceptability was very good. The ReZoom and the ReStor gave good intermediate vision which was very gratifying.

At present we have restricted ourselves to the ReZoom and the ReStor while the Preziol has been kept for those who cannot afford the otherwise, extremely (for India) costly IOLs. Interestingly, though the Preziol is a 2 stage IOL, still

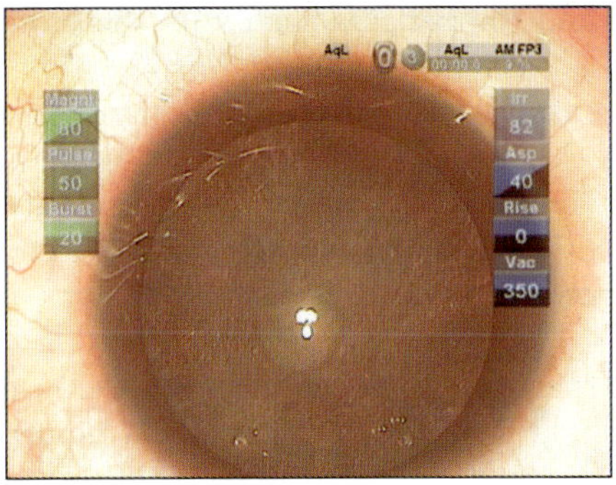

Figure 3: Central cataract in a 6 year old child

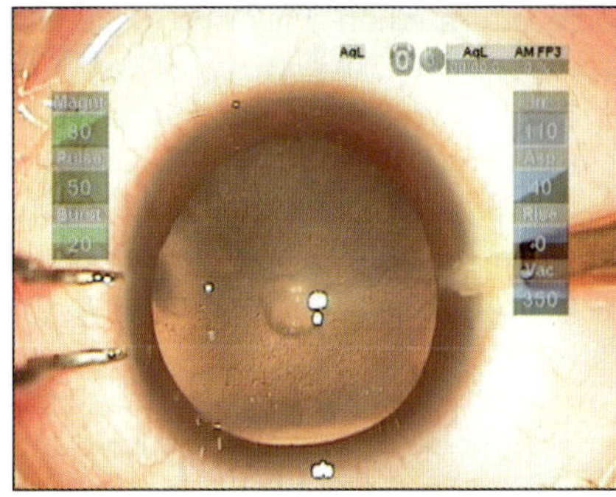

Figure 4: 0.8 mm diamond side port at 9.00 o'clock

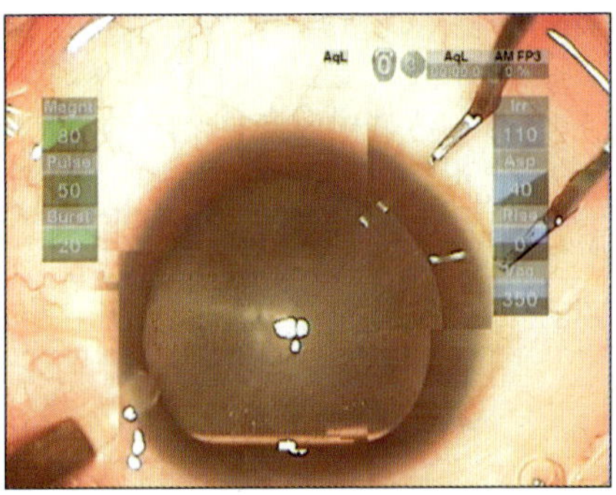

Figure 5: 0.8 mm diamond side port at 2.00 o'clock

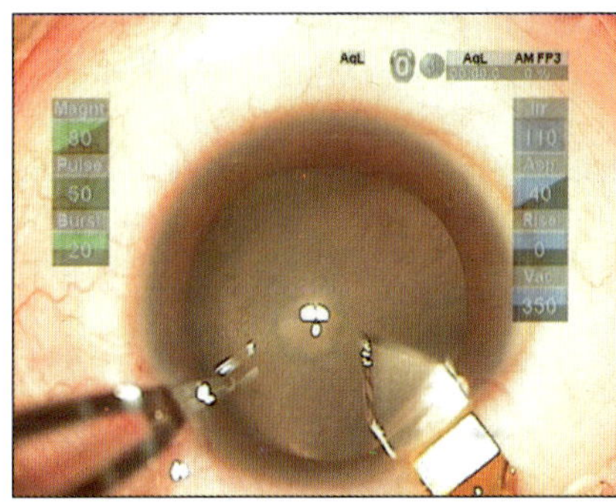

Figure 6: A 2.8 mm tunnel is made. Not the length of the square tunnel

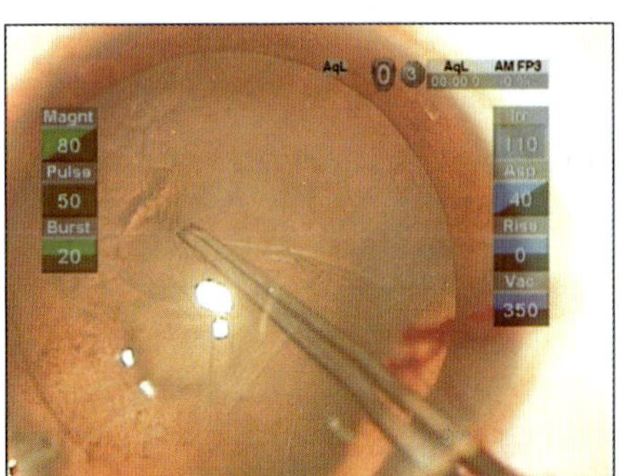

Figure 7: Commencing rhexis with the sharp tipped Utrata forceps

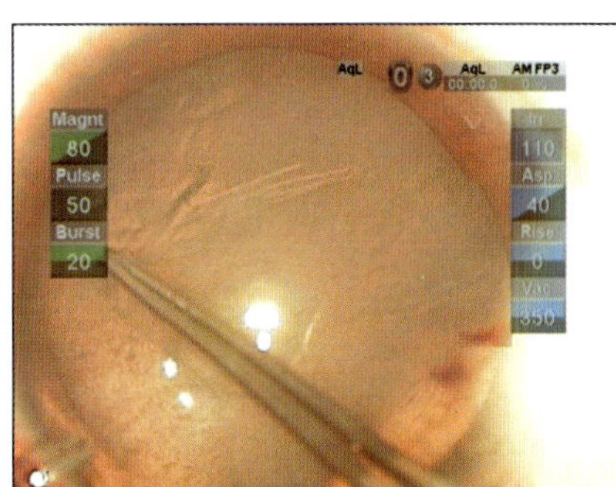

Figure 8: Completion of the rhexis. Note the almost 90 degree direction of the pull on the capsule

some intermediate vision is existent too and the patients even with the more economical implant are quite satisfied.

The AcrySof ReSTOR ® Intraocular Lens has a patented optic design using apodization, diffraction and refraction technologies.

Apodization is a gradual reduction or blending of the diffractive step heights. The apodized diffractive optic design gives it the ability to focus light correctly on the retina for images at various distances without mechanical movement of the lens.

Apodization optimally manages light energy delivered to the retina because it distributes the appropriate amount of light to near and distant focal points, regardless of the lighting situation.

Apodization based diffractive optics are designed to improve image quality while minimizing visual disturbances. The result is an increased range of quality vision that delivers a high level of spectacle freedom.

The ReZoom ™ Multifocal Lens has a patented lens design called Balanced View Optics ™ Technology. This lens design creates multiple focal points so patients can see well at a variety of distances, be it near, mid-distance, or far.

The ReZoom ™ Multifocal Lens has carefully proportioned visual zones that provide it with the ability to provide patients with vision at varying distances.

Each ReZoom ™ Multifocal Lens is divided into five different zones with each zone designed for different light and focal distances.

Unlike other earlier multifocal lens designs, (Array) the ReZoom ™ Multifocal Lens has proportioned the size of its zones to provide for good vision in a range of light conditions

Perioperative Routine and Selection of Anesthetic Agents

There is no need to separate children and parents as this is a very trying time for both. Too early an separation leads to a distraught mother and a crying unhappy non cooperative child.

Ideally children may receive clear liquids 4 hr before surgery without increasing the risk of aspiration.!

Though many institutions routinely use premedication for young children (between 18 months and 5 years of age) before ophthalmic procedures we have never found it necessary.

Both inhalational and intravenous general anesthetic techniques have been used successfully for pediatric cataract surgery. However, with the exception of a history of malignant hyperthermia, most general anesthesia in young children undergoing cataract surgery is done with an inhalational agent. Isoflurane has widely replaced halothane as the induction agent of choice in children. It possesses a less offensive odor than other volatile agents, is less stimulating to the airway, and lacks the arrhythmogenic properties of halothane.

Nitrous oxide, traditionally used with volatile anesthetics, may increase postoperative nausea and vomiting. The cause-and-effect relationship between nausea/vomiting and nitrous oxide remains controversial.

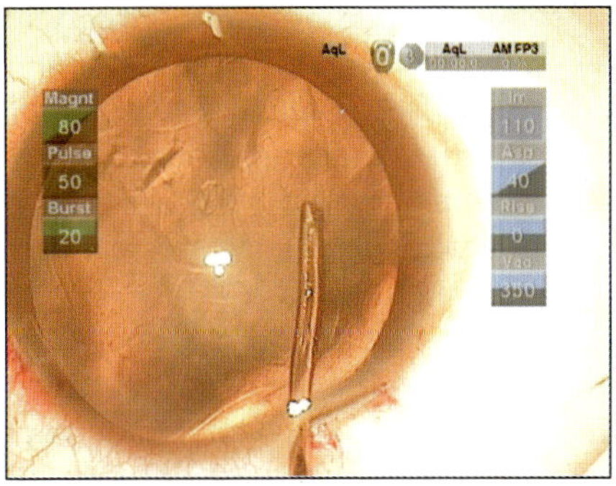

Figure 9: Application of the viscoelastic. Since AquaLase will be utilized, the hydrodissection is not done

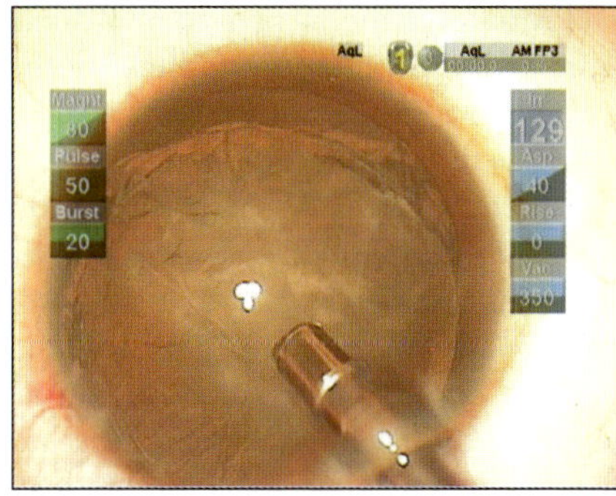

Figure 10: AquaLase grooving off the nuclear mass in the center

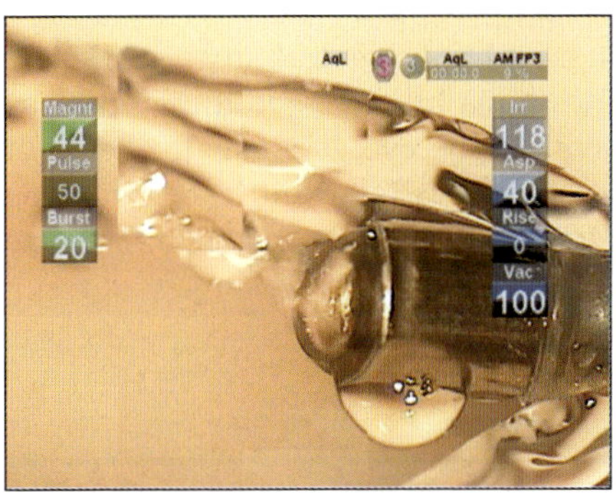

Figure 11: The AquaLase tip showing the polymer tip and the pulsed fluid flow

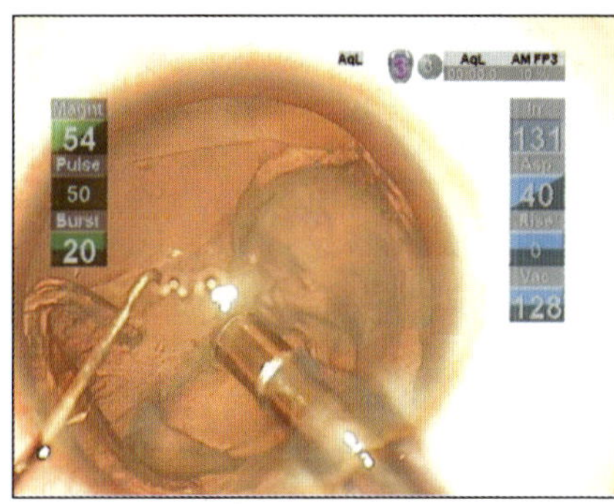

Figure 12: Note the nuclear mass enfolded and being AquaLased off

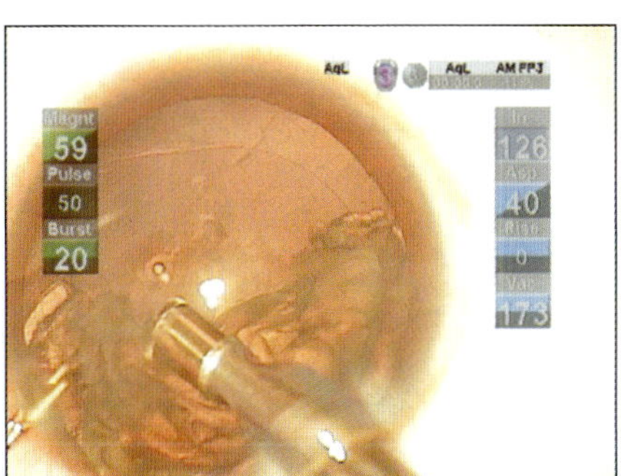

Figure 13: AquaLase working on the nuclear fragments

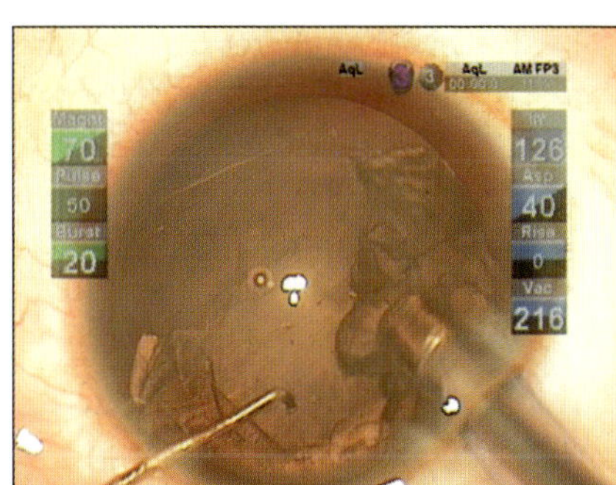

Figure 14: AquaLasing the final remnants

Propofol is the intravenous induction agent of choice for cataract surgery in older pediatric patients and those with preoperative intravenous access. Propofol is an isopropyl phenol that has a rapid onset and offset of action. It is used for the induction and maintenance of anesthesia or sedation. Intravenous injection of a therapeutic dose of propofol produces hypnosis rapidly with minimal excitation. Propofol is also believed to have antiemetic properties. It effectively produces hypnosis of short duration with minimal "hangover."

We usually combine it with ketamine hydrochloride, a dissociative anesthetic that can be used for the induction and maintenance of anesthesia. However ketamine hydrochloride does causes an increase in IOP, which should be kept in mind when following patients with glaucoma.

During anesthesia, even in patients whose IOP is usually normal, an increase in pressure can produce catastrophic effects. And may lead to prolapse of the iris and lens and loss of vitreous. Therefore, proper control of IOP is critical. We usually supplement the anesthesia with a1.5 cc sub Tenon block and let the eye soften for 3 minutes which obviates much of the risk of inhalation or injectable anesthesia.

Bell's phenomenon is an useful indicator an can be seen at any time during anesthesia when the patient's depth of anesthesia has changed.It manifests as upward (or sometime downward) movement of the eye. It is usually a sign of being light, although the patient is not awake. It is an indicator that the anesthesiologist should be prepared to "deepen" the anesthesia to facilitate surgery.

Oculocardiac Reflex

The oculocardiac reflex is stimulated by pressure on the globe and/or by traction on the extraocular muscles, the conjunctiva, or the orbital structures. The afferent limb is trigeminal and the efferent limb is vagal. Although the oculocardiac reflex is commonly associated with bradycardia, virtually any dysrhythmia, including ventricular tachycardia and asystole, may be seen.

It must be remembered that Children have increased vagal tone and, therefore, are more likely to present with the reflex. If a dysrhythmia appears, the surgeon to cease the manipulation and check that the depth of anesthesia and ventilatory status are adequate. Usually, the heart rate and rhythm return to baseline within 20 sec. If the reflex becomes a problem, atropine should be given intravenously.

Surgical Technique

A well made surgical tunnel is mandatory for babies and young children. It is important that the tunnels be made well. The first step is to make two 0.8 mm tunnels at 9.00 o'clock and 2.00 o'clock. The tunnels are made by applanating the scleral surface so that the tunnels are longer than they are broad. The next step is to fill the eye with an OVD (Ophthalmic Viscosurgical device). The best in the opinion of the authors is Viscoat By Alcon. The next best is Healon 5. The

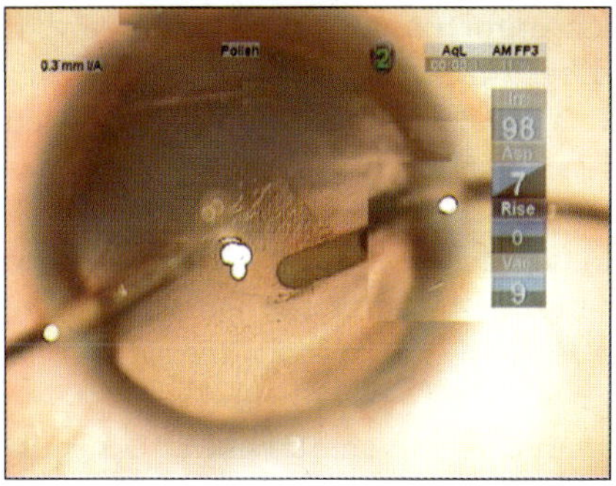

Figure 15: Polishing the posterior capsule

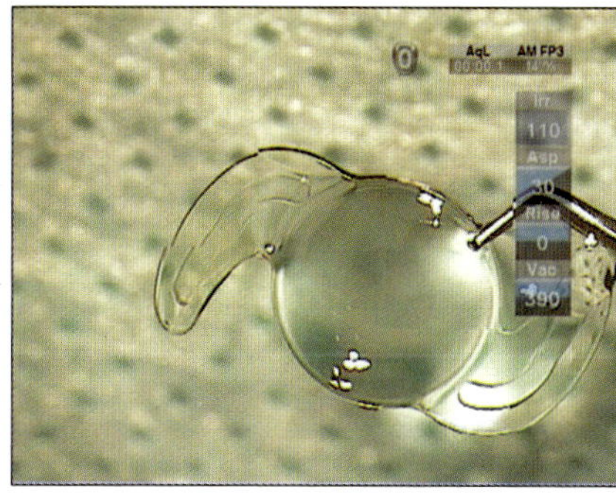

Figure 16: Preziol IOL (Care Group). Note the two zone optics

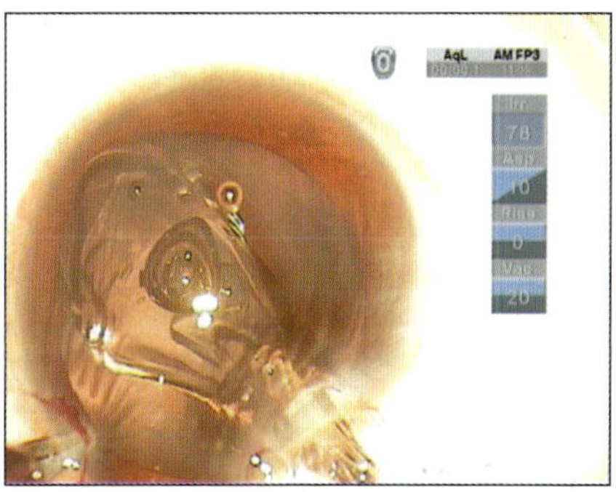

Figure 17: Lens being injected into the eye. Note the smooth slow entry, slipping under the edge of the rhexis

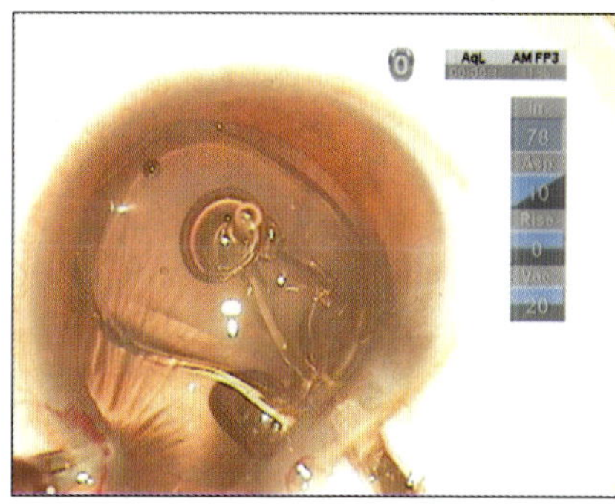

Figure 18: IOL injected using the sleeve and injector

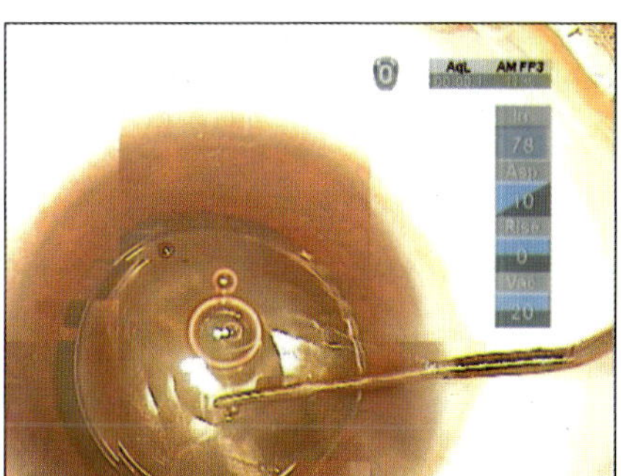

Figure 19: IOL rotated into place

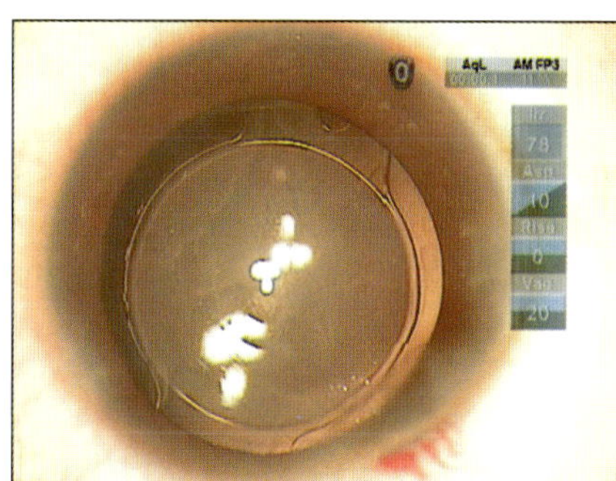

Figure 20: The final picture with the IOL well centered

most economical is methylcellulose which unfortunately runs out freely. If Methylcellulose is to be utilized it should be frozen (kept under the freezer). Methylcellulose increases its viscosity by a factor of 3 if frozen and does not run out at all. However once it warms up it runs again freely.

The next step is to carefully 'construct' the corneal incision. Refill OVD. Once again taking a 2.8mm diamond blade (ideal for children) applanated it to the sclera and then advance. Only enter the tunnel after the length is more than the breadth. *Be careful when removing the blade not to incise the sides of the tunnel.*

Rhexis in young children is best commenced with a sharp bent 27 G needle as the capsule is tough and does not give way easily and then continue the rhexis with a capsule forceps refilling the OVD at regular intervals. Do remember in children that the tendency is for the rhexis to increase. So plan for a 5 mm rhexis, and it invariably becomes bigger. If the eye is soft, after a block, rhexis is far easier. To do a rhexis in a tight eye is foolish as it will run away.

Hydrodissection under the rhexis is done with a blunt tipped side ported 24 G cannula. That way accidental injury to the capsule is avoided if the chamber suddenly shallows. The Hydrodissection is started at the 7.00 o'clock position and fluid injected slowly in all the clock hours. Usually the nucleus will tumble out if the cataract is soft.

The authors use the Alcon AquaLase which uses bursts of warmed water as a routine in children. It has a polymer blunt tip which protects the capsule. It is essential not to increase the suction too much. Usually all the cortex can be easily removed with the AquaLase but if any is left behind it can be easily removed with a I/A bimanual system.

AquaLase polishing if the capsule is essential. It leaves a very clean capsule. If not available than manual polishing of the capsule is compulsory.

Refill the chamber with the OVD of your choice and inject in the IOL.

The Intraocular implant is [placed in its folder being careful to be sure that it is properly sited and then injected into the eye using the proprietary injector. The 2.8 mm incision is more than adequate for both the Rezoom and the ReStor IOl and even the Preziol which has its own disposable injector.

The pupil is narrowed with a miotic (Intracameral pilocarpine 1 % with no preservative works well.) The pupil must be brought down to less than 4 mm prior leaving the case as in a child any sudden pressure will lead to the IOL being captured in the iris.

Up to the age of 4 years we do a posterior rhexis, but that to only after implanting the IOL, after ascertaining that the pressure and the anesthesia is very stable. The PCCC is followed by a short core anterior vitrectomy. The vitrectomy is an essential part of the procedure. Reports mention almost 63% of PCCC close by secondary membrane formation if core vitrectomy is not carried out. Usually following the AquaLase polishing the capsules are very clear. We prefer to delay doing the Posterior capsulotomy if the conditions are not ideal and prefer to enter via after 3 months when the IOL has had a good chance to stabilize.

After the age of 4 we prefer to simply do a Yag capsulotomy as a more stable procedure.

The chamber following surgery must reform with saline, and stay fromed on the table. If the chamber immediately flattens, it is prudent to take a single 10/0 Vicryl buried stitch at the site of the corneal incision.

An exceptional cleaning of the anterior chamber should be done. Meticulous removal of even slight traces of blood from anterior chamber at the end of surgery is must.

Epithelial cell metaplastic activities uses the intact anterior vitreous face, as well as surface of IOL as scaffolding, also RBCs are source of fibrosis.

Postoperative treatment is fairly simple. We do not permit the mother to handle a infant or even a small child's eyes under any circumstance. The mother is taught to place the drops in the inner corner of the eye and simply pat the child on the abdomen gently and wait. The moment the eye opens the drops go in. The child lids are very tight and very closely apposed to the eye. Any forcible effort only leads to the drops being literally "wipered" off. Previously we used to use Tobramycin, now replaced by Moxifloxacin eye drops tid with Prednisolone eye drops tid.

It is coupled with oral steroids. Oral drops of Betamethasone, 10 drops, b.i.d for children under 3 years of age, t.i.d for upto 5 years of age and q.i.d for over for a month. This usually takes care of any inflammation. We do not use mydriatics, but prefer to use a drop of 1% pilocar once a day for a month. In this regime, we never get lens capture, get perfectly centered pupils and do not have any inflammation.

Posterior Rhexis and Vitrectomy

There have been many publications since the time that Gimbel taught that a PCCC with a optic capture is the way to go. If the eye is soft, and the child is under GA with a positive pressure insufflations, doing a PCCC is easy. However if the anesthesia is not perfect and the eye is a bit tight, an attempt at PCCC often leads to a tear with vitreous in the A/C which means that the stability of the IOL is immediately at risk.

Statistics

We have done, 157 eyes, 65 are bilateral, 27 are unilateral of over the last 41/2 years starting from February of 2002. The results have been very gratifying. The maximum multifocal IOLs have been with the Array with the next highest, the Preziol. The only reason being that they were available earlier. We have nor restricted ourselves to the Rezoom and the Restor with the Preziol for the unaffording.

The visual results have been excellent in the bilateral group with 88% of them achieving 6/12 or better with the maximum correction and N8 easily. The unilateral group consisted of some who are bilateral but have not yet had the surgery done in the other eye. Again the results are excellent but the unilateral cataract with no or negligible cataract in the second eye have all achieved an maximum result of 6/18, 4 of whom are 6/24. which is reasonable considering that unilateral cataracts invariably do not do as well due to a latent amblyopia. Interestingly, the near vision is N8 which shows the near vision seems to be better than the distance in these unilateral cataracts. 9 eyes had to be re-operated to center the IOL.

Table 1: Multifocal IOLs implanted

Unilateral or bilateral				
Unilateral	*%*	*Bilateral*	*%*	*Total Children*
27	29.3	65	70.7	92

Total eyes 27 + 130 (65*2) = 157 eyes

Table 2: Age at implantation

Age at Implantation	*No*	*%*
2-3 years	27	17.2
4-6 years	47	29.9
7-9 years	38	24.2
10-12 years	45	28.7

Table 3: Complications n = 157

Complication	*No*	*%*
Corneal abrasion	03	1.9
Shallow A/C	11	7.0
Iritis Mild	12	7.6
Iritis severe	03	1.9
Raised IOP.Temp	15	9.6
Raised IOP.needed surgery	02	1.3
Hyphema	07	4.4
IOL decentrage requiring surgery	09	5.7

Table 4: Type of IOL implanted

Type of IOL implanted	*Manufacturer*	*No*	*%*
Preziol	(Care Group)	40	25.4
Array	(AMO)	74	47.2
ReZoom	(AMO)	36	23.0
ReStor	(Alcon)	7	4.4

- In conclusion. It would seem from a 41/2 year study which we are still evaluating that a primary Multifocal IOL is the way to go in infants and your pediatric cataracts.
- Regrettably Children are brought too late, parents and doctors are not aware of cataract. There are still too many opinions regarding whether an IOL should be placed in a small child, let alone a multifocal IOL, and invariably the parents are skeptical about surgery.
- Too many opinions, wastes precious time. Equally unfortunate is the concept in India of waiting till the cataract is mature to the level that one cannot see one's finger in adults. It is this concept which they apply to the child not realizing that it will, in the long run affect the rehabilitation of the child.
- It is also important to calculate the power as precisely as possible and if there is residual ametropia… correct with glasses or contact lenses as may prove necessary and consider the option of doing an Excimer laser at a later date after the child grows up.

The aim is to get as perfect a visual result as possible and to make the child achieve good vision with no additional visual props which would affect the child's ability to compete in the world of today.

Index

A

B

C

D

E

J

K

L

M

N

R

S

X

Z